Danilo Jankovic · Regional Nerve Blocks and Infiltration Therapy

I dedicate this book to my wife, Lydia, and my children Lara and Aleks.
Their love, support, and encouragement have made the book possible.

Danilo Jankovic
Regional Nerve Blocks and Infiltration Therapy
Textbook and Color Atlas

3rd Edition, fully revised and expanded

Consultant on English Edition

William Harrop-Griffiths
MA, MB, BS, FRCA
Consultant Anaesthetist
St Mary's Hospital, Paddington, London

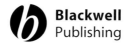
Blackwell Publishing

© 2004 by ABW Wissenschaftsverlag GmbH, Berlin
English language edition published by Blackwell Publishing Ltd
Blackwell Publishing, Inc., 350 Main Street, Malden, Massachusetts 02148-5020, USA
Blackwell Publishing Ltd, 9600 Garsington Road, Oxford OX4 2DQ, UK
Blackwell Publishing Asia Pty Ltd, 550 Swanston Street, Carlton, Victoria 3053, Australia

The right of the Author to be identified as the Author of this Work has been asserted in accordance with the Copyright, Designs and Patents Act 1988.

All rights reserved. No part of this publication may be reproduced, stored in a retrieval system, or transmitted, in any form or by any means, electronic, mechanical, photocopying, recording or otherwise, except as permitted by the UK Copyright, Designs and Patents Act 1988, without the prior permission of the publisher.

First published in German 1997
Second Edition published in English 2001
Third Edition published in English 2004

Library of Congress Cataloging-in-Publication Data

Jankovic, Danilo.
 [Regionalblockaden und Infiltrationstherapie. English]
 Regional nerve blocks and infiltration therapy : textbook and color atlas / Danilo Jankovic.– 3rd ed., fully rev. and expanded / consultant on English ed., William Harrop-Griffiths.
   p. ; cm.
 Rev. ed. of: Regional nerve blocks / Danilo Jankovic, Christopher Wells. 2nd ed. 2001.
 Includes bibliographical references and index.
 ISBN 1-4051-2263-3 (hardback)
 1. Conduction anesthesia. 2. Conduction anesthesia–Atlases.
 [DNLM: 1. Anesthesia, Conduction–methods–Atlases. 2. Anesthetics, Local–administration & dosage–Atlases. 3. Nerve Block–methods–Atlases. 4. Pain–drug therapy–Atlases. WO 517 J33r 2004a] I. Harrop-Griffiths, William. II. Jankovic, Danilo. Regionalblockaden. English. III. Title.

 RD84.J366 2004
 617.9'64-dc22
                              2004011189

ISBN 1-4051- 2263-3

A catalogue record for this title is available from the British Library

Set in Germany by Goldener Schnitt, Sinzheim
Printed and bound in Germany by Bosch Druck, Landshut

Commissioning Editor: Stuart Taylor
Development Editor: Katrina Chandler

For further information on Blackwell Publishing, visit our website:
http://www.blackwellpublishing.com

The publisher's policy is to use permanent paper from mills that operate a sustainable forestry policy, and which has been manufactured from pulp processed using acid-free and elementary chlorine-free practices. Furthermore, the publisher ensures that the text paper and cover board used have met acceptable environmental accreditation standards.

Foreword

Just over 35 years ago, I became interested in the use of neural blockade for the relief of pain during and after surgery and became convinced that this was a superb treatment option for appropriately selected patients. Despite the wonderful advances in general anaesthesia and development of much improved systemic analgesia, I have not changed my view of the important role of neural blockade in the treatment of acute pain. Initiatives in the United States of America to make pain a "fifth vital sign" have focussed attention on the need for improved pain management, and the availability of as wide as possible a choice of options for patients. I have proposed that the relief of acute pain should be viewed as a "human right". In this context, there are a significant number of patients who will not obtain effective pain relief without access to potent neural blockade techniques. Such techniques are described in a very concise and beautifully illustrated manner in this text.

The management of cancer pain and chronic non-malignant pain represents a much more major challenge than the treatment of acute pain. However, here again the judicious use of neural blockade techniques can make the world of difference to the effective management of a substantial number of patients. It is a great pity that in some clinics there has been a disconnection between those providing non-invasive methods of management and those with the knowledge and technical skill to provide effective and safe neural blockade techniques. The effective and safe performance of neural blockade methods requires the requisite knowledge of anatomy, physiology and pharmacology followed by carefully supervised training with the assistance of clear and concise texts and reviews. Again, this textbook by Jankovic provides an excellent basis for those wishing to become skilled in this field. In parallel with the execution of such skill and knowledge, the other key ingredient is an appropriate collaboration with colleagues who can provide the other dimensions of patient care to ensure the best possible outcome in the treatment of cancer pain and chronic non-malignant pain. Such an approach is necessary in order to avoid at one end of the spectrum almost complete neglect of neural blockade techniques and at the other end of the spectrum an overuse with neglect of alternative methods.

The author of this text is a very highly skilled practitioner of regional nerve blocks and, like the author, this text is very practically orientated. The descriptions of anatomy are highly relevant to the regional blocks described and the illustrations are amongst the best that I have seen. I have no doubt that the readers will find this text extremely valuable in their clinical practice aimed at the relief of acute, chronic and cancer pain.

Professor Michael J. Cousins AM
MB BS MD FANZCA FRCA FFPMANZCA FAChPM (RACP)
Professor & Director
Pain Management Research Institute
University of Sydney

Preface to the third edition

The extremely gratifying response to the first and second editions of this book has encouraged me to meet the strong demand for further training in the technique of regional blocks by providing a substantially expanded, thoroughly checked and augmented edition. Thanks to the translations of the second edition into English, Italian and Spanish, I have received comments and suggestions on the book from all over the world, and I have taken these into account in the present edition. Just under four years since the publication of the second edition, I am therefore presenting this handbook in an expanded and revised form, including a much larger number of topics. As always, the focus has been on educational aspects.

The following groups of topics have been **added**:

- Regional block techniques have been expanded and supplemented in accordance with the most recent findings in the field of regional anesthesia, particularly in the area of the brachial plexus and the lumbosacral plexus. The same applies to the section on neuraxial anesthesia.
- The chapter on regional anesthesia in ophthalmology is completely new. Chapters on percutaneous epidural neuroplasty and intravenous regional anesthesia have also been newly added, as well as one on the ganglion impar.
- As the important field of infiltration therapy techniques has been seriously and unjustly neglected in clinical practice, I have given it particular attention. After all, anesthetists and orthopedists, as well as physicians working in other specialties, all depend on this type of precise injection in everyday practice.
- The treatment of myofascial trigger points is also extremely important and requires specialized knowledge that is presented here. Quite specific injections into the most important trigger points are now presented in detail in this new edition, according to the regions of the body concerned (jaw, shoulder region, arm, gluteal region, etc.). The clinical signs and treatment of myofascial pain syndromes are also presented in precise detail. For example, intra-articular injections have been added, and the most important techniques involved are described.

I would like to express my thanks to colleagues and friends who have contributed to this edition: Prof. James Heavner, Prof. Gabor Racz, Prof. André van Zundert, and Prof. Battista Borghi. Thanks also go to my colleagues and friends, Prof. E. Freye and Prof. N. Körber, for advice, information, and ideas that have contributed to the success of this book.

I am grateful to Mr. H. Kreuzner, Dip. Eng., for his tremendous patience and expertise during our intensive collaboration and for the outstanding photographic work that resulted. Thanks also go of course to my son Aleks in this connection, who worked tirelessly and with tremendous commitment in producing and arranging the photographs. Last but not least, my thanks therefore also go to the members of my family, who have again supported me with all their strength and considerateness.

I would like to express my gratitude for the help with the English edition to my colleague and friend Professor William Harrop-Griffiths.

I am grateful to the staff at the publishers, particularly Matthias Franzke and Milena Schaeffer-Kurepkat, for their constant support and expert assistance.

Danilo Jankovic   Cologne, August 2004

Preface to the first edition

This book presents a practical summary of the most important block techniques used in diagnostic and therapeutic and local anesthesia in the upper body. This work is based on my many years' experience in clinical practice.

The book is aimed at the many specialist disciplines whose work involves pain therapy. This includes anesthetists, orthopedic surgeons, general surgeons, neurosurgeons, ENT surgeons, radiologists and fascia maxillary surgeons. The techniques presented here in the illustrations and text are an essential component of the modern multidisciplinary approach to pain therapy. Each individual block is discussed step by step and the way in which it is carried out is rendered easier to grasp through the use of specially developed record forms and checklists. At the same time. the physician concerned is informed about the relevant regulations that need to be observed. The focus is on the description and discussion of potential complications – how to recognize them quickly. how to prevent them and how to treat them in a timely fashion. I recommend those unfamiliar with this branch of pain therapy start by familiarizing themselves thoroughly with the anatomy of the region and the pharmacological properties of the most frequently used local anesthetics.

The underlying concept for this book was the idea of presenting, in a clear and practical fashion, ways of carrying out ablock with optimal efficacy while at the same time ensuring the patient's complete safety.

Special thanks go to my teacher, Prof. Hans Ulrich Gerbershagen. I would also like to thank the numerous colleagues and friends who have provided advice, information and ideas – particularly Dr. Günter Datz for his tremendous assistance, as weil as my colleagues in my immediate area of work, particularly Ms. Gabriele Haarmann and Mr. Peter Kaufmann. Thanks also go to my family for their understanding, patience and support.

Last, but not least, I should like to express my gratitude to the publishers, Blackwell Science, for their helpful collaboration and for the excellent design and presentation of the book.

I shall welcome and gratefully take account of any suggestions, tips and constructive criticism from readers of this book.

Danilo Jankovic   Cologne, December 1996

Contents

Foreword......V

Preface to the third edition......VI

Preface to the first edition......VII

1 Regional nerve blocks and infiltration therapy in clinical practice......1

Head and neck region

2 Regional anesthesia in ophthalmology......19
  André van Zundert, Danilo Jankovic
3 Occipital nerves......30
4 Trigeminal nerve......33
5 Infiltration of trigger points in the muscles of mastication......55
6 Cervicothoracic ganglion (stellate ganglion)......59
7 Superior cervical ganglion......69
8 Deep (and superficial) cervical plexus......76
9 Brachial plexus......82
  Interscalene block......83
  Supraclavicular perivascular (subclavian perivascular) block......96
  Vertical infraclavicular block......99
  Axillary block......106

Shoulder region

10 Suprascapular nerve......125
11 Subscapular nerve blocks
   Infiltration of subscapular muscle trigger points ("frozen shoulder")......128
12 Rotator cuff muscles
   Injection techniques in the myofascial trigger points......133
13 Shoulder region: intra-articular injections
   Intra-articular injection into the shoulder joint......138
   Intra-articular injection into the acromioclavicular joint......139

Elbow and hand region

14 Peripheral nerve blocks in the elbow region......143
15 Peripheral nerve blocks in the wrist region......146
16 Elbow and wrist
   Infiltration of myofascial trigger points and intra-articular injections......149
17 Intravenous regional anesthesia (IVRA)......159
18 Intravenous sympathetic block with guanethidine (Ismelin®)......164

Thorax, abdomen, lumbar and sacral spinal region

Thorax
19 Thoracic spinal nerve blocks......171

Lumbar spinal region
20 Lumbar paravertebral somatic nerve block 186
21 Lumbar sympathetic block 191

Abdomen
22 Celiac plexus block 199

Lumbosacral region
23 Iliolumbosacral ligaments 206
24 Ganglion impar (Walther ganglion) block 210
25 Infiltration of the piriform trigger points ("piriform syndrome") 214

Lower extremity

Anatomy of the lumbar plexus, sacral plexus and coccygeal plexus 218

Lumbar plexus blocks: introduction
26 Inguinal femoral paravascular block ("three-in-one" block) 220
27 Psoas compartment block (Cheyen access) 226
28 Sciatic nerve block 230

Blocking individual nerves in the lumbar plexus
29 Femoral nerve 238
30 Lateral femoral cutaneous nerve 241
31 Obturator nerve 243
32 Ilioinguinal and iliohypogastric nerves 246
33 Blocking peripheral nerves in the knee joint region 248
34 Blocking peripheral nerves in the ankle joint region 254

Neuraxial anesthesia

35 Neuraxial anatomy 263

Spinal anesthesia
36 Spinal anesthesia 272
37 Complications of spinal anesthesia 285
38 Continuous spinal anesthesia (CSA) 293
39 Continuous spinal anesthesia (CSA) in obstetrics 299
40 Chemical intraspinal neurolysis with phenol in glycerol 301

Epidural anesthesia
41 Lumbar epidural anesthesia 305
42 Thoracic epidural anesthesia 327
43 Epidural anesthesia in obstetrics 333
44 Lumbar epidural anesthesia in children 341
45 Epidural steroid injection 346
46 Combined spinal and epidural anesthesia (CSE) 355

Caudal epidural anesthesia
47 Caudal anesthesia in adult patients 361
48 Caudal anesthesia in children 376
49 Percutaneous epidural neuroplasty 381
    James E. Heavner, Gabor B. Racz, Miles Day, Rinoo Shah
50 Adjuncts to local anesthesia in neuraxial blocks 391

References 397

Subject index 419

Contributing authors

Chapter 2

Prof. André van Zundert
Catharina Hospital
Dept. of Anesthesiology, ICU & Pain Clinic
Michelangelolaan 2
5623 EJ Eindhoven
Netherlands

Chapter 28

For the subgluteal access route

Prof. Battista Borghi
Coordinator, International Orthopedic Anesthesia Club
Chief of Anesthesia Research Unit
Istituti Orthopedici Rizzoli
40136 Bologna
Italy

Chapter 49

Prof. James Heavner, DVM, PhD
Professor of Anesthesiology and Physiology
Director, Anesthesia Research
Texas Tech University Health Sciences Center
Lubbock, TX 79430
USA

Prof. Gabor Racz, MD
Professor and Chair Emeritus, Dept. of Anesthesiology
Director of Pain Services
Texas Tech University Health Sciences Center
Lubbock, TX 79430
USA

1 Regional nerve blocks and infiltration therapy in clinical practice

Introduction

Regional anesthesia means the interruption of impulse conduction in the nerves using specific, reversibly acting drugs (local anesthetics). This interruption of impulse conduction can be carried out in every region of the body in which the nerves are accessible for external injection.

The indications for regional anesthesia include:
1. Clinical anesthesia
Particularly in the fields of traumatology, orthopedics, urology, and gynecology, as well as in large-scale abdominal surgery with continuous procedures for epidural or spinal anesthesia.
2. Obstetrics
3. Postoperative analgesia
There is no postoperative analgesia procedure that is more appropriate than regional anesthesia. This field also includes the classic indications for a combination of local anesthetics with opioids or other substances.
Optimal patient care can only be achieved using a multimodal approach (effective pain therapy, early mobilization, early enteral nutrition, and emotional and psychological care). Effective pain therapy (e.g. with catheter analgesia procedures) plays a central role here, as it can substantially reduce the perioperative stress response (Table 1.1).
4. Pain therapy
In 1979, a commission set up by the International Association for the Study of Pain (IASP) defined pain as "… an unpleasant sensory and emotional experience, linked to actual or potential tissue damage".
Acute pain is caused by stimulation of pain receptors. This stimulation is transient, and sets in motion biologically useful protective mechanisms. Ideally, pain can be relieved by treating the cause. Chronic pain is regarded as a pathological response on the part of the

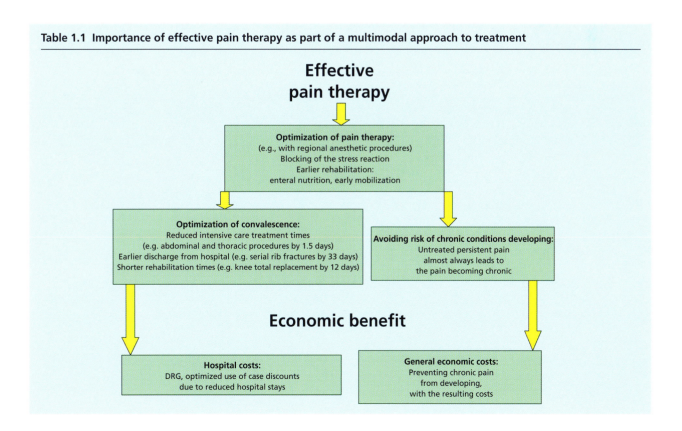

Table 1.1 Importance of effective pain therapy as part of a multimodal approach to treatment

body. It arises due to constant stimulation of nociceptive afferents, or can develop as neuropathic pain after injury or damage to the peripheral nociceptive system [5, 6, 17].

Chronic pain can often lead to alterations in patients' living habits, physical abilities, and personality, and requires a coordinated interdisciplinary approach. This in turn presupposes a clear diagnosis, based on a full general history and pain history, physical examination and functional assessment of the patient's musculature, locomotor apparatus, autonomic nervous system, and neurological and angiological situation.

In addition to medical treatment for pain, nerve blocks have a firmly established place in pain therapy – alongside physical and manual procedures, neurological and neurosurgical methods, physiotherapy and the psychosocial management of patients. In quantitative terms, regional anesthesia procedures play only a minor part in the management of chronic pain, but qualitatively they can produce very good results when used with the correct indications.

Nerve blocks in surgery and pain therapy
(Table 1.2)

The application of the anesthesiological methods described in the subsequent chapters of this book for temporary interruption of stimulus conduction in a nerve or nerve plexus requires the use of strictly established indications and the implementation of a coordinated therapeutic approach. In principle, these blocks can be administered for surgery, diagnosis, prognosis, and therapy [3].

Table 1.2 Important rules to observe when administering regional anesthesia or therapeutic nerve blocks

Before the block

Patient
1. **Preoperative information**
   – Explain the procedure
   – Discuss potential side effects and complications
   – Advise the patient about what to do after the procedure
   – Document the discussion
2. **Determine the patient's neurological status**
   – Exclude neurological abnormalities
3. Exclude **contraindications**
4. Avoid **premedication** in outpatients (particularly in blocks in which there is an increased risk of intravascular injection – e.g. stellate ganglion or superior cervical ganglion)

Anatomy, complications, side effects
1. With rarely used regional blocks, the **anatomic** and **technical** aspects should always be studied again beforehand
2. Detailed knowledge of potential **complications** and **side effects** of a regional block and how to avoid them
3. **Ability to control** potential complications and side effects
4. Select the **correct block techniques**
5. **Manual skill** and **good training** on the part of the anesthetist

Preparation

1. Ensure **optimal positioning** of the patient
2. Always secure **intravenous access**
3. Check that **emergency equipment** is complete and fully functioning
4. **Added vasopressors** are **contraindicated** in pain therapy
5. Observe **sterile precautions**

Safety standards when injecting larger doses of local anesthetics

1. Carry out **aspiration tests** before and during the injection
2. Administer a **test dose**
3. Inject local anesthetics in **incremental doses** (several test doses)
4. Maintain **verbal contact** with the patient
5. **Cardiovascular monitoring**
6. Keep careful **notes** of the block

Surgical blocks are administered with high-dose local anesthetics for targeted isolation of a specific body region in order to carry out an operation.

Diagnostic blocks using low-dose local anesthetics are appropriate for the differential diagnosis of pain syndromes. They allow the affected conduction pathways to be recognized and provide evidence regarding the causes of the pain. Diagnostic blocks can also be used to clarify the question of whether the source of the pain is peripheral or central.

Prognostic blocks allow predictions to be made regarding the potential efficacy of a longer-term nerve block, neurolysis or surgical sympathectomy. They should also be used to prepare the patient for the effects of a permanent block.

Therapeutic blocks are used in the treatment of a wide variety of pain conditions. Typical examples of these are post-traumatic and postoperative pain, complex regional pain syndrome (CRPS) types I and II (reflex sympathetic dystrophy and causalgia), joint mobilization, post-herpetic neuralgia and tumor pain.

Nerve blocks and chronic pain [11]

A **multimodal treatment approach** to chronic pain is essential for successful treatment. The use of nerve blocks as part of this approach presupposes that the following steps have been taken:
- careful analysis of the pain;
- correct diagnosis and establishment of the indication;
- assessment of the pain chronicity stage;
- well-selected patient groups.

Important preconditions for the application of nerve blocks in chronic pain include:
- a good knowledge of anatomy;
- attention to and control of potential side effects and complications;
- choice of the correct block techniques;
- manual skill and good training on the part of the therapist.

The most important tasks facing us include conducting more double-blind, randomized and well-controlled studies on the use of nerve blocks in chronic pain conditions, and developing a consistent standard for carrying out nerve blocks. The answers to two questions need to be found:
- selection criteria to identify which patients are suitable for nerve blocks;
- the number of nerve blocks to be used in the treatment of chronic pain.

Technical requirements

Carrying out temporary nerve blocks and regional anesthetic procedures in surgery and pain therapy requires the appropriate basic technical equipment and experience in the use of all of the instruments concerned.

The conditions for patient positioning, the aseptic conditions required, and the syringes, needle types and other supplies needed are discussed alongside the individual block techniques described in this book.

Complete and properly functioning equipment must be available both for primary care and in case of adverse events and complications, as well as treatment monitoring.

Accessories for primary care

Emergency equipment (Figs. 1.1 and 1.2)
- Intubation and ventilation facilities;
- oxygen source (breathing apparatus);
- ventilation bag with two masks (large, medium);
- Guedel tubes nos. 3, 4, 5;
- Wendel tubes nos. 26–32;
- endotracheal tubes nos. 28–36;
- tube clamp, blocker syringe (10 mL);
- laryngoscope with batteries (replacement batteries and replacement bulbs), spatula;
- Magill forceps, mouth wedge, 1 tube 2% lidocaine gel;
- suction device;
- infusion equipment;
- two sets of infusion instruments;
- five plastic indwelling catheters
- syringes (2 mL, 5 mL, 10 mL), plaster, gauze bandages.

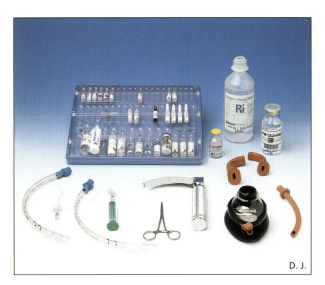

Fig. 1.1 Emergency equipment

Chapter 1

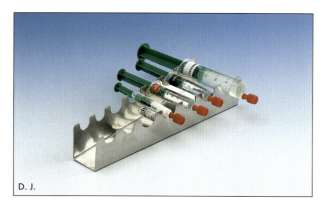

Fig. 1.2 Emergency drugs

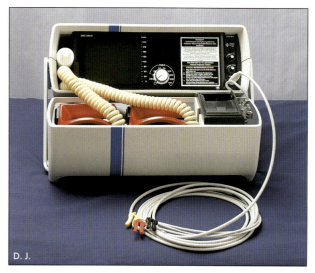

Fig. 1.3 Defibrillator

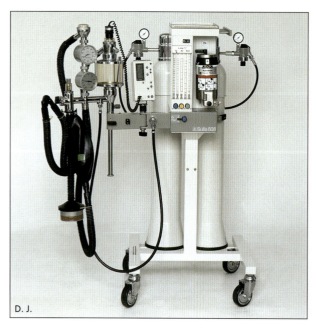

Fig. 1.4 Anesthetic machine

■ *Infusion solutions*
– 1 bottle each of Ringer's solution, plasma expander, 8.4% sodium bicarbonate (100 mL)

■ *Defibrillator* (Fig. 1.3)
■ *Drugs for emergency treatment*

When blocks are being administered, a sedative (Valium®), a vasopressor (ephedrine) and a vagolytic (atropine) should be available for immediate injection. All other emergency medications should also be on hand:
– 5 ampoules of atropine
– 2 ampoules of Alupent® (orciprenaline)
– 2 ampoules of Akrinor® (cafedrine–theodrenaline hydrochloride)
– 3 ampoules 0.1% Suprarenin® (epinephrine) (1 : 1000)
– 2 prepared syringes of Suprarenin® (1 : 10 000, 10 mL)
– 2 ampoules of dopamine
– 1 ampoule 10% calcium gluconate
– 1 ampoule dimetindene maleate (Fenistil®)
– prednisolone (Solu-Decortin®) (50 mg, 250 mg, 1000 mg)
– 5 ampoules 0.9% sodium chloride
– 2 ampoules 2% lidocaine
– 3 ampoules diazepam (Valium®) (10 mg)
– 2 ampoules midazolam (Dormicum®) (5 mg)
– 1 ampoule clonazepam (Rivotril®) (1 mg)
– 1 injection bottle thiopental sodium
– 2 ampoules etomidate (Hypnomidate®)
– 2 ampoules propofol (Disoprivan®)
– 2 ampoules succinylcholine (suxamethonium chloride)

Anesthetic machine
For neuraxial anesthesia, ganglion blocks, intravenous regional anesthesia and plexus anesthesia, an anesthesia trolley with facilities for intubation is also required (Fig. 1.4).

Monitoring
■ Electrocardiogram (ECG)
■ Pulse oximeter (Fig. 1.5)
■ Electrostimulator (e.g., HNS 11, B. Braun Melsungen, Germany; Fig. 1.6). Peripheral nerve stimulation is a valuable aid in clinical practice and has considerable advantages in combination with an atraumatic catheter technique.
■ Temperature sensor, touch-free miniature infrared skin thermometer (e.g., M.U.S.S. Medical, Hamburg, Germany) (Fig. 1.7)

The treatment of side effects and severe complications – e.g., after inadvertent intravascular, epidural, or subarachnoid injection of a local anesthetic – is discussed here together with the individual block techniques.

Local anesthetics in regional anesthesia and pain therapy

Local anesthetics produce reversible blockage of sodium channels in the nerve-cell membrane, thereby interrupting stimulus conduction.

Chemical structure and physicochemical properties [17]

All local anesthetics in common clinical use have three characteristic molecular sections in their chemical structure:

An aromatic residue, which basically determines the lipophilic properties of the agent. Substitutions in the aromatic group allow the pKa and lipid solubility of the substance to be influenced.

An intermediate chain, which in local anesthetics of the ester type (Table 1.3) contains a relatively unstable ester bond (CO–O) that can be broken down hydrolytically by pseudocholinesterases. Local anesthetics of the amide type (Table 1.4) are much more stable, since the amide bond (NH–CO) in their intermediate chain cannot be broken down in plasma. The length of the chain between the aromatic residue and the substituted amino group has an influence on the intensity of effect of the local anesthetic. The agent's protein-binding capacity and lipid solubility can be altered by substitution in the intermediate chain.

A substituted amino group, the protonization of which determines the ratio of the cationic to the basic form. Only the free base is capable of penetrating lipoprotein membranes. However, to be able to affect the nerve membrane, the local anesthetic must be available as a cation. The type of amino group substitution affects the distribution coefficient, the plasma protein binding and the intensity and duration of the drug's action.

Clinical significance of the physicochemical properties

Local anesthetics differ with regard to their molecular weight, their lipid and water solubility, pKa and protein-binding characteristics. These factors in turn have a substantial influence on the potency of the drug's local anesthetic effect on the onset of the effect and on its duration (Tables 1.5a, 1.5b).

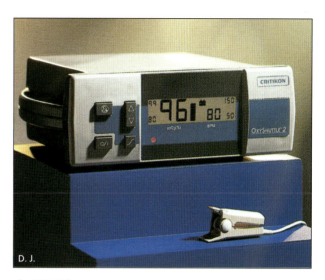

Fig. 1.5 Pulse oximeter

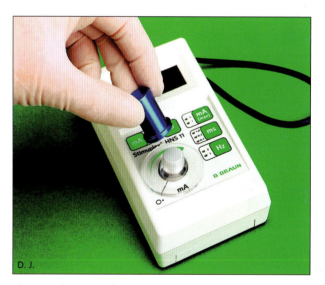

Fig. 1.6 Electrostimulator

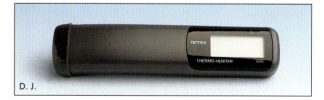

Fig. 1.7 Temperature sensor

Local anesthetic potency [4]

The combined effect of factors such as protein binding, stereoisomeric structure and lipophilia determine the potency of a local anesthetic agent. To achieve a blocking effect, the local anesthetic has to diffuse across the

Table 1.3 Local anesthetics with an ester bond

Aromatic residue / Intermediate chain / Substit. amino group	Name	Year introduced
(Cocaine structure)	Cocaine	1884
H₂N–C₆H₄–CO–O–C₂H₅	Benzocaine	1900
H₂N–C₆H₄–CO–O–CH₂–CH₂–N(C₂H₅)₂	Procaine	1905
C₄H₉(H)N–C₆H₄–CO–O–CH₂–CH₂–N(CH₃)₂	Tetracaine	1930
H₂N–C₆H₃(Cl)–CO–O–CH₂–CH₂–N(C₂H₅)₂	Chloroprocaine	1955

Table 1.4 Local anesthetics with an amide bond

Aromatic residue / Intermediate chain / Substit. amino group	Name	Year introduced
2,6-(CH₃)₂–C₆H₃–NH–CO–CH₂–N(C₂H₅)₂	Lidocaine	1944
2,6-(CH₃)₂–C₆H₃–NH–CO–(N-methylpiperidine)	Mepivacaine	1957
2-CH₃–C₆H₄–NH–CO–CH(CH₃)–NH–C₃H₇	Prilocaine	1960
2,6-(CH₃)₂–C₆H₃–NH–CO–(N-butylpiperidine)	Bupivacaine	1963
2,6-(CH₃)₂–C₆H₃–NH–CO–CH(C₂H₅)–N(C₃H₇)(C₂H₅)	Etidocaine	1972
thiophene(CH₃, CO-OCH₃)–NH–CO–CH(CH₃)–NH–C₃H₇	Carticaine	1974
2,6-(CH₃)₂–C₆H₃–NH–CO–(N-propylpiperidine)	Ropivacaine	1996
2,6-(CH₃)₂–C₆H₃–NH–CO–(N-butylpiperidine)	Levobupivacaine	2000

cell membrane into the interior of the cell (importance of lipophilia for membrane diffusion) so that, from the cytosol (appropriate hydrophilic properties), it can occupy the sodium channel in its then protonated form (Table 1.6). A high degree of lipophilia is associated with good membrane permeation, and a high degree of hydrophilia is associated with good solubility in the cytosol. Local anesthetics therefore have to have both of these properties in a favorable ratio.

However, the clinical distinction that is made in local anesthetics between those of mild potency (procaine), medium potency (lidocaine, prilocaine, mepivacaine), and high potency (ropivacaine, bupivacaine, levobupivacaine, etidocaine) does not conform to these correlations in all respects.

The onset of effect in the isolated nerve, at physiological pH, depends on the pKa value of the local anesthetic. The lower this value is, the more local anesthetic base can diffuse toward the membrane receptors, and the shorter the time will be to the onset of the nerve block. Higher concentrations of local anesthetic accelerate onset.

The duration of effect depends on the dosage and concentration of the local anesthetic, its binding to the membrane receptors (protein-binding capacity), and its reabsorption from the tissue into the blood.

Regional nerve blocks and infiltration therapy in clinical practice

Table 1.5a Physicochemical and pharmacological parameters

Agent	Molecular weight	pKa (25°)	Distribution coefficient (lipid/water)	Protein binding (%)	Potency in vitro (isolated nerve)
Procaine	236	8.9	0.02	5,8	1
Lidocaine	220	7.7	2.9	64–70	4
Mepivacaine	234	7.7	0.9	77–80	3–4
Prilocaine	246	7.6	0.8	55	3–4
Bupivacaine	288	8.1	27.5	95	16
Etidocaine	276	7.7	141	95	16
Ropivacaine	274	8.1	9	95	16
Levobupivacaine	288	8.09	27.5	97	16

Table 1.5b Local anesthetic potency and duration of effect

Low — Procaine
Medium — Lidocaine, Mepivacaine, Prilocaine
High — Bupivacaine, Levobupivacaine, Etidocaine, Ropivacaine

Equipotent concentrations

Medium-duration local anesthetics have more or less the same clinical potency (except perhaps for lidocaine – due to stronger vasodilation, this local anesthetic is resorbed more readily from the site of action, and this can affect the duration and intensity of the block).

Equipotent concentrations of long-acting local anesthetics cannot be demonstrated in the same way, since the three local anesthetics mentioned have completely different block profiles: etidocaine (highest lipophilic capacity) produces a mainly motor block, ropivacaine has a mainly sensory effect, and bupivacaine has both motor and sensory effects. Anesthetic concentrations of bupivacaine and ropivacaine are equipotent (one to one).

Block profile (Table 1.7)

The block profile shows the relation between sensory and motor block. Physicochemical properties determine the block profile. At high anesthetic concentrations – so far as these are toxicologically permissible – the excess quantity of the agent can also block fibers not primarily affected (motor or sensory fibers). On the other hand, the block profile is not altered by low concentrations. A reduced motor block is obtained at the cost of reduced analgesic quality, and this is why opioid supplementation is usually necessary with dilute concentrations of local anesthetic.

Incompatibility

Local anesthetics can precipitate after dilution with alkaline solutions, and should therefore not be diluted with or injected simultaneously with sodium bicarbonate.

Side effects and systemic effects

(Tables 1.8 and 1.9)
When assessing the safety and tolerability of a local anesthetic, account needs to be taken not only of its

Table 1.6 Chemical requirements of a local anesthetic. Local anesthetics must combine lipophilic and hydrophilic properties in a favorable ratio with each other. Hydrophilia = soluble in cytosol, lipophilia = overcoming the cell membrane

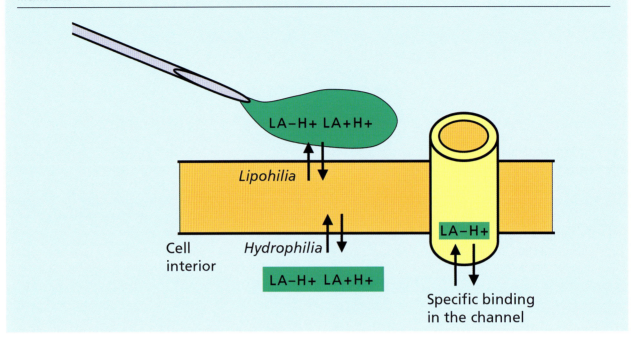

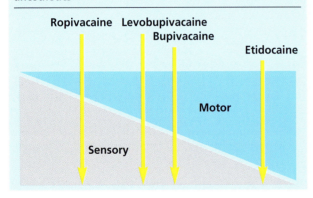

Table 1.7 Relative block profile of long-acting local anesthetics

Table 1.8 Toxicity of clinical dosages of local anesthetics

Local anesthetic	Central nervous system	Heart
Lidocaine	++	+
Mepivacaine	++	+
Prilocaine	+	+/−
Bupivacaine	+++	++++++ *
Levobupivacaine	++	++++
Ropivacaine	++(+)	+++

* Clinical dose can be equivalent to a lethal dose when incorrectly administered.

central nervous and cardiovascular effects, but also of its allergenic potential and of toxic degradation products that may form as it is metabolized.

Systemic effects

Adverse systemic effects of local anesthetics can occur when their plasma concentration is high enough to affect organs with membranes that can be irritated.
Toxic plasma levels can be reached as a result of:
– Inadvertent intravascular or intrathecal/epidural injection;
– Overdosing, particularly in areas with good perfusion and correspondingly high resorption;
– Failure to adjust the dosages (mg/kg body weight), particularly in patients with hepatic or renal disease.

The severity of intoxication depends on the absolute plasma level, as well as on the strength of the local anesthetic's effect. While anesthetic dosages of short-acting local anesthetics (prilocaine, mepivacaine, lidocaine) can trigger clear CNS symptoms in a range extending to generalized cramp, cardiotoxic reactions are also possible with long-acting local anesthetics. In particular, cases of cardiac arrest have been reported with bupivacaine with comparatively small intravascular injections (50 mg; not treatable in half of the cases). Cardiac symptoms and cardiac arrest can also occur with ropivacaine after inadvertent intravascular injections. However, these can be treated effectively and only occur at higher dosages. The following sequence of increasing systemic toxicity applies to the most frequently used local anesthetics: procaine < prilocaine < mepivacaine < lidocaine < ropivacaine < levobupivacaine < bupivacaine.

CNS toxicity: Central reactions predominate in terms of frequency and clinical significance. The symptoms of these are listed in Table 1.9 in order of severity and toxicity. For speedy and appropriate treatment, it is important to observe and react immediately when even the preconvulsive signs of CNS intoxication are seen – particularly numbness of the tongue and perioral region. Since the symptoms of CNS toxicity occur either immediately after injection of the local anesthetic (intravascular injection) or within the first half hour (overdose), constant verbal contact must be maintained with the patient during this period.

Cardiovascular toxicity: toxic effects on the cardiovascular system usually occur after the administration of very high doses. They are seen in the form of conduction disturbances in the autonomic cardiac and vascular nerve fibers, depression of cardiac function, and peripheral vasodilation (Tables 1.8 and 1.9).

> Immediate treatment measures in cases of CNS and CVS intoxication are described in detail in the section on complications in Chapter 6.

Substance-specific side effects [17]

One specific side effect of prilocaine is the increased methemoglobin level caused by the metabolite o-toluidine. Clinically, cyanosis, headache, cardiac palpitation and vertigo can be expected at methemoglobin levels of 10–20%, and loss of consciousness, shock and death when the level is 60% or more. This does not call into question the beneficial toxicological properties of prilocaine, since clinically relevant methemoglobinemia can only occur at dosages of more than 600 mg, which is much more than clinically used doses of mepivacaine or lidocaine. A clinically harmful methemoglobin level can be treated within a few minutes by the intravenous administration of 2–4 mg/kg toluidine blue (or alternatively, 1–2 mg/kg methylene blue). Because of this specific side effect, prilocaine is not indicated in patients with congenital or acquired methemoglobinemia, in patients who are anemic or have a history of heart disease, in obstetrics (e.g., for pudendal nerve or paracervical block), or in children under the age of 6 months.

Allergenic potential

There are no reliable data regarding the frequency of allergic reactions after the administration of local anesthetics. There is no doubt that these are extremely rare, although the symptoms can range from allergic dermatitis to anaphylactic shock. Occasional cases of allergic reactions to ester local anesthetics have been reported, and the preservative substances which the various preparations contain (e.g., parabens) and the antioxidant sodium bisulfide in epinephrine-containing solutions are also under discussion as potential causes. In patients with suspected intolerance of local anes-

Table 1.9 Symptoms of intoxication due to local anesthetics

Central nervous system	Cardiovascular system
Stimulation phase, mild intoxication	
Tingling of lips, tongue paresthesias, perioral numbness, ringing in the ears, metallic taste, anxiety, restlessness, trembling, muscle twitching, vomiting	Cardiac palpitation, hypertonia, tachycardia, tachypnea, dry mouth
Stimulation phase, moderately severe intoxication	
Excitation phase, moderate toxicity	
Speech disturbance, dazed state, sleepiness, confusion, tremor, choreoid movements, tonic–clonic cramp, mydriasis, vomiting, polypnea	Tachycardia, arrhythmia, cyanosis and pallor, nausea and vomiting
Paralytic phase, severe toxicity	
Stupor, coma, irregular breathing, respiratory arrest, flaccidity, vomiting with aspiration, sphincter paralysis, death	Severe cyanosis, bradycardia, drop in blood pressure, primary heart failure, ventricular fibrillation, hyposystole, asystole

Table 1.10 Functional distinctions between nerve fibers

Fiber type	Function
A_α	Motor, touch, pressure, depth sensation
A_β	Motor, touch, pressure, depth sensation
A_γ	Regulation of muscle tone
A_δ	Pain, temperature, touch
B	Preganglionic sympathetic function
C	Pain, temperature, touch, postganglionic sympathetic function

Table 1.11 Overview of drugs

Drug	Potency	Duration of effect	Toxicity	Half-life	V_{diss}
Lidocaine	1 (Ref.)	2 h	1 (Ref.)	96′	91
Mepivacaine	1	2–3 h	1.2	114′	84
Prilocaine	1	2–3 h	0.5	93′	261

Recommended maximum doses without epinephrine, according to specialist information:

Lidocaine	Mepivacaine	Prilocaine
200 mg	300 mg	400 mg

thetics, intracutaneous testing with 20 µL of the agent can be conducted. When the result is positive, subcutaneous provocation tests at increasing dosages (0.1 mL diluted to 1 : 10 000, 1 : 1000, and 1 : 10; undiluted at 0.1 mL, 0.5 mL, and 1 mL) can be considered. When these tests are being carried out, it is vital to prepare all the necessary safety measures in case of a severe reaction.

Selection of suitable substances for regional block

When surgical interventions are being carried out under regional anesthesia, priority must go to shutting off both sensory and motor systems, and knowledge of the expected length of the operation is vital to the choice of anesthetic. The onset of effect and the toxicity of the drug used play important parts, but not decisive ones. In the context of pain therapy, in which the fast-conducting A delta fibers and the slow-conducting C fibers (Table 1.10) are the target of the block, toxicity is much more important than the duration of the effect.

In diagnostic and therapeutic blocks, in which there is a risk of intravascular injection – e.g., in a stellate ganglion block or superior cervical ganglion block – prilocaine should be selected, as it is the medium-duration local anesthetic with the lowest toxicity (mepivacaine or lidocaine are alternatives) (Table 1.11).

Bupivacaine has an important role in regional blocks, being a longer-duration local anesthetic that provides high-quality analgesia and an easily controlled motor block. Its anesthetic potency is about four times that of local anesthetics with medium-duration effects (such as prilocaine). When the lower dosage required in pain therapy than in regional anesthesia is taken into account, bupivacaine can be used for practically all pain therapy procedures in spite of its relatively high toxicity.

Ropivacaine is the most recently introduced long-duration local anesthetic in the amino-amide series. The differential block is even more marked than with bupivacaine, and the drug is associated with much lower CNS toxicity and cardiac toxicity. These characteristics make it particularly suitable for regional anesthesia procedures in which higher dosages or concentrations are required. Ropivacaine provides good quality analgesia while largely maintaining motor activity (up to 80% of patients have no measurable motor block on the Bromage scale). At a dosage of 2 mg/mL, the drug is therefore the local anesthetic of choice for epidural obstetric analgesia and for postoperative analgesia (Table 1.7). With its pharmacological profile, ropivacaine is the first local anesthetic with primarily analgesic effects, and it is therefore particularly suitable for pain therapy indications.

Every anesthetist and pain therapy physician who uses anesthetic methods for temporary interruption of stimulus conduction in a ganglion, nerve or neural plexus should be familiar with the properties and potential applications of the following agents.

Short-acting local anesthetics

Procaine (Novocaine®)

Class of drug: Local anesthetic of the ester type.
Single threshold dose: 500 mg without epinephrine in adults.
LD_{50} (mouse): 52.2–60.0 mg/kg body weight i.v.
Plasma half-life: < 0.14 h.
Latency: Medium.
Duration of effect: 0.5–1 h, depending on the area of application and the concentration used.
Metabolism: Procaine is broken down in plasma by pseudocholinesterase into *p*-aminobenzoic acid – a naturally occurring component of folic acid synthesis – and into diethylaminoethanol. The metabolites are excreted in the urine or broken down in the liver.
Tolerability and control: Procaine is one of the local anesthetics that have the lowest toxicity. Due to its short half-life, procaine is easily controlled.

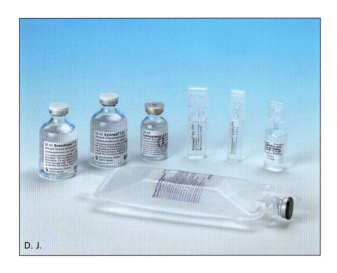

Clinical uses: It is not so much its local anesthetic potency that predominates in procaine, but rather its muscle-relaxing properties and vasodilatory effect – which are of primary importance in infiltration therapy and trigger-point treatment.

In the therapeutic field, very good results can be obtained with superior cervical ganglion block. However, procaine's high allergenic potency in comparison with amide local anesthetics argues against its use.

Dosage: Procaine is administered at concentrations of 0.5–2%. Precise dosages are described in the relevant sections of this book.

2-Chloroprocaine

2-Chloroprocaine, an ester local anesthetic, is a chlorinated derivative of procaine and is most rapidly metabolized local anesthetic currently used. Although the potency of chloroprocaine is relatively low, it can be used for epidural anesthesia in large volumes in a 3% solution because of its low systemic toxicity. The duration of action is between 30 and 60 minutes. This agent enjoyed its greatest popularity for epidural analgesia and anesthesia in obstetrics because of the rapid onset and low systemic toxicity in both mother and fetus. However, frequent injections are needed to provide adequate pain relief in labor and it is more usual to establish analgesia with chloroprocaine and then change to a longer acting agent such as ropivacaine or bupivacaine.

The use of chloroprocaine declined because of reports of prolonged neurological deficit following accidental subarachnoid injection. This toxicity was ascribed to the sodium meta-bisulfite used in the past as preservative. However there are no reports of neurotoxicity with newer preparations of chloroprocaine which contain disodium ethylenediaminetetraacetic acid (EDTA) as the preservative. Nevertheless these preparations are not recommended for intrathecal administration. However, since then, a number of reports of back pain have appeared. The incidence of back pain appears to be related to the large volume (greater than 40 ml) of drug injected. Chloroprocaine has also proved of value for peripheral nerve blocks and epidural anesthesia when the duration of surgery is not expected to exceed 30 to 60 minutes.

Tetracaine

Tetracaine is a **long-acting amino ester**. It is significantly more potent and has a longer duration of action than procaine or 2-chloroprocaine. Tetracaine remains a very popular drug for spinal anesthesia in the United States. This drug possesses excellent topical anesthetic properties, and solutions of this agent were commonly used for endotracheal surface anesthesia. Because of its slow onset and high toxicity, tetracaine is rarely used in peripheral nerve blocks.

Medium-term local anesthetics

Lidocaine (Xylocaine®, lignocaine)

(Tables 1.5a, 1.8, 1.11)

Class of drug: Lidocaine is a medium-duration local anesthetic of the amide type.

Single threshold dose: 200 mg without epinephrine in adults/70 kg body weight. After injection of a maximum dose, subsequent injections should not be given for 90 min. The second dose must not exceed a maximum of half of the first dose.

LD_{50} (mouse): 31.2–62.2 mg/kg body weight i.v.

Plasma half-life: ca. 1.6 h.

Latency: Fast.

Duration of effect: 1–2 h, depending on the area of application and the concentration used.

Metabolism: Lidocaine is metabolized in hepatic microsomes. Only about 3% of the drug is excreted unchanged via the kidney.

Tolerability and control: Lidocaine is one of the local anesthetics with moderate relative toxicity. It is characterized by a medium-term duration of effect and good distribution characteristics.

Lidocaine causes vasodilation, which may be less than that of procaine. When the medium-duration local anesthetics are compared, the strengths of the associated vasodilatory effects show the following sequence: lidocaine > mepivacaine > prilocaine. Lidocaine is therefore often used with epinephrine.

Clinical uses: Lidocaine is widely used in clinical practice, particularly in neural and segmental therapy. It is also suitable for infiltration anesthesia, for peripheral nerve block, for epidural anesthesia, and for mucosal surface anesthesia (2% gel, Emla®).

Dosage: Lidocaine is mainly administered as a 0.5–1% (1.5)% solution. Specific doses are given in the relevant chapters of this book.

Emla® cream

Emla® (a mixture of 2.5% lidocaine and 2.5% prilocaine) is a topical local anesthetic that penetrates intact skin and reaches an anesthetic depth of up to 5 mm. The onset of effect is approximately 1 h. When the effect takes place, the vessels in the skin show vasoconstriction initially, followed by vasodilation when higher concentrations are reached. This form of administration of this local anesthetic mixture has proved particularly useful in pediatric anesthesia before intravenous access placement, and for minor surgical procedures on the skin surface.

Lidocaine plaster

Lidocaine, administered in various forms (i.v., i.m. or transdermally) relieves pain associated with post-herpetic neuralgia (PHN) [1, 12, 13]. The analgesia is based on the blockade of neuronal sodium channels. However, intravenous administration of lidocaine can lead to plasma concentrations associated with antiarrhythmic effects. Topical application of lidocaine in the form of a gel or plaster avoids high plasma concentrations. This type of lidocaine plaster was developed in the USA, where it has been licensed since 1999 for pain treatment in post-herpetic neuralgia (Lidoderm®, Endo Pharmaceuticals Ltd., Chadds Ford, PA). The plaster consists of a soft, stretchable polyester base connected to an adhesive layer that contains 5% lidocaine. The plaster is 10 × 14 cm in size.

The systemic absorption of lidocaine has been shown in preclinical and clinical studies to be minimal (3%) in both volunteers and patients with PHN. Treatment with lidocaine plaster has been investigated in comparison with a placebo in three randomized, double-blind clinical studies including a total of 217 patients with PHN [7, 14, 15]. A significant reduction in pain intensity and allodynia was observed. Lidocaine plaster therefore represents a treatment option with a relatively low risk of adverse systemic events or drug interactions [8].

In Europe, clinical testing of the plaster for use in post-herpetic neuralgia is currently taking place, and its licensing for this indication can be expected within the next two or three years.

Mepivacaine (Scandicaine®, Meaverine®)

(Tables 1.5a, 1.8, 1.11)

Class of drug: Mepivacaine is a medium-duration local anesthetic of the amide type.

Single threshold dose without epinephrine in adults (70 kg body weight): 200 mg in the ENT field, 300 mg in other applications.

LD_{50} (mouse): 40.3 ± 3.2 mg/kg body weight i.v.

Plasma half-life: ca. 1.9 h.

Latency: Fast.

Duration of effect: 1–3 h, depending on the area of application and the concentration used.

Metabolism: Mepivacaine is metabolized in the hepatic microsomes.

After intravenous administration, up to 16% of the agent is excreted unchanged via the kidney. Degradation in the liver mainly produces m-hydroxymepivacaine and p-hydroxymepivacaine. These metabolites are conjugated with glucuronic acid and excreted in the urine. Another metabolite, pipecolylxylidide, collects in bile and passes through the enterohepatic circulation with its degradation products. No 2,6-xylidine is produced when mepivacaine is metabolized, and there is no evidence that either the agent or its metabolites have mutagenic or carcinogenic properties.

Tolerability and control: Mepivacaine is another of the local anesthetics with moderate relative toxicity. It is characterized by a medium-term duration of effect, with good distribution properties and some vasodilatory effect.

Clinical uses: Mepivacaine is the local anesthetic of choice when a medium-duration effect is required for diagnostic and therapeutic blocks in pain therapy – particularly in outpatients. It is suitable for infiltration anesthesia, intravenous regional anesthesia, peripheral nerve block and ganglion block, and for epidural anesthesia. Mepivacaine cannot be recommended in the obstetrics due to its long elimination half-life in the neonate.

Dosage: Mepivacaine is mainly used as a 1% (1.5%) or 0.5% solution. Specific doses are given in the relevant chapters of this book.

Prilocaine (Xylonest®)

(Tables 1.5a, 1.8, 1.11)

Class of drug: Prilocaine is a medium-duration local anesthetic of the amide type.

Single threshold dose: 600 mg (with or without vasopressor) in adults/70 kg body weight.

LD_{50} (mouse): 62 mg/kg b.w. i.v.

Plasma half-life: ca. 1.5 h.

Latency: Fast.

Duration of effect: 2–3 h, depending on the area of application and the concentration used.

Metabolism: Prilocaine is mainly metabolized in hepatic microsomes, but also in the kidney and lungs. During degradation, the metabolite ortho-toluidine is produced. At doses higher than 600 mg, the body's reduction systems may become exhausted. At doses higher than 800 mg, noticeable methemoglobinemia can be expected (see the section on substance-specific side effects). Fast elimination from the blood leads to low systemic toxicity.

Tolerability and control: Among the amide local anesthetics, prilocaine shows the best ratio between anesthetic potency and toxicity. Due to its high distribution volume and marked absorption in the lungs, plasma levels are significantly lower than those of mepivacaine and lidocaine (by a factor of 2–3). It has a medium-term duration of effect.

Clinical uses: Due to its comparatively low toxicity, prilocaine is particularly suitable for regional anesthesia techniques that require a single injection of a large volume or a high anesthetic dosage. The increasing use of prilocaine (2% isobaric solution) for spinal anesthesia is relatively new. Comparative studies in recent years have shown good tolerability, while transient neurological symptoms (TNS; see Chapter 37) were observed more often with lidocaine and mepivacaine. Prilocaine – like other medium-duration agents – is not suitable for continuous blocks. Due to the possibility of raised methemoglobin levels, prilocaine should not be used in anemic patients, children under the age of 6 months, or in obstetrics.

Dosage: Depending on the area of application, a 0.5–2% solution is used. Specific doses are given in the relevant chapters of this book.

Long-acting local anesthetics

Ropivacaine (Naropin®)

(Tables 1.5a, 1.7, 1.11)

Class of drug: Local anesthetic of the amide type, pure S-enantiomer.

Single threshold dose:
Anesthesia:
Epidural: 0.5–1%, 200 mg;
Plexus blocks: 0.75%, 300 mg;
Conduction and infiltration anesthesia: 0.5–0.75%, 225 mg;
Injection at myofascial trigger points: 0.2% (1–2 mL per trigger point).

Continuous procedures: 0.2%, up to 14 mL/h. Increased doses may be required during the early postoperative period – up to 0.375%, 10 mL/h (maximum 37.5 mg/h). When it is administered over several days, the resulting concentrations are well below potentially toxic plasma levels.

A dosage of 300 mg should be regarded as a guideline value, as this dosage has been confirmed as tolerable by various pharmacological studies.

LD_{50} (mouse): ca. 11.0–12.0 mg/kg b.w. i.v.
Plasma half-life: ca. 1.8 h.
Duration of effect: Epidural anesthesia ca. 7 h (analgesia); ca. 4 h (motor block), 10 mg/mL.
Plexus anesthesia (brachial plexus, lumbosacral plexus): 9–17 h, 7.5 mg/mL.
Infiltration anesthesia: postoperative analgesia after inguinal herniorrhaphy > 7 h (5–23 h), 7.5 mg/mL.
Peripheral nerve blocks in pain therapy: 2–6 h (0.2–0.375 mg/mL).

Latency: Medium (decreasing latency at increasing concentrations).

Metabolism: Ropivacaine is metabolized in the liver, mainly through aromatic hydroxylation. Only about 1% of the drug is excreted unchanged in the urine. The main metabolite is 3-hydroxyropivacaine.

Tolerability: Ropivacaine provides relatively low toxicity for a long-term local anesthetic. Compared with bupivacaine, it has a lower arrhythmogenic potential, and the margin between convulsive and lethal doses is wider. Ropivacaine has more favorable receptor kinetics ("fast in – medium out") in cardiac sodium channels, and in comparison with bupivacaine has only slight depressant effects on the energy metabolism of the mitochondria in cardiac muscle cells.

Clinical uses: The first clinical tests were carried out in 1988. Ropivacaine (Naropin®) has been in use since 1996. It is the first local anesthetic with a primary analgetic effect and is therefore of particular interest in pain therapy (postoperative and obstetric, as well as therapeutic blocks). In comparison with bupivacaine, it has fewer toxic side effects (CNS and, in particular, cardiac toxicity). High doses are needed before toxic effects develop. CNS symptoms appear well before cardiac symptoms, which in the clinical situation provides time for the local anesthetic injection to be stopped and for early treatment steps to be taken. In an animal model, the chances of successful resuscitation were also found to be better than with bupivacaine (90% vs. 50%) [9]. In addition, ropivacaine shows marked differential blocking in epidural analgesia and peripheral blocks. With a good quality of analgesia, up to 80% of patients have no measurable motor block on the Bromage scale. Epidural combinations (e.g., with sufentanil, dosage range 0.5–1 µg/mL) are possible. In view of the increased use of peripheral blocks and infiltrations at painful trigger points, evidence of higher muscular tissue tolerance in comparison with bupivacaine is also of interest [19].

The relatively low toxicity of ropivacaine means that high concentrations can be given (e.g., 10 mg/mL solution for epidural anesthesia) – providing more intense motor block, a higher success rate and better quality analgesia than 0.5% bupivacaine, for example (see Table 1.6).

Dosage: Ropivacaine is administered at concentrations of 2 mg/mL (0.2%), 7.5 mg/mL (0.75%), and 10 mg/mL (1%). Use for continuous epidural infusion has been approved (Naropin® 2 mg/mL polybag, 100 and 200 mL infusion solution). Cumulative daily doses of up to 675 mg (see specialist information) are well tolerated in adults. Precise information on doses is given in the following chapters.

Levobupivacaine (Chirocaine®)

(Tables 1.5a, 1.7, 1.8)

Class of drug: Local anesthetic of the amide type. A pure S-enantiomer of bupivacaine.

Single threshold dose without epinephrine in adults: 150 mg.

LD_{50} (mouse): 10.6 mg/kg b.w.

Plasma half-life: 80 ± 22 min. Plasma protein binding of levobupivacaine in humans has been assessed in vitro, and was more than 97% at concentrations of 0.1–1.0 µg/mL.

Latency: Medium (between ropivacaine and bupivacaine).

Duration of effect: 8–24 h, depending on the area of application and the concentration used.

Metabolism: Levobupivacaine is extensively metabolized, and unaltered levobupivacaine is not found in the urine or feces. 3-Hydroxylevobupivacaine, one of the principal metabolites of levobupivacaine, is excreted via the urine as a glucuronic acid and sulfate ester conjugate. In-vitro studies have shown that levobupivacaine is metabolized via CYP3A4 isoforms and CYP1A2 isoforms into desbutyl-levobupivacaine or 3-hydroxylevobupivacaine. The studies showed that the degradation of levobupivacaine and bupivacaine is similar. After intravenous administration of levobupivacaine, the recovery rate within 48 h averaged ca. 95%, quantitatively measurable in urine (71%) and feces (24%). There is evidence of in-vivo racemate formation with levobupivacaine.

Tolerability and control: Experimental animal studies have demonstrated a lower risk of CNS and cardiovascular toxicity with levobupivacaine than with bupivacaine. In volunteers, fewer negative inotropic effects were observed after intravenous administration of more than 75 mg levobupivacaine in comparison with bupivacaine. QT interval changes only occurred in a very few cases.

Clinical uses: There is little experience as yet with levobupivacaine in clinical practice. The numbers of published controlled clinical studies are also comparatively small. Available in-vitro, in-vivo, and controlled patient studies comparing levobupivacaine and bupivacaine have shown similar potency for neural blocks. After epidural administration of levobupivacaine, the same quality of sensory and motor block as with bupivacaine was seen. However, a significant differential block, as provided by ropivacaine, cannot be expected, as the drug has the same degree of lipophilia as bupivacaine. Levobupivacaine has not been approved for use in Germany.

Dosage: 0.125–0.75%. Precise information on doses is given in the following chapters.

Bupivacaine (Carbostesin®, Marcaine®)

(Tables 1.5a, 1.7, 1.8)

Class of drug: Local anesthetic of the amide type.

Single threshold dose: 150 mg without epinephrine in adults.

LD_{50} (mouse): 7.8 ± 0.4 mg/kg b.w. i.v.

Plasma half-life: ca. 2.7 h.

Latency: Medium.

Duration of effect: 2.5–20 h, depending on the area of application and the concentration used. A mean duration of effect of 3–6 h can be assumed.

Metabolism: Bupivacaine is broken down in hepatic microsomes at a high rate. The predominant metabolization involves dealkylation to pipecolylxylidide (desbutyl-bupivacaine). There is no evidence that either the agent or its metabolites have mutagenic or carcinogenic properties.

Tolerability and control: Bupivacaine is one of the local anesthetics that has a high relative toxicity. Its anesthetic potency is about four times greater than that of mepivacaine. It is characterized by a slower onset of effect and by a long duration of effect.

Clinical uses: Bupivacaine is indicated as a long-duration local anesthetic, particularly for regional anesthesia in the surgical field, in postoperative analgesia, and in therapy for various pain conditions.

It is suitable for infiltration anesthesia, peripheral nerve block, ganglion block and plexus block, as well as all forms of neuraxial anesthesia.

The marked cardiac toxicity of bupivacaine has been known since publications dating from the late 1970s, and severe and fatal adverse effects are still reported. Strict observation of safety standards is therefore of fundamental importance for the safe use of this drug at high doses.

Dosage: Depending on the indication, bupivacaine is administered as a 0.125–0.5% solution. A 0.75% solution is still being marketed. Higher concentrations are not required in pain therapy. Specific doses are given in the following chapters.

Examination and patient preparation

Before regional anesthesia, the same type of examination of the patient should be carried out as for general anesthesia. Contraindications must be excluded, as well as neurological abnormalities, and when there are relative contraindications – e.g., hemorrhagic diathesis, stable systemic neurological disease or local nerve damage – a careful assessment of the risk–benefit ratio needs to be made.

Particular attention needs to be given to anatomical relationships, palpation of the landmarks and precise localization and marking of the needle insertion point.

To ensure cooperation, the patient should be given detailed information about the aim of the block, its technical performance and possible or probable paresthesias and their significance. The patient should also be informed about potential adverse effects and complications of the block, and outpatients in particular should be familiarized with guidelines on behavior after anesthesia. The patient information session should be documented using a consent form signed by the patient.

In general, premedication and the administration of sedatives or analgesics should be avoided, particularly in outpatient pain therapy. Constant verbal contact should be maintained with the patient during the block, so that potential side effects or complications can be recognized immediately. In addition, any sedation that is not adjusted individually can lead to respiratory and circulatory complications, which may be mistaken for the early symptoms of local anesthetic toxicity.

Documentation of treatment

The patient history, including investigations at other centers, and diagnostic results should be documented just as carefully as the preparation, implementation, and success of the block. The checklists and record forms used in our own pain center have been adapted for each individual block technique, and are included in the following chapters.

Head and neck region

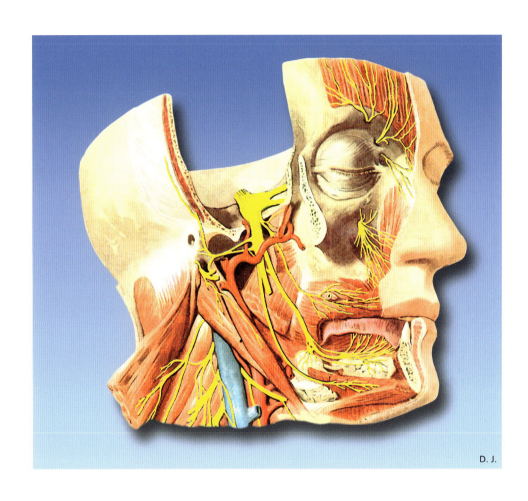

2 Regional anesthesia in ophthalmology

André van Zundert, Danilo Jankovic

The pioneering work of Koller (1884) on the anesthetic effect of cocaine in the context of ophthalmic surgery was the historical starting-point for local and regional anesthesia [8].

Anatomy of the eye [2, 5, 10, 12]

The eyeball or **bulbus oculi** is embedded in the orbit, and is covered by the eyelids (Fig. 2.2). The length of the orbit varies substantially (42–54 mm). The eyeball makes up approximately one-quarter (7 mL) of the total volume of the orbit. The remainder of the orbit is filled with fatty tissue, vessels, the lacrimal gland, nerves, connective tissue, and the extraocular muscles. The orbit is form by two compartments, an **extraconal** space and an **intraconal** space, surrounded by the four rectus muscles. Injected local anesthetics are easily able to pass the barrier between the two compartments by diffusion.

The superior eyelid, the **palpebra superior**, and the inferior eyelid, the **palpebra inferior**, form the boundaries of the palpebral fissure, the **rima palpebrarum**. This ends at the medial angle of the eye, the **angulus oculi medialis**, with a bulge that encloses the lacrimal caruncle or **caruncula lacrimalis**.

The inner wall of the eyelids is covered by the conjunctiva (**tunica conjunctiva**) (Fig. 2.1). Closure of the eyelids is carried out by the **orbicularis oculi muscle** (facial nerve), and raising of the upper lid is carried out by the **levator palpebrae superioris muscle** (oculomotor nerve; Figs. 2.2 and 2.3). The **lacrimal gland** lies above the lateral angle of the eye (Fig. 2.2), and is divided into an orbital part and a palpebral part by the tendon of the **levator palpebrae superioris muscle**. The orbit, covered with periosteum (periorbita), is filled with a fatty tissue body, the retrobulbar fat, in which the eyeball, optic nerve and eye muscles are embedded (Fig. 2.2).

The movements of the eyeball are made possible by six muscles – four straight ones and two oblique ones: the **superior rectus muscle, inferior rectus muscle, medial rectus muscle** (oculomotor nerve), lateral rectus muscle (abducent nerve), **superior oblique muscle** (trochlear nerve), and **inferior oblique muscle** (oculomotor nerve; Fig. 2.3).

On the anterior surface of the eyeball, the **bulbus oculi**, lies the transparent **cornea**. Underneath this is the **crystalline lens** of the eye, which is located in front of the **iris**, with its central opening, the **pupil**. The optic nerve exits on the posterior surface of the eyeball, slightly medial to the optic axis (Fig. 2.5). A distinction is made between three different spaces in the eye: the **anterior chamber of the eyeball**, bounded by the cornea, the iris and the lens; the **posterior chamber of the eyeball**, which encircles the lens in a ring-like shape; and the **postremal chamber of the eyeball**, which contains the **vitreous body** (corpus vitreum; Fig. 2.5).

The eye has two different vascular systems: the **ciliary arteries** and the **central retinal artery**. All of the vessels originate from the **ophthalmic artery** (Fig. 2.4). The vascular system in the posterior ciliary arteries not only serves to supply blood, but is also important for maintaining intraocular pressure and tension in the eyeball. The large vessels (ophthalmic artery and vein) and the nerve fascicles are concentrated in the area of the posterior pole of the eye. The highest risk of injury is therefore during puncture of the posterior third of

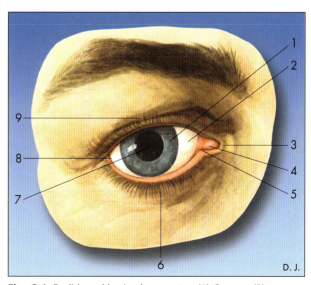

Fig. 2.1 Eyelids and lacrimal apparatus. (1) Cornea, (2) conjunctiva, (3) medial angle of the eye, (4) lacrimal caruncle, (5) lacrimal papilla, (6) inferior eyelid, (7) pupil, (8) lateral angle of the eye, (9) superior eyelid

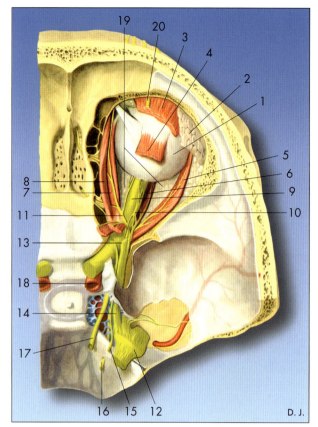

Fig. 2.2 Anatomy of the eye. (1) Eyeball, (2) lacrimal gland, (3) levator palpebrae superioris muscle, (4) superior rectus muscle, (5) lateral rectus muscle, (6) inferior rectus muscle, (7) medial rectus muscle, (8) superior oblique muscle, (9) optic nerve, (10) ciliary ganglion, (11) nasociliary nerve, (12) trigeminal ganglion, (13) frontal nerve, (14) ophthalmic nerve, (15) trochlear nerve, (16) abducent nerve, (17) oculomotor nerve, (18) internal carotid artery, (19) retrobulbar fat, (20) supraorbital nerve

ciliary ganglion, a tiny collection of nerve cells, lies in the posterior part of the orbit between the optic nerve and the lateral rectus muscle (Fig. 2.2). The sensory and sympathetic roots of the ciliary ganglion are provided by the nasociliary nerve and the neural network around the internal carotid artery, but do not always connect to the ciliary ganglion. Their fibers can reach the eye directly via the ciliary nerves. The sympathetic fibers, which are already postganglionic after they have switched to the cervical sympathetic trunk ganglia, can accompany the ophthalmic artery and its branches on the way to their destination. Stimuli from the cornea, iris, choroid and intraocular muscles are conducted in the sensory fibers.

Anatomy relevant to injections

- The average distance between the orbital margin and the ciliary ganglion is approximately 38 mm (ranging between 32 and 44 mm). In cadaver studies, Karampatiakis et al. [7] found that when a retrobulbar block was carried out with a needle 40 mm long, the needle tip would reach the posterior optic nerve in 100% of cases; even with needles 35 mm long, the covering of the optic nerve would be touched in 18% of cases.

> To protect the posterior pole of the eye and the ciliary ganglion, the block needle should be no more than 32 mm in length.

- The eyeball has an average longitudinal diameter of 23.5 mm (over 25 mm in severely myopic patients, increasing the risk of injury). The greatest risk of injury when carrying out a block is when the needle is introduced superior to or superomedial to the orbit. By contrast, when the direction of the gaze is straight ahead, the needle can be introduced with little risk at the inferolateral orbital margin and advanced parallel to the orbital floor up to the level of the posterior eyeball.

Physiology

The physiological pressure in the interior of the eye is between 10 and 20 mmHg. It is higher in patients with a large-diameter eyeball and in the recumbent position; it is higher in the morning than in the evening, and increases during coughing, physical exertion, and vomiting. An increased $P{co_2}$ or a reduced $P{o_2}$ increases the pressure inside the eye. Inhalation anesthetics, as well as barbiturates, neuroleptic agents, opioids, and propofol, among other substances, lead to a reduction in intra-ocular pressure, while laryngoscopy and intubation

the orbit, ca. 32–44 mm from the orbital margin. The **ciliary ganglion** is also located in this area, as well as the neighboring cranial nerves as they pass to the extraocular eye muscles (Fig. 2.2).

The orbital structures and their soft-tissue coverings mainly receive their sensory supply from the ophthalmic nerve. Branches of the maxillary nerve are also involved (see Chapter 4, Trigeminal nerve).

The nerve fibers in the retina pass in fascicles to the optic disk, in which they fuse to form the **optic nerve** and leave the eyeball. The **optic nerve** is surrounded by meninges. The dural sheath and arachnoid sheath show a gradual transition to become the sclera (Fig. 2.2). The **sclera** is ca. 0.8–1.0 mm thick and provides relatively little resistance to needle perforation.

The fascial sheath of the eyeball (vagina bulbi) is referred to as the **Tenon capsule**. It is a fibrous, elastic layer of connective tissue that surrounds the eyeball and the external eye muscles in the anterior orbit. The

– as well as drugs such as ketamine and muscle relaxants – have the opposite effect. The anterior and posterior chambers of the eye contain 250 μL of an aqueous liquid (rate of synthesis ca. 2.5 μL/min).

Anesthesia in eye surgery

Indications
- Regional anesthesia for **intraocular procedures** (e.g., cataract operations, vitrectomies, etc.):
  - Anesthesia of the eyeball, eyelid, conjunctiva
  - Retrobulbar (intraconal) or peribulbar (extraconal) anesthesia
  - Sub-Tenon anesthesia
  - Surface anesthesia
- **Extraocular procedures** (e.g. in strabismus) are usually carried out with the patient under general anesthesia.

Preoperative examination
Ophthalmological procedures are usually carried out in older people, and are associated with few risks. The great majority of diagnostic and surgical procedures in the eye can be safely carried out on an outpatient basis and usually with regional anesthesia. Independently of the type of anesthesia selected, a preoperative visit should be made. An information discussion with the patient is an absolute necessity.

Analgesia and sedation [4, 14]
It is recommended that one of the following drugs is given immediately before carrying out regional anesthesia:
- Midazolam 1 mg (+ remifentanil 0.33 μg/kg)
- Propofol 0.5 mg/kg

Deep sedation should not accompany regional anesthesia; the patient should be capable of cooperating.

Preparations
Place the patient in a comfortable position. Nasal oxygen administration should be carried out routinely. Continuous monitoring (pulse oximetry, ECG monitoring, blood-pressure monitoring) and intravenous access are necessary. An intravenous infusion is not obligatory. Before the procedure, the effect of the regional anesthesia administered should be checked (motility testing).

Characteristics of an ideal eye block
- The block should be carried out with the smallest possible volume of the local anesthetic.
- Analgesia and akinesia of the eyeball (the latter is not always necessary).

Regional anesthesia in ophthalmology

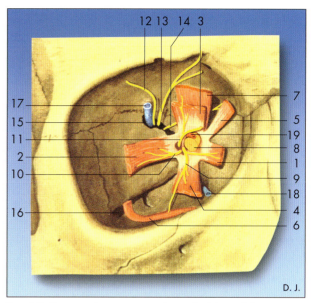

Fig. 2.3 Eye: muscles, nerves, and vessels. (1) Medial rectus muscle, (2) lateral rectus muscle, (3) superior rectus muscle, (4) inferior rectus muscle, (5) superior oblique muscle, (6) inferior oblique muscle, (7) levator palpebrae superioris muscle, (8) optic nerve, (9) oculomotor nerve, (10) abducent nerve, (11) nasociliary nerve, (12) lacrimal nerve, (13) frontal nerve, (14) trochlear nerve, (15) superior orbital fissure, (16) inferior orbital fissure, (17) superior ophthalmic vein, (18) inferior ophthalmic vein, (19) ophthalmic artery

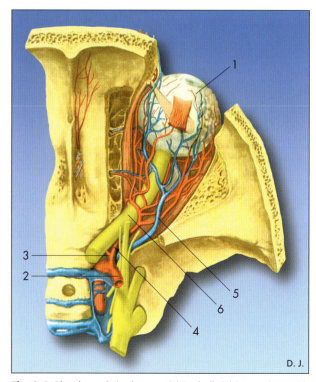

Fig. 2.4 Blood supply in the eye. (1) Eyeball, (2) internal carotid artery, (3) central retinal artery, (4) ophthalmic artery, (5) superior ophthalmic vein, (6) optic nerve

Chapter 2

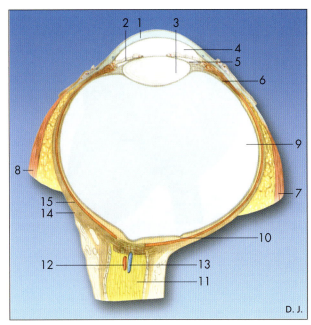

Fig. 2.5 Horizontal section through the eyeball. (1) Cornea, (2) iris, (3) lens, (4), anterior chamber of the eyeball, (5) posterior chamber of the eyeball, (6) ciliary body, (7) lateral rectus muscle, (8) medial rectus muscle, (9) vitreous body, (10) central retinal fovea, (11) optic nerve, (12) central retinal artery, (13) central retinal vein, (14) sclera, (15) chorioid

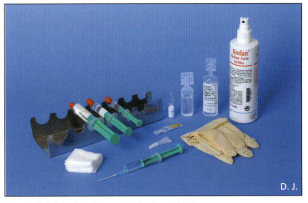

Fig. 2.6 Materials for a retrobulbar block

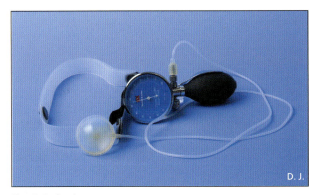

Fig. 2.7 Oculopressor

- No pain during the operation.
- No significant complications.

Techniques of conduction and infiltration anesthesia

Retrobulbar block (intraconal anesthesia)
[2, 10, 12, 16]

Indications
Intraocular procedures (e.g., cataract surgery, vitrectomies).

Preparations
See above.

Materials (Fig. 2.6)
Atkinson (23 G, 11/4´) 0.60 × 32 mm needle, retrobulbar/peribulbar. Syringe 5 mL, swab, compresses, disinfectant, sterile precautions, local anesthetic (or alternatively: curved or bent needle – e.g., Strauss needle).
Sharp versus blunt needle tip: blunt needles are better in patients with high-grade myopia, with a longitudinal diameter of the eyeball of more than 25 mm. However, sharp tips provide a better feel when advancing the needle.

Patient positioning
The best position for the patient is semi-recumbent (45°).

Injection technique
Depending on the anesthetist's preferences, two puncture methods are possible: usually transcutaneous, through the lower eyelid (Fig. 2.8a) or, more rarely, transconjunctival (Fig. 2.8b).
The block needle is introduced in the 7 o'clock position on the right or the 5 o'clock position on the left. The eye should be gazing upward and to the contralateral side, and the eyeball can be delicately pushed in a medial and cranial direction using a free finger. The needle is directed initially at a slight angle toward the orbital floor (2–3°) under the eyeball. The needle is introduced along the bony floor of the orbit toward the back in the direction of the root of the nose and at an angle of less than 45° to the skin. Moving the eyeball inward and upward results in tensing of the inferior oblique muscle, which is thereby pulled out of the injection area.
At the end of the injection, the needle exits between the inferior rectus muscle and the lateral rectus muscle into the space lying temporal to the optic nerve, in which the ciliary ganglion is located.

- The needle must not be advanced against hard resistance.
- The injection of the local anesthetic should be carried out slowly, in incremental doses, after prior aspiration.
- After the injection, an oculopressor should be placed for ca. 5–10 min, at a pressure of ca. 20–30 mmHg (Fig. 2.7). This allows better distribution of the local anesthetic as well as providing prophylaxis against hematoma.

Motility testing of the eye must be carried out before the procedure (Fig. 2.12).

Dosage [6]
- Oxybuprocaine HCl 0.4% for surface anesthesia if the transconjunctival access route is chosen.
- 3–5 mL local anesthetic (e.g., 0.75% ropivacaine, 0.5% bupivacaine, 2% prilocaine, 2% mepivacaine, 2% lidocaine) or combinations of these.
- Possible adjuncts to the local anesthetic:
- Epinephrine (5 µg/mL or 1 : 200 000; see Chapter 50, Adjuncts to local anesthesia)
- Hyaluronidase (150 IU; Hylase®, Pharma Dessau, Germany) [6]

The addition of hyaluronidase to local anesthetics leads to improved diffusion and thus to a faster onset. This provides very good conditions for surgical procedures in the eye.

Side effects and complications [16]
- Hemorrhage in the very well vascularized orbit, with a frequency of 0.7–1.7% (known as "compartment syndrome"), can lead to blindness.
- Conjunctival hemorrhage (20–100%).
- Retinal detachment and vitreous hemorrhage after perforation of the eyeball can lead to loss of vision.
- Subperiosteal hemorrhage due to contact between the needle and the orbital floor.
- Chemosis (25–40%) due to fast injection of larger volumes of a local anesthetic.
- Perforation of the eyeball and intraocular injections can occur, particularly in severely myopic patients. To avoid these, patients should gaze straight ahead throughout the block procedure.
- Injury to the optic nerve or intraneural injection (immediate blindness).
- Subarachnoid injection is a severe complication (see Chapter 37, p. 285).
- Intravascular injection, with serious CNS intoxication (see Chapter 1, p. 9 and Chapter 6, p. 65).
- Oculocardiac reflex: bradycardia due to the vasovagal reflex is observed in younger and frail patients and may be seen both during the block procedure and also intraoperatively.
- Injury to the extraocular muscles (usually the inferior oblique muscle or inferior rectus muscle) can lead to muscle necrosis, contractions, or disturbances of healing.

Peribulbar block (extraconal anesthesia) [1, 10]

If there is a fear of complications due to retrobulbar injection in certain patients (e.g., severely myopic patients with a long eyeball), extensive anesthesia and partial akinesia can also be achieved using a peribulbar block for procedures in the anterior part of the eye. In this case, the local anesthetic can be injected extraconally. Several technical variations of peribulbar, periocular and

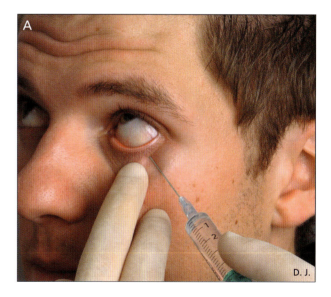

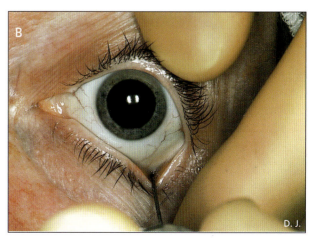

Fig. 2.8 Retrobulbar block.
(A) Transcutaneous access, (B) transconjunctival access

extraconal anesthesia have been described. The method most often used today is a "two-injection technique."

Materials
(See retrobulbar block.)
Peribulbar needle, 25 G, 0.50 × 30 mm.

> ■ The injections are carried out transcutaneously through the lower eyelid or upper eyelid.
> ■ The patient's gaze should be directed straight ahead with both techniques.

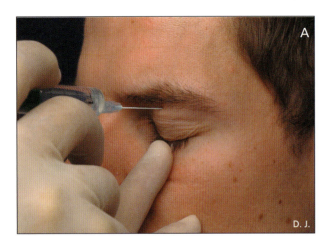

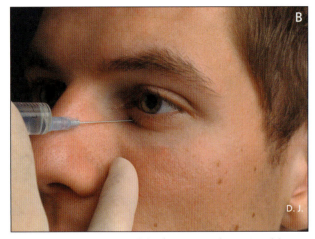

Fig. 2.9 Peribulbar block. (A) Inferotemporal injection, (B) superior extraconal injection

Injection technique
The areas selected for puncture are those that are least well perfused with blood.
- Inferior, extraconal, or inferotemporal injection (injection depth up to a maximum of 25 mm). The superior orbital fissure serves as a landmark (Fig. 2.9a).
- Superior, extraconal injection (just medial to the medial angle of the eyelid). The anterior lower orbital margin serves as a landmark (Fig. 2.9b).

Dosage
Slow injection of 3–5 mL local anesthetic per puncture point (see retrobulbar anesthesia).
After the injection, an oculopressor should be used for ca. 10 min (Fig. 2.7). This allows better extraconal–intraconal diffusion of the injected local anesthetic.

Disadvantages
- In peribulbar anesthesia, injuries to the trochlea or superior oblique muscle can occur. Some authors therefore recommend avoiding upper supranasal injection. However, this can lead to poorer results with the block.
- Larger amounts of local anesthetic are needed to achieve adequate extraconal–intraconal diffusion (increased intra-ocular pressure).
- Slower times to onset.
- There is a higher failure rate with peribulbar anesthesia in comparison to retrobulbar anesthesia (10–20%).

Complications
- Perforation of the eyeball (1 : 12 000 – 16 000 cases)
- Peribulbar hemorrhage
- Eyelid ecchymosis

Sub-Tenon block [3, 11, 13, 15]
In the sub-Tenon block, the sub-Tenon capsule is separated from the sclera and elevated. After opening and introduction of a special blunt sub-Tenon needle, the local anesthetic is injected into the sub-Tenon space. This method represents an alternative to the two methods described above, in which potential complications such as eyeball perforation can be avoided.

Preparations
See retrobulbar block.

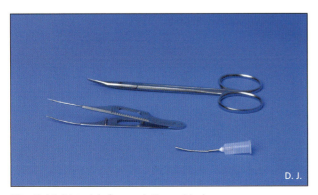

Fig. 2.10 Materials for a sub-Tenon block

Materials (Fig. 2.10)
An eyelid speculum (e.g., Barraquer's), Moorfield forceps, blunt Westcott scissors, blunt sub-Tenon needle, 5-mL syringe, solution for surface anesthesia of the conjunctiva (oxybuprocaine 0.4%), local anesthetic, hyaluronidase (15–150 IU/mL), 5% aqueous iodine solution to clean the conjunctiva.

> N.B. before the procedure:
> - Should be conducted with sterile precautions
> - Surface anesthesia of the conjunctiva with 0.4% oxybuprocaine drops (inferonasal part)
> - Cleaning of the conjunctiva with a 5% aqueous iodine solution
> - Delicate placement of an eyelid speculum

Procedure (Fig. 2.11)
- The conjunctiva and the Tenon capsule adhering to it (between the medial rectus muscle and the inferior rectus muscle) are elevated with the forceps ca. 5–7 mm away from the corneal limbus (inferonasal point).
- The conjunctiva and Tenon space are opened using Westcott scissors.
- Blunt preparation of the channel to the posterior sub-Tenon space then follows. The sclera should be visible.
- The blunt sub-Tenon needle is introduced into the posterior sub-Tenon space. Resistance is felt during this procedure (the posterior sub-Tenon capsule and the sclera are close together).
- Slow injection of the local anesthetic is then carried out.
- After the injection, an oculopressor is placed for ca. 5–10 min (Fig. 2.7).
- Motility checking of the eye then follows.

Dosage
2–4 mL of local anesthetic (e.g., 0.75% ropivacaine, 0.5% bupivacaine, 2% prilocaine, 2% mepivacaine, 2% lidocaine).
Combination with hyaluronidase (15–150 IU/mL) is recommended in order to improve the diffusion of the local anesthetic.

Potential complications
This method is associated with few potential complications, which include:
- Subconjunctival injection (chemosis). Prophylaxis: addition of hyaluronidase and use of an oculopressor after the block.
- Perforation of the sclera.
- Subconjunctival hemorrhage.
- Adverse cardiovascular events.

Advantages
- Complications occur extremely rarely.

Disadvantages
- Eyelid akinesia is variable and depends on the volume of local anesthetic injected.
- About 10% of patients require supplementation with an additional block of the facial nerve (4%), surface anesthesia (2.6%) or retrobulbar block (0.8%).
- Pain during injection.

Anticoagulation and ocular block
In patients who are taking anticoagulant medication, coagulation parameters (INR) should be checked before the procedure. Long needles with sharp tips increase the risk of hemorrhage. Smaller needles and single-shot injections appear to be safer, and the sub-Tenon technique is apparently safer still [9].

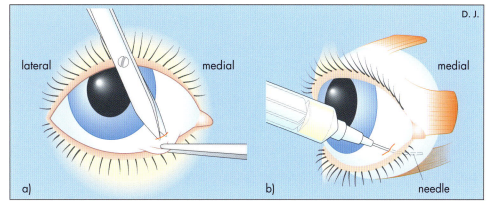

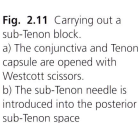

Fig. 2.11 Carrying out a sub-Tenon block.
a) The conjunctiva and Tenon capsule are opened with Westcott scissors.
b) The sub-Tenon needle is introduced into the posterior sub-Tenon space

Chapter 2

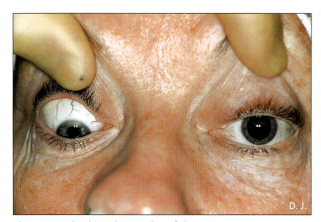

Fig. 2.12 Checking the motility of the eye

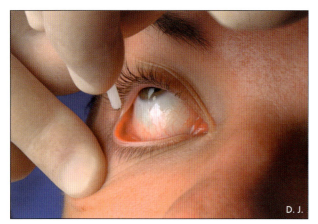

Fig. 2.13 Surface anesthesia

Local or surface anesthesia

Local anesthetic solutions in droplet form (known as non-akinetic methods of ocular anesthesia) can be applied externally if the surgeon requires only small incisions for procedures in the anterior part of the eye. Drip anesthesia is used in more extensive procedures as an additional method of infiltration and block anesthesia. Resorption of the local anesthetic through the mucosa is extremely fast. The introduction of oxybuprocaine represented a substantial advance in ocular anesthesia. This agent causes only a mild burning sensation, and has neither hyperemic nor vasoconstrictive effects. In addition, it has no effect on the pupil and only causes mild loosening of the corneal epithelium. With the patient gazing upward and with the head tilted backward, the drops are introduced into the conjunctival sac (Fig. 2.13).

This procedure cannot be generally recommended and is reserved for highly motivated and non-anxious patients. It is not suitable for deaf patients or patients with or speech difficulties.

Additional blocks for eyelid akinesia

Facial nerve block

In the majority of intraocular procedures, it is necessary to prevent eyelid movement (orbicularis oculi muscle). This can be achieved by a distal infiltration block of the nerve endings of the facial nerve that provide the motor supply to the orbit.

Anatomy (Fig. 2.14)
The seventh cranial nerve carries motor fibers for the muscles of facial expression, and – in the intermediate nerve, a nerve fascicle emerging separately from the brain stem – gustatory fibers and visceral efferent secretory (parasympathetic) fibers. Both sections of nerve pass through the internal acoustic meatus and emerge as a neural trunk in the facial canal. The geniculate ganglion is located at the bend in the nerves in the petrous bone. The facial canal then courses via the tympanic cavity and turns caudally toward the stylomastoid foramen, through which the nerve exits from the skull. In the parotid gland, it divides into its end branches (parotid plexus). Before entering the parotid gland, the facial nerve gives off the posterior auricular nerve and

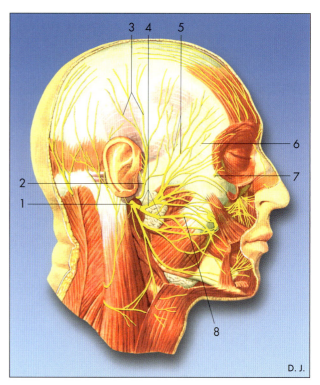

Fig. 2.14 Anatomy of the facial nerve. (1) Facial nerve, (2) auriculotemporal nerve, (3) superficial temporal branches, (4) parotid plexus, (5) temporal branches, (6) zygomaticotemporal branch of zygomatic nerve, (7) zygomaticofacial branch of zygomatic nerve, (8) buccal branches of facial nerve

Regional anesthesia in ophthalmology

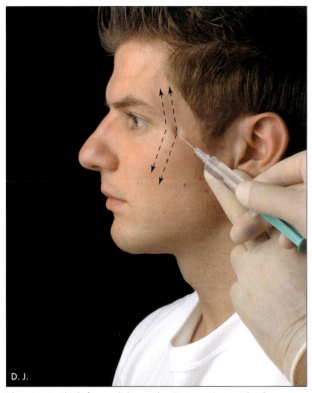

Fig. 2.15 Block for eyelid anesthesia. Van Lint method

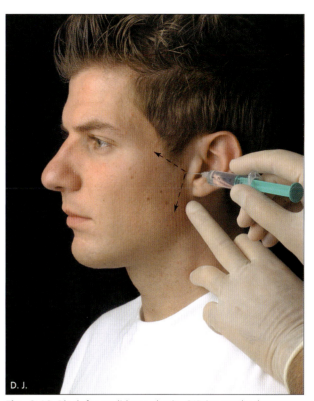

Fig. 2.16 Block for eyelid anesthesia. O'Brien method

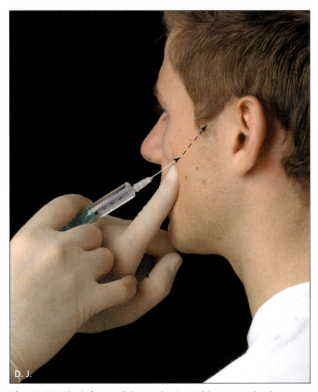

Fig. 2.17 Block for eyelid anesthesia. Atkinson method

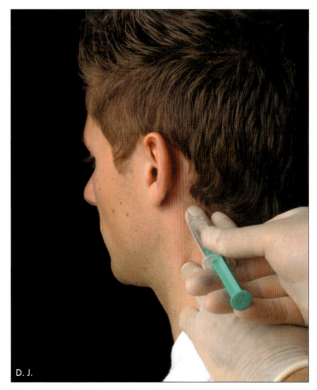

Fig. 2.18 Block for eyelid anesthesia. Nadbath–Rehmann method

branches to the posterior belly of the digastric muscle and to the stylohyoid muscle. From the parotid plexus emerge the temporal branches, zygomatic branches, buccal branches, and marginal mandibular branch, and the cervical branch to the platysma. These branches supply the muscles of facial expression.

Block techniques
The facial nerve can be blocked using various techniques along its course to the orbit.

Van Lint method (Fig. 2.15)
The injection is carried out temporally from the exterior margin of the eyelid, or classically just below it temporally. A 23-G needle 30–40 mm long is initially introduced until bone contact is made. After careful aspiration, the injection is carried out medially and downward, and then medially and upward. Fan-shaped injection is carried out as the needle is advanced (dosage: 1.5–2 mL local anesthetic).

O'Brien method (Fig. 2.16)
The facial nerve trunk is blocked just above the condylar process of the mandible. It is helpful for the patient to open and close the mouth. After palpation of the condylar process of the mandible, a 25-G needle 30–40 mm long is introduced until bone contact is made, and 1 mL local anesthetic is injected. The needle is then withdrawn, followed by injections first in the caudal direction and then in the cranial direction (dosage: 2–3 mL local anesthetic).

Atkinson method (Fig. 2.17)
A 23-G needle 30–40 mm long is introduced below the exterior angle of the eye at the level of the zygomatic arch and is moved upward and outward (dosage: 3 mL local anesthetic).

Nadbath–Rehmann method (Fig. 2.18)
The blocking of the main trunk of the facial nerve is carried out directly underneath the mastoid process. A 25-G needle 30 mm long is introduced vertically to a depth of 1.5–2 cm (dosage: 2–3 mL local anesthetic).

Block of peripheral branches of the trigeminal nerve

See Chapter 4.

Conduction anesthesia for intraocular procedures

Block ☐ Right ☐ Left

Name: _____ Date: _____
Diagnosis: _____
Premedication: ☐ No ☐ Yes _____

Purpose of block:	☐ Surgery
Needle:	☐ ___ G ☐ Sharp ☐ Blunt
	☐ Other ☐ ___ G ___ mm long
i. v. access:	☐ Yes
Monitoring:	☐ ECG ☐ Pulse oximetry
Ventilation facilities:	☐ Yes (equipment checked)
Emergency equipment (drugs):	☐ Checked
Patient:	☐ Informed

Position: ☐ Supine ☐ Sitting ☐ Semi-sitting
Approach: ☐ Retrobulbar ☐ Peribulbar ☐ Sub-Tenon
☐ Surface anesthesia ☐ Other (facial nerve, trigeminal nerve)

Sedoanalgesia before block:
☐ Midazolam ___ mg ☐ Propofol ___ mg/kg
☐ Remifentanil ___ µg/kg ☐ Other _____

Local anesthetic: ___ mL ___ % _____
Addition to injection solution: ☐ No ☐ Yes

Patient's remarks during injection:
☐ None ☐ Pain ☐ Paresthesias ☐ Warmth

Objective block effect after 15 min:
☐ Akinesia ☐ Mydriasis ☐ Exophthalmos ☐ Incomplete block

Monitoring after block: ☐ < 1 h ☐ > 1 h
Time of discharge: _____

Complications: ☐ None
☐ Yes (hematoma, intravascular injection, other)
_____

VISUAL ANALOG SCALE

0 10 20 30 40 50 60 70 80 90 100

Special notes:
_____
_____
_____
_____

Record and checklist

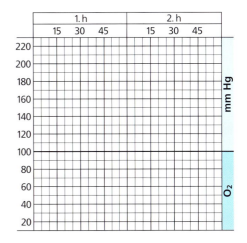

3 Occipital nerves
Greater occipital nerve
Lesser occipital nerve

Anatomy

After exiting from the lower edge of the obliquus capitis inferior muscle, the second cervical spinal nerve divides into anterior and posterior branches.

The anterior branches of the first four cervical spinal nerves form the cervical plexus, which is covered by the sternocleidomastoid muscle. The superficial branches of the cervical plexus, which penetrate the cervical fascia and pass to the skin, include the sensory **lesser occipital nerve** (anterior branch from C2 and C3). This emerges at the posterior edge of the sternocleidomastoid muscle, above its midpoint. It ascends steeply along the splenius capitis muscle and divides into several branches (Fig. 3.1). The areas it supplies include the skin on the upper exterior side of the neck, the upper part of the auricle and the adjoining skin of the scalp.

The posterior branch of the second cervical spinal nerve passes in a dorsal direction around the obliquus capitis inferior muscle and runs between the occipitovertebral muscles and the semispinalis capitis muscle. Here it divides into three branches: an ascending branch, which supplies the longissimus capitis muscle; a descending branch, which anastomoses with the posterior branch of C3 (the third occipital nerve); and the medial **greater occipital nerve** (posterior branch of C2).

The sensory greater occipital nerve passes in a cranial direction, goes through the semispinalis capitis muscle and trapezius muscle and reaches the skin about 2–3 cm away from the midline in the area of the superior nuchal line. It gives off several branches toward the top of the head and extends laterally as far as the ear. The course of its branches follows the branches of the occipital artery.

Blocks of the greater and lesser occipital nerves

Indications

Blocks of the **greater** and **lesser occipital nerves** are carried out for prognostic, diagnostic and therapeutic

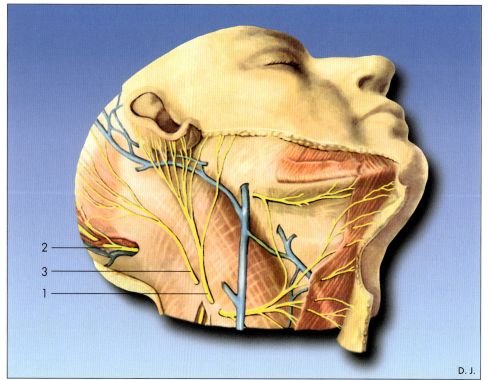

Fig. 3.1 Nerves supplying the surface of the back of the head:
(1) great auricular nerve,
(2) greater occipital nerve and occipital artery,
(3) lesser occipital nerve

purposes in patients with painful conditions in the region of the back of the head.

Diagnostic
- Differential diagnosis of pain at the back of the head – e.g., in suspected tumors of the posterior cranial fossa.

Therapeutic
- Occipital neuralgia characterized by pain in the suboccipital area and back of the head [5].

> Neuralgia of the occipital nerves caused by compression is anatomically almost impossible. The origin of the neuralgia must under all circumstances be identified. The cause is often degenerative change – e.g., in the vertebral column, or muscle tension with irritation of the nerve roots. There may also be articular disease or tumors in the second and third cervical dorsal roots. In whiplash injuries, consideration can be given to activation of the numerous myofascial trigger points – e.g., in the area of the cervical musculature, masticatory muscles and sternocleidomastoid, trapezius, occipitofrontal and suboccipital muscles – and simultaneous treatment of these is possible [6].

> Genuine occipital neuralgia is extremely rare.

Specific contraindications
None.

Procedure

Preparations
Check that the emergency equipment is complete and in working order. Sterile precautions, skin prep.

Materials
Syringes (2 mL), fine 26-G needles (2.5 cm), disinfectant, swabs for compression (Fig. 3.2).

Patient positioning
Sitting, with head tilted forward slightly.

Landmarks
Occipital artery, inferior nuchal line: one-third of the distance between the external occipital protuberance and the foramen magnum.

Occipital nerves

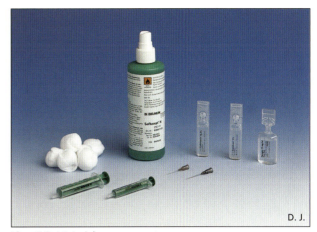

Fig. 3.2 Materials

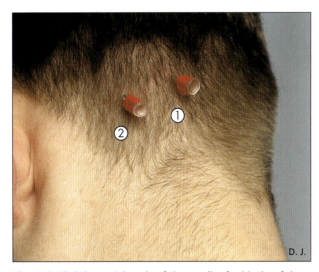

Fig. 3.3 Slightly cranial angle of the needles for blocks of the greater occipital nerve (1) and lesser occipital nerve (2)

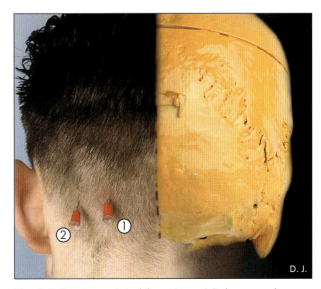

Fig. 3.4 Puncture points: (1) greater occipital nerve and (2) lesser occipital nerve

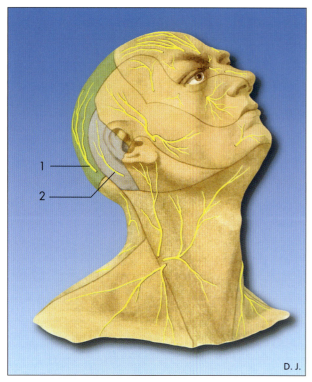

Fig. 3.5 Areas supplied by the greater occipital nerve (1) and lesser occipital nerve (2)

Injection techniques
Greater occipital nerve
The needle is inserted about 2.5 cm from the midline, directly medial to the easily palpable occipital artery. It is advanced at a slightly cranial angle (Fig. 3.3) between the insertions of the trapezius and semispinalis muscles until bone contact is made. After minimal withdrawal and aspiration, the local anesthetic is injected.

Lesser occipital nerve
The injection is carried out about 2.5 cm lateral to the puncture point described above (Fig. 3.4). Bone contact is also sought at a slightly cranial angle and the needle is withdrawn a little, followed by aspiration and injection.

Spread of the blocks
The areas supplied are illustrated in Figure 3.5.

> There are close anatomical connections both with the trigeminal nerve and with the third occipital nerve. The third occipital nerve in particular is often anesthetized as well.

Dosage
Diagnostic
0.5–1 mL local anesthetic – e.g. 0.5–1% prilocaine, mepivacaine, or lidocaine.

Therapeutic
1–1.5 mL local anesthetic – e.g. 0.75% ropivacaine, 0.5% bupivacaine (0.5% levobupivacaine), often with 1–2 mg dexamethasone added.

> Higher doses should be avoided due to the high vascular perfusion and resultant rapid absorption.

Block series
When there is evidence of improvement in the symptoms, 8–12 blocks are indicated.

Complications
Inadvertent intra-arterial injection may occur, extremely rarely.

Treatment measures
See Chapter 6, p. 66.

4 Trigeminal nerve

Anatomy

The trigeminal nerve, the largest of the cranial nerves, exits from the pons with a small motor root (the portio minor) and a large sensory root (portio major).

In the semilunar cavity of the dura mater, the sensory root expands to become the trigeminal ganglion (semilunar ganglion). The motor root runs along the medial side of the ganglion to the mandibular nerve.

The trigeminal ganglion lies on the dorsal surface of the petrous bone. The three main branches originate from its anterior margin (Fig. 4.1): the **ophthalmic nerve, maxillary nerve** and **mandibular nerve.**

Ophthalmic nerve

The optic branch is purely sensory and passes lateral to the cavernous sinus and abducent nerve to the superior orbital fissure. It draws sympathetic fibers from the internal carotid plexus and in turn gives off sensory fibers to the oculomotor nerve, trochlear nerve and abducent nerve. Before entering the fissure, the ophthalmic nerve branches into the lacrimal nerve, nasociliary nerve and frontal nerve.

The **frontal nerve** runs along the levator palpebrae superioris muscle to behind the center of the orbital cavity. There it divides into the **supraorbital nerve,** which passes to the supraorbital notch, and the **supratrochlear nerve**, which runs in a medial direction toward the trochlea.

The branches of the supratrochlear nerve supply the upper eyelid, the root of the nose and the adjoining skin of the forehead (upper end branch), as well as the skin and conjunctiva of the medial canthus (lower end branch).

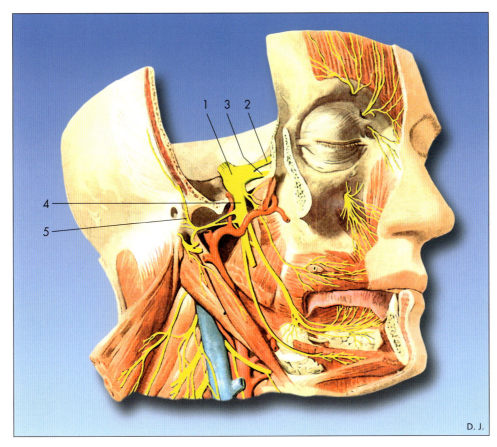

Fig. 4.1 Sensory supply to the face.
(1) Trigeminal ganglion,
(2) ophthalmic nerve,
(3) maxillary nerve,
(4) mandibular nerve and
(5) auriculotemporal nerve

Chapter 4

Maxillary nerve

The second branch of the trigeminal nerve is also purely sensory. It emerges from the skull through the round foramen and enters the pterygopalatine fossa.

From here, it gives off the zygomatic nerve to the orbit and the pterygopalatine nerves – two very short nerves that connect with the **pterygopalatine (sphenopalatine) ganglion** (Fig. 4.11).

As a continuation of its trunk, the infraorbital nerve penetrates through the inferior orbital fissure to the base of the orbit, to the infraorbital groove and infraorbital canal. After passing through the infraorbital foramen, it reaches the facial surface of the maxilla. Here it divides into three groups of branches, which supply the side of the nose, the lower eyelid and the upper lip.

Mandibular nerve

As the largest branch of the trigeminal nerve, the mandibular nerve contains the sensory parts of the trigeminal ganglion and takes up the motor root of the trigeminal nerve.

After passing through the oval foramen, the mandibular nerve forms a short, thick nerve trunk, on the medial side of which lies the **otic ganglion.** In its later course, the mandibular nerve divides into an anterior trunk with mainly motor fibers and a posterior trunk with nerve branches and end fibers mainly consisting of sensory fibers. The most important nerves and areas of supply in the posterior trunk are:

– **Mental nerve** (skin and mucosa of the lower lip and chin)
– **Inferior alveolar nerve** (molar and premolar teeth of the mandible)
– **Lingual nerve** (floor of the mouth, mucosa of the anterior two-thirds of the tongue)
– **Auriculotemporal nerve** (ear, skin and fascia of the temple)

The sensory branch of the anterior trunk, the **buccal nerve,** supplies the skin and mucosa in the area of the buccinator muscle.

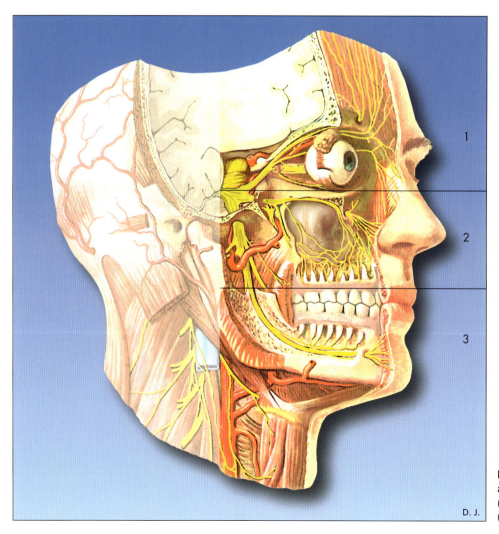

Fig. 4.2 (1) Supraorbital and supratrochlear nerves, (2) infraorbital nerve, (3) mental nerve

Trigeminal nerve

Blocks of the supraorbital and supratrochlear nerves

The end branches of these two nerves provide the sensory supply for the skin of the forehead, top of the nose and the skin and conjunctiva of the medial canthus (Fig. 4.2).

Indications
Diagnostic
- Differential diagnosis of hyperalgesic zones – e.g. the frontal part of the occipitofrontalis muscle

Therapeutic
- Trigeminal neuralgia of the first branch and post-herpetic neuralgia
- Postoperative and post-traumatic pain
- Minor surgical interventions (note higher doses) along the surface of the innervated area – e.g. removal of cysts and atheromas, wound care

Specific contraindications
None.

Procedure

Preparations
Check that the emergency equipment is complete and in working order. Sterile precautions.

Materials
2-mL syringes, fine 26-G needles (25 mm), disinfectant, swabs for compression (Fig. 4.3).

Skin prep
For all blocks.

Patient positioning
Supine.

Landmarks
Supraorbital foramen, upper angle of the orbit.
Supraorbital nerve: palpation of the supraorbital foramen at the orbital margin.
Supratrochlear nerve: palpation of the upper angle of the orbit on the medial side of the root of the nose.

Injection techniques
Supraorbital nerve
After palpation of the supraorbital foramen, a swab is laid on the eyelid to prevent uncontrolled spread of the local anesthetic. The needle is introduced as far as the supraorbital foramen (bone contact), slightly withdrawn, and after aspiration the injection is carried out slowly (Fig. 4.5).

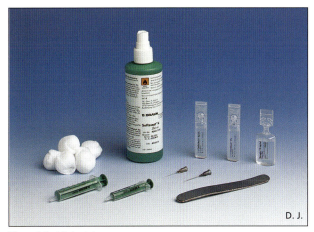

Fig. 4.3 Materials

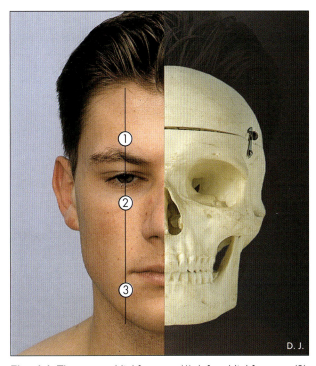

Fig. 4.4 The supraorbital foramen (1), infraorbital foramen (2) and mental foramen (3) lie on a single line running about 2.5 cm lateral to the midfacial line and passing through the pupil

Supratrochlear nerve
After palpation of the upper angle of the orbit, a swab is laid on the eyelid to prevent uncontrolled spread of the local anesthetic. The needle is introduced at the upper internal angle of the orbit (Fig. 4.6) and minimally withdrawn after bone contact. Slow injection of the local anesthetic follows after careful aspiration.

Chapter 4

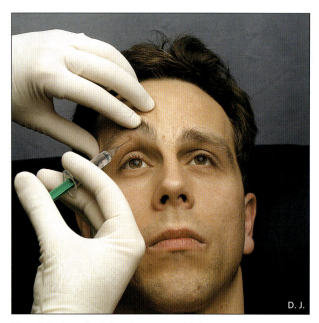

Fig. 4.5 Anesthetizing the supraorbital nerve

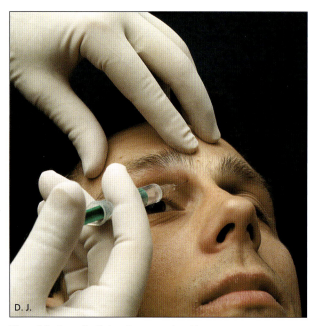

Fig. 4.6 Anesthetizing the supratrochlear nerve

> It is not necessary to elicit paresthesias. Look for bone contact, withdraw the needle slightly, aspirate and inject.

Dosage
Diagnostic
0.5–1 mL local anesthetic – e.g. 0.5–1% prilocaine, mepivacaine, lidocaine.

Therapeutic
0.5–1 mL local anesthetic – e.g. 0.5–0.75% ropivacaine, 0.25–0.5% bupivacaine.

Surgical
Up to 5 mL local anesthetic.
Shorter procedures: e.g. 1% prilocaine or 1% mepivacaine.
Longer procedures: 0.75% ropivacaine, 0.5% bupivacaine (0.5% levobupivacaine).

Side effects
Possible hematoma formation (prophylactic compression).

> After the injection, carry out thorough compression (massaging in) to prevent hematoma formation and to encourage the local anesthetic to spread.

Complications
Risk of blood vessel and nerve damage with injections into the foramina and bone channels.

> No injections should be made into the supraorbital foramen due to the risk of nerve injury.

Blocks of the infraorbital nerve

The infraorbital nerve, the end branch of the maxillary nerve, emerges about 1 cm below the middle of the lower orbital margin through the infraorbital foramen (Figs. 4.2, 4.35).

Indications
Diagnostic
- Differential diagnosis of trigger zones

Therapeutic
- Trigeminal neuralgia in the second branch and post-herpetic pain
- Facial pain in the innervation area of the infraorbital nerve, post-traumatic pain and pain after dental extraction
- Minor surgical procedures on the surface of the area of distribution (note higher dosages)

Specific contraindications
None.

Procedure

Preparation and materials (Fig. 4.3)

Skin prep
For all blocks.

Patient positioning
Supine.

Landmarks
Infraorbital foramen, orbital margin (Figs. 4.2 and 4.4).

Extraoral injection
Palpation of the infraorbital foramen, about 1 cm below the middle of the lower orbital margin.

Intraoral injection
Palpation of the lower orbital margin.

Injection techniques
Extraoral injection
After palpating the infraorbital foramen, the needle is introduced cranially just below the palpation point until bone contact is made (Fig. 4.7) and then withdrawn slightly.

Intraoral injection
The center of the lower orbital margin is palpated and marked with the middle finger. The upper lip is raised with a spatula or with the thumb and index finger. The needle is introduced above the second premolar tooth toward the infraorbital foramen, until bone contact is made, and then withdrawn slightly (Fig. 4.8).

> For both of these techniques, it is important that slow injection of the local anesthetic should only be carried out after careful aspiration. Afterwards, thorough compression should be carried out to prevent hematoma formation and to obtain better distribution of the local anesthetic.

> No injections should be made into the infraorbital canal due to the risk of nerve injury.

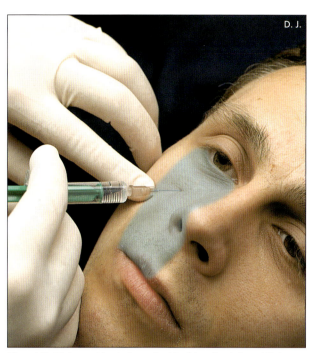

Fig. 4.7 Extraoral technique for blocking the infraorbital nerve

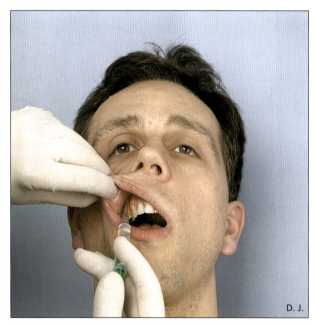

Fig. 4.8 Intraoral technique for blocking the infraorbital nerve

Dosages
Diagnostic
0.5–1 mL local anesthetic – e.g. 0.5–1% prilocaine, mepivacaine, lidocaine.

Therapeutic (extraoral technique)
0.5–1 mL local anesthetic – e.g. 0.5–0.75% ropivacaine, 0.5% bupivacaine (0.5% levobupivacaine).

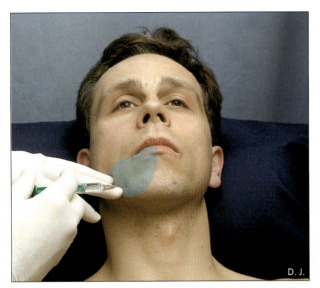

Fig. 4.9 Extraoral technique for blocking the mental nerve

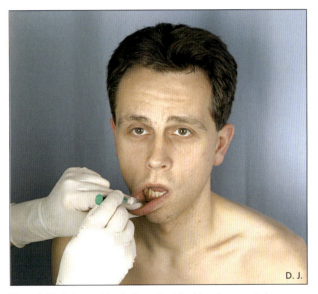

Fig. 4.10 Intraoral technique for blocking the mental nerve

Surgical
Up to 5 mL local anesthetic extraorally.
Shorter procedures: 1% prilocaine or 1% mepivacaine.
Longer procedures: 0.75% ropivacaine, 0.5% bupivacaine (0.5% levobupivacaine).
Intraorally: 2–3 mL local anesthetic.

Side effects
Potential hematoma formation (prophylactic compression).
If the needle is advanced too far, penetration of the orbit can occur.
Symptom: temporary double vision.

Complications
Injection into the bone canal carries a risk of nerve damage.

Blocks of the mental nerve

The mental nerve, the sensory end branch of the mandibular nerve, emerges from the mental foramen at the level of the second premolar (Fig. 4.2).
It provides the sensory supply of the skin and mucosa of the lower lip and chin (Fig. 4.37).

Indications
Diagnostic
- Differential diagnosis of trigger points and hyperalgesic zones

Therapeutic
- Trigeminal neuralgia of the third branch
- Post-traumatic pain and pain in the innervation area of the mental nerve
- Dental treatment of canine tooth, first premolars and incisors of the lower jaw
- Post-dental extraction pain (intraoral technique)
- Surgical procedures on the surface of the lower lip (note higher dosages)

Specific contraindications
None.

Procedure

Preparation and materials (Fig. 4.3)

Skin prep
In all blocks.

Patient positioning
Supine.

Landmarks
Mental foramen (Figs. 4.2 and 4.4).

Extraoral and intraoral injection
Palpation of the mental foramen at the level of the second premolar.

Injection techniques
Extraoral injection
After palpation of the mental foramen, the needle is inserted about 2.5 cm lateral to the midline (Fig. 4.9) until bone contact is made.

Intraoral injection
After palpation of the mental foramen, the lower lip is pressed downward using a spatula. The needle is inserted between the first and second premolars, into the lower reflection of the oral vestibule, in the direction of the neurovascular bundle (Fig. 4.10).

> For both of these techniques, it is important that slow injection should only be carried out after careful aspiration. Afterward, thorough compression should be carried out to prevent hematoma formation and to obtain better distribution of the local anesthetic.

Dosage
Diagnostic
0.5–1 mL local anesthetic – e.g. 0.5–1% prilocaine, mepivacaine, lidocaine.

Therapeutic (extraoral technique)
0.5–1 mL local anesthetic – e.g. 0.5–0.75% ropivacaine, 0.5% bupivacaine (0.5% levobupivacaine).

Surgical
Up to 5 mL local anesthetic extraorally.
Shorter procedures: 1% prilocaine or 1% mepivacaine.
Longer procedures: 0.75% ropivacaine, 0.5% bupivacaine (0.5% levobupivacaine).
Intraorally: 2–3 mL local anesthetic.

Side effects
Potential hematoma formation (prophylactic compression).

Complications
Injection into the bone canal carries a risk of nerve damage.

> Injections should never be made into the mental canal, due to the risk of nerve injury.

Blocks of the maxillary nerve and pterygopalatine ganglion

The maxillary nerve emerges from the skull through the round foramen. It connects with the pterygopalatine (sphenopalatine) ganglion in the pterygopalatine fossa (Fig. 4.11). The nerve and ganglion are responsible for sensory and autonomic supply to the central area of the face and head.

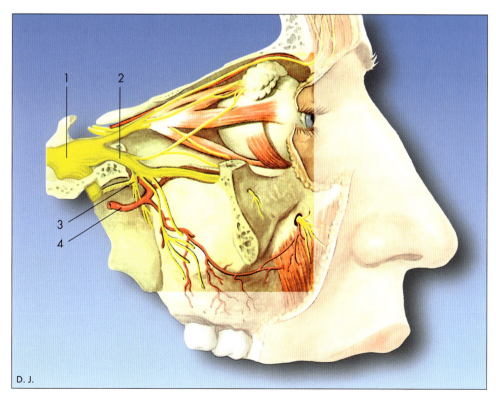

Fig. 4.11 (1) Trigeminal ganglion (Gasserian ganglion) and (2) pterygopalatine fossa with the maxillary nerve, (3) pterygopalatine ganglion and (4) maxillary artery

Indications
Diagnostic
- Differential diagnosis of facial pain

Therapeutic
- Trigeminal neuralgia in the second branch, postherpetic neuralgia
- Cluster headache [6], histamine headache, Sluder's neuralgia [19]
- Facial pain in the area of supply
- Pain in the eye region (iritis, keratitis, corneal ulcer), root of the nose, upper jaw and gums
- Postoperative pain in the area of the maxillary sinus and teeth
- Pain after dental extraction

Neural therapy
- Hay fever, vasomotor rhinitis
- Diseases of the oral mucosa
- Localized paresthesias

Specific contraindications
Bleeding diathesis, anticoagulation treatment.

Procedure

These blocks should only be carried out only with appropriate experience. It is absolutely necessary to have a detailed discussion with the patient before the procedure.

Preparations
Check that the emergency equipment is complete and in working order. Sterile precautions. Intravenous access.

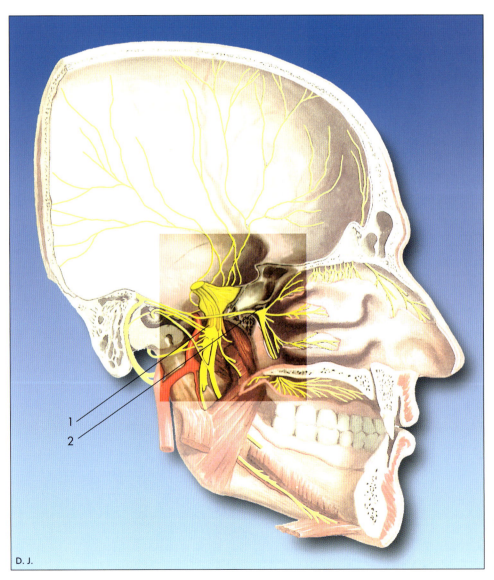

Fig. 4.12 Nerves and ganglia in the vicinity: (1) otic ganglion, (2) pterygopalatine ganglion

Materials
2-mL syringe, 22-G needle (40 mm) for the intraoral technique, 5-mL and 10-mL syringe, 23-G needle (60 mm) for the extraoral technique. Disinfectant, spatula for the intraoral technique, compresses, cooling element available, emergency drugs (Fig. 4.13).

Skin prep
In all blocks.

Intraoral technique

Patient positioning
The patient should be sitting, leaning back slightly and with the head tilted back.

Landmarks
Posterior edge of the upper seventh tooth (second maxillary molar) (Fig. 4.14).

Injection technique
Using a 22-G needle (40 mm), the puncture is made medial to the posterior edge of the upper seventh tooth (second maxillary molar) through the greater palatine foramen. The needle is introduced at an angle of about 60°. The vicinity of the ganglion is reached at a depth of 3.5–4 cm. The greater palatine canal is about 3.4 cm long in adults.
After careful aspiration at various levels, the local anesthetic is injected (Fig. 4.15).

> Intraoral access is associated with fewer complications.

Dosage
Therapeutic
Intraorally: 1–2 mL local anesthetic – e.g. 0.75% ropivacaine, 0.5% bupivacaine (0.5% levobupivacaine).

Extraoral technique

Above the zygomatic arch (suprazygomatic technique)

> Injection above the zygomatic arch is much more elegant and more comfortable for the patient.

Patent positioning
Sitting, with face to the side and with the mouth slightly opened. Alternative: supine.

Landmarks
Center of the upper margin of the zygomatic arch.

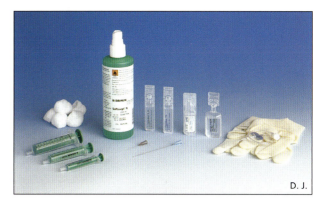

Fig. 4.13 Materials

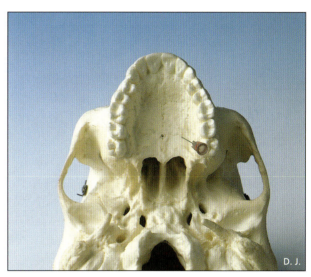

Fig. 4.14 Intraoral technique: orientation

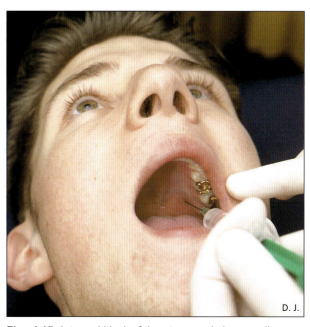

Fig. 4.15 Intraoral block of the pterygopalatine ganglion

Chapter 4

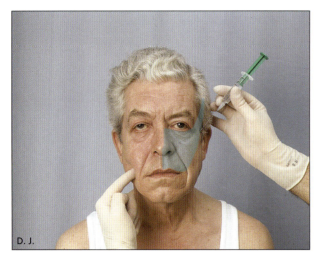

Fig. 4.16 Orientation for injections above the zygomatic arch

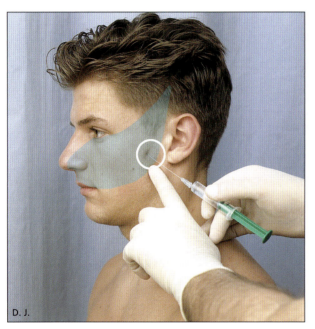

Fig. 4.17 Extraoral technique beneath the zygomatic arch (mandibular fossa)

Injection technique
A skin injection is made directly above the middle of the zygomatic arch. A 6-cm long needle is introduced at an angle of ca. 45° in the direction of the pterygopalatine fossa (contralateral molar teeth) (Fig. 4.16). After paresthesias have been elicited in the area of the nostril, the upper lip and the cheek, the needle is withdrawn slightly and aspirated carefully at various levels, and the local anesthetic is administered slowly in several small doses. Repeated aspiration at various levels must be carried out during this procedure.

> Separate blocking of the maxillary nerve and pterygopalatine region is rarely possible with this method.

Below the zygomatic arch (infrazygomatic technique)

Patient positioning
Supine or sitting, face to the side with the mouth slightly open.

Landmarks
Mandibular fossa.

Injection technique
The most important requirement for carrying out this block successfully is accurate location of the mandibular fossa between the condylar and coronoid processes of the mandible.
It is helpful for the patient to open and close the mouth. After skin infiltration, a 6-cm needle is introduced at an angle of 45° in the direction of the back of the eyeball (Fig. 4.17).
After ca. 4–4.5 cm, the lateral part of the pterygoid process is reached and the needle is withdrawn slightly and lowered into the pterygopalatine fossa (about 0.5 cm medial to the pterygoid). After the paresthesias described above have been elicited and after careful aspiration at various levels, the local anesthetic is carefully injected in several small doses.
If pain occurs in the region of the orbit, the procedure should be stopped.

Dosage
Diagnostic
Up to 5 mL local anesthetic – e.g. 0.5% prilocaine, mepivacaine, lidocaine.

Therapeutic
Extraorally: 5–10 mL local anesthetic – e.g. 0.5% ropivacaine, 0.25% bupivacaine (0.25% levobupivacaine). In acute conditions, with 1–2 mg dexamethasone added.

Surgical
Extraorally: 5–10 mL local anesthetic – e.g. 0.75% ropivacaine, 0.5% bupivacaine (0.5% levobupivacaine), 1% prilocaine, 1% mepivacaine.

Block series
A sequence of six to eight blocks is recommended for the extraoral technique.

Side effects

- Transient visual weakness (extremely rare).
- Horner's syndrome, extremely rare and usually with high doses. There are connections with the superior cervical ganglion via the pterygoid canal, deep petrosal nerve and greater superficial petrosal nerve.
- Hematoma in the cheek or orbital cavity due to blood vessel puncture (Figs. 4.18 and 4.19).
Immediate outpatient treatment: alternating ice-pack and heparin ointment, depending on the spread of the hematoma, for ca. 1 h. This can be continued at home, with the patient also taking coated Reparil® tablets (sodium aescinate) if appropriate. Resorption of the hematoma, which is harmless but visually uncomfortable for the patient, occurs within 2 weeks at the most.

Complications

- Intravascular injection (maxillary artery and maxillary vein; Fig. 4.27).
- Epidural or subarachnoid injection (Fig. 4.28).

Both of these complications are extremely rare. Immediate treatment: see Chapter 6, p. 66f.

> The maxillary artery and vein lie in the immediate vicinity.

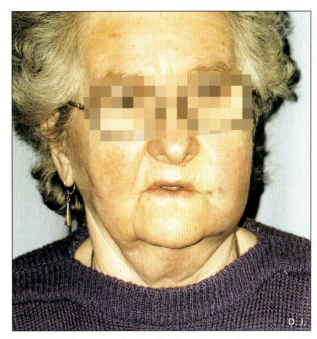

Fig. 4.18 Hematoma in the cheek: status on the second day after injection and immediate treatment

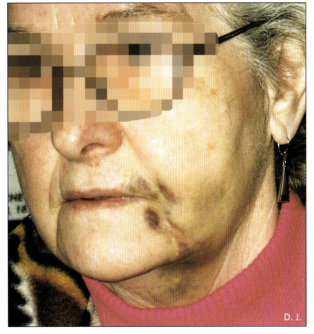

Fig. 4.19 Hematoma in the cheek: 7 days after injection

Record and checklist

Maxillary nerve and pterygopalatine ganglion
Block no. ☐ Right ☐ Left

Name: _____ Date: _____

Diagnosis: _____

Premedication: ☐ No ☐ Yes _____

Purpose of block:		☐ Diagnostic	☐ Therapeutic
Needle:	☐ 22 G	☐ 40 mm long	☐ 60 mm long
i.v. access:		☐ Yes	☐ No
Monitoring:		☐ ECG	☐ Pulse oximetry
Ventilation facilities:		☐ Yes (equipment checked)	
Emergency equipment *(drugs)*:		☐ Checked	
Patient:		☐ Informed	

Position: ☐ Supine ☐ Sitting
Approach: ☐ Above the zygomatic arch ☐ Intraoral
☐ Below the zygomatic arch (mandibular fossa)

Local anesthetic: _____ ml _____ % _____
Test dose: _____ ml
Addition to
injection solution: ☐ No ☐ Yes _____

Patient's remarks during injection:
☐ None ☐ Pain ☐ Paresthesias ☐ Warmth
Nerve region _____ _____ _____

Objective block effect after 15 min:
☐ Cold test ☐ Temperature measurement right ____°C left ____°C
☐ Numbness (V$_2$)

Monitoring after block: ☐ < 1 h ☐ > 1 h
Time of discharge _____

Complications: ☐ None
☐ Yes (hematoma, intravascular, injection, other)
_____

Subjective effects of the block: Duration: _____
☐ None ☐ Increased pain
☐ Reduced pain ☐ Relief of pain

VISUAL ANALOG SCALE

|||||||||||||||||||||||||||||||||||||||||||||||||||||||||||||
0   10   20   30   40   50   60   70   80   90   100

Special notes:
_____
_____
_____
_____
_____
_____

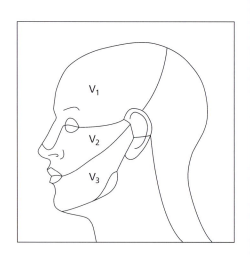

© Copyright ABW Wissenschaftsverlag 2004,
Jankovic, Regional nerve blocks and infiltration therapy, 3rd edition

Nasal block of the pterygopalatine ganglion

The pterygopalatine (sphenopalatine) ganglion, which lies in the pterygopalatine fossa (sphenomaxillary fossa), is triangular in shape; extending to ca. 5 mm, it is the largest neuronal conglomerate outside of the brain. The ganglion has three types of nerve fiber and is connected to the trigeminal nerve via sensory fibers. It is linked to the facial nerve, internal carotid plexus and superior cervical ganglion via sympathetic fibers; the motor fibers have parasympathetic (visceromotor) connections. There is also direct contact between the anterior horn of the spinal cord and the neurohumoral axis (adenohypophysis) [15, 21].

Indications
Greenfield Sluder [19] drew attention to the significance of this ganglion as long ago as 1903. In 1918, he described a number of symptoms capable of being treated by injection or topical application of a local anesthetic or cocaine, with the associated anesthesia of the pterygopalatine ganglion: headache; pain in the eyes, mouth, or ears; lumbosacral pain, arthritis, glaucoma and hypertension. Similar observations were reported by Ruskin [17], Byrd and Byrd [5] and Amster [1].
More recent studies [3, 8, 14, 16] have shown that nasal local anesthesia of the ganglion can be used with good success rates in the treatment of:
- Acute migraine
- Acute or chronic cluster headache
- Various types of facial neuralgia
- Tumor pain in the nasal and pharyngeal area

Specific contraindications
None.

Procedure

Materials (Fig. 4.20)
2-mL syringe, plastic part of a plastic indwelling catheter (for self-administration in tumor pain), nasal speculum, applicators (cotton buds).

Patient positioning
Supine or sitting, with head tilted back.

Application
An applicator soaked in local anesthetic – e.g. 2% lidocaine gel or a 4% aqueous lidocaine solution – preferably a cotton bud – is carefully advanced along the inferior nasal concha as far as the posterior wall of the nasopharynx (Fig. 4.21) and left in place for 20–30 min (Fig. 4.22).
In patients with cancer pain, the plastic part of a plastic indwelling catheter can be advanced as far as possible into the nasal cavity, and the local anesthetic – e.g. 0.5% bupivacaine – can be instilled with a 2-mL syringe. The block can be carried out bilaterally.

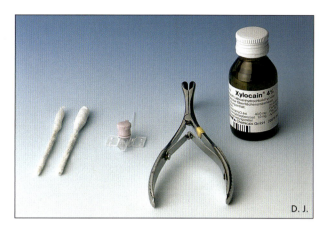

Fig. 4.20 Materials

> To prevent trauma, the applicator should not be advanced forcefully if resistance is encountered.

Dosage
Local anesthetics: 2% lidocaine gel, 1.5–2 mL 4% lidocaine (aqueous solution) or 1.5–2 mL bupivacaine. Disadvantage: the onset of effect is slightly slower.

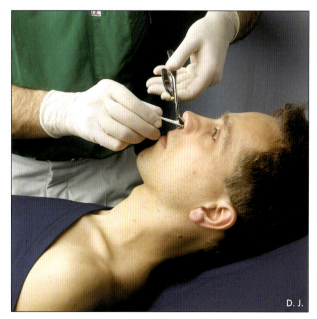

Fig. 4.21 Nasal application

Chapter 4

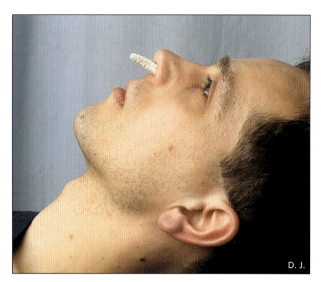

Fig. 4.22 The anesthetic should be allowed 20–30 min to take effect

10% cocaine: at a dosage of 0.2–0.4 mL, there is no reason to fear adverse CNS effects [3]. Advantage: very fast onset of effect.
If the recommended doses are used, there is no difference between these substances with regard to effectiveness and resorption.

Block series
In acute pain, one or two applications are recommended. In chronic conditions, one to three applications can be given over a period of up to 3 weeks.
In cancer pain, applications may be indicated three times per day over a longer period.

Side effects
The method is not very invasive and has minimal side effects. Effects that may occur include: a sense of pressure in the nose, sneezing, short-term lacrimation due to irritation of branches of the lacrimal gland, a bitter taste and slight numbness in the oral and pharyngeal cavity.

Complications
Very occasionally, toxic effects may occur as a result of absorption of the local anesthetic into very well vascularized tumor tissue. In long-term treatments, erosions may sometimes lead to spinal absorption of the local anesthetic. To prevent this, periodic rinsing with a physiological saline solution can be carried out.

Block of the mandibular nerve and otic ganglion

After passing through the oval foramen, the mandibular nerve forms a short, thick nerve trunk, with the otic ganglion lying on the medial side of it. Its most important branches (Fig. 4.23) are the buccal nerve, lingual nerve, inferior alveolar nerve, mental nerve and auriculotemporal nerve.

Indications
Diagnostic
- Differential diagnosis of trigeminal neuralgia (anterior two-thirds of the tongue) and glossopharyngeal neuralgia (posterior third of the tongue)

Therapeutic
- Tinnitus (the otic ganglion has connections with the chorda tympani, the nerves of the pterygoid canal and the medial pterygoid nerve)
- Trigeminal neuralgia in the third branch
- Trismus after dental extraction
- Dental surgery and maxillary surgery (higher dosages required)
- Temporomandibular joint dysfunction syndrome (in collaboration with an orthodontist), if infiltration of the trigger points of the temporalis muscle, lateral pterygoid muscle and masseter muscle is unsuccessful

Specific contraindications
Bleeding diathesis, anticoagulation treatment.

Procedure

This block should only be carried out only with appropriate experience. It is absolutely necessary to have a detailed discussion with the patient before the procedure.

Preparation and materials (Fig. 4.13)

Skin prep
In all blocks.

Patient positioning
Supine, with face to the side.

Landmarks
Mandibular fossa, zygomatic arch, tragus (the needle insertion point lies ca. 2 cm laterally, Fig. 4.24).

Injection technique
After skin infiltration, a 60-mm needle is introduced into the skin perpendicularly (Fig. 4.25).

Trigeminal nerve

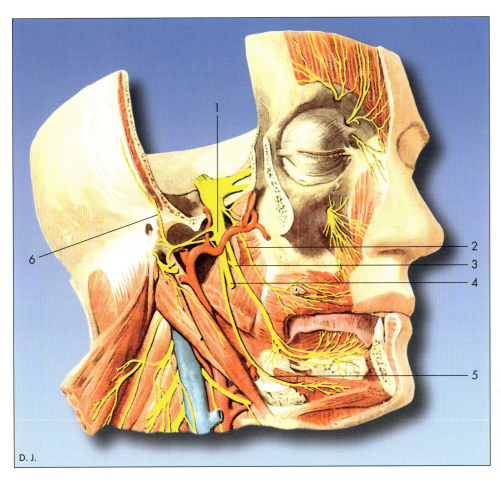

Fig. 4.23 Distribution areas of: (1) mandibular nerve; (2) buccal nerve; (3) lingual nerve; (4) inferior alveolar nerve; (5) mental nerve; (6) auriculotemporal nerve

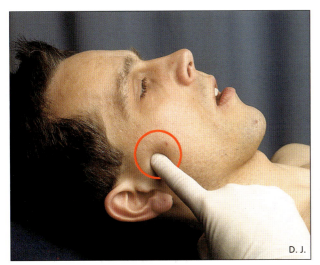

Fig. 4.24 The most important requirement is that the mandibular fossa should be identified precisely. It lies between the condylar process and the coronoid process of the mandible and is easiest to localize when the patient opens and closes his or her mouth

Fig. 4.25 Needle insertion technique: the needle is directed at an angle of 90°

Paresthesias in the lower jaw region, lower lip and lower incisors occur when the needle reaches a depth of ca. 4–4.5 cm.

After paresthesias have clearly developed, the needle is withdrawn slightly, aspirated carefully at various levels and the local anesthetic is slowly injected in several

47

small doses. Aspiration should be repeated several times at different levels as this is done.
There is a delayed onset of the desired effect in the area of the auriculotemporal nerve.

> The middle meningeal artery and maxillary artery lie in the immediate vicinity.

> If contact is made with the pterygoid process when the needle is being introduced, withdraw the needle 0.5–1 cm and redirect dorsally.

Distribution of the block
The area supplied by the mandibular nerve is shown in Figure 4.32.
The otic ganglion (Fig. 4.26), which lies directly under the oval foramen, is always anesthetized along with the nerve.

Dosage
Diagnostic
Up to 5 mL local anesthetic – e.g. 5% prilocaine, mepivacaine, lidocaine.

Therapeutic
5–10 mL local anesthetic – e.g. 0.5% ropivacaine, 0.25% bupivacaine (0.25% levobupivacaine).
In acute conditions, with 1–2 mg dexamethasone added.

Surgical
10 mL local anesthetic – e.g. 0.75% ropivacaine, 0.5 bupivacaine, 1% prilocaine, 1% mepivacaine.

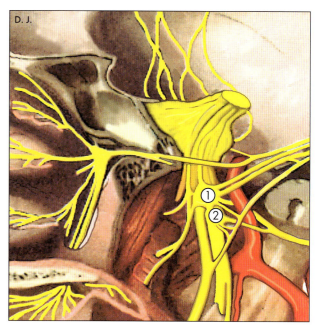

Fig. 4.26 There are close anatomical connections between the otic ganglion (1) and the mandibular nerve (2)

Block series
A series of six to eight blocks is recommended. When there is evidence of symptomatic improvement, further blocks can also be carried out.

Side effects
- Transient facial paralysis caused by injecting too superficially.
- Hematoma in the cheek due to vascular puncture. These harmless hematomas can take up to two weeks to resolve.
Immediate treatment: see the section on blocks of the maxillary nerve and pterygopalatine ganglion, Figs. 4.18 and 4.19.

Complications
- Intravascular injection (middle meningeal artery and maxillary artery, Fig. 4.27).
- Epidural or subarachnoid injection (Fig. 4.28). Immediate treatment: see Chapter 6, p. 67.

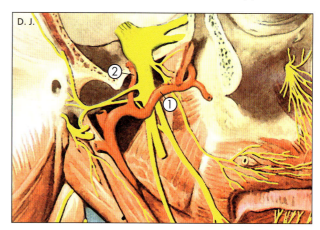

Fig. 4.27 Risk of intravascular injection: (1) maxillary artery, (2) middle meningeal artery

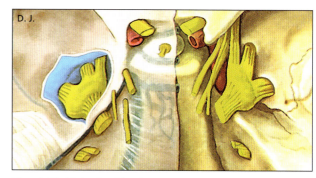

Fig. 4.28 Risk of epidural or subarachnoid injection

Mandibular nerve and otic ganglion
Block no. ☐ Right ☐ Left

Record and checklist

Name: _____ Date: _____
Diagnosis: _____
Premedication: ☐ No ☐ Yes _____

Purpose of block:		☐ Diagnostic	☐ Therapeutic
Needle:	☐ 22 G	☐ 50 mm long	☐ 60 mm long
i.v. access:		☐ Yes	☐ No
Monitoring:		☐ ECG	☐ Pulse oxymetry
Ventilation facilities:		☐ Yes (equipment checked)	
Emergency equipment (drugs):		☐ Checked	
Patient:		☐ Informed	

Position: ☐ Supine ☐ Sitting
Approach: ☐ Mandibular fossa

Local anesthetic: _____ ml _____ % _____
Testdose: _____ ml
Addition to
injection solution: ☐ No ☐ Yes _____

Patient's remarks during injection:
☐ None ☐ Pain ☐ Paresthesias ☐ Warmth
Nerve region _____

Objective block effect after 15 min:
☐ Cold test ☐ Temperature measurement right ____°C left ____°C
☐ Numbness (V_3)
Monitoring after block: ☐ < 1 h ☐ > 1 h
Time of discharge _____

Complications: ☐ None
☐ Yes (hematoma, intravascular injection, other)
_____

Subjective effects of the block: Duration: _____
☐ None ☐ Increased pain
☐ Reduced pain ☐ Relief of pain

VISUAL ANALOG SCALE

|0 | 10 | 20 | 30 | 40 | 50 | 60 | 70 | 80 | 90 | 100|

Special notes:
_____
_____
_____
_____

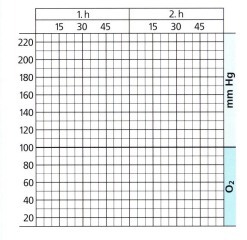

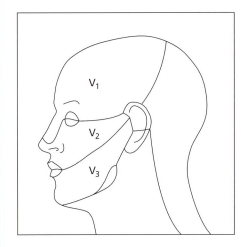

Chapter 4

Gasserian ganglion block

The trigeminal ganglion (semilunar ganglion, Gasserian ganglion) lies on the dorsal surface of the petrous bone. The intracranial Gasserian ganglion lies medially in the middle cranial fossa, lateral to the cavernous sinus, internal carotid artery and cranial nerves III–VI, and posterior and superior to the oval foramen, through which the mandibular nerve exits from the intracranial cavity (Fig. 4.29). All of these structures can be injured when the ganglion is blocked. The average size of the ganglion is ca. 1–2 cm.

Part of the ganglion (the posterior two-thirds) is located within the trigeminal cave (Meckel cavity), a duplication of the dura that encloses the ganglion. The oval foramen is a channel ca. 5 mm long and its largest diameter is ca. 8 mm.

Indications

Local anesthetics
Diagnostic, before neurodestructive procedures.

Neurodestructive procedures
Neurodestructive methods – particularly radiofrequency lesions of the ganglion, and more rarely glycerol rhizolysis, alcohol injection, corticosteroid injection, or balloon compression of the ganglion – are used in pain conditions that are unbearable and cannot be influenced using other conservative measures:
- Cancer pain
- Trigeminal neuralgia
- Cluster headache
- Pain in the eye region
- Post-herpetic neuralgia

Specific contraindications
Local infection, sepsis, hemorrhagic diathesis, anticoagulation treatment, significantly increased intracranial pressure.

Procedure

This block should only be carried out by highly experienced specialists. A very good knowledge of anatomy, manual skill, radiographic guidance when conducting the procedure, and strictly aseptic conditions are required. It is necessary to have a detailed discussion with the patient before the procedure.

Premedication
This method is painful, and preoperative administration of 0.05 mg fentanyl is therefore recommended.

Preparations
The completeness and functioning of the emergency equipment should be checked. Sterile precautions. Intravenous access, ECG monitoring, ventilation facilities, pulse oximetry.

Materials
A fine 22-G spinal needle 80 mm long, 2-mL and 5-mL syringes, disinfectant, sterile compresses, emergency medication, intubation kit, and cooling element should be ready to hand.

Skin prep
In all blocks.

Patient positioning
Supine; the head is raised with a cushion.

Landmarks (Fig. 4.30)
– Medial edge of the masseter muscle, ca. 3 cm lateral from the angle of the mouth at the level of the second molar tooth.
– Ipsilateral pupil.

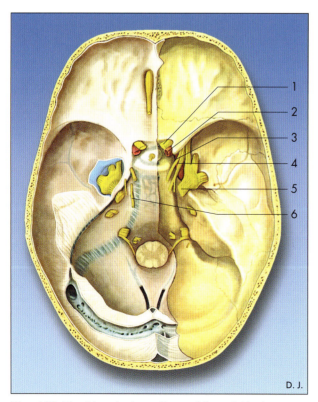

Fig. 4.29 The trigeminal ganglion and the neighboring cranial nerves and internal carotid artery. (1) Optic nerve, (2) internal carotid artery, (3) oculomotor nerve, (4) trochlear nerve, (5) trigeminal nerve, (6) abducent nerve

Trigeminal nerve

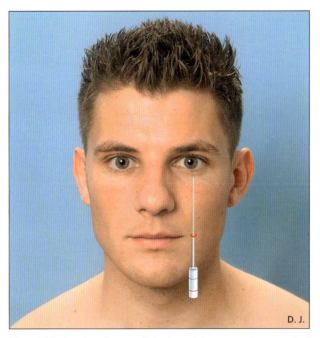
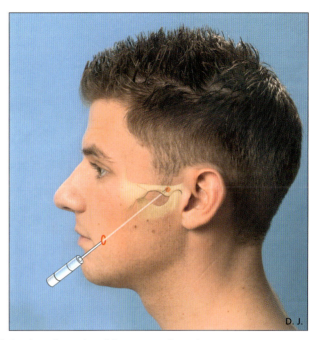

Fig. 4.30 Landmarks: medial edge of the masseter muscle, ipsilateral pupil, center of the zygomatic arch

– Center of the zygomatic arch and articular tubercle (external acoustic meatus).

The following should be noted during puncture:
- The operator should stand on the side on which the block is being carried out.
- Radiographic guidance for the puncture is indispensable.
- An intraoral location should be excluded after introduction of the needle (risk of contamination).
- There is a risk of perforating the dural cuff (subarachnoid injection).
- Frequent aspiration and fractionated injection of the smallest possible fractions (blood, CSF?).

Needle insertion technique
Local anesthesia at the needle insertion site is carried out ca. 3 cm from the angle of the mouth (medial edge of the masseter muscle). The patient is asked to gaze straight ahead and focus on a marked point on the wall. The needle should be directed toward the forward-gazing pupil when seen from the front and toward the articular tubercle of the zygomatic arch or external acoustic meatus when viewed from the side (Fig. 4.30).
The needle is then introduced at the level of the second molar tooth, through the previous skin injection in the direction indicated. An intraoral location of the needle must be excluded (risk of contamination). After 4.5–6 cm, bone contact should be made (infratemporal surface of the large wing of the sphenoid bone, directly in front of the upper boundary of the oval foramen; Fig. 4.31). The needle is now withdrawn slightly, and the path to the oval foramen (ca. 1–1.5 cm away from the first bone contact; Fig. 4.31) is probed millimeter by millimeter by advancing and withdrawing

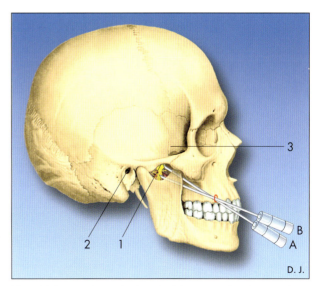

Fig. 4.31 Injection point (level of the second molar tooth). Needle position A: bone contact – infratemporal. Needle position B: entrance into the oval foramen. (1) Zygomatic arch, (2) external acoustic pore, (3) temporal fossa

Chapter 4

the needle. If the tip of the needle is located in the oval foramen, the patient will report pain and paresthesias in the area of distribution of the mandibular nerve (mandible). The needle is now slowly advanced for a further 0.5–1 cm. A small test dose of 0.1–0.2 mL local anesthetic is carefully administered. The remaining dose of 1–1.5 mL is injected in small fractions with constant aspiration. Particular attention should be given to possible subarachnoid or intravascular positioning of the needle. The sensory distribution of the block is shown in Figure 4.32.

Dosage
1–2 mL local anesthetic – e.g. 1% lidocaine, 0.5–0.75% ropivacaine, or 0.5% bupivacaine.

Complications
Subarachnoid injection (total spinal anesthesia) (Fig. 4.28)
Immediate measures: see Chapter 6, p. 67.
Important prophylactic measures:
- Very good knowledge of anatomy
- Precise execution of the procedure (radiographic guidance)
- Careful dosage
- Constant aspiration and injection in the tiniest fractions of 0.1 mL local anesthetic (several test doses)
- No time pressure

Intravascular injection (Fig. 4.27)
Intravascular injection (middle meningeal artery) is always possible (in this highly vascularized region).

Hematoma in the cheek or orbit due to vascular puncture (Figs. 4.18 and 4.19)
Immediate measures: see p. 43.

Transient visual weakness or blindness
Optic nerve; extremely rare.

Trigeminal nerve: comparison of analgesia zones

Figures 4.33 to 4.37 provide schematic illustrations of the areas supplied by the individual nerves. During blocks, the anesthetic spread may overlap.

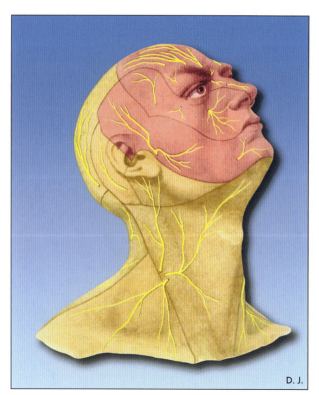

Fig. 4.32 Sensory deficit after blocking of the trigeminal ganglion

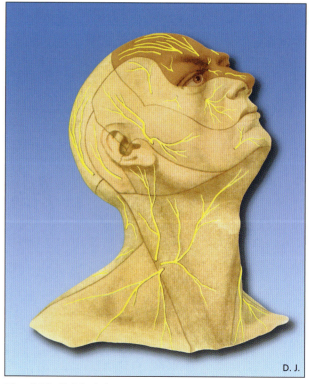

Fig. 4.33 Ophthalmic nerve

Trigeminal nerve

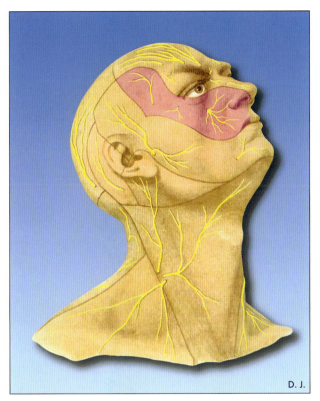
Fig. 4.34 Maxillary nerve

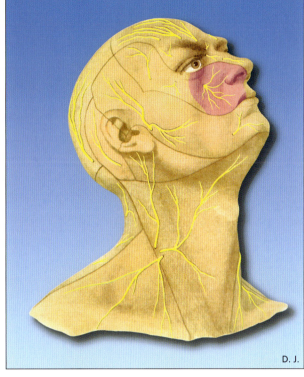
Fig. 4.35 Infraorbital nerve

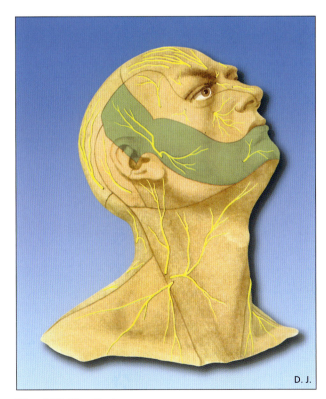
Fig. 4.36 Mandibular nerve

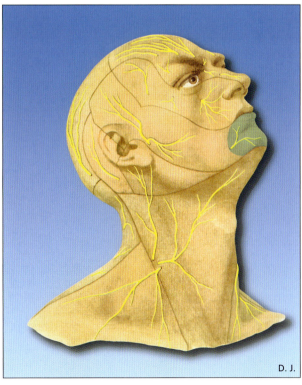
Fig. 4.37 Mental nerve

Record and checklist

Trigeminal ganglion (Gasserian ganglion)
Block ☐ Right ☐ Left

Name: _____ Date: _____
Diagnose: _____
Premedication: ☐ No ☐ Yes _____

Purpose of block:	☐ Diagnostic	☐ Therapeutic
Needle:	☐ 22 G	☐ 80 mm long ☐ 100 mm long
i.v. access:		☐ Yes
Monitoring:	☐ ECG	☐ Pulse oximetry
Ventilation facilities:		☐ Yes (equipment checked)
Emergency equipment *(drugs)*:	☐ Checked	☐ X-ray
Patient:		☐ Informed

Position: ☐ Supine ☐ Other

Local anesthetic: _____ ml _____ % ☐ Fractionated
Test dose: _____ ml
Addition to injection solution: ☐ No ☐ Yes _____
☐ Radiofrequency lesion
☐ Neurolysis _____ ml _____ %
☐ Other _____

Patient's remarks during injection:
☐ None ☐ Pain ☐ Paresthesias ☐ Warmth
Nerve region _____ _____ _____

Objective block effect after 15 min:
☐ Cold test ☐ Temperature measurement right ____°C left ____°C
☐ Numbness (V₁, V₂, V₃)
Monitoring after block: ☐ < 1 h ☐ > 1 h
Time of discharge _____

Complications: ☐ None ☐ Amblyopia ☐ Hematoma ☐ Dural puncture
☐ Intravascular injection ☐ Postdural puncture headache
☐ Subarachnoidal injection ☐ Respiratory disturbance
☐ Total spinal anesthesia ☐ Neurological complications
_____

Subjective effects of block: Duration: _____
☐ None ☐ Increased pain
☐ Reduced pain ☐ Relief of pain

VISUAL ANALOG SCALE

0   10   20   30   40   50   60   70   80   90   100

Special notes: _____
_____

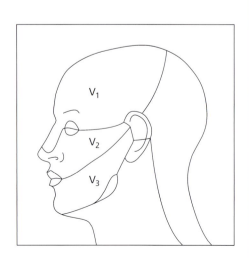

© Copyright ABW Wissenschaftsverlag 2004,
Jankovic, Regional nerve blocks and infiltration therapy, 3rd edition

5 Infiltration of trigger points in the muscles of mastication

Temporomandibular joint pain–dysfunction syndrome

This chapter describes injection techniques in the three clinically most relevant muscles of the temporomandibular joint – the masseter muscle, temporalis muscle, and lateral pterygoid muscle.
It was dental specialists who carried out most of the research that led to the recognition of the muscular components of the general craniomandibular pain syndrome. These syndromes are often associated with definite signs of temporomandibular joint dysfunction. In 1969, Laskin [1] presented the classic definition of the myofascial pain–dysfunction (MPD) syndrome. For this diagnosis, he required that only one of the following requirements should be met:
1. Unilateral pain, usually in the ear or in the preauricular area.
2. Pressure pain in the muscles of mastication.
3. A creaking or cracking noise in the temporomandibular joint.
4. Restricted opening of the mouth.

A lack of clinical or radiographic evidence of organic changes in the temporomandibular joint is characteristic. Targeted injections into identified trigger points (TrPs) have an important role as a supplementary measure in addition to other corrective dental measures, stretching exercises, sprays, etc.

Masseter muscle ("trismus muscle")

The anatomic insertions of the masseter muscle are located in the zygomatic arch and maxilla at the top and on the external surface of the ramus of the mandible and angle of the mandible at the bottom (Fig. 5.1).
Symptoms of active trigger points in this muscle (occluder) are marked **restriction of mouth opening (trismus), dental pain** (lower and upper molar teeth), and **unilateral tinnitus** (deeper muscle; Fig. 5.1).

Procedure

Materials
Sterile precautions, 25-G needle 25 mm long, 2-mL and 5-mL syringes, swabs, local anesthetic.

Injection technique
Superficial layer of the muscle
The trigger points in the middle and lower belly of the muscle are located using what is known as "pincer-grip palpation" with the mouth open and the jaw supported, so that they can be held between the fingers (Fig. 5.2). The needle is advanced until bone contact is made (mandible) and then withdrawn 1–2 mm (Fig. 5.3). The injection is carried out after aspiration.

Deeper layer of the muscle
This layer lies on the posterior part of the ramus of the mandible. The mouth is opened wide and the depression directly underneath the head of the mandible in front of the external auditory canal is palpated (Fig. 5.4).

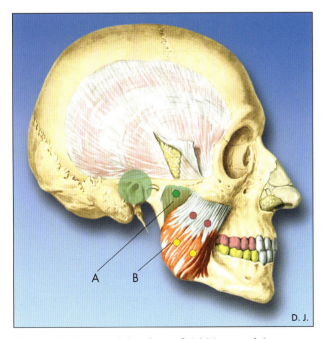

Fig. 5.1 (1) The deep (A) and superficial (B) parts of the masseter muscle.
Myofascial trigger points with referred pain (into the upper and lower molar teeth and deep into the ear).
Illustration adapted from Travell and Simons [3]

Chapter 5

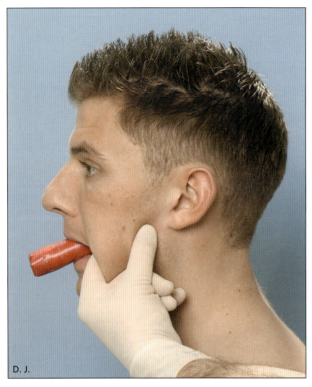

Fig. 5.2 Masseter muscle. Palpation using what is known as the "pincer grip." Searching for trigger points in the superficial part of the muscle

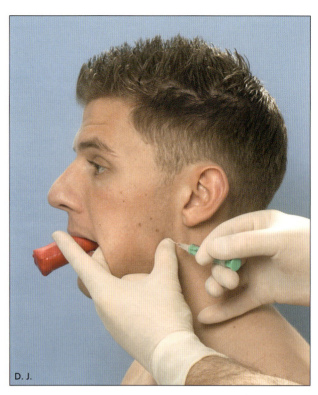

Fig. 5.3 Masseter muscle. Injection into the superficial part of the muscle

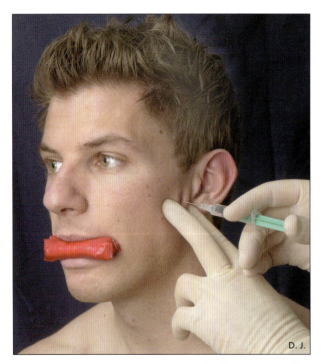

Fig. 5.4 Masseter muscle. Injection into the deeper part of the muscle

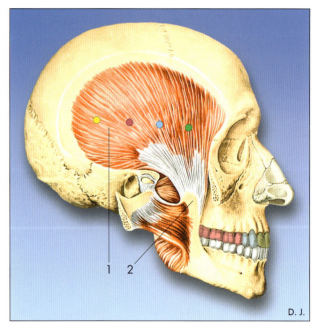

Fig. 5.5 (1) Temporal muscle. Myofascial trigger points with referred pain (temporal headache and maxillary dental pain). (2) Coronoid process.
Illustration adapted from Travell and Simons [3]

Dosage
0.5–1 mL local anesthetic per TrP – e.g. 0.2–0.5% ropivacaine, 0.5% procaine, 0.5% lidocaine.

Temporal muscle ("temporal headache and maxillary dental pain")

The anatomic insertions of the temporal muscle (occluder) are at the temporal bone at the top and on the fascia of the temporal fossa, and on the coronoid process of the mandible at the bottom. Four trigger points have been described (Fig. 5.5). The symptoms include **temporal headache** and **dental pain** in the maxillary teeth.

Procedure

Materials
Sterile precautions, 25-G needle 25 mm long, 2-mL and 5-mL syringes, swabs, local anesthetic.

Injection technique
The patient is asked to open the mouth slightly to relax the muscles. Pulsation in the temporal artery is palpated. One finger is kept constantly on the artery to avoid inadvertent injection, while the other finger palpates and fixes the TrP. The needle is introduced obliquely until bone contact is made, and then withdrawn by 1 mm. After aspiration, the local anesthetic is injected (Fig. 5.6).
After infiltration and massaging of the injected area, a cooling spray and passive stretching of the muscle are applied. This is followed by warm packing and then active jaw movements.

Dosage
0.5–1 mL local anesthetic per TrP – e.g. 0.2–0.5% ropivacaine, 0.5% procaine, 0.5% lidocaine.

Lateral pterygoid muscle ("pain radiating deep into the temporomandibular joint")

Anatomy
The upper part inserts anteriorly at the sphenoid bone and posteriorly at the articular disk and temporomandibular joint capsule. The lower part inserts anteriorly at the lateral pterygoid plate and posteriorly at the neck of the mandible (Fig. 5.7).

Symptoms
The lateral pterygoid muscle (jaw opening) transfers pain deep into the **temporomandibular joint** and to

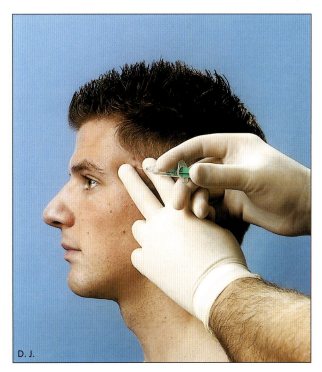

Fig. 5.6 Temporal muscle. Injection into trigger point 1

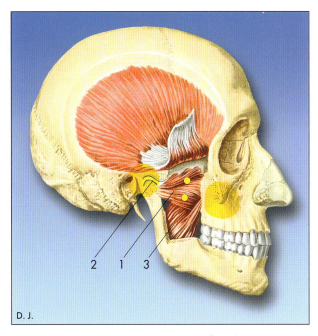

Fig. 5.7 (1) Lateral pterygoid muscle. Myofascial trigger points with referred pain (yellow; maxilla and temporomandibular joint). (2) Articular disk, (3) medial pterygoid muscle. *Illustration adapted from Travell and Simons* [3]

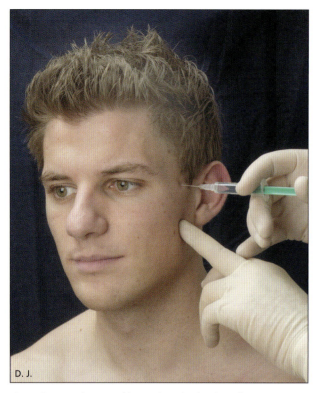

Fig. 5.8 Lateral pterygoid muscle. Injection into the upper part of the muscle

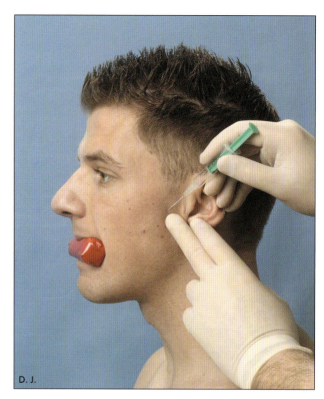

Fig. 5.9 Lateral pterygoid muscle. Injection into the lower part of the muscle

the **maxillary sinus region** (Fig. 5.7). The pain is always combined with functional disturbances of the joint. The muscle's trigger points are the most important myofascial cause of referred pain in the area of the temporomandibular joint (this myofascial syndrome is often confused with temporomandibular joint arthritis).

Procedure

Materials
Sterile precautions, 23-G needle 40 mm long, 2-mL and 5-mL syringes, swabs, local anesthetic.

Extraoral injection technique

A good knowledge of the anatomy is a prerequisite for carrying out this injection, as the full extent of the muscle cannot be palpated extraorally.

Upper part
A vertical puncture is made in an easily palpable depression just above the zygomatic arch and, after aspiration, infiltration is carried out up to a depth of 1.5–2 cm (Fig. 5.8).

Lower part
The patient is asked to open the mouth wide. The needle's path lies through the masseter muscle. The needle is introduced through the mandibular notch at an angle of ca. 45° in the direction of the upper molar teeth at a depth of ca. 3–4 cm (Fig. 5.9). After aspiration, the injection is carried out.

Dosage

1–2 mL local anesthetic per TrP – e.g. 0.2–0.5% ropivacaine, 0.5% procaine, 0.5% lidocaine.

6 Cervicothoracic ganglion (stellate ganglion)

Anatomy

There are two sympathetic trunks arranged paravertebrally that belong to the peripheral autonomic nervous system. In the area of the neck, these include four sympathetic trunk ganglia on each side, serving as cholinergic switchpoints: the **superior** and **middle cervical ganglia**, the **vertebral ganglion** and the **cervicothoracic ganglion** (Fig. 6.1).

The **cervicothoracic ganglion** (stellate ganglion) at the level of C7–T1 arises from the fusion of the lowest cervical ganglion (7th and 8th cervical ganglion) with the highest thoracic ganglion (1st and/or 2nd thoracic ganglion).

The immediate vicinity of the ganglion is dominated by the first rib, the pleura and the brachial plexus. The ganglion lies ventral to the vertebral artery, medial and dorsal to the common carotid artery and the jugular vein, and lateral to the esophagus and trachea. It is separated from the transverse processes of the 6th and 7th cervical vertebrae by the longus colli muscle (Fig. 6.2).

It receives afferent fibers from the white rami communicantes of the 1st and 2nd thoracic nerves and gives off gray rami communicantes to the 1st (and 2nd) thoracic nerves and the 8th (and 7th) cervical nerves.

The stellate ganglion is connected to the neighboring ganglia, the brachial plexus, the cranial intercostal nerves and the phrenic nerve, and to the vagus nerve and recurrent laryngeal nerve (Fig. 6.3). Fibers from the gray rami communicantes also supply the heart and great vessels (subclavian, carotid, vertebral, inferior thyroid and intercostal arteries), the esophagus and the trachea, as well as the thymus gland (Fig. 6.4).

The size and development of the stellate ganglion are subject to considerable variation. Average sizes of between 25 mm (15–50 mm) × 3–10 mm × 5 mm have been reported (Fig. 6.5) [17, 18, 25]. This corresponds to the size of the superior cervical ganglion and is much more voluminous than the middle cervical ganglion. On the other hand, the stellate ganglion is only developed in 80% of patients; some authors [17,18] have only been able to identify it in 38% of individuals studied.

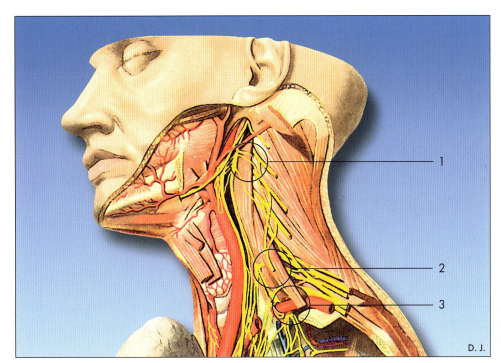

Fig. 6.1 The cervical ganglion trunk: (1) superior cervical ganglion, (2) middle cervical ganglion and (3) cervicothoracic ganglion

Stellate ganglion block

Indications
Block of the stellate ganglion is a useful method of pain therapy in patients with perfusion disturbances in the areas of the head, neck, upper extremities and upper thoracic wall.
The following indications have been described in the literature:

- Vasospastic diseases in the areas of the face, shoulder and arm.
- Arterial dysfunctions: Raynaud–Burger syndrome, anterior scalene syndrome, Volkmann's ischemic contracture.
- Venous dysfunctions: thrombophlebitis, postphlebitic edema.
- Combined dysfunctions – e.g. lymphedema after mastectomy.
- Head: intracranial vascular spasms, facial paralysis, vertigo, central post-stroke syndrome (contralateral block!).
- Eye: central vein thrombosis, occlusion of the central retinal artery.
- Nose: vasomotor rhinitis.
- Ear: Ménière's disease [10, 11, 13, 24], sudden deafness [15], tinnitus.

Our own results in the treatment of tinnitus show that up to 8 weeks after the start of the disease, 80% of patients can be successfully treated using 2–10 blocks over a period of 1–6 weeks. Up to 12

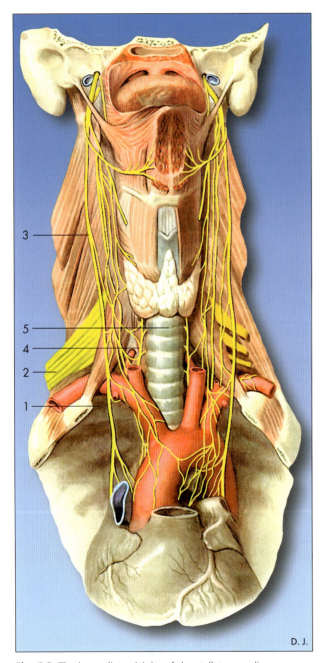

Fig. 6.2 The immediate vicinity of the stellate ganglion: (1) pleura, (2) brachial plexus, (3) vagus nerve, (4) recurrent laryngeal nerve, (5) trachea

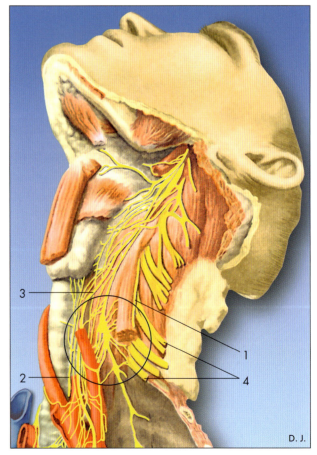

Fig. 6.3 Close anatomical connections in the ganglion trunk include those to (1) the phrenic nerve, (2) the recurrent laryngeal nerve, (3) the vagus nerve and (4) the brachial plexus

weeks after the start of the disease, the success rate with 10–16 blocks, spread over a period of 6 weeks, was only 35%. If the condition had been present for more than 6 months, block treatment was unsuccessful.

- Traumatic cerebral edema [9].
- Complex regional pain syndrome (CRPS) in the area of the face, neck and arm [35].
- Phantom pain.
- Hyperhidrosis.
- Joint stiffness.
- Positive effect on the immune system [21].
- Acute herpes zoster and zoster neuralgia in the head and neck region.

A trigeminal and cervical localization is reported in ca. 25% of cases. Good to very good results are obtained with stellate ganglion block in acute zoster (with opioids added if necessary [8]).

In assessing the success rates reported in the literature, it should be noted whether a distinction has been made between acute and chronic herpes zoster. The 85% success rate reported by Colding [4] when treatment was initiated within 3 weeks of the start of disease confirms the results reported by other authors [5, 29, 32, 36]. Milligan and Nash [23] regard 1 year after the start of disease as being the limit for treatment with stellate ganglion block. The results of their block series – freedom from pain in 22% of patients – are therefore not comparable.

Our own results [15] in the treatment of zoster neuralgia: up to 12 weeks after the start of disease, the success rate with 7–19 blocks, spread over a period of 3–10 weeks, was 80%. If the disease had started 6 months or more previously, the results were varied and unsatisfactory.

Specific contraindications

Grade 2 atrioventricular (AV) block, contralateral pneumothorax, recent thrombolytic therapy after myocardial infarction or pulmonary embolism, anticoagulation treatment, severe asthma/emphysema (if appropriate, priority can be given to block of the superior cervical ganglion here; see Chapter 7), paralysis of the contralateral phrenic nerve or recurrent laryngeal nerve. In addition, blocks should never be carried out bilaterally at the same time.

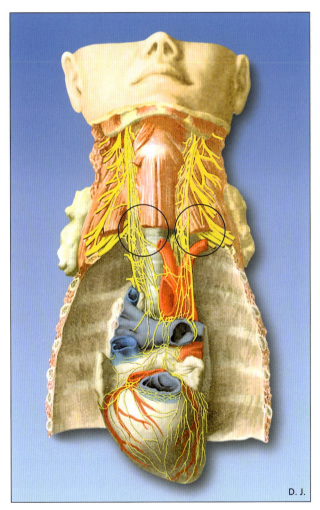

Fig. 6.4 Fibers from the gray rami communicantes supply the heart, esophagus, airways and thymus

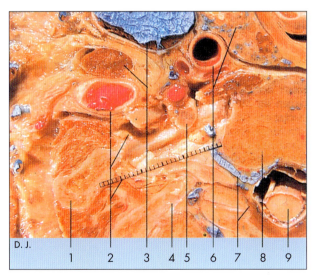

Fig. 6.5 The immediate vicinity of the ganglion (transverse section). (1) First rib, (2) subclavian artery and scalenus anterior muscle, (3) jugular vein, (4) second rib, (5) cervicothoracic ganglion, (6) common carotid artery and thyroid gland, (7) T2 intervertebral artery and zygapophyseal joint, (8) T2 vertebral body, (9) spinal medulla. The average size of the cervicothoracic ganglion is 25 mm × 3–10 mm × 5 mm

Chapter 6

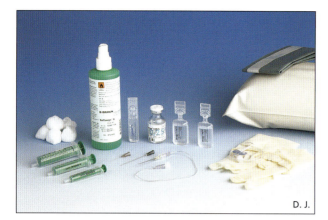

Fig. 6.6 Materials

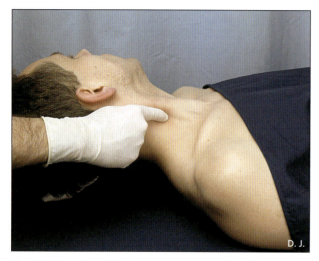

Fig. 6.7 Palpation of the transverse process of the 6th vertebra

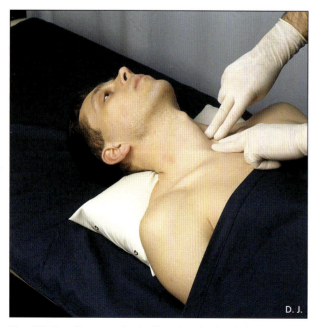

Fig. 6.8 Two-finger method of locating the level of C7

Procedure

The paratracheal anterior technique is the currently accepted standard. This block should only be carried out by experienced pain therapists. A detailed discussion should be held with the patient before the procedure.

Preparations
Check that the emergency equipment is complete and in working order. Sterile precautions, skin prep. Intravenous access, ECG monitoring, ventilation facilities, pulse oximetry.
Avoid premedication. The patient must remain responsive at all times so that any possible side effects or complications will be apparent immediately.

Materials
Fine 26-G needles 2.5 cm long for local anesthesia, 5-mL syringe, 10-mL syringe, 22-G needle (3 cm or 5 cm long, depending on the patient's anatomy) with injection tube (immobile needle), intubation kit, emergency drugs, cushions for positioning, disinfectant (Fig. 6.6).

Skin prep
In all blocks.

Patient positioning
Supine, with neck extended.

Landmarks
Sternocleidomastoid muscle, common carotid artery, jugular fossa, transverse processes of the 6th or 7th cervical vertebra.
1. The 6th cervical vertebra is palpated. For this purpose alone, the patient rotates the head toward the opposite side (Fig. 6.7).
2. For palpation of the site between the larynx and the sternocleidomastoid muscle, a cushion is placed under the shoulder blades and the head is tilted back. The patient must not swallow, speak, cough, or move, and is asked to breathe with the mouth slightly open in order to relax the neck muscles (Fig. 6.8).
3. The index and middle fingers are moved between the trachea and sternocleidomastoid muscle to locate the pulse in the common carotid artery. This is displaced laterally together with the medial margin of the sternocleidomastoid muscle (Fig. 6.9). The transverse process is now identified. Usually, the transverse process of C6 is easily palpated at the level of the cricoid, or the transverse process of C7 can be located using the two-finger method (Fig. 6.8).

Injection technique

> The injection can be made at the level of C6 or C7. The transverse process of the sixth cervical vertebra is easier to palpate; the distance from the pleura is greater and there is less danger of puncturing the vertebral artery. Block at the level of C7 can extend as far as T3, with a reduced dose of local anesthetic. However, the likelihood of injuring the pleura or puncturing the vertebral artery is greater here.

After skin infiltration, the needle is introduced vertical to the skin at this point and advanced until bone contact is made with the transverse process (Figs. 6.9 and 6.10). The transverse process is reached at a depth of 2–4 cm, depending on the anatomy.

After bone contact has been made, the needle is withdrawn about 1 mm and with careful aspiration at various levels, an initial test dose of 1 mL of the local anesthetic is injected.

> If there is no bone contact, or if paresthesias in the brachial plexus are elicited, the needle must be withdrawn and corrected medially. If the transverse process is still not reached, the direction of the needle should be carefully corrected caudally or cranially.

After approximately 1 min, slow injection of the remaining dose can be carried out.

> A single test dose by no means guarantees correct positioning of the needle. The remaining dose must never be injected quickly and carelessly. It must be administered slowly in small quantities (several test doses) with constant aspiration.

Effect of the block

Characteristic unilateral symptoms of a stellate ganglion block are: conjunctival injection, increased tear production, swelling of the nasal mucosa, reddening, hyperthermia and anhidrosis in the affected side of the face. At higher doses, hyperthermia and anhidrosis in the region of the shoulder and arm can occur.

Horner's syndrome is regarded as the clinical sign of a successfully conducted block. In 1869, the ophthalmologist Johann Friedrich Horner described the triad of

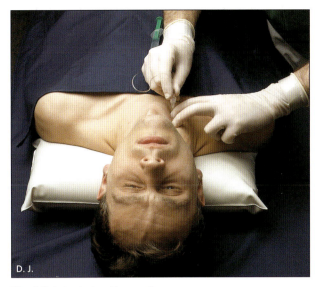

Fig. 6.9 Introducing the needle

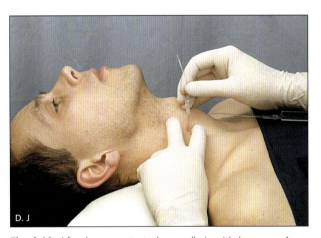

Fig. 6.10 After bone contact, the needle is withdrawn ca. 1 mm. The injection is carried out after aspiration at various levels

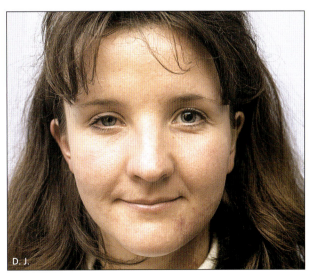

Fig. 6.11 Horner's syndrome: ptosis, miosis and enophthalmos

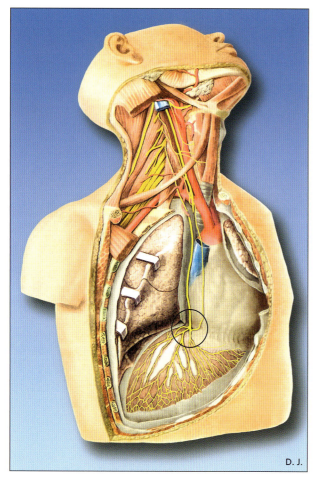

Fig. 6.12 Course of the phrenic nerve

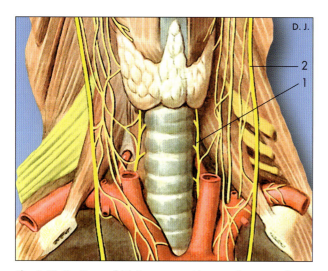

Fig. 6.13 Positions of (1) the recurrent laryngeal nerve and (2) the vagus nerve

ptosis, meiosis and enophthalmos as a sequela of paralysis of the sympathetically innervated ocular muscles (Fig. 6.11).

> Horner's syndrome is not necessarily a sign of complete block of the stellate ganglion. Two effects of the block need to be distinguished:
> - After ca. 1–2 min, Horner's syndrome develops as a result of cerebral (facial) spread. This can be achieved with a low dose of the local anesthetic.
> - Complete block, including the shoulder and arm region, requires a higher dose and the local anesthetic needs to spread as far as T4.
>
> This complete cervicothoracic sympathetic block is only obtained after ca. 15-20 min. Horner's syndrome occurs not only after stellate ganglion block, but is also characteristic of all blocks of the cervical sympathetic trunk.

Dosage

"Low dose" for indications in the head region (cerebrofacial effects) [3, 9, 15, 30]:
2–4 mL local anesthetic – e.g. 0.375–0.5% ropivacaine, 0.25–0.5% bupivacaine (0.25–0.5% levobupivacaine), or 1% prilocaine, 1% mepivacaine, 1% lidocaine.

"Medium high dose" for indications in the shoulder and arm region [3, 6, 12, 25, 30, 33, 35]:
10–15 mL local anesthetic – e.g. 0.2–0.375% ropivacaine, 0.25% bupivacaine (0.25% levobupivacaine), or 0.5% prilocaine, 0.5% mepivacaine, 0.5 lidocaine.
In acute pain, 1–3 mg morphine, 0.0125–0.025 mg fentanyl [8, 22, 34], or 0.03 mg buprenorphine with local anesthetic, or in a physiological saline solution.

Block series
If the clinical picture being treated does not show temporary improvement after the second block, there is no point in carrying out a series of treatments. Otherwise, for all the indications mentioned, a series of 6–10 blocks can be carried out. In difficult cases (e.g. herpes zoster ophthalmicus), further blocks can also be carried out when there is a visible trend toward improvement.

Side effects
Hematoma formation (harmless).
Persistent coughing [27].

Block of the following nerves:
- Phrenic nerve (Fig. 6.12), main symptom: dyspnea with normal auscultation findings.
- Vagus nerve (Fig. 6.13), main symptom: tachycardia, hypertension.
- Recurrent laryngeal nerve (Fig. 6.13), main symptom: foreign-body sensation in the throat, hoarseness. It should be noted here that in ca. 43% of cases, anastomoses with the cervicothoracic ganglion are found [17, 18].
- Brachial plexus: a partial brachial plexus block may occur if the local anesthetic spreads into the area of the roots of C6–T1.

When giving consent, the patient must be clearly informed about the possibility of these adverse effects – most of which do not require any treatment.

Complications
Intravascular injection
Intravascular injections are extremely rare when the correct technique is used. In particular, there is a risk of injection into the vertebral artery (the diameter of which is ca. 0.3 mm larger on the left side than on the right). More rarely, there is a risk of puncturing the carotid artery, the inferior thyroid artery, or the first intercostal artery (Fig. 6.14).

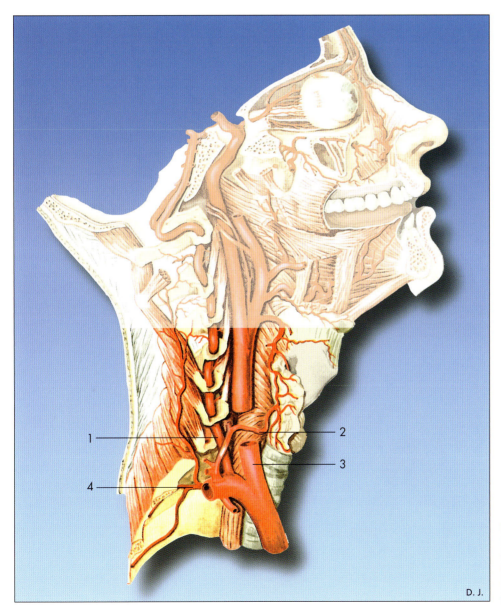

Fig. 6.14 Risk of intravascular injection into
(1) the vertebral artery,
(2) the inferior thyroid artery,
(3) the carotid artery and
(4) first intercostal artery

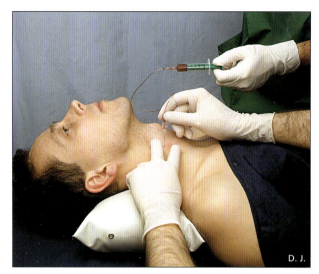

Fig. 6.15 Inadvertent intra-arterial injection has to be avoided, since even small amounts of local anesthetic are sufficient to cause CNS intoxication

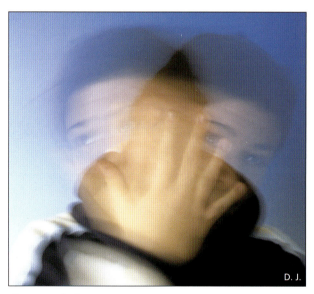

Fig. 6.16 Blackout

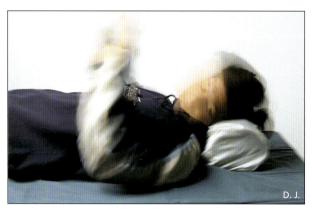

Fig. 6.17 Tonic–clonic seizure

Most complications arise when the local anesthetic is administered without prior bone contact.

Bilateral block of the stellate ganglion is contraindicated, since bilateral paresis of the recurrent laryngeal or phrenic nerves would be life-threatening.

CNS intoxication
Intravascular administration (Fig. 6.15), overdosage and/or rapid vascular uptake of the local anesthetic can quickly lead to toxic CNS reactions. Symptoms include:

- Sudden vertigo, pressure in both ears and in the head.
- Brief blackouts, not usually requiring treatment (Fig. 6.16).
- Reversible "locked-in syndrome" with brief apnea and inability to move or respond to external stimuli [7]. The patient remains conscious and is hemodynamically stable, and vertical eye movement is maintained.
Treatment: constant verbal contact, oxygen administration, support for breathing (with mask ventilation if necessary), cardiovascular monitoring, diazepam if necessary (0.05 mg/kg body weight, i.v.).
- Tonic–clonic seizure: a very serious complication (Fig. 6.17). Without immediate and correct treatment is given, this can lead to cerebral injury or even death.
Treatment: thiopental (1–2 mg/kg b.w. – routinely ca. 150 mg – i.v. carefully dosed), to prevent additional cardiovascular or CNS depression. Sedation with diazepam (10–20 mg). Oxygen administration (mask), support for breathing. The airways must be kept free, if necessary with succinylcholine (60–80 mg) to make intubation easier. Vasopressor administration to support the circulation. Leg elevation, fluid volume replacement. Cardiovascular monitoring; cardiopulmonary resuscitation if necessary.

Preconvulsive signs of toxic reactions are a numb sensation on the lips and tongue, vertigo, metallic taste, drowsiness, ringing in the ears, visual disturbances, slurred speech, muscle tremor, nystagmus.

Effects on the cardiovascular system
Toxic effects on the cardiovascular system only occur after very high doses of local anesthetic, manifesting as a drop in blood pressure, bradycardia, circulatory collapse and cardiac arrest.

Cervicothoracic ganglion (stellate ganglion)

Treatment: leg elevation, fluid volume replacement, oxygen administration, vasopressor administration if needed, cardiopulmonary resuscitation if needed.

Epidural or subarachnoid injection [31]
There is a risk of perforating the dural membrane if the needle is inserted too medially (Fig. 6.18). Cerebrospinal fluid (CSF) pressure is very low in the cervical area and it is almost impossible to aspirate CSF. High epidural anesthesia or high spinal anesthesia is extremely rare. It can lead to bradycardia, hypotension and possibly to respiratory arrest and loss of consciousness. The first signs are: heaviness in the limbs, sweating, dyspnea, apprehension and anxiety.

Treatment: immediate endotracheal intubation, ventilation with 100% oxygen, rapid volume infusion, atropine i.v. in bradycardia, vasopressor administration if needed.

> After a stellate block has been carried out, the patient must be monitored for 60 min. In the outpatient department, medium-duration local anesthetics (e.g. prilocaine, mepivacaine, or lidocaine) are preferable.

Pneumothorax
The incidence of this complication is extremely low when the paratracheal technique is used. If it occurs at all, it usually produces a small pneumothorax that resolves spontaneously (Fig. 6.19). If there is a suspicion of a pneumothorax, a chest radiograph is required after 4–6 h.

Esophageal perforation or tracheal perforation
Extremely rare. Puncture of the esophagus (Fig. 6.19) causes a bitter taste during the injection. Careful follow-up is indicated if there is any suspicion.

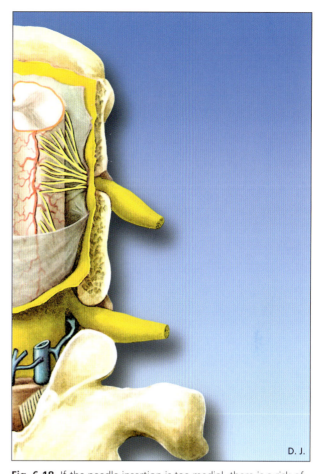

Fig. 6.18 If the needle insertion is too medial, there is a risk of epidural or subarachnoid injection

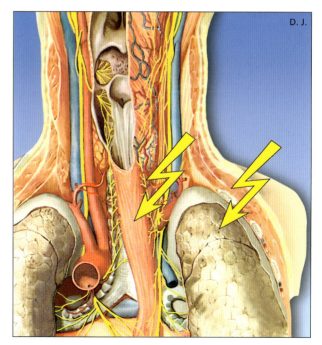

Fig. 6.19 Risk of pneumothorax (C7!); risk of esophageal perforation

Record and checklist

Cervicothoracic ganglion (stellate ganglion)

Block no. ☐ Right ☐ Left

Name: _____ Date: _____

Diagnosis: _____

Premedication: ☐ No ☐ Yes _____

Purpose of block: ☐ Diagnostic ☐ Therapeutic
Needle: ☐ 22 G ☐ 40 mm long ☐ 50 mm long
i.v. access: ☐ Yes
Monitoring: ☐ ECG ☐ Pulse oximetry
Ventilation facilities: ☐ Yes (equipmet checked)
Emergency equipment (drugs): ☐ Checked
Patient: ☐ Informed

Position: ☐ Supine ☐ Neck extended
Approach: ☐ Paratracheal ☐ C6 ☐ C7
 ☐ Other _____

Local anesthetic: _____ ml _____ % _____
Test dose: _____ ml
Addition to
injection solution: ☐ No ☐ Yes _____
Patient's remarks during injection:
 ☐ None ☐ Pain ☐ Paresthesias ☐ Warmth
Nerve region _____ _____ _____

Objective block effect after 15 min:
 ☐ Cold test ☐ Temperature measurement right ____°C left ____°C
Horner's syndrome: ☐ Yes ☐ No
Segment affected: ☐ C2 ☐ C3 ☐ C4 ☐ C5 ☐ T ____
Monitoring after block: ☐ < 1 h ☐ > 1 h
 Time of discharge _____

Complications: ☐ None
 ☐ Yes (intravascular, epidural, subarachnoid injection; other) _____
Side effects: ☐ None
 ☐ Yes (recurrent laryngeal nerve, phrenic nerve, vagus) _____

Subjective effects of the block: Duration: _____
 ☐ None ☐ Increased pain
 ☐ Reduced pain ☐ Relief of pain

VISUAL ANALOG SCALE

|||||||||||||
0 10 20 30 40 50 60 70 80 90 100

Special notes: _____
_____
_____

© Copyright ABW Wissenschaftsverlag 2004,
Jankovic, Regional nerve blocks and infiltration therapy, 3rd edition

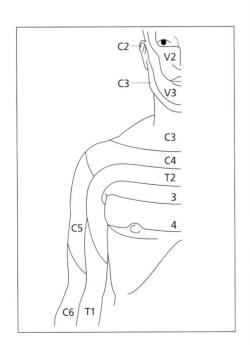

7 Superior cervical ganglion

Anatomy

The superior cervical ganglion arises from the fusion of three or four upper cervical ganglia. It lies medial to the vagus trunk, in front of the longus capitis muscle and behind the internal carotid artery, in the angle of the vertebrae and transverse processes of the second and third cervical vertebrae (Figs. 7.1 and 7.2). In the literature, its long, flat, or spindle-like extension is described as being 14–43 mm in length, 6–8 mm in breadth, and 3–5 mm in depth [8, 9] (Fig. 7.3). The superior cervical ganglion is thought to contain 760 000–1 000 000 nerve fibers in all, 5000–12 000 of which are preganglionic. Some 5000 of these fibers are myelinated [8, 9]. This underlines its importance as a switchpoint with numerous double or triple connections to neighboring ganglia, nerves, and vessels. The superior cervical ganglion takes its preganglionic fibers mainly from the spinal nerves coursing thoracically, with only a few being drawn from the neighboring cervical nerve roots. An unknown number of these preganglionic fibers pass through the ganglion toward the higher carotid ganglia, without switching. **Rami communicantes** connect the superior cervical ganglion with numerous organs, vessels, muscles, bones, joints, the last four cranial nerves, the vertebral plexus, and also with the phrenic nerve. It supplies the upper cervical spinal nerves with **gray rami communicantes**, and it sends off vascular fibers to the internal and external carotid arteries. **Autonomic branches** pass from the ganglion to the larynx, pharynx, heart, and – together with vascular plexuses – to the salivary and lacrimal glands, to the hypophysis, thyroid, and other glands. There are also contacts with the middle cervical ganglion and to the tympanic plexus. There are connections with the

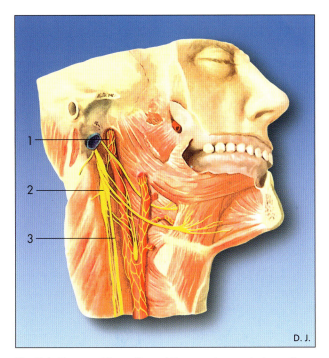

Fig. 7.1 Topographic position of the superior cervical ganglion: (1) glossopharyngeal nerve, (2) superior cervical ganglion, (3) vagus nerve. The superior cervical ganglion has an average size of: 26.6 mm (14–43 mm) × 7.2 mm × 3.4 mm

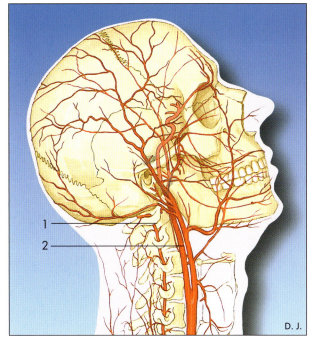

Fig. 7.2 Arteries in the immediate vicinity of the ganglion: (1) vertebral artery and (2) internal carotid artery

Chapter 7

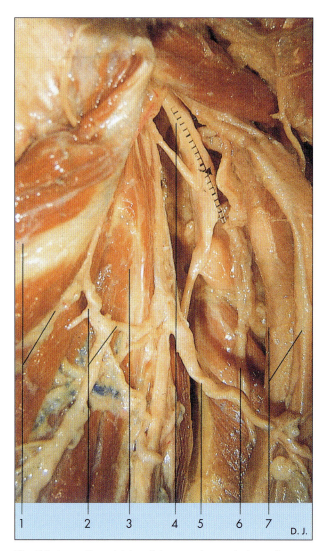

Fig. 7.3 Immediate vicinity of the superior cervical ganglion: (1) sternocleidomastoid muscle, repositioned dorsally, and the accessory nerve, (2) anastomosis between the C2 vertebral branch and nerve XII, (3) scalenus medius muscle, (4) superior cervical ganglion, (5) hypoglossal nerve, (6) external branch of the superior laryngeal nerve, (7) neurovascular fascicle, repositioned anteriorly

pterygopalatine ganglion via the nerve of the pterygoid canal, deep petrosal nerve, and greater superficial petrosal nerve. A variable number of fibers from the superior cervical ganglion pass to the inferior ganglion of the vagus nerve, to the hypoglossal nerve and to the posterior root of the ansa cervicalis [8, 9]. The superior cervical cardiac nerve may be absent, more often on the right side. In these cases, it is replaced by a branch of the vagus nerve from the external branch of superior laryngeal nerve.

Blocks of the superior cervical ganglion

Indications
The areas of application are partly identical to those for the stellate block, but due to its marked cerebrofacial effects, the superior cervical ganglion block is particularly suitable for the head and facial region – although controlled studies are still lacking here.

Therapeutic
- Migraine [5], cluster headache, headaches of cervical origin
- Complex regional pain syndrome (CRPS) in the head region
- Perfusion disturbances, vasospastic diseases
- Central post-stroke syndrome (contralateral block!)
- Facial pain
- Vertigo (of vertebral origin)
- Peripheral facial paralysis
- Trigeminal neuralgia in the 1st and 2nd branches
- Post-herpetic neuralgias* (otic, ophthalmic)
- Sudden deafness,* tinnitus*
- Hyperhidrosis in the head region.

Neural therapy
- Asthma, urticaria, vasomotor rhinitis, etc.

Specific contraindications
Grade 2 atrioventricular (AV) block, recent antithrombotic therapy after myocardial infarction or pulmonary embolism, anticoagulation treatment, contralateral paresis of the phrenic nerve or recurrent laryngeal nerve.
Simultaneous bilateral block.

Procedure

Lateral extraoral technique

This block should only be carried out by an experienced anesthetist. The patient should have a full explanation of the procedure before it is carried out.

Preparations
Check that the emergency equipment is complete and in working order. Sterile precautions. Intravenous access, ECG monitoring, pulse oximetry, ventilation facilities.

---
* The explanations given in Chapter 6, p. 61, also apply here.

Superior cervical ganglion

Materials
5-mL syringe, 23-G needle (60 mm), intubation kit, emergency drugs, disinfectant (Fig. 7.4).

Skin prep
In all blocks.

Patient positioning
Supine, with the head turned about 30–40° to the opposite side.

Landmarks
Mastoid process, angle of the mandible, medial margin of the sternocleidomastoid muscle (Fig. 7.5). The angle of the mandible and the mastoid are marked with the index and middle finger. From the anterior margin of the mastoid process, a vertical line is drawn downward; about 1 cm above the angle of the mandible, a horizontal mark is applied. The intersection of these two lines defines the injection point (Fig. 7.6).

Injection technique
After skin infiltration, a 6-cm long needle is introduced in the direction of the contralateral mastoid at a craniodorsal angle of about 20° (Fig. 7.7). In normal anatomy, bone contact is made at about 3.5–5 cm, and careful aspiration is carried out at various levels after the needle has been minimally withdrawn. Only then can a test dose of 0.5 mL of the local anesthetic be administered.

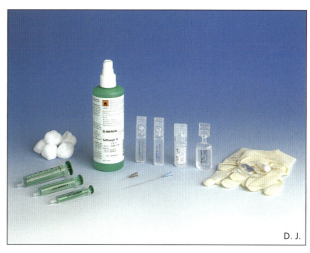
Fig. 7.4 Materials

After about 1 min, slow injection of the remaining dose can be carried out. The patient's upper body is then raised.

A single test dose by no means guarantees correct positioning of the needle. The remaining dose must never be injected quickly or carelessly. It must be administered slowly in small quantities (several test doses) with repeated aspiration.

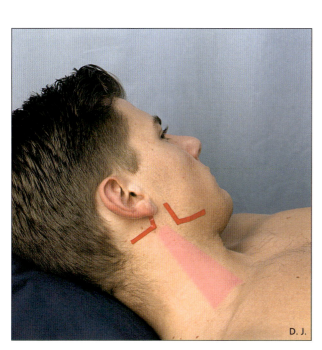
Fig. 7.5 Landmarks for locating the needle insertion position. Angle of the mandible, mastoid, medial margin of the sternocleidomastoid muscle

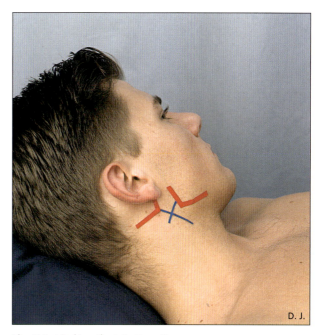
Fig. 7.6 Marking the injection site

Chapter 7

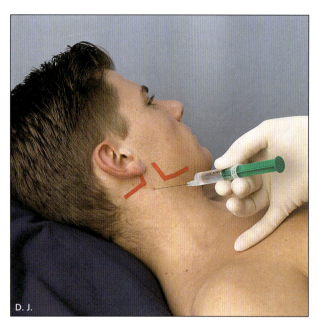

Fig. 7.7 Craniodorsal puncture in the direction of the contralateral mastoid

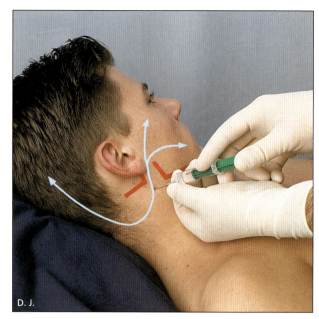

Fig. 7.8 Characteristic directions of radiation during the injection

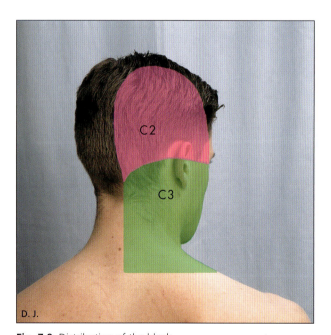

Fig. 7.9 Distribution of the block

Effects of the block
Characteristic signs of a successful block are radiation and a warm sensation in the area of the back of the head, ear, eyes and corner of the mouth and the ipsilateral half of the face (Figs. 7.8 and 7.9). Conjunctival injection, increased tear production and ipsilateral nasal congestion are equally characteristic, as is Horner's syndrome – which is by no means restricted to stellate block, but occurs in all blocks of the sympathetic cervical trunk.

Dosage
Therapeutic
5 mL local anesthetic – e.g. 0.5–1% procaine, 0.5–1% prilocaine, 0.5–1% lidocaine, 0.2% ropivacaine, 0.125% bupivacaine (0.125% levobupivacaine).

Block series
A series of 6–10 blocks is appropriate for all indications. In difficult cases (e.g. herpes zoster), additional blocks can also be carried out when there is evidence of improvement.

Side effects
Hematoma formation (harmless).
Block of the following nerves:
- Phrenic nerve, main symptom: dyspnea
- Recurrent laryngeal nerve, main symptoms: foreign-body sensation in the neck and hoarseness
- Vagus nerve, main symptoms: tachycardia, hypertension

If the the needle direction is incorrect, the patient will complain of pain and will resist the injection. In this case, the needle must be withdrawn to the subcutaneous tissues so that its position can be corrected.

Superior cervical ganglion

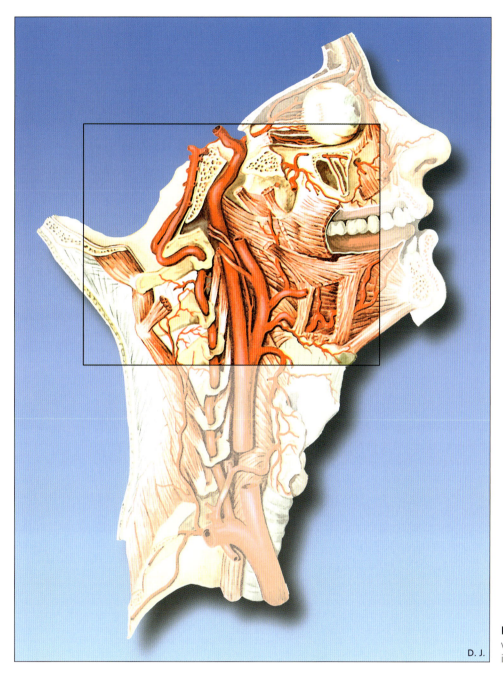

Fig. 7.10 Course of the vertebral artery and risk of intra-arterial injection

- Glossopharyngeal nerve, main symptoms: numbness in the posterior third of the tongue, paresis of the pharyngeal muscles
- Partial anesthesia of the cervical plexus
- Persistent coughing

When giving consent, the patient must be informed about these adverse effects and prepared for them.

Complications

Most complications arise when the local anesthetic is administered without prior bone contact.
Bilateral block of the superior cervical ganglion is contraindicated, since bilateral paralysis of the recurrent laryngeal nerve or phrenic nerve is life-threatening.

Intravascular injection
There is a particular risk of injection into the vertebral artery (Fig. 7.10), the diameter of which is about 0.3 mm wider on the left side than on the right. Intra-arterial administration of a local anesthetic can produce toxic reactions very quickly.
For the symptoms and treatment, see Chapter 6, p. 65.

Epidural or subarachnoid injection
There is a risk of perforating the dural membrane. Cerebrosbinal fluid (CSF) pressure is very low in the cervical area, and it is almost impossible to aspirate CSF. The resultant high epidural anesthesia or high spinal anesthesia can lead to bradycardia, a drop in blood pressure, and possibly to respiratory arrest and loss of consciousness.
For treatment, see Chap.6, p.67.

> Due to the potential complications, the patient must be monitored after the injection has been carried out – for at least 30 min after procaine administration and at least 60 min after administration of ropivacaine or bupivacaine.

Superior cervical ganglion blocks in pain therapy or as an option in depressive conditions
In my own clinical experience over many years with superior cervical ganglion block series (10–12 on average), there have been surprisingly good results in a large number of patients. These observations principally concern patients with pain-associated depression in chronic pain conditions (various types of headache, migraines, facial pain, post-nucleotomy pain, fibromyalgia, etc.). In the superior cervical ganglion block, the usual volume of 5 mL local anesthetic (e.g. 1% procaine) covers neighboring nerves such as the vagus nerve, for example. The superior cervical ganglion is often barely distinguishable from the vagus nerve. Left-sided vagus stimulation with an implantable electrode has been successfully used since 1938 to treat various neurological diseases such as epilepsy [1, 2], treatment-resistant depression [12–14], anxiety states [15], sleep disturbances [15], and other conditions. Dysfunction of the autonomic nervous system is almost always present as an accompanying symptom of depression [3]. The long-term analgetic effect of vagus stimulation was demonstrated in a study by Kirchner et al. [7]. Like the anti-epileptic and antidepressive action of vagus stimulation, this is probably due to neurobiochemical effects. For example, patients receiving vagus stimulation of the cerebrospinal fluid show a significant increase in norepinephrine and serotonin levels and a significant decrease in proalgetic excitatory amino acids such as aspartate and glutamate. The same group of authors report marked symptomatic improvement during vagus stimulation in a patient with chronic tension headache. In this context, answers will have to be found in the future to the following questions: What role does the superior cervical ganglion play in this? Is the functioning of the superior cervical ganglion more important than that of the vagus nerve? It should not be forgotten that the superior cervical ganglion is the last station at which information from the body can be modulated before entering the CNS.

Superior cervical ganglion

Block no. ☐ Right ☐ Left

Name: _____ Date: _____
Diagnosis: _____
Premedication: ☐ No ☐ Yes _____

Purpose of block:	☐ Diagnostic	☐ Therapeutic
Needle: ☐ 23 G	☐ 50 mm ☐ 60 mm ☐ _____	
i.v. access:	☐ Yes	
Monitoring:	☐ ECG	☐ Pulse oximetry
Ventilation facilities:	☐ Yes (equipment checked)	
Emergency equipment (drugs):	☐ Checked	
Patient:	☐ Informed	

Position: ☐ Supine ☐ Head to contralateral side
Approach: ☐ Extraoral (direction of C2 vertebra)

Local anesthetic: _____ mL _____ % _____
Test dose: _____ mL
Addition to
injection solution: ☐ No ☐ Yes _____
Patient's remarks during injection:
☐ None ☐ Pain ☐ Paresthesias ☐ Warmth
Nerve region _____

Objective block effect after 15 min:
☐ Cold test ☐ Temperature measurement right _____°C left _____°C
Horner's syndrome: ☐ Yes ☐ No
Segments affected: ☐ C2 ☐ C3 ☐ C4 ☐ C5 (numbness, warmth)
Monitoring after block: ☐ < 1 h ☐ > 1 h
Time of discharge _____

Complications:
☐ None ☐ Yes (intravascular, epidural, subarachnoid injection; other) _____

Side effects:
☐ None ☐ Yes (recurrent laryngeal nerve, phrenic nerve, vagus nerve, glossopharyngeal nerve ...) _____

Subjective effects of the block: Duration: _____
☐ None ☐ Increased pain
☐ Reduced pain ☐ Relief of pain

VISUAL ANALOG SCALE

0 10 20 30 40 50 60 70 80 90 100

Special notes:
_____
_____

© Copyright ABW Wissenschaftsverlag 2004,
Jankovic, Regional nerve blocks and infiltration therapy, 3rd edition

Record and checklist

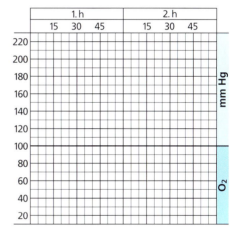

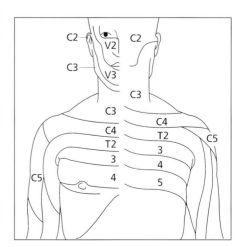

8 Deep (and superficial) cervical plexus

Anatomy

The anterior branches of the four upper cervical spinal nerves (C1 to C4) form the **cervical plexus** (Fig. 8.1), which is covered by the sternocleidomastoid muscle. The branches of the cervical plexus carry motor, sensory, proprioceptive and autonomous fibers and divide into superficial cutaneous branches penetrating the cervical fascia and deeper muscular branches that mainly innervate the joints and muscles.

The **cutaneous branches** of the cervical plexus are the lesser occipital nerve, great auricular nerve, transverse cervical (colli) nerve and the supraclavicular nerves (Fig. 8.2).

The **lesser occipital nerve** (from C2 and C3) passes on the splenius capitis muscle to its insertion area, where it fans out into several branches and supplies the skin on the upper side of the neck and upper part of the auricle and the adjoining skin of the scalp. The largest plexus branch is usually the **great auricular nerve** (from C2 and C3), which passes upward behind

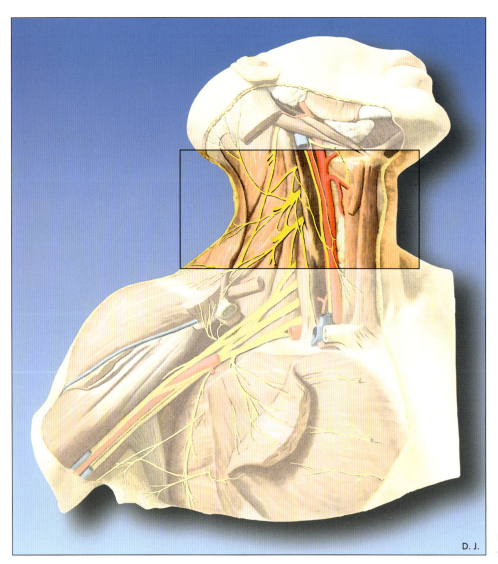

Fig. 8.1 Anatomy of the deep cervical plexus

Deep (and superficial) cervical plexus

the external jugular vein and divides into a posterior and an anterior end branch. The posterior branch supplies the skin lying behind the ear and the medial and lateral surfaces of the lower part of the auricle. The anterior branch supplies the skin in the lower posterior part of the face and the concave surface of the auricle. The **transverse cervical nerve** (from C2 and C3) passes almost horizontally over the external surface of the sternocleidomastoid muscle in an anterior direction toward the hyoid bone, divides into superior and inferior branches and supplies the skin over the anterolateral side of the neck between the mandible and the sternum. The common trunk of the **supraclavicular nerves** (from C3 and C4) appears at the posterior margin of the sternocleidomastoid muscle, just below the transverse cervical nerve, passes downward and divides into anterior, medial and posterior supraclavicular nerve branches. The areas supplied by the supraclavicular nerves include the skin over the caudal part of the neck and the skin above the shoulders and the lateral upper chest, as well as the skin covering the anterior part of the deltoid muscle and occupying the acromial region.

The **muscular branches** of the cervical plexus include segmentally arranged nerve branches supplying the deeper anterior neck muscles (the rectus capitis anteri-

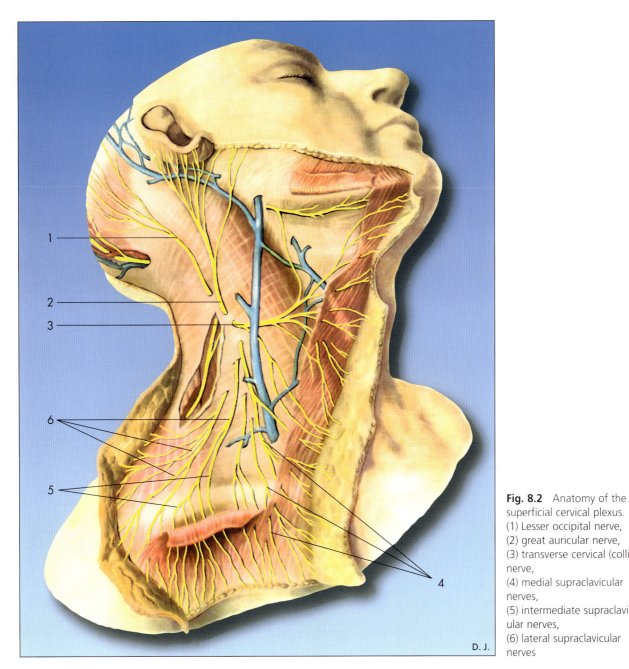

Fig. 8.2 Anatomy of the superficial cervical plexus. (1) Lesser occipital nerve, (2) great auricular nerve, (3) transverse cervical (colli) nerve, (4) medial supraclavicular nerves, (5) intermediate supraclavicular nerves, (6) lateral supraclavicular nerves

or and lateralis, longus colli, longus capitis and intertransverse, scalenus anterior and medius and levator scapulae), as well as the inferior descending cervical nerve, the trapezius branch and the phrenic nerve. The **inferior descending cervical nerve** (from C2 and C4) gives off several fibers to the carotid and jugular neural plexus and joins with the superior descending cervical nerve to form the ansa cervicalis. The area supplied includes the sternothyroid muscle, sternocleidomastoid muscle, thyrohyoid muscle, geniohyoid muscle and omohyoid muscle.

The **trapezius branch** appears at the surface just below the accessory nerve and passes to the trapezius muscle. The **phrenic nerve** (from C4 and C3/5) is the motor nerve for the diaphragm, but it also contains sensory and sympathetic fibers that supply the fibrous pericardium, mediastinal pleura and the central part of the diaphragmatic pleura as the nerve courses through the thorax. Connections have been described between the phrenic nerve (left or right branch) or the phrenic plexus and the following structures: inferior and middle cervical ganglion, subclavian plexus, pulmonary plexus, inferior vena cava, esophagogastric junction, cardiac end of the stomach, hepatic portal, suprarenal cortex, etc.

Block of the deep cervical plexus

Indications
Diagnostic
- Localization and differentiation of various types of neuralgia

Therapeutic
- Post-herpetic neuralgia
- Occipital and cervicogenic headache
- Torticollis

Surgical
In combination with a block of the superficial cervical plexus:
- Carotid endarterectomy [1, 2]
- Excision of cervical lymph nodes
- Plastic surgery in the area of innervation

Specific contraindications
Grade 2 atrioventricular (AV) block, anticoagulant treatment, contralateral paresis of the phrenic nerve or recurrent laryngeal nerve.
Simultaneous bilateral blocks.

Procedure

This block should only be carried out by experienced anesthetists. It is absolutely necessary to have a detailed discussion with the patient before the procedure.

Preparations
Check that the emergency equipment is complete and in working order. Sterile precautions. Intravenous access, ECG monitoring, pulse oximetry, ventilation facilities.

Materials
5-mL syringes, 10-mL syringes, three fine 22-G needles (5 cm), intubation kit, emergency drugs, disinfectant (Fig. 8.3).

Skin prep
in all blocks.

Patient positioning
Supine, with the head tilted slightly backward and turned about 45° to the opposite side.

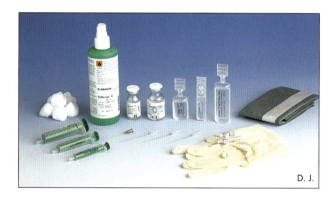

Fig. 8.3 Materials

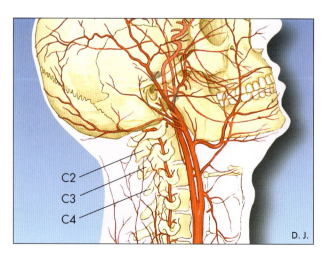

Fig. 8.4 Landmarks: transverse processes of C2 to C4

Deep (and superficial) cervical plexus

Landmarks
Posterior edge of the sternocleidomastoid muscle, caudal part of the mastoid process, Chassaignac's tubercle (C6), transverse processes of C2, C3, C4 and C5 (Figs. 8.4 and 8.6).

The patient is asked to turn the head toward the opposite side and to lift it slightly, making the posterior edge of the sternocleidomastoid apparent.

The transverse process of C6 and the caudal tip of the mastoid process are located. A line is drawn from the mastoid process along the posterior edge of the sternocleidomastoid muscle to the level of C6 (Figs. 8.5 and 8.6). The transverse process of C2 is palpated and marked on the skin. This lies about 1.5 cm caudal to the mastoid process and about 0.5–1 cm dorsal to the marked line. The transverse processes of C3, C4 and C5 are also palpated and marked. The distances between them are each ca. 1.5 cm, and like C2 they lie about 0.5–1 cm dorsal to the marked line.

Injection technique
The aim is to block the anterior branches of the cervical plexus in the groove of the transverse process.

After thorough skin prep, skin infiltration is carried out at the marked areas of C2, C3 and C4 and the needles are introduced (Fig. 8.6). To do this, the anaesthetist stands at the patient's head. In the sequence C2 to C4, the needles are directed perpendicular to the skin and advanced slightly caudal (ca. 30°) to the transverse process. In normal anatomy, the distance from the transverse processes to the skin varies between 1.5 and 3.5 cm. After clear bone contact and minimal withdrawal of the needle, careful aspiration needs to be carried out at various levels.

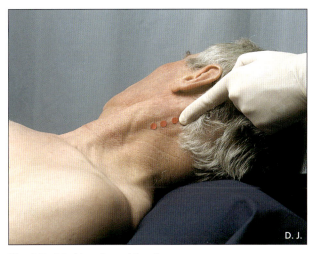
Fig. 8.5 Marking the guiding lines

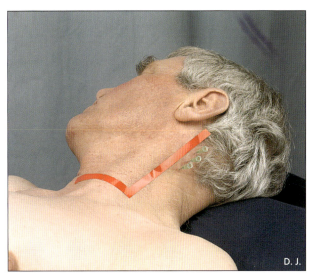
Fig. 8.6 Needle insertion in the area of the transverse processes of C2, C3 and C4

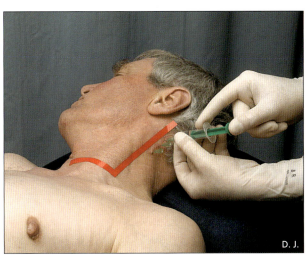
Fig. 8.7 Injection after aspiration

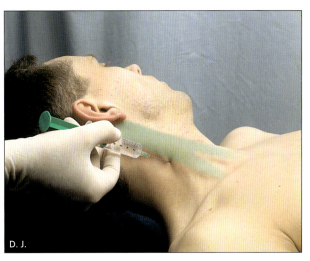
Fig. 8.8 Superficial cervical plexus block

> The tip of the needle must reach the groove of the transverse process in order to ensure good anesthesia.

Only then may the local anesthetic be injected in several small doses, with repeated aspiration (Fig. 8.7).

> An injection should never be carried out without definite bone contact. The local anesthetic must be slowly administered in small amounts (several test doses) and with repeated aspiration.

> If the needle slips along the transverse process and enters an intervertebral foramen, there is a risk of dural puncture.

Effects of the block
If the local anesthetic spreads in the direction of the superior cervical ganglion and/or the cervicothoracic ganglion, Horner's syndrome may develop (see Chapter 6, p. 63).

Block series
If there is improvement after two treatment sessions, a series of 8–12 therapeutic blocks is indicated.

Dosage
Diagnostic
2 mL local anesthetic per segment – e.g. 1% prilocaine, mepivacaine, lidocaine.

Therapeutic
3 mL local anesthetic per segment – e.g. 0.2–0.375% ropivacaine, 0.125–0.25% bupivacaine (0.125–0.25% levobupivacaine).

Surgical
30 mL local anesthetic:
0.75% ropivacaine or 0.25–0.5% bupivacaine (0.25–0.5% levobupivacaine) mixed with 1% prilocaine or 1% mepivacaine.
Of this: 10 mL for fan-like injection into the superficial cervical plexus (center of the posterior edge of the sternocleidomastoid muscle, Figs. 8.2 and 8.8) and 20 mL for anesthesia of the deep cervical plexus.

Side effects
Simultaneous block of the following nerves:
- Phrenic nerve, main symptom: unilateral paralysis of diaphragmatic movement
- Recurrent laryngeal nerve, main symptoms: hoarseness and foreign-body sensation in the throat
- Glossopharyngeal nerve, main symptoms: numbness in the final third of the tongue, paralysis of the pharyngeal muscles
- Vagus nerve, main symptoms: tachycardia, hypertension
- Partial block of the upper part of the brachial plexus

> When giving consent, the patient must be informed about these adverse effects and prepared for them.
> The patient must be monitored for 60 min after the block has been performed.

Complications
Intravascular injection
There is always a risk of intravascular injection due to the rich vascular supply in this area. Particular attention should be given to avoiding puncture of the vertebral artery. Toxic reactions may occur after intravascular administration of local anesthetics, and the symptoms and treatment of these are outlined in Chapter 6, p. 65.

Epidural or subarachnoid injection
When the needle slides along the transverse process and enters an intervertebral foramen, there is a risk of dural puncture and subarachnoid injection of local anesthetic. This can lead to a high spinal or high epidural block. The clinical picture and management of this complication is covered in Chapter 6, p.67.

Deep cervical plexus

Block no. ☐ Right ☐ Left

Record and checklist

Name: _____ Date: _____
Diagnosis: _____
Premedication: ☐ No ☐ Yes _____
Neurologial abnormalities: ☐ No
☐ Yes (which?) _____

Purpose of block:	☐ Diagnostic	☐ Therapeutic
Needle: ☐ 22 G	☐ 40 mm ☐ 50 mm	☐ 60 mm
i.v. access:	☐ Yes	
Monitoring:	☐ ECG	☐ Pulse oxymetry
Ventilation facilities:	☐ Yes (equipment checked)	
Emergency equipment (drugs):	☐ Checked	
Patient:	☐ Informed	

Position: ☐ Supine ☐ Head to contralateral side
Needle technique: 3-needle technique (C2, C3, C4)

Local anesthetic: _____ mL _____ % _____ per segment
Addition to
injection solution: ☐ No ☐ Yes _____
Patient's remarks during injection:
☐ None ☐ Pain ☐ Paresthesias ☐ Warmth
Nerve region _____ _____ _____

Objective block effect after 15 min:
☐ Cold test ☐ Temperature measurement right _____°C left _____°C
Horner's syndrome ☐ Yes ☐ No
☐ Sensory (C2, C3, C4, C5) ☐ Motor
Segments affected: _____ (numbness, warmth)
Monitoring after block: ☐ < 1 h ☐ > 1 h
Time of discharge _____

Complications:
☐ None ☐ Yes (intravascular, epidural, subarachnoid Injection)
Side effects:
☐ None ☐ Yes (Horner's syndrome, phrenic nerve, recurrent
laryngeal nerve, brachial plexus ...) _____

Subjective effects of the block: Duration: _____
☐ None ☐ Increased pain
☐ Reduced pain ☐ Relief of pain

VISUAL ANALOG SCALE

|||||||||||
0 10 20 30 40 50 60 70 80 90 100

Special notes: _____

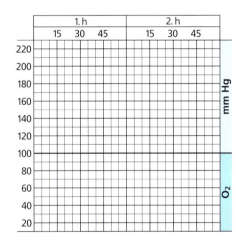

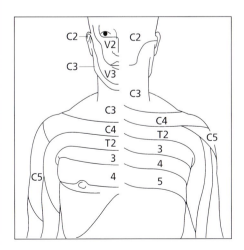

9 Brachial plexus
Interscalene block
Supraclavicular perivascular (subclavian perivascular) block
Vertical infraclavicular block
Axillary block

Anatomy

The brachial plexus arises from the union of the spinal nerve roots of C5, C6, C7, C8 and T1 and it often also contains fine fibers from the fourth cervical nerve and second thoracic nerve.

After they have left their intervertebral foramina, the roots of the plexus appear in the interscalene groove between the scalenus anterior and scalenus medius muscles and they join together there to form the primary cords or **trunks** (Fig. 9.1). The upper roots (C5, C6) form the **superior trunk**, the roots of C7 continue as the **middle trunk** and the **inferior trunk** arises from the roots of C8 and T1. After passing through the interscalene groove, the primary cords of the plexus, lying close together, move towards the first rib. The suprascapular nerve and subclavian nerve already branch off from the superior trunk here, in the posterior triangle of the neck above the clavicle. When crossing the first rib, the trunks of the plexus lie dorsolateral to the subclavian artery and are enclosed along with the artery by a connective-tissue sheath. The plexus runs through under the middle of the clavicle, following the course of the subclavian artery, into the tip of the axilla. As it does so, each of the primary cords divides into the **anterior** (ventral) **divisions** and **posterior** (dorsal) **divisions**. These supply the ventral flexor muscles and the dorsal extensor muscles of the upper extremity.

In the axilla itself, the nerve cords regroup and separate into the individual nerves (Fig. 9.2).

The ventral branches of the superior and middle trunk combine to form the **lateral cord** (fasciculus lateralis, C5, C6, C7; Fig. 9.3).

The following nerves emerge from this:
- Musculocutaneous nerve
- Median nerve (lateral root)
- Lateral pectoral nerve

All of the dorsal branches of the three trunks form the **posterior cord** (fasciculus posterior, C5–8, T1). The end branches of this (Fig. 9.3) are the:
- Radial nerve
- Axillary nerve
- Thoracodorsal nerve
- Inferior subscapular nerve
- Superior subscapular nerve

The ventral branches of the inferior trunk continue as the **medial cord** (fasciculus medialis, C8, T1). The following nerves (Fig. 9.3) emerge from this:
- Ulnar nerve
- Median nerve (medial root)
- Medial pectoral nerve
- Medial antebrachial cutaneous nerve
- Medial brachial cutaneous nerve

Introduction

The classical blocks of the brachial plexus using Hirschel's [19] (axillary approach) and Kulenkampff's [23] (supraclavicular block) anesthesia have been continuously developed and supplemented with additional access routes (Fig. 9.4). As representative techniques for a multitude of clinical procedures for plexus anesthesia, the axillary perivascular block [3, 18, 74], sub-

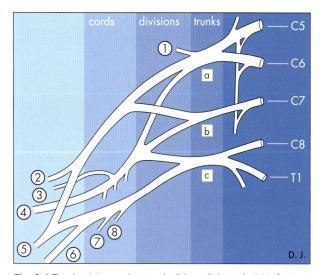

Fig. 9.1 Trunks: (a) superior trunk, (b) medial trunk, (c) inferior trunk, divisions and cords of the brachial plexus. (1) Suprascapular nerve, (2) musculocutaneous nerve, (3) axillary nerve, (4) radial nerve, (5) median nerve, (6) ulnar nerve, (7) medial antebrachial cutaneous nerve, (8) medial brachial cutaneous nerve

clavian perivascular block using the Winnie and Collins technique [73], Winnie's interscalene block [70, 74] and Raj's infraclavicular approach [41] may be mentioned. All of the blocks of the brachial plexus are based on the concept that the nerve plexus lies within a perivascular and perineural space in its course from the transverse processes to the axilla. Like the epidural space, this space limits the spread of the local anesthetic and conducts it to the various trunks and roots. Within the connective tissue sheath, the concentration and volume of the local anesthetic used determine the extent of the block's spread.

Apart from technical aspects, the main differences between the various block procedures are that the injection is made into the interscalene space, the subclavian space, the infraclavicular space, or the axillary space – leading to different focuses for the block.

In this chapter, four techniques that are among the standard methods for plexus anesthesia will be described: the interscalene, subclavian perivascular, infraclavicular and axillary blocks of the brachial plexus.

All four procedures have well-known advantages in contrast with general anesthesia:

- They can be used on an outpatient basis.
- Use in patients with a full stomach, high-risk and emergency patients and patients who are anxious about general anesthesia.
- Absence of side effects such as nausea and vomiting.
- Absence of postoperative pulmonary complications.
- Excellent postoperative pain control, particularly with the use of long-term local anesthetics (continuous procedures).
- Sympathetic block with vasodilation, better perfusion and faster recovery of traumatized extremities.

Certain points should always be observed when preparing for this procedure:

- Contraindications must be excluded.
- The anatomic relationships in each patient must be precisely studied and studied again for repeated blocks.
- Neurological abnormalities must be excluded.
- The procedure must be explained to the patient in detail in order to ensure cooperation.
- The patient must be placed in a comfortable position during the intervention.
- All patients should be informed of possible side effects and complications; outpatients in particular must also be advised of what they should and should not do after anesthesia or pain treatment.

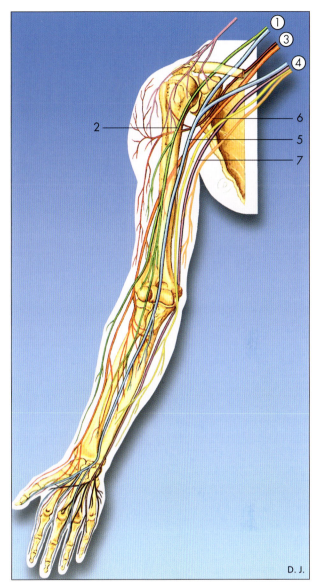

Fig. 9.2 Regrouping of the nerve cords in the area of the axilla and their distal distribution. (1) Lateral cord, (2) musculocutaneous nerve, (3) posterior cord, (4) medial cord, (5) median nerve, (6) radial nerve, (7) ulnar nerve

Interscalene block

Indications

Surgical

- Clavicle, shoulder, upper arm [1, 56] (the exception is the medial aspect):
  As a "single-shot" administration or continuous regional anesthesia [17, 37, 61] or in combination with basic general anesthesia.

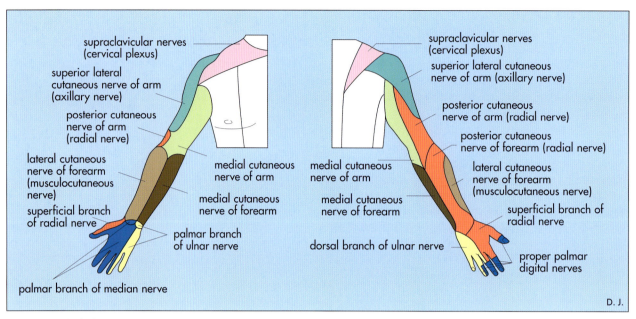

Fig. 9.3 Brachial plexus, cutaneous innervation

In combination with basic general anesthesia, the administration of 20–25 mL 0.75% ropivacaine or 20 mL 0.5% bupivacaine allows a marked reduction in the dosage of the general anesthetic and, in our own experience, leads to excellent postoperative pain control.
- Reduction of shoulder dislocation.

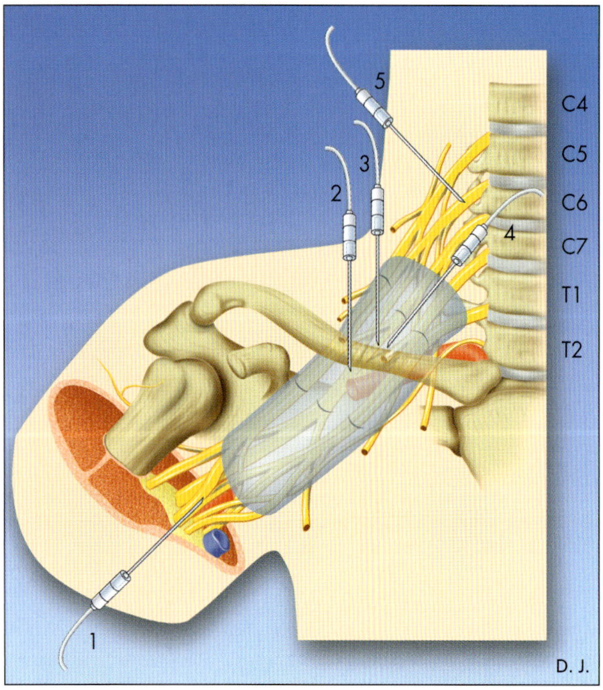

Therapeutic
- Shoulder and upper arm pain ("frozen shoulder"): humeroscapular periarthritis, muscles of the rotator cuff, post-stroke pain (ca. 70% of patients have severe shoulder pain). The aim of the block is to allow pain-free and successful physiotherapy.
- Mobilization of the shoulder.
- Shoulder arthritis.
- Post-herpetic neuralgia in the innervation area.
- Lymphedema after breast amputation.
- Vascular diseases and injuries, with continuous block in the acute stage.
- Complex regional pain syndrome (CRPS), type I (sympathetic reflex dystrophy) and type II (causalgia):
  If abduction of the arm is possible, an axillary block is preferable here (see p. 106).
- Postamputation pain – e.g. after disarticulation.
- Tumor-related pain:
  Continuous administration (e.g. in Pancoast tumor and neuropathic tumor pain [65]) is an alternative to repeated single applications here. The therapeutic effect of additional opioid administration has been evaluated in the literature [21, 64]. The period of treatment is limited. It can provide supplementation to oral opioid administration, but it cannot replace it.

Fig. 9.4 Various access routes for blocking the brachial plexus: (1) axillary block, (2) infraclavicular block, (3) Kulenkampff supraclavicular block, (4) Winnie and Collins subclavian perivascular block, (5) Winnie interscalene block

Contraindications

Specific
- Infection or malignant disease in the neck.
- Infection of the skin in the puncture area.
- Contralateral paresis of the phrenic or recurrent laryngeal nerves.
- Anticoagulation treatment.
- Distorted anatomy – e.g. due to prior surgical interventions or trauma to the neck.

Relative
The decision should be taken after carefully weighing up the risks and benefits:
- Hemorrhagic diathesis.
- Stable systemic neurological diseases.
- Local nerve injury (as there may be doubt whether the cause is surgery or anesthesia).
- Severe chronic obstructive pulmonary disease.

Procedure

Interscalene technique (Winnie's anterior route)

"Single-shot" technique

This block should only be carried out by experienced anesthetists or under their supervision. It is absolutely necessary to have a detailed discussion with the patient before the procedure.

Preparations
Check that the emergency equipment is present and in working order. Sterile precautions. Intravenous access, ECG monitoring, pulse oximetry, intubation kit, emergency medication, ventilation facilities.

Materials (Figs. 9.5 and 9.6)
Paresthesia technique
Plexufix® 25-mm (38–50-mm) long 24-G (45°) needle with "immobile needle" injection lead (B. Braun Melsungen).

Electrostimulation
- Stimuplex® HNS 11 nerve stimulator (B. Braun Melsungen).
- Stimuplex D® 50-mm 22-G (15°) needle with "immobile needle" injection lead (B. Braun Melsungen).

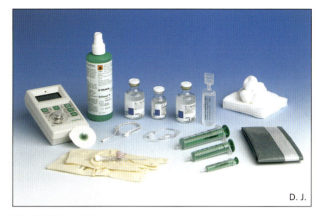

Fig. 9.5 Materials

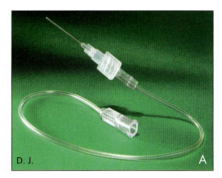 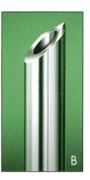

Fig. 9.6a, b 24-G needle, short-beveled

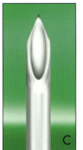 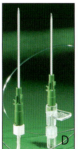 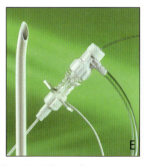

Fig. 9.6c Single-shot technique: Stimuplex® D needle
Fig. 9.6d Continuous technique: Contiplex® D needle
Fig. 9.6e Continuous technique: Tuohy continuous needle

Continuous technique*
Anterior technique
- Contiplex D® set: 50-mm 22-G (15°) needle (B. Braun Melsungen) with Contiplex ® catheter

or
- Contiplex®–Tuohy continuous set: 38(–52)-mm 18-G Tuohy needle with Contiplex ® catheter

---

* If technical difficulties arise, the catheter and Tuohy puncture needle are always removed simultaneously. A catheter must never be withdrawn through a Tuohy puncture needle that remains in place (because of catheter shearing).

Chapter 9

Posterior technique
- Contiplex D® set: 80(–110)-mm 18-G (15°) needle with Contiplex ® catheter
- Contiplex®–Tuohy continuous set: 102-mm 18-G Tuohy needle with Contiplex ® catheter
- Syringes: 2, 10 and 20 mL.
- Local anesthetics, disinfectant, swabs, compresses, sterile gloves and drape.

Skin prep
In all blocks.

Patient positioning
Supine, with the head turned to the opposite side.

Landmarks
Sternocleidomastoid muscle, interscalene groove between the scalenus anterior and scalenus medius muscles (Fig. 9.7), transverse process (C6), external jugular vein.

Location of the puncture site
To locate the injection site, the patient's arm is drawn in the direction of the knee (Fig. 9.8). The patient is asked to turn the head to the opposite side and to lift it slightly (ca. 20°), so that the posterior edge of the sternocleidomastoid muscle becomes evident (Fig. 9.9). The transverse process (C6) is palpated at the lateral edge of the sternocleidomastoid muscle. For confirmation (pleura) and guidance, the pulsation of the subclavian artery (at the lower end of the interscalene groove) and the upper

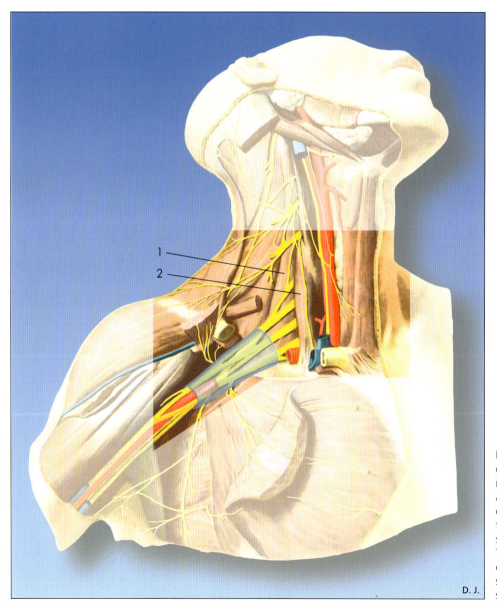

Fig. 9.7 The interscalene groove. Scalenus medius muscle (1) and scalenus anterior muscle (2). Injection of the local anesthetic into the proximal neurovascular sheath of the brachial plexus. The plexus is located in a kind of "sandwich" between the scalenus anterior muscle and scalenus medius muscle

edge of the clavicle can also be palpated and their distance from the injection site can be estimated (Fig. 9.10).

Posterior to the sternocleidomastoid muscle, the scalenus anterior muscle is palpated. The interscalene groove between the scalenus anterior and scalenus medius muscles is felt with "rolling fingers" and located (Fig. 9.11). The injection site in the interscalene groove lies at the level of the cricoid, opposite the transverse process of C6 (Chassaignac's tubercle). The external jugular vein often crosses the level of the cricoid cartilage here (Fig. 9.12). When there are anatomical difficulties, it is helpful for the patient to inhale deeply or to try and blow out the cheeks. The scalene muscles then tense up and the interscalene groove becomes more easily palpable.

Injection technique
The traditional technique first described by Winnie is a classic paresthesia technique. After disinfection of the puncture area, draping and skin infiltration, the injection site is isolated using the index and middle fingers. The injection needle is advanced between the fingers in the direction of the transverse process (C6). The direction of insertion runs medially and ca. 30–40° caudally, as well as slightly posteriorly (Fig. 9.13).The index and middle finger continue to palpate the interscalene groove.
When the needle is positioned superficially, paresthesias usually occur in the area of the elbow, index finger and thumb. Paresthesias in the shoulder region also frequently occur. These result from stimulation of the suprascapular nerve, which is often located in the connective tissue sheath [3].

> When the anatomy is normal and no paresthesias are elicited after ca. 2–2.5 cm, the needle position needs to be corrected.

Once the paresthesias have been elicited, the correct positioning of the needle is checked by aspirating at various levels and quickly injecting an initial dose of the local anesthetic (2–3 mL). The patient will experience a brief pain (pressure paresthesia) due to expansion of the perivascular space. During further injection of the local anesthetic, aspiration has to be repeated after every 4–5 mL. Pressure from the index or middle finger allows the direction of spread of the local anesthetic to be guided during the injection. After successful injection, the entire area is massaged in order to ensure even distribution of the local anesthetic. This also provides hematoma prophylaxis.

Locating the interscalene groove:

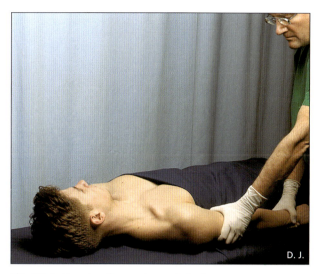

Fig. 9.8 1. Drawing the arm towards the knee

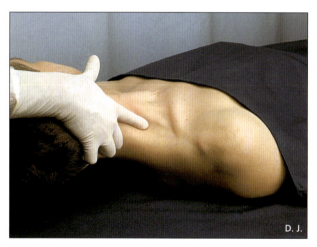

Fig. 9.9 2. Turning the head to the opposite side and raising it slightly

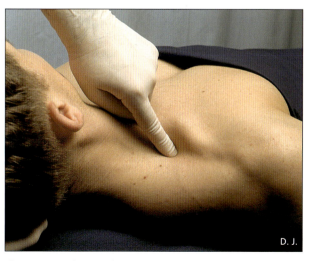

Fig. 9.10 3. Palpating the clavicle and subclavian artery

Chapter 9

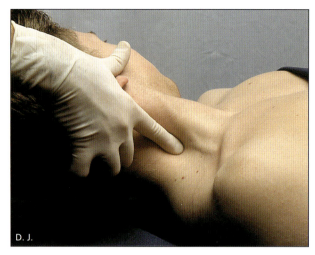

Fig. 9.11 4. Palpating the interscalene groove with "rolling" fingers

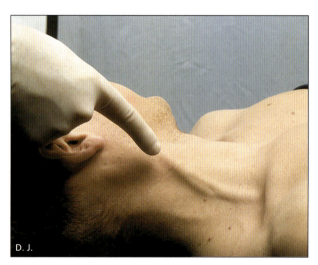

Fig. 9.12 Position of the external jugular vein

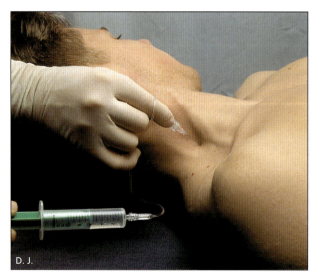

Fig. 9.13 Injection in the direction of the transverse process of C6

The patient must be informed about the expected paresthesias and their significance.

Electrostimulation
Stimulation current of 1–2 mA and 2 Hz is selected for a stimulus duration of 0.1 ms.
The injection needle is advanced in the direction of the transverse process (C6). After the motor response from the relevant musculature (biceps brachii muscle – musculocutaneous nerve and/or deltoid muscle – axillary nerve [51, 62] or twitching of the distal arm muscles), the stimulant current is reduced to 0.2–0.3 mA. Slight twitching suggests that the stimulation needle is in the immediate vicinity of the nerve. After aspiration, injection of a local anesthetic is carried out in incremental doses. During the injection, the twitching slowly disappears.

Dosage
Surgical
"Single-shot" administration:
40 mL local anesthetic is sufficient for an adequate block of the brachial plexus and caudal part of the cervical plexus. In the literature [13, 25, 47, 61, 70], the doses administered vary from 30 mL to 50 mL. A mixture of 20 mL 0.75% ropivacaine or 0.5% bupivacaine (0.5% levobupivacaine) with 20 mL 1% prilocaine (1% mepivacaine) has proved its value very well in practice (in our own experience). This leads to a fast onset and long duration.
25 mL local anesthetic – e.g. 1% prilocaine (1% mepivacaine), in combination with 5–10 mg diazepam i.v. for reducing a dislocated shoulder.
20–25 mL local anesthetic – e.g. 0.75% ropivacaine or 0.5% bupivacaine (0.5% levobupivacaine), in combination with basic general anesthesia for surgical interventions in the area of the shoulder and clavicle. This leads to very good postoperative pain control.
20 mL local anesthetic is sufficient to block the lower part of the cervical plexus and the upper part of the brachial plexus. The brachial plexus is only incompletely anesthetized with this amount and block of the ulnar nerve territory is often deficient.

Therapeutic
"Single-shot" administration (block series):
10 mL local anesthetic – e.g. 0.2% ropivacaine or 0.125–0.25% bupivacaine (0.125–0.25% levobupivacaine) in shoulder and upper arm pain, shoulder arthritis, post-stroke pain, lymphedema after mastectomy.
10–20 mL local anesthetic – e.g. 0.2–0.375% ropivacaine or 0.25% bupivacaine (0.25% levobupivacaine)

in post-herpetic neuralgia, vascular diseases and injuries, complex regional pain syndrome (CRPS) types I and II, post-amputation pain.

25 mL local anesthetic – e.g. 1% prilocaine or 1% mepivacaine in combination with 5–10 mL diazepam i. v. to mobilize the shoulder.

If there is evidence of symptomatic improvement, a series of 8–12 blocks can be carried out.

Continuous interscalene block – anterior technique (adapted from Meier)

Skin prep
In all blocks.

Patient positioning
(See the steps for locating the puncture site under "Interscalene block – 'single-shot' technique," p. 87).

Landmarks (Fig. 9.14a)
- Superior thyroid notch
- Posterior edge of the sternocleidomastoid muscle
- Posterior scalene groove
- External jugular vein
- Transition from the middle to lateral third of the clavicle.

Technique [31]
After identification of the posterior edge of the sternocleidomastoid muscle at the level of the superior thyroid notch, the block needle (55-mm Contiplex® D or Contiplex®–Tuohy needle, 38 or 52 mm) is introduced at an angle of 30° caudally and slightly laterally, in the direction of the transition from the middle to the lateral third of the clavicle (Fig. 9.14b). A stimulation current of 1–2 mA and 2 Hz is selected with a stimulus duration of 0.1 ms. After a motor response from the relevant musculature (twitching in the biceps brachii muscle – musculocutaneous nerve and/or deltoid muscle – axillary nerve is regarded to be as reliable as twitching of the distal muscles [51, 62]), the stimulation current is reduced to 0.2–0.3 mA. Slight twitching suggests that the stimulation needle is in the immediate vicinity of the nerve. The catheter is advanced approximately 3 cm beyond the end of the cannula or needle (Fig. 9.15). After removal of the cannula or needle, fixation of the catheter and placement of a bacterial filter, and after careful aspiration and injection of a test dose, the bolus administration of the local anesthetic follows.

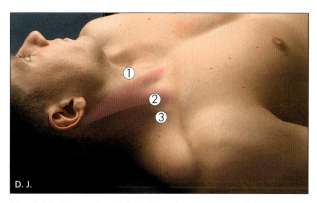

Fig. 9.14a Interscalene block (anterior access route). The posterior edge of the sternocleidomastoid muscle at the level of the superior thyroid notch. (1) Superior thyroid notch, (2) posterior edge of the sternocleidomastoid muscle, (3) external jugular vein and posterior scalene groove

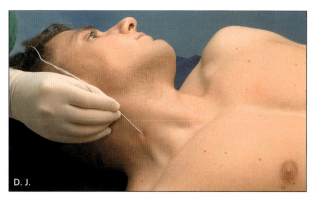

Fig. 9.14b Introducing the puncture needle at an angle of ca. 30° to the skin, caudally and laterally in the direction of the transition from the middle to the lateral third of the clavicle

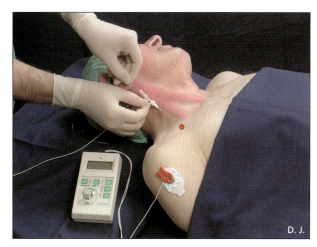

Fig. 9.15 Interscalene block (continuous technique). Introducing the catheter through a Tuohy needle

Chapter 9

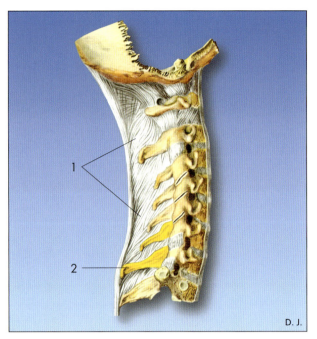

Fig. 9.16 Interscalene block, posterior access route.
Landmarks: spinous processes of C6 and C7 (vertebra prominens).
(1) nuchal ligament, (2) vertebra prominens

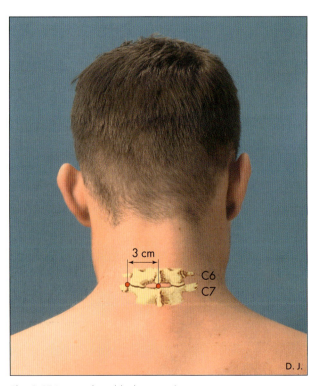

Fig. 9.17 Interscalene block, posterior access route.
Puncture site: the mid-point between the spinous processes of C6 and C7 is marked. The puncture site is located ca. 3 cm lateral and paravertebral to this

Continuous interscalene block – posterior technique (Pippa technique)

The posterior cervical paravertebral block of the brachial plexus is an alternative to Winnie's anterior route. This method was first described by Kappis in 1912, and was republished by Pippa in 1990 as a "loss of resistance" technique [33, 44, 65]. The availability of electrical nerve stimulation has made this access route to the brachial plexus more important.

Indications and contraindications
(See anterior interscalene block, p. 83.)

Procedure

This block should only be carried out by experienced anesthetists or under their supervision. An detailed discussion with the patient is an absolute necessity.

Preparation
(See anterior interscalene block, p. 85.)

Materials
(See anterior interscalene block, p. 85.)

Skin prep
In all blocks.

Patient positioning
Sitting, with the neck flexed (to relax the cervical muscles) and supported by an assistant (the lateral recumbent position can be used as an alternative).

Landmarks
- Spinous processes of the sixth (C6) and seventh (C7 – vertebra prominens) cervical vertebrae (Fig. 9.16).
- The mid-point between the spinous processes of C6 and C7 is marked. The puncture site is located approximately 3 cm lateral to this point (Fig. 9.17).
- Level of the cricoid cartilage (target direction).

> It is absolutely necessary to note the following points during this puncture procedure:
> - Electrical nerve stimulation is the method of choice.
> - After puncture, the needle should be passed towards the lateral edge of the cricoid cartilage.

Brachial plexus

- Contact with the transverse process (C7) is made after ca. 3.5–6 cm (depending on the anatomy).
- The transverse process is approximately 0.5–0.6 cm thick.
- There is a risk of perforating the dural sheath if the puncture is carried out too medially (epidural or subarachnoid injection).
- There is a risk of pneumothorax.
- Frequent aspiration should be carried out and the injection should be made in incremental doses (blood, CSF?)
- Note any contractions in the biceps brachii muscle (musculocutaneous nerve), deltoid muscle (axillary nerve), or index finger and thumb.

Technique

Disinfection of the puncture area, draping and skin infiltration. After an incision with a stylet, the needle is introduced at the sagittal level and perpendicular to the skin, aiming approximately for the level of the ipsilateral cricoid cartilage(Fig. 9.18). The needle passes the major cervical muscles (trapezius, splenius cervicis and levator scapulae; Fig. 9.19) on the way to the transverse process (C7). It is absolutely necessary to avoid any deviation in a medial direction from the sagittal level. At a depth of ca. 3.5–6 cm, contact is made with the transverse process of C7. The needle is withdrawn slightly, the injection direction is corrected slightly cranially, and one advances past the transverse process a further 1.5–2 cm deeper. Stimulation current of 1–2 mA and 2 Hz is selected with a stimulus durationof 0.1 ms. After the motor response from the relevant musculature (biceps brachii muscle and/or deltoid, or muscles of the index finger and thumb), the current is reduced to 0.3–0.5 mA. The catheter is advanced approximately 3 cm beyond the end of the needle or cannula. After removal of the needle or cannula, fixation of the catheter and placement of a bacterial filter, and after careful aspiration and injection of a test dose, the bolus administration of the local anesthetic follows.

Dosage

40 mL local anesthetic (see above) is commonly used for the procedure. As a subsequent 24-hour infusion for postoperative analgesia:
- 0.2% ropivacaine, **6–14 mL/h** (max. 37.5 mg/h)
- 0.25% bupivacaine [17] (0.25% levobupivacaine), **0.25 mg/kg b.w./h**

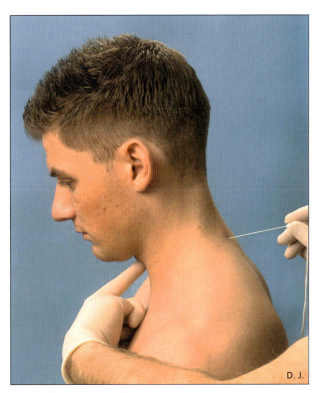

Fig. 9.18 Interscalene block, posterior access route. Puncture technique: the needle is introduced at the sagittal level and perpendicular to the skin in the direction of the ipsilateral cricoid cartilage

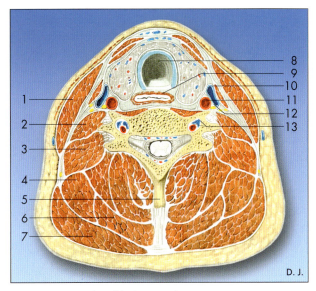

Fig. 9.19 Interscalene block, posterior access route. Puncture technique: the needle passes the strong cervical muscles (trapezius muscle, splenius cervicis muscle, and levator scapulae muscle). (1) Sternocleidomastoid muscle, (2) scalenus anterior muscle, (3) scalenus medius and scalenus posterior muscles, (4) levator scapulae muscle, (5) spine of the sphenoid bone, (6) splenius capitis and splenius cervicis muscles, (7) trapezius muscle, (8) trachea, (9) esophagus, (10) internal jugular vein, (11) common carotid artery, (12) vagus nerve, (13) vertebral artery and vein

Chapter 9

- 0.125% bupivacaine (0.25% levobupivacaine), **0.125 mg/kg b.w./h**, combined with opioids if appropriate [37]

> Individual adjustment of the dosage and period of treatment is necessary. The following information is therefore only intended to provide guidance.

Distribution of the blocks
The complete distribution of the anesthesia is shown in Fig. 9.20.

Interscalene block

Side effects
Simultaneous anesthesia of the following nerves and ganglia (Fig. 9.21):
- Vagus nerve, main symptoms: tachycardia, hypertension.
- Recurrent laryngeal nerve, main symptoms: hoarseness and foreign-body sensation in the throat.
- Phrenic nerve, main symptoms: unilateral paralysis of diaphragmatic movement and simulation of pneumothorax, particularly with continuous blocks [13, 37]. An ipsilateral block of the phrenic nerve has been observed as a side effect after an interscalene block in nearly 100% of patients [63].
- Cervicothoracic (stellate) ganglion, with Horner's syndrome.
- Bronchospasm [59].
- Contralateral anesthesia [14].
- Bilateral distribution of the local anesthetic [28].
- Reversible "locked-in" syndrome [11].

> The patient must be warned of these potential adverse events.

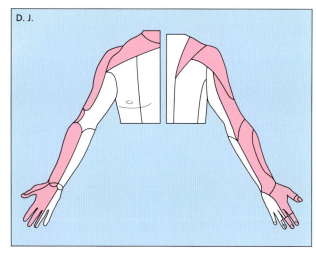

Fig. 9.20 The nerve areas most frequently blocked 15 min after administration of the block with bupivacaine [20]

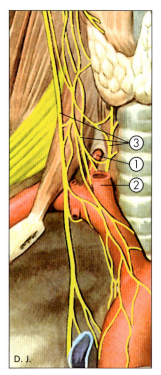

Fig. 9.21 The most important nerves and vessels in the injection area: (1) vertebral artery, (2) carotid artery, (3) laryngeal, vagus and phrenic nerves

Complications
Nerve injuries
Traumatic nerve injuries are an extremely rare complication of this technique [2, 61].
Prophylaxis: Only needles with short-beveled tips should be used. Intraneural positioning should be excluded. Vasopressor additives should be avoided. This procedure should not be performed in adult patients under general anesthesia. For details, see p. 106 in the section on axillary blocks.

Intravascular injection [11]
There is a particular risk of intravascular injection into the vertebral artery (Fig. 9.21) or other cervical vessels. This can very quickly lead to toxic reactions. For the symptoms and treatment, see Chapter 6, p. 65.

Epidural or subarachnoid injection [24, 43, 57]
Epidural injection of the local anesthetic can lead to high epidural block, and subarachnoid administration can lead to a total spinal block. Both complications are

significant and life-threatening, and require immediate treatment (see Chapter 6, p. 67).
Prophylaxis: injection with short needles and introduction of the needle in a caudal direction.

CNS toxicity
Overdose and/or intravascular diffusion of the local anesthetic can, in extremely rare cases, lead to CNS toxicity (see Chapter 6, p. 66).

Pneumothorax
When the technique is carried out correctly, this complication is unlikely. The needle is advanced at a safe distance from the dome of the pleura.

Pressure on the carotid artery
Extremely rare and transient. Caused by the volume of the injection [50].

Record and checklist

Interscalene block of the brachial plexus
„Single-shot"-technique ☐ Right ☐ Left

Name: _____ Date: _____
Diagnosis: _____
Premedication: ☐ No ☐ Yes _____

Neurological abnormalities: ☐ No
                             ☐ Yes (which?) _____

Purpose of block: ☐ Surgical ☐ Diagnostic ☐ Therapeutic
i. v. access: ☐ Yes
Monitoring: ☐ ECG   ☐ Pulse oxymetry
Ventilation facilities: ☐ Yes (equipment checked)
Emergency equipment (drugs)   ☐ Checked
Patient: ☐ Informed

Position: ☐ Supine   ☐ Head to contralateral side
Needle type: ☐ Plexufix® ☐ 25 mm ☐ 50 mm
                ☐ Stimuplex® D ____ mm ☐ Other _____

Puncture technique: ☐ Interscalene groove located ☐ Level C6
                    ☐ Paresthesias ☐ Electrostimulation
Nerve region _____

Local anesthetic: _____ ml _____ % _____
(in incremental doses)
Addition: ☐ Yes _____ µg/mg ☐ No
Patient's remarks during injection:
☐ None   ☐ Paresthesias   ☐ Warmth
☐ Pain triggered (intraneural location?) _____
Nerve region _____

Objective block effect after 15 min:
☐ Cold test   ☐ Temperature measurement right ___°C left ___°C
☐ Sensory   ☐ Motor
Monitoring after block: ☐ < 1 h   ☐ > 1 h
                Time of discharge: _____

Complications:
☐ None   ☐ Intravascular ☐ Epidural/subarachnoid ☐ Pneumothorax
Side effects::
☐ None   ☐ Hematoma   ☐ Phrenic nerve ☐ Recurrent laryngeal nerve
☐ Horner's syndrome

Subjective effects of the block: Duration: _____
☐ None   ☐ Increased pain   ☐ Reduced pain   ☐ Relief of pain

VISUAL ANALOG SCALE

|||||||||||
0   10   20   30   40   50   60   70   80   90   100

Special notes: _____

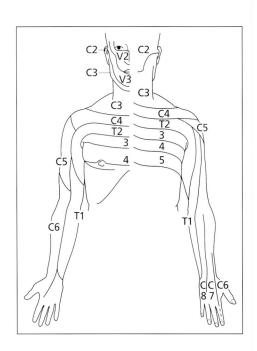

© Copyright ABW Wissenschaftsverlag 2004,
Jankovic, Regional nerve blocks and infiltration therapy, 3rd edition

Interscalene block of the brachial plexus
Continuous technique   ☐ Right   ☐ Left

Purpose of block:	☐ Surgical	☐ Therapeutic
i. v. access:	☐ Yes	
Monitoring:	☐ ECG	☐ Pulse oxymetry
Ventilation facilities:		☐ Yes (equipment checked)
Emergency equipment (drugs)		☐ Checked
Patient:		☐ Informed
Position:	☐ Supine	☐ Other
Puncture technique:	☐ Electrostimulation	
Access route:	☐ Anterior	☐ Posterior
Needle type:	☐ Contiplex® D ___ mm ___ G	☐ Tuohy ___ mm ___ G
	☐ Other _____	

Puncture technique: ☐ Interscalene groove located   ☐ Level C6
                                 ☐ Paresthesias   ☐ Electrostimulation

Nerve region _____ _____

Catheter: ☐ Advanced _____ cm
Aspiration test: ☐ Carried out
Bacterial filter: ☐ Placed
Bolus administration: _____ mL _____ % _____
(in incremental doses)
Addition to
injection solution: ☐ No   ☐ Yes _____ μg/mg

Patient's remarks during injection:
☐ None   ☐ Paresthesias   ☐ Warmth
Pain triggered (intraneural location?) _____
Nerve region _____

Objective block effect after 15 min:
☐ Cold test   ☐ Temperature measurement: right ___ °C left ___ °C
☐ Sensory   ☐ Motor
☐ Continuous monitoring _____

☐ Infusion for postoperative analgesia
Local anesthetic: _____ % _____ ml/h
☐ Addition to LA: _____ mg _____ μg _____

Patient-controlled anesthesia PCA
Local anesthetic: _____ %
Addition _____
☐ Baseline rate _____ ml/h _____
☐ Bolus administration _____ ml
☐ Lockout interval _____ min

Complications:
☐ None   ☐ Intravascular   ☐ Epidural/subarachnoid   ☐ Pneumothorax

Side effects:
☐ None   ☐ Hematoma   ☐ Phrenic nerve
☐ Recurrent laryngeal nerve   ☐ Horner's syndrome

Subjective effects of the block: Duration: _____
☐ None   ☐ Increased pain   ☐ Reduced pain   ☐ Relief of pain

VISUAL ANALOG SCALE

|0   10   20   30   40   50   60   70   80   90   100|

Record and checklist

Name: _____
Date: _____
Diagnosis: _____
Premedication: ☐ No ☐ Yes _____

Neurolocial abnormalities: ☐ No
☐ Yes (which??) _____

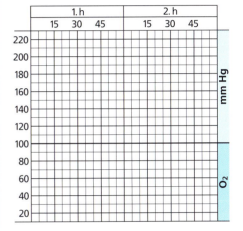

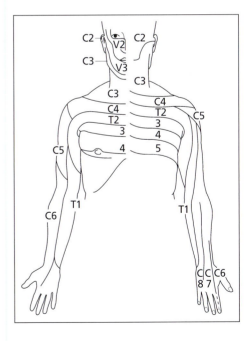

Special notes:

_____
_____
_____

© Copyright ABW Wissenschaftsverlag 2004,
Jankovic, Regional nerve blocks and infiltration therapy, 3rd edition

Supraclavicular perivascular (subclavian perivascular) block

Definition
Injection of a local anesthetic into the area of the brachial plexus trunks in the caudal part of the interscalene groove, in its most compact part above the clavicle. This technique was first described by Winnie and Collins [73].

Indications
Surgical
Operations in the upper arm, forearm and hand.

Therapeutic
None.

Contraindications
Specific
- Infections or malignant diseases in the area of the throat and neck.
- Infection of the skin in the injection area.
- Contralateral paresis of the phrenic nerve or recurrent laryngeal nerve.
- Anticoagulant treatment.
- Distorted anatomy – e.g. due to prior surgical interventions or trauma in the area of the throat and neck.
- Severe chronic obstructive pulmonary disease.
- Contralateral pneumothorax.

Relative
The decision should be taken after carefully weighing up the risks and benefits:
- Hemorrhagic diathesis.
- Stable systemic neurological diseases.
- Local nerve injury (as there may be doubt whether the cause is surgery or anesthesia).

Procedure

This block should only be carried out by experienced anesthetists or under their supervision. Patients should receive full information before the procedure.

Preparations and materials
(See the section on the interscalene block, Figs. 9.5 and 9.6.)

Technique
Locating the injection site
The most important landmarks are:
- The interscalene groove, with its caudal part in the supraclavicular fossa (see the section on the interscalene block, steps for location, Figs. 9.8–9.12). The process of locating the site is often difficult when the caudal part of the interscalene groove is covered by the omohyoid muscle. During the injection, particular attention should be given to the course of the scalenus medius muscle (Fig. 9.22).
- The subclavian artery, which is located in the immediate vicinity of the plexus trunks. The arterial pulse is the most important mark for the injection.
- The midpoint of the clavicle. The injection point is located ca. 1.5–2 cm lateral to the clavicular head of the sternocleidomastoid muscle and 2 cm above the clavicle.
- The course of the external jugular vein as far as the supraclavicular fossa.

> The close anatomical relationships in this block are characterized by the trunks of the brachial plexus, the subclavian artery, the first rib and the dome of the pleura (Fig. 9.23; cf. Chapter 6, Fig. 6.2).

Injection technique
- After clear palpation of the subclavian artery, the tip of the left index finger is placed directly over the pulsation.
- The hub of an injection needle with a short-beveled tip is fixed between the index finger and the thumb of the right hand (Fig. 9.24).
- The needle is introduced in a caudal direction along the long axis of the body, near the scalenus medius muscle. The needle hub almost touches the skin of the throat, with the shaft lying parallel to the skin.

> The dome of the pleura is located immediately medial to the first rib. It is therefore absolutely essential to avoid a posteromedial injection, due to the risk of pneumothorax.

- Perforation of the fascia is confirmed by a "fascial click," and it is accompanied by paresthesias. The patient is asked to say "now" when paresthesias are experienced and to describe their location precisely. Paresthesias elicited below the shoulder, particularly in the innervation area of the median nerve, are important here. Paresthesias in the shoulder area indicate stimulation of the suprascapular nerve and are less important, since this nerve often lies outside the neurovascular sheath.

Brachial plexus

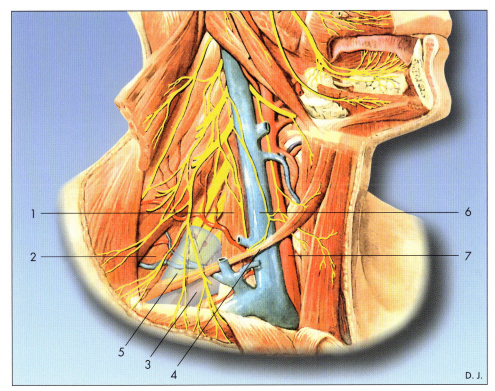

Fig. 9.22 Interscalene groove, with the brachial plexus.
(1) Scalenus anterior muscle,
(2) scalenus medius muscle,
(3) subclavian artery,
(4) omohyoid muscle,
(5) neurovascular sheath,
(6) internal jugular vein,
(7) common carotid artery

- After paresthesias have been elicited, correct positioning of the needle is checked by aspiration at various levels and an initial dose of local anesthetic (2–3 mL) is quickly injected. The increased pressure within the perivascular space causes pain for the patient (known as pressure paresthesia). During the injection of local anesthetic, aspiration must be repeated after each 4–5 mL. The index finger of the left hand should apply pressure above the needle in order to prevent the local anesthetic from spreading cranially (Figs. 9.25, 9.26).
- After successful injection, the entire area is massaged to ensure even distribution of local anesthetic. This also serves for hematoma prophylaxis.

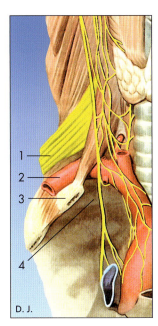

Fig. 9.23 (1) Brachial plexus, (2) subclavian artery, (3) first rib, (4) dome of the pleura

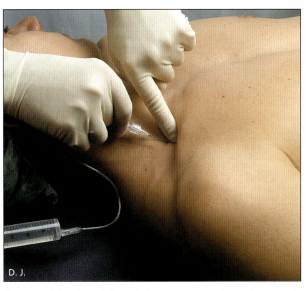

Fig. 9.24 Palpation of the subclavian artery and introduction of the needle

97

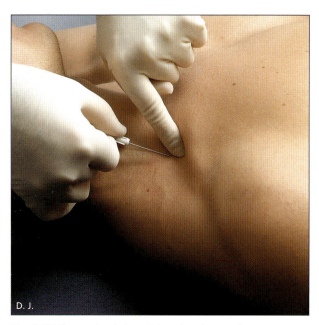

Fig. 9.25 Electrostimulation. Advancing the needle

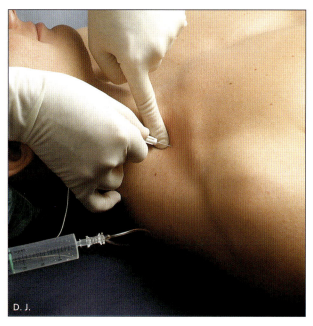

Fig. 9.26 Electrostimulation. Injection

Electrostimulation
A stimulation current of 1–2 mA and 2 Hz is selected with a stimulus duration of 0.1 ms, and the needle is advanced in the direction of the brachial plexus trunks (Fig. 9.25). After the motor response from the relevant musculature, the current is reduced to 0.2–0.3 mA (Fig. 9.26). Slight twitching suggests that the stimulation needle is in the immediate vicinity of the nerve. After aspiration, injection of a local anesthetic is carried out in incremental doses. During the injection, the twitching slowly disappears.

Problem situations
- If the needle is positioned too far anteriorly in the vicinity of the scalenus anterior muscle, the subclavian artery may be punctured. This is definite evidence that the needle is located in the perivascular space.
The needle is withdrawn to lie subcutaneously and then introduced dorsolaterally, in the vicinity of the scalenus medius muscle, until paresthesias are elicited.
- If no paresthesias are elicited, then the needle has missed all three trunks of the brachial plexus lying and it will come into contact with the first rib (protective function, preventing pleural puncture).
The needle is withdrawn to a subcutaneous position and its direction is corrected by about 1 cm dorsally, closer to the scalenus medius muscle.
- When a tourniquet is applied, an additional block of the intercostobrachial nerve (T2) and medial brachial cutaneous nerve is sometimes required. For this purpose, the arm is abducted about 90° and 5 mL of local anesthetic is injected directly above the pulsations of the axillary artery.

Dosage
Surgical
40 mL local anesthetic
- 0.75% ropivacaine
- 0.5% bupivacaine (0.5% levobupivacaine)
- 1% prilocaine
- 1% mepivacaine

Distribution of the block
The complete distribution of the anesthesia is shown in Fig. 9.27.

Side effects
Concomitant block of the following nerves and ganglia:

The patient must be informed about the expected paresthesias and their significance. If severe pain occurs during the injection (intraneural location), the injection should be stopped immediately and the position of the needle should be changed.

- Vagus nerve, recurrent laryngeal nerve, phrenic nerve.
- Stellate ganglion (see section on interscalene block, p. 92).

The patient must be warned of these possible adverse effects.

Complications
- Pneumothorax (0.5–6%; Fig. 9.28).
- Neural injury (see section on axillary block, p. 111).
- Intravascular injection (see Chapter 6, section on stellate ganglion, p. 65).
- CNS intoxication (see section on axillary block of the brachial plexus, p. 112).

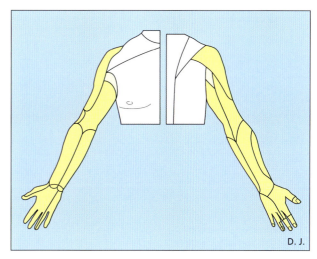

Fig. 9.27 Distribution of the block. The most frequently blocked nerve areas 15 min after initiating a block with bupivacaine [20]

Vertical infraclavicular block (Kilka, Geiger and Mehrkens technique)

With the traditional infraclavicular block of the brachial plexus [41], an alternative access route was sought that would provide a more effective alternative to the axillary route [52, 67]. The aim of this technique was to achieve a more complete distribution of the anesthesia and a faster onset, allowing better tolerance of the tourniquet and dispensing with the need for special positioning of the arm, while facilitating catheter techniques [22, 30].

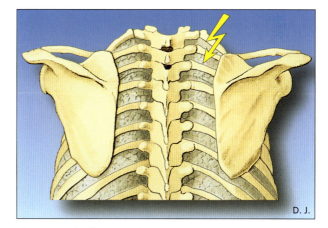

Fig. 9.28 Risk of pneumothorax

Indications and contraindications
(See axillary block, p. 106.)

Additional contraindications
- Chest deformities.
- Distorted anatomy (e.g. a dislocated and healed clavicular fracture, prior surgical procedures, or trauma in the puncture area).
- Foreign bodies in the puncture area (subclavian central venous line, cardiac pacemaker, etc.).

Procedure

This block should only be carried out by experienced anesthetists or under their supervision. Full prior explanation for the patient is mandatory.

Preparations
(See interscalene block, p. 85.)

Materials (Fig. 9.6)
Stimuplex® neurostimulator HNS 11 (B. Braun Melsungen).

"Single-shot" technique
Stimuplex D® 40(–55)-mm 22-G (15°) needle (B. Braun Melsungen), or
Tuohy 38(–52)-mm 18-G needle (B. Braun Melsungen).

Continuous technique
Contiplex D® set: 55-mm 18-G (15°) needle (B. Braun Melsungen) with Contiplex® catheter.
Contiplex®–Tuohy continuous set: 38(–52)-mm 18-G Tuohy needle with Contiplex® catheter.
Syringes: 2, 10, 20 mL.
Local anesthetics, disinfectant, swabs, compresses, sterile gloves and drape.

Chapter 9

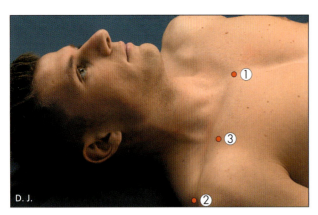

Fig. 9.29 Vertical infraclavicular block. Landmarks: (1) middle of the jugular fossa, (2) ventral process of the acromion, (3) puncture site

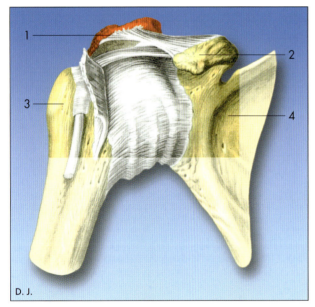

Fig. 9.30 Vertical infraclavicular block. The precise location of the ventral acromion (1) is very important. The immobile acromion can be distinguished from the mobile humeral head by passive movement of the ipsilateral upper arm. (2) Coracoid process, (3) humerus, (4) scapula

Skin prep
In all blocks.

Patient positioning
Supine, with the hand on the side being blocked lying relaxed on the abdomen.

Landmarks
- Center of the suprasternal notch.
- Anterior acromion.
- Infraclavicular fossa.
- The course of the brachial plexus should be studied again (see interscalene block, steps for locating the puncture site, Figs. 9.8–9.12).

Locating the puncture site
The line between the suprasternal notch and the anterior acromion is halved (Fig. 9.29). Precise location of the anterior acromion is very important (the immobile acromion can be distinguished from the mobile humeral head by passive movement of the upper arm; Fig. 9.30). The plexus lies at a depth of ca. 3 cm lateral to the axillary artery and vein. The first rib provides some protection against puncture of the pleura.

The following points must be observed during the puncture procedure:
- Electrical nerve stimulation is the method of choice.
- The anesthetist should stand at the patient's head (this provides better control of any needle deviation, particularly in the medial direction).
- Caution should be exercised if a depth of 3 cm is reached without any motor response from the relevant musculature (risk of pneumothorax!).
- The needle should never be directed medially (possible injury to the subclavian artery and vein).
- Peripheral muscle contractions (flexion or extension of the first to third fingers – radial and median nerves) are regarded as a promising response to the stimulation.
- Aspiration of blood means that the puncture is too far medial.
- If severe pain occurs during the injection (intraneural location), the injection should be stopped immediately and the position of the needle should be corrected.
- Before and during the injection (after each 4–5 mL), aspiration should be performed.

Technique

"Single-shot" technique

After disinfection of the puncture area and draping, skin infiltration should be carried out **directly below the clavicle** (Fig. 9.31). A skin incision is made with a stylet at the puncture site so that the needle can be introduced easily. The electrostimulation needle is advanced **strictly perpendicular to the surface the patient is resting on** (Figs. 9.32 and 9.33). A stimulation current of 1–2 mA and 2 Hz is selected with a stimulus duration of 0.1 ms. After the motor response from the relevant musculature, the stimulation current is reduced to 0.3–0.5 mA. The plexus is located at a depth of ca. 3–4 cm. Slight twitching suggests that the stimulation needle is in the immediate vicinity of the plexus. After aspiration, injection of a local anesthetic is carried out in incremental doses. During the injection, the twitching slowly disappears.

Dosage

Surgical

40–50 mL local anesthetic – e.g. 0.5–0.75% ropivacaine or 0.5% bupivacaine (0.5% levobupivacaine). A combination of 0.5–0.75% ropivacaine or 0.5% bupivacaine (0.5% levobupivacaine) with 1% prilocaine or 1% mepivacaine has proved very successful in practice.

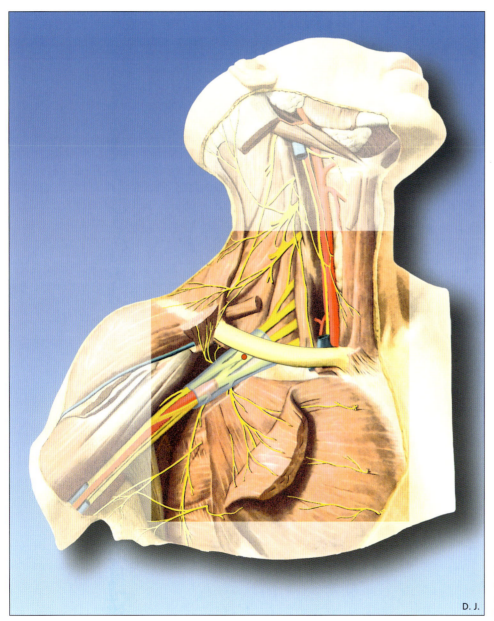

Fig. 9.31 Vertical infraclavicular block. Puncture is carried out directly underneath the clavicle

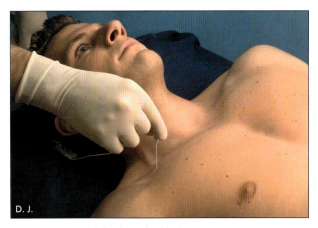

Fig. 9.32 Vertical infraclavicular block.
Puncture: the needle is introduced strictly perpendicular to the surface the patient is resting on

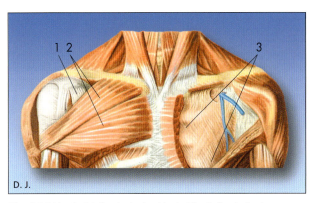

Fig. 9.33 Vertical infraclavicular block. The infraclavicular region, with (1) the pectoralis minor muscle, (2) the pectoralis major muscle, (3) the pectoral fascia (deep layer)

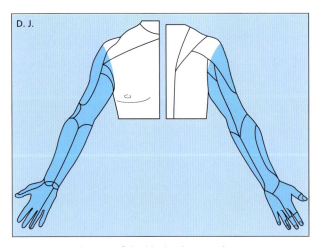

Fig. 9.34 Distribution of the block. The neural areas most frequently blocked 15 min after administration of the block

Therapeutic
15–20 mL local anesthetic – e.g. 0.2–0.375% ropivacaine or 0.125–0.25% bupivacaine (0.125–0.25% levobupivacaine).

Distribution of the block
The complete distribution of the anesthesia is shown in Fig. 9.34.

Continuous technique
The Tuohy or Contiplex plastic indwelling catheter should be advanced as slowly as possible. A stimulation current of 1–2 mA and 2 Hz is selected with a stimulus duration of 0.1 ms. After the motor response from the relevant musculature is seen, the stimulation current is reduced to 0.2–0.3 mA. Slight twitching suggests that the stimulation needle is in the immediate vicinity of the nerve. The opening of the Tuohy needle should be directed toward the course of the neurovascular sheath of the plexus (Fig. 9.4). The catheter is advanced approximately 3 cm beyond the end of the needle or cannula (Fig. 9.35). As the needle's angle of puncture is not parallel to the neurovascular sheath, some springy resistance can often be expected when advancing the catheter. Initial administration of 5–10 mL 0.9% saline is recommended. After removal of the needle or cannula, fixation of the catheter and placement of a bacterial filter, and after careful aspiration and injection of a test dose, the bolus administration of the local anesthetic follows.

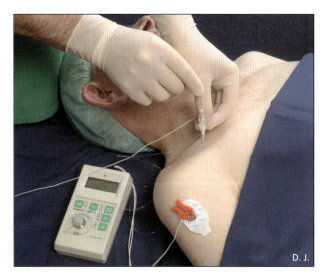

Fig. 9.35 Vertical infraclavicular block (continuous technique). Introduction of the catheter

Dosage

Test dose and bolus administration
Test dose: 3–5 mL local anesthetic – e.g. 0.5–0.75% ropivacaine or 0.25–0.5% bupivacaine (0.25–0.5% levobupivacaine).
Bolus administration: 20–40 mL local anesthetic – e.g. 0.5–0.75% ropivacaine or 0.25–0.5% bupivacaine (0.25–0.5% levobupivacaine).

Maintenance dose

> Individual adjustment of the dose and period of treatment is absolutely necessary. The following information is therefore only intended to provide guidance.

Continuous infusion
Infusion of the local anesthetic via the plexus catheter should be started approximately 1 h after the bolus administration. Administering a test dose is obligatory. The following dosages have proved their value in practice:
6–15 mL/h 0.2% ropivacaine (max. 37.5 mg/h).
8–18 mL/h (usually 10–14 mL/h) 0.125% bupivacaine (0.125% levobupivacaine).
6–16 mL/h (usually 8–10 mL/h) 0.25% bupivacaine (0.25% levobupivacaine).
If necessary, the infusion can be supplemented with bolus doses of 5–10 mL 0.5–0.75% ropivacaine or 0.25–0.5% bupivacaine (0.25–0.5% levobupivacaine).

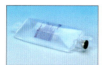

Patient-controlled analgesia (PCA)
Baseline rate of **4 mL/h** 0.2% ropivacaine or 0.125% bupivacaine (0.125% levobupivacaine).
Bolus administration of **3–4 mL** 0.2% ropivacaine or 0.125% bupivacaine (0.125% levobupivacaine).
Lockout interval of 15–20 min.

Side effects
- Hematoma formation.
- Horner's syndrome (rare).

Complications
- Pneumothorax (Fig. 9.36) [35].
  Prophylaxis: not directing the needle medially.
- Intravascular injection (see axillary block, p. 112)
- CNS toxicity (see axillary block, p. 112)
- Nerve injury (see axillary block, p. 111)

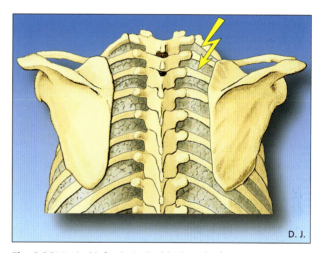

Fig. 9.36 Vertical infraclavicular block. Risk of pneumothorax

Record and checklist

Infraclavicular block of the brachial plexus
„Single-shot"-technique   ☐ Right   ☐ Left

Name: _____ Date: _____

Diagnosis: _____

Premedication: ☐ No   ☐ Yes _____

Neurological abnormalities: ☐ No
                                ☐ Yes (which?) _____

Technique: ☐ Vertical infraclavicular   ☐ Other

Purpose of block: ☐ Surgical   ☐ Therapeutic
i. v. access: ☐ Yes
Monitoring: ☐ ECG   ☐ Pulse oximetry
Ventilation facilities: ☐ Yes (equipment checked)
Emergency equipment (drugs):   ☐ Checked
Patient: ☐ Informed

Position: ☐ Supine
Needle type: ☐ Stimuplex® D ____ mm (15°) ☐ Other _____

Puncture technique: ☐ Electrostimulation

Local anesthetic: _____ ml _____ % _____
(in incremental doses)

Addition to
injection solution: ☐ No   ☐ Yes _____ µg/mg

Patient's remarks during injection:
☐ None   ☐ Paresthesias   ☐ Warmth
Pain triggered (intraneural location?) _____
Nerve region _____

Objective block effect after 15 min:
☐ Cold test   ☐ Temperature measurement: right____°C   left____°C
☐ Sensory   ☐ Motor

Monitoring after block: ☐ < 1 h   ☐ > 1 h
                          Time of discharge _____

Complications: ☐ None   ☐ Signs of intoxication   ☐ Pneumothorax
☐ Hematoma   ☐ Neurological injury (median nerve, ulnar nerve, radial nerve)

Subjective effects of the block: Duration: _____
☐ None   ☐ Increased pain   ☐ Reduced pain   ☐ Relief of pain

VISUAL ANALOG SCALE

0 10 20 30 40 50 60 70 80 90 100

Special notes:
_____
_____
_____

© Copyright ABW Wissenschaftsverlag 2004,
Jankovic, Regional nerve blocks and infiltration therapy, 3rd edition

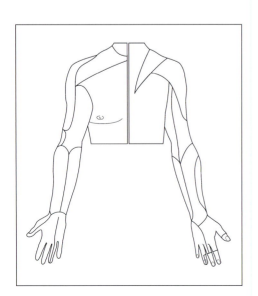

Infraclavicular block of the brachial plexus
Continuous technique   ☐ Right   ☐ Left

Technique: ☐ Vertical infraclavicular   ☐ Other

Purpose of block: ☐ Surgical   ☐ Therapeutic
i. v. access: ☐ Yes
Monitoring: ☐ ECG   ☐ Pulse oximetry
Ventilation facilities: ☐ Yes (equipment checked)
Emergency equipment *(drugs)*:   ☐ Checked
Patient: ☐ Informed

Position: ☐ Supine
Puncture technique: ☐ Electrostimulation
Needle type   ☐ Contiplex® D ___ mm ___ G   ☐ Tuohy ___ mm ___ G
   ☐ Other _____
Catheter: ☐ Advanced _____ cm
Aspiration test: ☐ Carried out
Bacterial filter: ☐
Test dose: _____ mL _____ %
Bolus administration: _____ mL _____ %
(in incremental doses)
Addition to
injection solution: ☐ No   ☐ Yes _____ µg/mg
Patient's remarks during injection:
☐ None   ☐ Paresthesias   ☐ Warmth
☐ Pain triggered (intraneural location?) _____
Nerve region _____

Objective block effect after 15 min:
☐ Cold test   ☐ Temperature measurement: right ____ °C   left ____ °C
☐ Sensory   ☐ Motor
☐ Continuous monitoring

☐ Infusion for postoperative analgesia
Local anesthetic: _____ % _____ ml/h
Addition to LA: _____ mg _____ µg
Patient-controlled anesthesia (PCA)
Local anesthetic: _____ %
Addition: _____
☐ Baseline rate _____ mL/h
☐ Bolus administration _____ mL
☐ Lockout interval _____ min

Complications:
☐ None   ☐ Signs of intoxication   ☐ Pneumothorax
☐ Hematoma   ☐ Neurological injury (median nerve, ulnar nerve, radial nerve)

Subjective effects of the block: Duration: _____
☐ None   ☐ Increased pain   ☐ Reduced pain   ☐ Relief of pain
VISUAL ANALOG SCALE

|0 10 20 30 40 50 60 70 80 90 100|

© Copyright ABW Wissenschaftsverlag 2004,
Jankovic, Regional nerve blocks and infiltration therapy, 3rd edition

Record and checklist

Name: _____
Date: _____
Diagnosis: _____
Premedication: ☐ No   ☐ Yes _____

Neurological abnormalities: ☐ No
☐ Yes (which?) _____

Special notes: _____

Chapter 9

Axillary block

Single-shot techniques and block series

Indications
Surgical
- As a single-shot or continuous block [7, 26, 33, 45, 46, 55]. This is the method of choice for all general, vascular, neurosurgical or orthopedic procedures and manipulations in the arm below the elbow and in the hand region.

Diagnostic
- Postamputation pain.
- Complex regional pain syndrome (CRPS) types I and II.
- Checking (confirmation) of surgical sympathectomy.
- Differential diagnosis of peripheral and central pain.

Prophylactic
- As an alternative to cervicothoracic ganglion block, when a stellate block is contraindicated or cannot be carried out for technical reasons.

Therapeutic
- Following peripheral nerve injury, with causalgia development (see case 3, p. 121).
- Following surgical neurolysis, to improve postoperative reinnervation.
- Severe arterial spasm – e.g. after accidental intra-arterial injection of thiopental (or as a continuous block).
- Complex regional pain syndrome (CRPS) types I and II (see cases 1 and 2, pp. 120f).
- Rheumatic diseases.
- Wrist arthritis.
- Neuropathies – e.g. due to diabetes.
- Post-herpetic neuralgia.
- Post-amputation pain (block series in chronic pain conditions).
- Postoperative pain (in most cases, a preoperative block with a long-duration local anesthetic is sufficient).

Contraindications
Specific
- Infections (e.g. lymphangitis) or malignant disease in the arm.
- Anticoagulation treatment.
- Upper arm fractures or other conditions preventing abduction of the arm.
- Patient refusal.

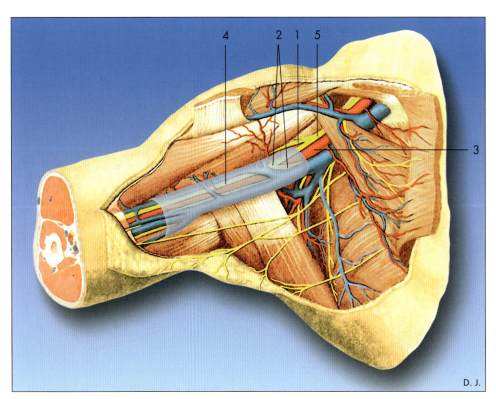

Fig. 9.37 Distal (axillary) neurovascular sheath.
(1) Musculocutaneous nerve,
(2) median nerve,
(3) axillary artery,
(4) ulnar nerve,
(5) lateral cord

Brachial plexus

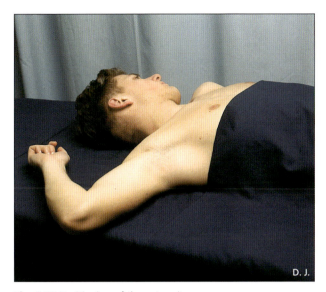

Fig. 9.38 Positioning of the extremity

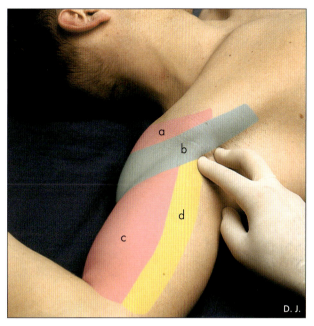

Fig. 9.39 Palpation of the axillary artery. (a) Deltoid muscle, (b) pectoralis major muscle, (c) biceps muscle, (d) coracobrachialis muscle

Relative
The decision should be taken after carefully weighing up the risks and benefits:
- Hemorrhagic diathesis.
- Stable systemic neural diseases.
- Local nerve injury (as there may be doubt whether the cause is surgery or anesthesia).

Procedure

This block should only be carried out by experienced anesthetists or under their supervision. The patient should be fully informed about the procedure.

Preparations and materials
(See section on interscalene block, p. 85; see Figs. 9.5 and 9.6).

Skin prep
In all blocks.

Patient positioning
Supine, with the upper arm abducted (90–100°) and the forearm flexed (90°) and rotated outward (Fig. 9.38).

Hyperabduction must be avoided. It obliterates the arterial pulsation, making palpation of the artery difficult and adversely affecting the distribution of the local anesthetic.

Landmarks
Axillary artery, deltoid muscle, pectoralis major muscle, biceps muscle, coracobrachialis muscle. The axillary fossa is delimited by the deltoid muscle and pectoralis major muscle above and by the biceps and coracobrachialis muscles below (Fig. 9.39). The axillary artery lies together with the ulnar nerve, median nerve and radial nerve, as well as the brachial and medial antebrachial cutaneous nerves in the neurovascular sheath. The sheath normally encloses the axillary vein as well, but not always.

Location of the injection site
The axillary artery is palpated as proximally as possible under the lateral edge of the pectoralis major muscle and is fixed with the index and middle fingers (Fig. 9.39).

The high proximal palpation and fixing of the axillary artery increases the likelihood of including the musculocutaneous in the block. This nerve leaves the axillary fossa together with the axillary nerve at the level of the coracoid process.

Injection technique

After disinfection of the entire axilla and draping, the skin is infiltrated immediately above the fixed artery. The skin at the injection site is incised with a stylet to

Chapter 9

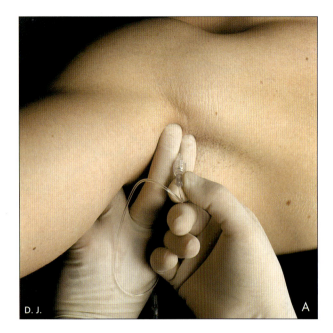

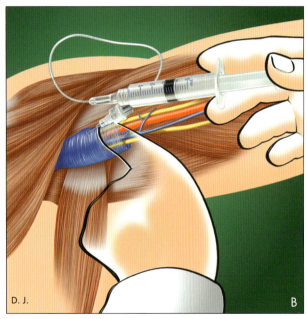

Fig. 9.40a, b Puncturing the neurovascular sheath

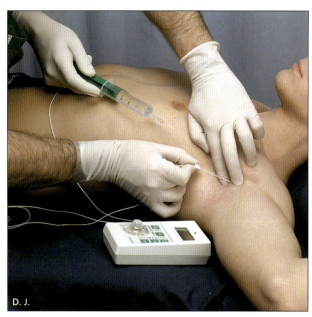

Fig. 9.41 Electrical nerve stimulation

"Fascial clicks"
Entry of the needle into the neurovascular sheath is confirmed by what are termed "fascial clicks." When needles with short-beveled tips are used, puncture of the connective tissue is easily felt and is often also audible.

Pulse-synchronous movement of the needle
Positioning of the needle tip in the immediate vicinity of the artery can be confirmed by pulse-synchronous movement of the needle, although this does not guarantee secure positioning in the neurovascular sheath and does not provide reliable evidence on its own.

Electrical nerve stimulation (Fig. 9.41)
Twitching of the relevant musculature to neural stimulation; this allows individual nerves to be targeted and located with ease, and nerve lesions are rarely produced. Patient cooperation is not required.

Technique
A stimulation current of 1–2 mA and 2 Hz is selected with a stimulus duration of 0.1 ms. After the motor response from the relevant musculature, the stimulation current is reduced to 0.2–0.3 mA. Slight twitching suggests that the stimulation needle is located in the immediate vicinity of the nerve. After aspiration, injection of a local anesthetic is carried out in incremental doses. During the injection, the muscle twitching slowly disappears.

make introduction of the needle easier. Winnie [69] recommends the use of an "immobile needle." This is slowly advanced proximally at an angle of ca. 15–30° in the direction of the neurovascular sheath (Fig. 9.40a, b).

Needle position
Before the injection, it must be confirmed that the neurovascular sheath has been reached and that the needle is securely positioned in the fascial compartment. The following techniques are suitable for this:

Paresthesias
It is not obligatory to produce paresthesias with this block technique. Due to the potential risk of nerve injury – Selander [47, 49] reports post-block neuropathies in 2.8% of cases, while other authors [66, 68] only report occasional complications – paresthesias should be avoided if possible. On the other hand, it should be emphasized that in ca. 40% of cases, paresthesias are produced inadvertently [47, 49, 53], and these are a definite sign of correct needle positioning. The patient must be informed about these and must be able to report the occurrence of paresthesias immediately and describe their spread.

Arterial puncture technique
Aspiration of blood indicates that the needle is located in the axillary artery and therefore within the neurovascular sheath.

Injection
When the needle is securely located in the neurovascular sheath, repeated aspiration is carried out and the local anesthetic is injected slowly. A certain amount of pressure is needed for this, since the fascial cover creates resistance to the injection.
Aspiration must be repeated after each injection of 4–5 mL, no matter which technique is used.

Perivascular technique
In the perivascular technique [3, 18], all of the local anesthetic is distributed in the neurovascular sheath around the artery (perivascular).

Transarterial injection
This technique is being increasingly used due to its high success rate (89–99%) [6, 53, 72] and low complication rate, and its value has been particularly demonstrated with obese patients. After targeted puncture of the artery and blood aspiration (Fig. 9.42), the needle is withdrawn until no more blood can be aspirated.
Without creating paresthesias, 20 mL of local anesthetic is injected initially. The needle is then advanced to the opposite side of the artery and, after careful aspiration, the remaining volume (20 mL) is administered [61]. The following are variants of this procedure:

Single injection into a single compartment [6]
The entire dose of the local anesthetic is deposited behind the artery (posterior).

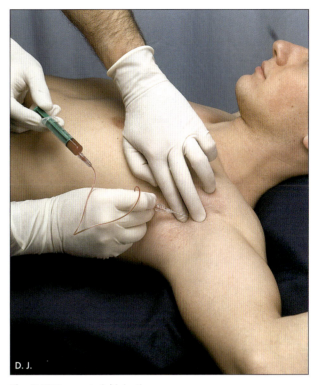

Fig. 9.42 Transarterial injection

Multiple injections into multiple compartments [53]
Half of the dose is injected behind the artery (posterior) and the other half is distributed according to the area to be operated on: in the ulnar and median nerve region (in front of the artery), radial nerve region (behind the artery) (Fig. 9.37).
Potential disadvantages of the transarterial technique are that persistent bleeding may reduce the quality of the anesthesia by diluting the local anesthetic, or that a hematoma may compress neighboring nerves and prevent access of the local anesthetic. As with all procedures, intravascular injection – into the axillary vein as well – is theoretically possible with this technique [15].

Distribution of the local anesthetic
To ensure optimal distribution of the local anesthetic, the neurovascular sheath is compressed with the fingers distal to the needle during the injection. Applying a tourniquet distal to the injection site is ineffective, since the muscle mass is little affected by this [71, 74]. After removal of the needle, compressing the axilla (3–5 min) (Fig. 9.43) and simultaneous massaging encourages improved distribution of the local anesthetic. It also serves for hematoma prophylaxis.

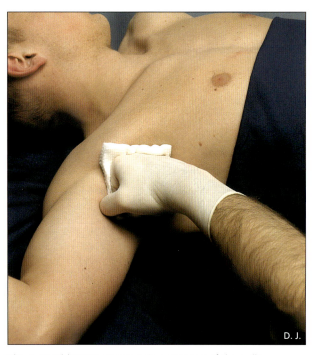

Fig. 9.43 Obligatory compression massage of the axilla

- The axillary artery should be palpated as high as possible, fixed between the index and middle fingers and punctured in a cranial direction.
- Only needles with short-beveled tips should be used, preferably an "immobile needle" with a short injection line.
- Correct positioning of the needle in the neurovascular sheath should be checked before the injection.
- Before and during the injection (after each 4–5 mL), aspiration should be carried out repeatedly.
- If severe pain occurs during the injection (intraneural position), the injection should be stopped at once and the position of the needle should be corrected.
- After the injection, compression massage of the axillary fossa should be carried out for 3–5 min.
- Avoid supplementation. An incomplete plexus block should not be supplemented with other additional peripheral nerve blocks, since this would mean paresthesias would not be available as warning signals [53, 72].
- Avoid paresthesias if possible.

Dosage
Surgical
40–50 mL local anesthetic – e.g. 0.75% ropivacaine or 0.5% bupivacaine (0.5% levobupivacaine).
A combination of 0.75% ropivacaine or 0.5% bupivacaine (0.5% levobupivacaine) with 1% prilocaine or 1% mepivacaine has proved its value in practice (in our own experience).
According to De Jong [8, 9, 10], **42 mL** local anesthetic is required to reach the musculocutaneous and axillary nerves. Other authors report the use of 30–50 mL. Opinions vary with regard to the addition of opioids [12, 21].

Diagnostic
20 mL local anesthetic – e.g. 0.2% ropivacaine, 0.125–0.25% bupivacaine (0.125–0.25% levobupivacaine), 0.5% prilocaine, 0.5% mepivacaine.

Prophylactic
10–20 mL local anesthetic – e.g. 0.2–0.375% ropivacaine, 0.125–0.25% bupivacaine (0.125–0.25% levobupivacaine).

Therapeutic
10 mL local anesthetic – e.g. 0.2–0.375% ropivacaine or 0.125–0.25% bupivacaine (0.125–0.25% levobupivacaine), in diabetic and other neuropathies and in rheumatic diseases.
10–15 mL local anesthetic – e.g. 0.2% ropivacaine or 0.125% bupivacaine (0.125% levobupivacaine), in wrist arthritis.
10–20 mL local anesthetic – e.g. 0.375% ropivacaine or 0.25% bupivacaine (0.25% levobupivacaine), in post-amputation pain, after surgical neurolysis and in post-herpetic neuralgia.
20 mL local anesthetic – e.g. 0.2–0.375% ropivacaine or 0.25–0.375% bupivacaine (0.25–0.375% bupivacaine), in complex regional pain syndrome (CRPS) types I and II.
20 mL local anesthetic – e.g. 0.75% ropivacaine or 0.5% bupivacaine (0.5% levobupivacaine), in severe arterial spasm – e.g. after accidental intra-arterial injection of thiopental.

Distribution of the block
After onset of the full effect – the latency period can be up to 30 min in the axillary block – the anesthesia completely covers the arm and hand from the elbow downwards, as well as much of the upper arm (Fig. 9.44).

Brachial plexus

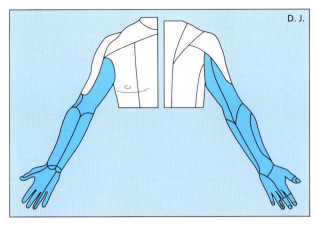

Fig. 9.44 The most frequently blocked nerve areas after axillary access, 15 min after initiating the block with bupivacaine [20]

Block series
A series of blocks usually consists of 8–12 treatments. When there is noticeable improvement in the symptoms, further blocks can also be carried out (see case reports, pp. 120f).

Side effects [7]
- Hematoma formation due to puncture of the axillary artery. Note the obligatory prophylactic compression.

The patient must be warned for these potential adverse effects in advance.

Complications
Nerve injury
Traumatic nerve injury is a rare complication. It can be caused by the use of sharp needles (lesions due to nerve puncture), by intraneural or microvascular injury (hematoma and its sequelae), prolonged ischemia, or by toxic effects of intraneurally injected local anesthetics [27, 47]. If functional neurological disturbances occur after surgical interventions, the following causes should be considered:
- Incorrect positioning of the arm during the operation (pressure, extension, rough manipulation).
- Direct surgical trauma.
- Injury due to tourniquet ischemia, manifesting as postoperative myalgia [53].
- Inadequate attention during postoperative care, particularly with regard to the positioning of the anesthetized arm. After the administration of long-term local anesthetics, paresthesias have been described with poor postoperative positioning [61].

Patients must be given the relevant information, especially in outpatient procedures.

From the anesthesiological point of view, the following points should be taken into account:

Prophylaxis
- Only needles with short-beveled tips should be used. During the injection, the needle should be introduced parallel to the nerve fascicle with the beveled angle in the longitudinal direction of the course of the nerve.
- Intraneural positioning of the needle should be excluded. If the patient reports severe pain during the injection, the injection should be stopped at once and the needle should be withdrawn.
- Vasopressor additives should be avoided. They are rarely indicated – and are even contraindicated in pain therapy – and may cause prolonged ischemia. They are also contraindicated in hypertonia, hyperthyroidism and arrhythmia [48, 49].
  In particular, reactions to epinephrine (restlessness, tachycardia, arrhythmia) may be confused with signs of overdose of local anesthetic.
- Avoid supplementation. An incomplete plexus block should not be supplemented with other additional peripheral nerve blocks, since this would mean paresthesias would not be available as warning signals [53, 72].
- Blocks should not be carried out in adult patients under general anesthesia.

Careful documentation
The following should be documented in every nerve block:
- Approach.
- Needle type.
- Local anesthetic used and additives, if any.
- Description of the paresthesias elicited.
- Any vascular puncture or injection pain.
- Hematoma formation.
- Any supplementation.
- Tourniquet duration.

Diagnosis and treatment
When there is the slightest suspicion of neurological injury, a detailed examination should be carried out and the diagnosis should be made by a neurologist. In the axillary plexus block, the median and ulnar nerves are the ones most often affected. The prognosis is generally very good. With neurological treatment and physiotherapy, restoration of function takes a few days, up to a maximum of a year ("tincture of time") [47, 53, 61, 66, 68].

Intravascular injection
There is a particular risk of injection into the axillary artery or axillary vein [15]. For symptoms and treatment, see Chapter 6, p. 65.
Prophylaxis: During slow injection, aspiration should be repeated after each 4–5 mL.

CNS toxicity
In very rare cases, overdose of local anesthetic, fast absorption of local anesthetic at the injection site, or inadvertent intravascular injection can lead to toxic reactions. These develop in the course of ca. 20 min after the injection, or much more quickly with intravascular administration.
- Early symptoms include a numb sensation in the lips and tongue, a metallic taste, sleepiness, vertigo, ringing in the ears, auditory disturbances, visual disturbances, slurred speech, muscular trembling and nystagmus.
- Generalized tonic–clonic seizures are the most dangerous cerebral complication, but these do not lead to brain damage or death of the patient provided immediate and correct treatment is given. For therapeutic procedures for CNS intoxication, see Chap. 6, p. 66.

Pseudoaneurysms
- Formation of a pseudoaneurysm of the axillary artery [16, 36, 75], accompanied by postoperative paresthesias and plexus paralysis.

Axillary block of the brachial plexus
„Single-shot"-technique   ☐ Right   ☐ Left

Record and checklist

Name: _____ Date: _____
Diagnosis: _____
Premedication: ☐ No   ☐ Yes _____

Neurological abnormalities: ☐ No
                              ☐ Yes (which?) _____

Purpose of block: ☐ Surgical   ☐ Diagnostic   ☐ Therapeutic
i. v. access: ☐ Yes
Monitoring: ☐ ECG   ☐ Pulse oximetry
Ventilation facilities: ☐ Yes (equipment checked)
Emergency equipment (drugs):   ☐ Checked
Patient: ☐ Informed

Position: ☐ Supine   ☐ Abducted upper arm (90-100°)
Needle type: ☐ Plexufix® 24 G (45°)   ☐ 25 mm   ☐ 50 mm
                  ☐ Stimuplex® D ____ mm
                  ☐ Other _____

Puncture techniquue: ☐ Perivascular   ☐ Paresthesias
                      ☐ Transarterial   ☐ Electrostimulation

Local anesthetic: _____ mL _____ % _____
(in incremental doses)
Addition to
injection solution: ☐ No   ☐ Yes _____ µg/mg

Patient's remarks during injection:
☐ None   ☐ Paresthesias   ☐ Warmth
Pain triggered (intraneural location?) _____
Nerve region _____

Objective block effect after 15 min:
☐ Cold test   ☐ Temperature measurement: right ___°C   left ___°C
☐ Sensory   ☐ Motor

Monitoring after block: ☐ < 1 h   ☐ > 1 h
                          Time of discharge _____

Complications: ☐ None   ☐ Signs of intoxication
☐ Hematoma   ☐ Neurological injuries (median nerve, ulnar nerve, radial nerve)

Subjective effects of the block: Duration: _____
☐ None   ☐ Increased pain   ☐ Reduced pain   ☐ Relief of pain

VISUAL ANALOG SCALE

|||||||||||||||||||||||||||||||||||||||||||||||||||||||
0   10   20   30   40   50   60   70   80   90   100

Special notes:
_____
_____

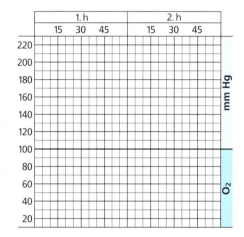

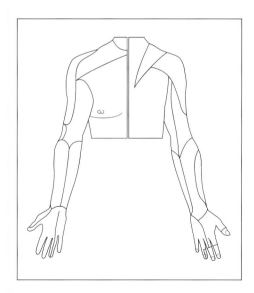

© Copyright ABW Wissenschaftsverlag 2004,
Jankovic, Regional nerve blocks and infiltration therapy, 3rd edition

Continuous axillary block

Indications
Surgical
- This is the method of choice as a continuous [26, 45, 46, 55] or single block in all general, vascular, neurosurgical or orthopedic interventions and manipulations in the arm below the elbow and in the hand region.

Prophylactic
- Postoperative analgesia.
- Prevention or reduction of post-amputation pain. It is recommended that the continuous block is started 2–3 days before the planned intervention, if possible.

Therapeutic
- After surgical reimplantation.
- Poor perfusion of the upper extremity.
- Arterial occlusive disease.
- Edema after radiotherapy (with additional corticoids).
- Post-amputation pain (in acute pain).
- Pain caused by trauma.

Specific and relative contraindications
The contraindications are similar to those for the single-shot block.

Procedure

This block should only be carried out by experienced anesthetists. Patients should receive full information before the procedure.

> Continuous administration requires continuous monitoring, daily checking of the catheter position, daily change of the bacterial filter and dressing, as well as an obligatory test dose before every subsequent injection.

Preparations
(See the section on the interscalene block, p. 85)

Materials (Fig. 9.45)
Stimuplex® HNS 11 nerve stimulator (B. Braun Melsungen).
Syringes (2 mL, 10 mL, 20 mL), catheter set (e.g. Contiplex® D or Contiplex®–Tuohy continuous set – e.g. B. Braun Melsungen; see Fig. 9.6c and d), drape, stylet, disinfectant, bacterial filters, cooled physiological saline.

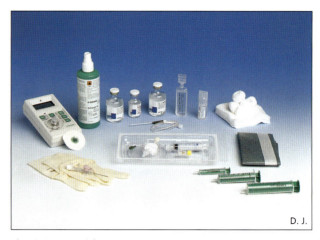

Fig. 9.45 Materials

Skin prep
In all blocks.

Patient positioning
As for the single-shot block.

Landmarks and location of the injection site
The anatomical orientation, with high proximal palpation and fixing of the axillary artery, is the same as for the single-shot block.

Injection technique
After careful skin prep of the axilla and draping, the skin is infiltrated immediately above the fixed artery. The skin is incised at the infiltration site and the needle is introduced at an angle of ca. 30° in the direction of the neurovascular sheath. To avoid vascular and neural injury, the needle should be advanced as slowly as possible and its bevel should be turned towards the axillary artery (Fig. 9.46).

Needle position
"Fascial clicks" and the loss of resistance technique [29] or electrical nerve stimulation [40, 54, 58] can be used to confirm that the neurovascular sheath has been reached and that the needle is positioned within the fascial compartment.

Introducing the catheter
When the injection needle is securely positioned in the neurovascular sheath, the metal stylet is fixed and the Teflon cannula is advanced over the needle as far as the mark. For this purpose, the needle is lowered to ca. 10–20°, to allow it to be advanced parallel to the artery as much as possible (Fig. 9.47).

After removal of the needle and aspiration, 5 mL of cold physiological saline is injected via the Teflon cannula. Any paresthesia, and low resistance during the injection in particular, will confirm correct positioning in the neurovascular sheath.

The catheter is introduced through the cannula as far as the 10-cm mark if possible (mark II), so as to avoid dislodgement (Fig. 9.48).

Injection of the local anesthetic
After removal of the cannula, fixation of the catheter and placement of a bacterial filter and after careful aspiration and injection of a test dose, bolus administration of the local anesthetic is carried out.

Dosage [5, 26, 45, 55]
The choice and dosage of the local anesthetic depend on the goal of treatment:
- Anesthesia for surgery with subsequent pain therapy.
- Analgesia for mobilization treatment.
- Sympatholytic treatment in peripheral perfusion disturbances.

Initial bolus administration
Test dose: 3–5 mL local anesthetic – e.g. 0.375–0.75 ropivacaine or 0.25–0.5% bupivacaine (0.25–0.5% levobupivacaine).
Bolus administration: 20–40 mL local anesthetic – e.g. 0.375–0.75% ropivacaine or 0.25–0.5% bupivacaine (0.25–0.5% levobupivacaine).

Maintenance dose

> Individual adjustment of the dosage and period of treatment is absolutely necessary. The following information therefore only serves for general guidance.

Intermittent administration
Every 5–6 h, 5–10 mL local anesthetic – e.g. 0.5–0.75% ropivacaine or 0.25–0.5% bupivacaine (0.25–0.5% levobupivacaine), after a prior test dose. Reduction of the dosage and/or dosage intervals depending on the clinical picture.

Continuous infusion
Infusion of the local anesthetic via the plexus catheter should be started ca. 1 h after the bolus administration. A test dose is obligatory.

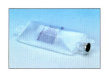

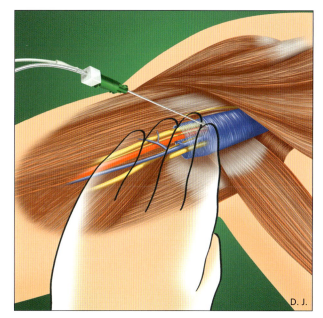

Fig. 9.46 Outlet angle of 30°

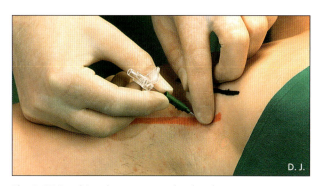

Fig. 9.47 Reaching the neurovascular sheath

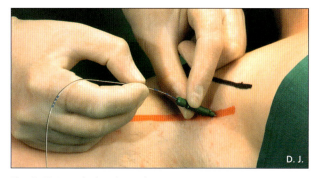

Fig. 9.48 Introducing the catheter

The following dosages have proved their value:
6–14 mL/h 0.2% ropivacaine (max. 37.5 mg/h)
8–18 mL/h (usually 10–14 mL) 0.125% bupivacaine (0.125% levobupivacaine), or: **4–16 mL (usually 8–10 mL)** 0.25% bupivacaine (0.25% levobupivacaine).

If necessary, the infusion can be supplemented with bolus doses of 5–10 mL 0.5–0.75% ropivacaine or 0.25–0.5% bupivacaine (0.25–0.5% levobupivacaine).

Patient-controlled analgesia (PCA)
Baseline rate of **6–8 mL/h** 0.2% ropivacaine.
Bolus administration of **4–6 mL** 0.2% ropivacaine.
Lockout interval of 20–30 min.

Side effects and complications
- Hematoma formation due to puncture of the axillary artery.
- Formation of a pseudoaneurysm on the axillary artery [16, 36, 75], accompanied by postoperative paresthesias and plexus paralysis.
- Traumatic nerve injury (extremely rare).
- Intravascular injection into the axillary artery or axillary vein [15] (extremely rare).
- CNS intoxication (very rare) due to local anesthetic overdose, rapid absorption at the injection site, or inadvertent intravascular injection.
- Bacterial colonization of the catheter, with or without local or systemic infection.
  Prophylaxis: daily exchange of the bacterial filter, limitation of the period of catheter placement [26, 55].
- Catheter dislodgement.
- Catheter leakage, particularly at infusion speeds of more than 15 mL/h.

Axillary block of the brachial plexus
Continuous technique ☐ Right ☐ Left

Purpose of block: ☐ Surgical ☐ Therapeutic
i. v. access: ☐ Yes
Monitoring: ☐ ECG ☐ Pulse oximetry
Ventilation facilities: ☐ Yes (equipment checked)
Emergency equipment (drugs): ☐ Checked
Patient: ☐ Informed

Position: ☐ Supine ☐ Abducted upper arm (90–100°)
Puncture technique: ☐ Electrostimulation
Needle type ☐ Contiplex® D ___ mm ___ G ☐ Tuohy ___ mm ___ G
 ☐ Other _____
Catheter: ☐ Advanced _____ cm
Aspiration test: ☐ Carried out
Bacterial filter: ☐
Test dose: _____ mL _____ %
Bolus administration: _____ mL _____ %
(in incremental doses)
Addition to
injection solution: ☐ No ☐ Yes _____ µg/mg
Patient's remarks during injection:
☐ None ☐ Paresthesias ☐ Warmth
Pain triggered (intraneural location?) _____
Nerve region _____

Objective block effect after 15 min:
☐ Cold test ☐ Temperature measurement: right ___ °C left ___ °C
☐ Sensory ☐ Motor
☐ Continuous monitoring

☐ Infusion for postoperative analgesia
Local anesthetic: _____ % _____ ml/h
Addition to LA: _____ mg _____ µg _____
Patient-controlled anesthesia (PCA)
☐ Local anesthetic: _____ %
☐ Addition: _____
☐ Baseline rate _____ mlLh _____
☐ Bolus administration _____ mL
☐ Lockout interval _____ min

Complications: ☐ None ☐ Signs of intoxication
☐ Hematoma ☐ Neurological injuries (median nerve, ulnar nerve, radial nerve)

Subjective effects of the block: Duration: _____
☐ None ☐ Increased pain ☐ Reduced pain ☐ Relief of pain

VISUAL ANALOG SCALE

|||||||||||||||||||||||||||||||||||||||||||||||||||||
0 10 20 30 40 50 60 70 80 90 100

Special notes:

© Copyright ABW Wissenschaftsverlag 2004,
Jankovic, Regional nerve blocks and infiltration therapy, 3rd edition

Record and Checklist

Name: _____
Date: _____
Diagnosis: _____
Premedication: ☐ No ☐ Yes _____

Neurological abnormalities: ☐ No
☐ Yes (which?) _____

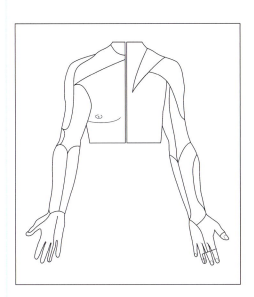

Interscalene, subclavian perivascular and axillary blocks of the brachial plexus: advantages and disadvantages

Interscalene block

Advantages
- Clear anatomical landmarks: interscalene groove, sternocleidomastoid muscle, transverse process (C6). Can therefore be carried out even with distorted anatomy – e.g. in obese patients.
- Patient cooperation is not absolutely necessary.
- No special positioning of the arm is required.
- Technically simple procedure.
- Due to the proximal injection at the level of C6, most of the plexus is anesthetized and the block can be carried out even in cases of infection or malignant disease in the arm. In addition, the caudal parts of the cervical plexus are included.
- Surgery and pain treatment are possible in the whole region of the shoulder and upper arm.
- Subsequent intraoperative injections are possible in extended interventions.
- The risk of pneumothorax is very low. The needle is advanced at a reasonable distance from the dome of the pleura.

Disadvantages
- It is necessary to produce paresthesias.
- The ulnar nerve territory is not always adequately anesthetized.
- The potential complications – although these are extremely rare – include: neural injury, epidural or subarachnoid injection, intravascular injection, CNS intoxication.

Subclavian perivascular block

Advantages
- Clear anatomical landmarks: caudal part of the interscalene groove, subclavian artery, midpoint of the clavicle.
- Injection of the local anesthetic is possible without repositioning the upper extremity.
- There is no risk of subarachnoid or epidural injection, nor of puncturing the vertebral artery.
- Infections in the arm do not represent a contraindication to this technique.

Disadvantages
- Risk of pneumothorax.
- Puncture of the subclavian artery is possible.
- Very rarely, applying a tourniquet requires an additional block of the intercostobrachial nerve (T2) and medial brachial cutaneous nerve.
- No applications in pain therapy.

Infraclavicular block

Advantages
- No positioning difficulties (e.g. in fractures, rheumatism).
- Precise positioning of the needle reduces the complication rate.
- More favorable distribution of the local anesthetic in the infraclavicular space (lower doses).
- The catheter is easily fixed, leading to a lower repositioning rate and unrestricted movement for the patient.
- Easy catheter maintenance.
- No influence on respiratory function [42].

Disadvantages
- Catheter placement is more difficult than with the axillary access route (the puncture angle is not parallel to the neurovascular sheath).
- Risk of pneumothorax.
- Possible incorrect intravascular positioning.
- Arterial pulsation is not available for guidance.

Axillary block

Advantages
- Clear anatomical landmarks: axillary artery.
- Easily conducted due to the superficial position of the neurovascular sheath. Can also be used in children and in patients with pulmonary problems or renal insufficiency (e.g. inserting an arteriovenous shunt).
- Also applicable as a continuous block.
- A safe method of anesthesia for surgery and pain therapy treatment, particularly in the forearm and hand.
- The following complications and side effects are excluded: pneumothorax, epidural or subarachnoid injection, concomitant block of the vagus, phrenic and recurrent laryngeal nerves or of the stellate ganglion.
- This is the method of choice for outpatients and emergency patients.

Disadvantages
- Abduction of the upper arm is required.
- The anesthesia is not sufficient for surgery on the shoulder or upper arm.
- The musculocutaneous nerve and/or axillary nerve are often not adequately anesthetized.
- Extremely rare but possible complications are: nerve injury, intravascular injection and CNS intoxication.

Plexus catheter in outpatients?

The catheter technique also allows plexus anesthesia to be used in operations lasting longer than the duration of local anesthetics. Independently of the surgical technique, postoperative blood perfusion disturbances almost always occur, particularly after microsurgical interventions – partly due to the body's reaction to the invasive procedure.

With continuous sympatholysis, the catheter technique allows substantial improvement in the perfusion of the operated arm. Continuous administration of local anesthetics and the consequent postoperative analgesia allow effective physiotherapy and therefore speedy mobilization of the operated arm.

In **inpatients**, continuous plexus block for appropriate indications is also an excellent anesthetic procedure in the context of acute pain therapy and sympatholysis. However, in this situation, the continuous method requires constant monitoring and checking that the technique is successful. This includes in particular:

- Daily checking of the catheter position, to ensure early recognition of intravascular dislocation or dislocation of the catheter from the neurovascular sheath.
- Daily exchanging of the bacterial filter and dressing, to keep the risk of bacterial colonization of the catheter and the associated risk of infection as low as possible.
- The need for continuous monitoring of the effectiveness of the block and for adjustment of the local anesthetic dose, if necessary, makes self-administration by the patient impossible.

In **outpatient** pain therapy, the use of a catheter for continuous plexus anesthesia is therefore rare and it is only possible with very cooperative patients.

Additional reasons why the present author has for many years preferred single injections in the context of block series are as follows:

- At the beginning of the therapy, the period of treatment that will be needed is often difficult to estimate and may extend (as the cases described on the following pages show) for 2–3 months. The frequency of treatment necessary during this period is more easily determined using single injections.
- Although complication-free catheter placement for 2–3 weeks (or up to 7 weeks in individual cases) has been reported in the literature [29], this is not sufficient and is associated with too many risks in outpatients.
- The goal of pain therapy blocks – e.g. in complex regional pain syndrome – is to allow physiotherapy and intensive exercise at home for the patient. Many patients find the catheter disturbing (with irritation and a foreign-body sensation) or even obstructive, and there is a risk of inadvertent dislodgement.

Chapter 9

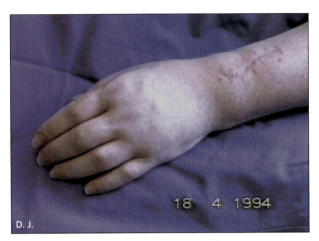

Fig. 9.49 Condition at admission on 18 April 1994

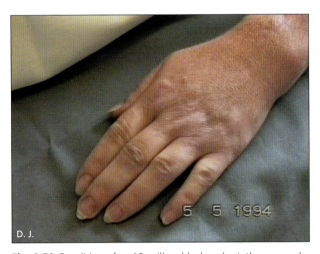

Fig. 9.50 Condition after 10 axillary blocks, physiotherapy and intensive home exercise

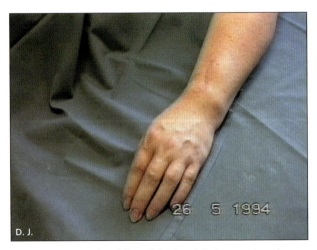

Fig. 9.51 Improved mobility of the hand during continued treatment

Example cases of axillary block of the brachial plexus

Case 1
Total number of blocks: 17.

Patient W. M., a 44-year-old woman
Ongoing pain after surgery for reduction of forearm fracture. After 2 months of unsuccessful treatment, including calcitonin therapy, the patient was referred to our outpatient pain department.

Findings on admission, 18 April 1994
Development of puffy edema (hand and distal part of the forearm), extreme pain when moving the hand, physiotherapy impossible (Fig. 9.49).

Therapy
Starting on the day of presentation, a 3-week series of 10 axillary plexus blocks in all (each dosage 20 mL 0.25% bupivacaine). After the blocks, the patient received physiotherapy and carried out intensive exercise at home [39, 60].
Due to marked improvement in the symptoms (Fig. 9.50), treatment was continued. During the subsequent 3 weeks, the patient received four blocks at a reduced dosage (10 mL 0.25% bupivacaine), with the physiotherapy and home exercises continuing. The mobility of the hand was significantly improved with these measures (Fig. 9.51).
Treatment was concluded with three blocks, again at a reduced dosage (10 mL 0.125% bupivacaine).

Final findings, 6 July 1994
Complete disappearance of symptoms.

Case 2
Total number of blocks: 23.

Patient G.H., a 46-year-old woman
Radius fracture in the right arm on 16 January 1994; removal of the external fixation on 17 March 1994, with incorrect hand position and development of puffy edema (hand and distal part of the forearm). After 3 months of unsuccessful treatment, the patient was referred to our outpatient pain department as therapy-resistant.

Findings on admission, 18 April 1994
Development of puffy edema, extreme pain, movement of the hand impossible, physiotherapy impossible (Fig. 9.52).

Therapy
Starting on the day of presentation, a 3-week series of 10 axillary plexus blocks (each dosage 20 mL 0.25% bupivacaine). Following the blocks, the patient received physiotherapy and carried out intensive exercises at home [39, 60].

Due to marked improvement in the mobility of the hand (Fig. 9.53) and a 60% reduction in pain, the treatment was continued after 5 May 1994. During the subsequent 3 weeks, the patient received five blocks at a reduced dosage (10 mL 0.25% bupivacaine). Physiotherapy and home exercise were continued and the pain reduction was increased up to 80% (Fig. 9.54).

Treatment was concluded with a further eight blocks (with reduction of the dosage to 10 mL 0.125% bupivacaine).

Final findings, 11 July 1994
Complete resolution of the edema, reduced pain and improvement in the mobility of the hand by more than 80% (Fig. 9.55). Partial contractures in the area of the little finger and ring finger. The patient was able to return to work.

Case 3
Total number of blocks: 29 (including four stellate blocks and four cervicobrachial plexus blocks).

Patient S. G. a 47-year-old woman
Humerus fracture after a bicycle accident on 28 September 1994. Emergency operation (with internal fixation). Wrist-drop with severe injury to the radial nerve and injury to the median nerve. Development of causalgia. On 6 December 1994, neurolysis of the radial nerve with subsequent deterioration in symptoms and edema formation. Three and a half months after the accident, the patient was referred to our outpatient pain department as therapy-resistant (calcitonin, antidepressants, physiotherapy) with a prognosis of "hopeless."

Findings on admission, 16 January 1995
In addition to the symptoms described above, there was the characteristic clinical picture of "frozen shoulder." Access to the axilla was therefore not possible in this patient (Fig. 9.56).

Therapy
At the patient's request, the calcitonin treatment and antidepressant administration were stopped. During the first 3 weeks, the patient received four blocks of the cervicothoracic (stellate) ganglion, followed by four blocks of the cervicobrachial plexus. There was no

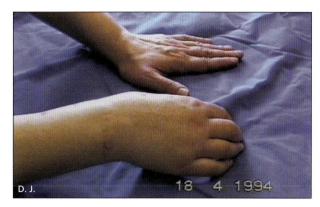
Fig. 9.52 Patient G.H. at admission

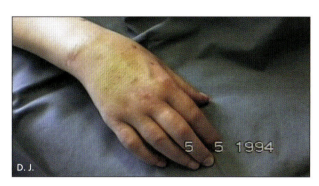
Fig. 9.53 Results of therapy after 10 blocks

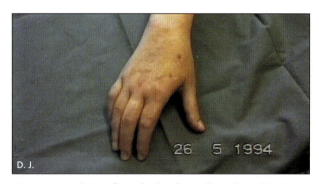
Fig. 9.54 Condition after a further five axillary plexus blocks

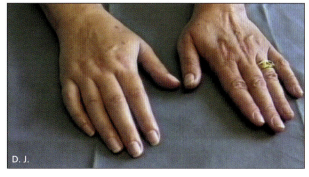
Fig. 9.55 Final findings on 11 July 1994: complete resolution of the edema. Pain reduction and increased mobility of the hand by more than 80%

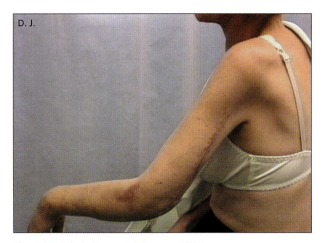

Fig. 9.56 Admission on 16 January 1995

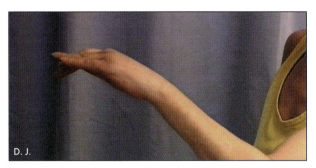

Fig. 9.57 Condition after six axillary blocks on 6 March 1995: resolution of the edema, partial mobility of the wrist

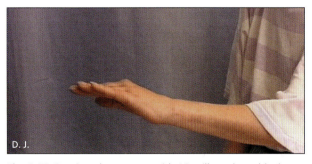

Fig. 9.58 Continued treatment with 15 axillary plexus blocks and continuing improvement in symptoms

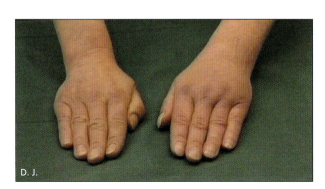 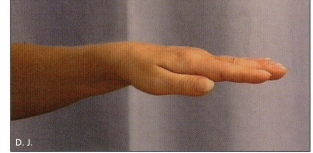

Figs. 9.59, **9.60** Condition at completion of treatment on 25 April 1995

improvement in the original symptoms. However, the mobility of the shoulder improved sufficiently to allow partial abduction of the arm, making it possible to carry out axillary plexus blocks.

On 15 February 1995, a 3-week series of six axillary blocks of the brachial plexus was started (each dosage 20 mL 0.25% bupivacaine).

Following the blocks, this very cooperative patient received physiotherapy and carried out intensive exercise at home [39, 60]. On 6 March 1995 (Fig. 9.57), her condition had already clearly improved: the edema had resolved and the wrist was partly mobile.

Treatment was continued with a further 15 blocks (each dose reduced to 10 mL 0.25% bupivacaine). The continued neurological follow-up confirmed increasing improvement in the reinnervation of the hand.

Physiotherapy and home exercises were continued, the mobility of the hand continually increased and the pain declined (Fig. 9.58).

Final findings, 25 April 1995

Complete resolution of the edema and "frozen shoulder." Almost complete absence of pain, mobility of the hand restored to about 85% (Figs. 9.59 and 9.60). Neurological follow-up showed 80% recovery. In March 1996, some of the internal fixation was removed.

Shoulder region

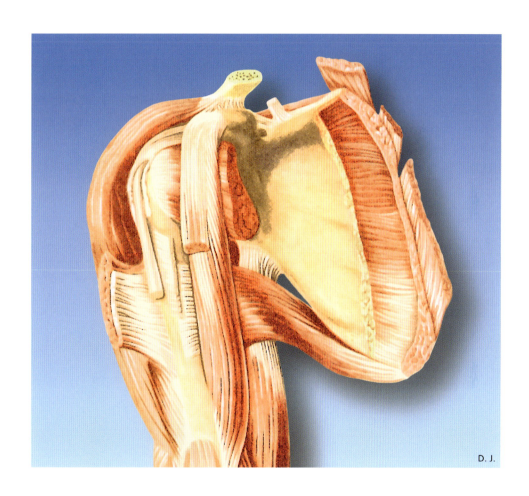

10 Suprascapular nerve

Anatomy

The suprascapular nerve receives fibers from the fifth and sixth cervical spinal nerves. It branches off from the superior trunk of the brachial plexus (Fig. 10.1) and courses through the supraclavicular fossa along the lateral edge of the plexus as far as the scapular notch. It enters the supraspinous fossa through the notch. Covered by the supraspinatus muscle, the suprascapular nerve passes to the neck of the scapula and under the transverse scapular ligament to the infraspinous fossa. It supplies the supraspinatus and infraspinatus muscles, and sends off fibers to the shoulder and acromioclavicular joint, as well as to the suprascapular vessels (Fig. 10.2).

Suprascapular nerve blocks

Indications
Diagnostic
- Painful conditions in the shoulder region and shoulder joint.

Therapeutic
- Rheumatic and degenerative diseases of the shoulder girdle.
- "Frozen shoulder," pseudoparetic shoulder, stiff shoulder (mobilization in shoulder ankylosis).
- Humeroscapular periarthritis after mechanical stress on the soft-tissue structures in the shoulder girdle, after immobilization of an arm, trauma, or surgery.
- Hemiplegia (shoulder–arm pain, increased load on the supraspinatus muscle or subluxation of the shoulder joint are reported in ca. 70% of cases).
- Tumor pain in the area of the shoulder girdle (the catheter technique is preferable here, even when treatment time is restricted). The block cannot replace oral medication, but may be useful in addition.
- Post-herpetic neuralgia.

Specific contraindications
Anticoagulant treatment.

Procedure

Prior discussion with the patient is an absolute necessity.

Preparations
Check that the emergency equipment is complete and in working order. Sterile precautions, intravenous access, intubation kit, emergency medication.

Materials
5-mL syringe, 10-mL syringe, 22-G needle (50 mm or 70 mm), swabs, disinfectant (Fig. 10.3).

Skin prep
In all blocks.

Patient positioning
Sitting, with the neck tilted forward comfortably (so-called "pharaoh posture").

Landmarks
Acromion, spine of scapula (Fig. 10.4). A line is drawn along the spine of the scapula between the acromion and the medial edge of the shoulder blade. A second line parallel to the line of the spinous processes of the vertebrae transects the connecting line. The injection site lies about 2.5–3 cm cranial to the intersection of the two straight lines (Fig. 10.5).

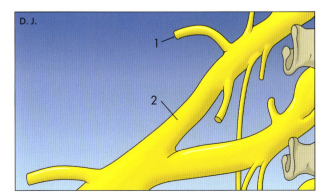

Fig. 10.1 Branching of the suprascapular nerve (1) from the superior trunk of the brachial plexus (2)

Chapter 10

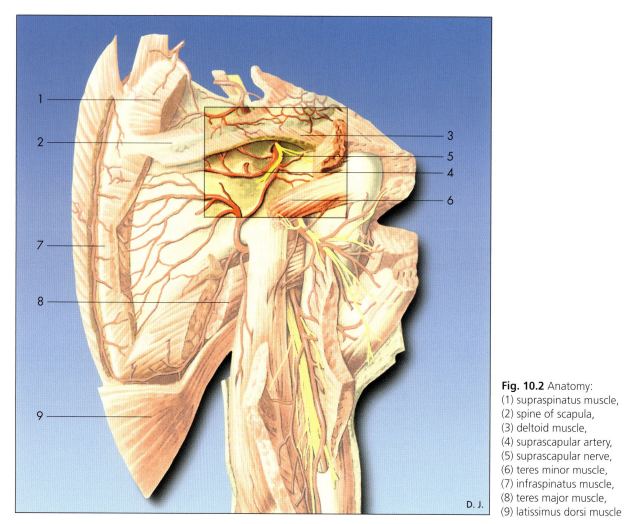

Fig. 10.2 Anatomy:
(1) supraspinatus muscle,
(2) spine of scapula,
(3) deltoid muscle,
(4) suprascapular artery,
(5) suprascapular nerve,
(6) teres minor muscle,
(7) infraspinatus muscle,
(8) teres major muscle,
(9) latissimus dorsi muscle

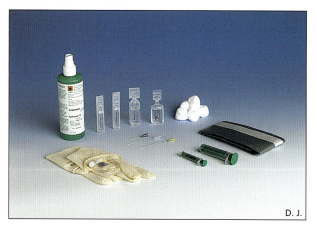

Fig. 10.3 Materials

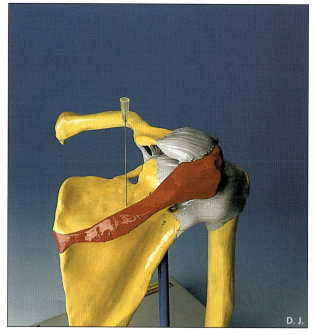

Fig. 10.4 Anatomical orientation

Injection technique

After skin prep, a needle 50 mm or 70 mm long, depending on the patient's anatomy, is slowly advanced perpendicular to the skin surface in the direction of the scapular notch (Fig. 10.6).

Depending on the anatomy, bone contact is made after 3.5–5 cm. The needle is then corrected medially and laterally, until the scapular notch is reached. After careful aspiration, the local anesthetic is slowly injected; aspiration must be repeated during the injection.

> During the injection, the patient usually experiences an aching sensation in the upper arm and shoulder joint. Targeted eliciting of paresthesias is not necessary, but they may occur unintentionally.

Dosage

Diagnostic
5 mL local anesthetic – e.g. 1% prilocaine or 1% mepivacaine.

Therapeutic
5–10 mL local anesthetic – e.g. 0.75% ropivacaine or 0.5% bupivacaine (0.5% levobupivacaine).
In acute conditions, 2–4 mg dexamethasone can be added in each of the first and second blocks.

Block series
If there is a trend toward improvement after the first and second treatment, a series of six to eight blocks is useful in all indications.

Side effects

If the dose is too large, transient weakness can occur in the supraspinatus and infraspinatus muscles, and outpatients in particular should be informed about this.

Complications

- Intravascular injection (suprascapular artery), extremely rare.
- Pneumothorax, extremely rare (Fig. 10.7).
  Prophylaxis: only advance the needle until bone contact is made.

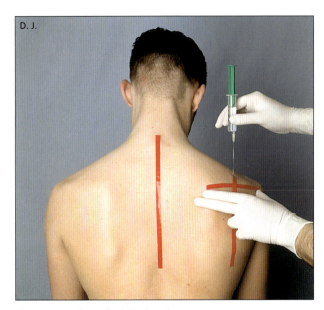

Fig. 10.5 Marking the injection site

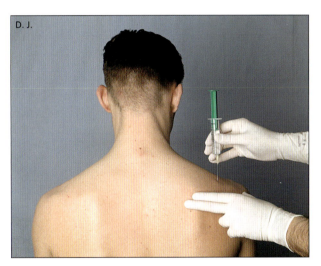

Fig. 10.6 Slow needle insertion in the direction of the scapular notch

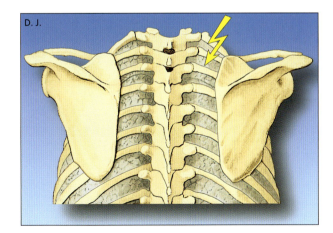

Fig. 10.7 To prevent pneumothorax, the needle should only be advanced until bone contact is made

11 Subscapular nerve blocks
Infiltration of subscapular muscle trigger points ("frozen shoulder")

Introduction

The activation of trigger points in the subscapular and other muscles in what is known as the "rotator cuff" and neighboring muscles (Table 11.1), and irritation of the neighboring nerves, create pain that has a classic distribution pattern [15]. The pattern involves pain during movement and at rest, with nocturnal exacerbation. "Frozen shoulder" or stiff shoulder is a descriptive term that should not be regarded as a diagnosis. "Frozen shoulder" is regarded by some authors as being the end stage of various shoulder diseases, while others regard it as being an independent, idiopathic disease.

The current clinical nomenclature includes three categories of "frozen shoulder": idiopathic "frozen shoulder"; adhesive capsulitis; and subacromial fibrosis [1, 15]. Other possible etiologies are: irritation of the acromioclavicular joint [1], compression of the suprascapular nerve [8], prolonged immobilization of the arm [4], cervical radiculopathy [4], muscular spasm [15], hemiplegia [7], myocardial infarction [3, 4], biceps tendinitis [1], and others. Some authors regard "frozen shoulder" as an algoneurodystrophic process [16], while others have identified similarities with the clinical picture of Dupuytren's contracture [6]. The key role of the subscapular muscle in the etiology of "frozen shoulder" is often emphasized [9]. There is no specific and standardized treatment for "frozen shoulder" syndrome. Active physiotherapy should be started as soon as possible in order to prevent adhesions from developing. Pain can be reduced by various supportive measures (ice or heat application, ultrasound, transcutaneous electric nerve stimulation (TENS), nonsteroidal anti-inflammatory drugs, opioids, local or systemic steroid administration, targeted injection at trigger points, etc.).

Mobilization and manipulation of the shoulder joint shows good results in the early stages of "frozen shoulder." Rhythmic stabilization exercises and therapeutic blocking of the suprascapular and subscapular nerves are recommended [7].

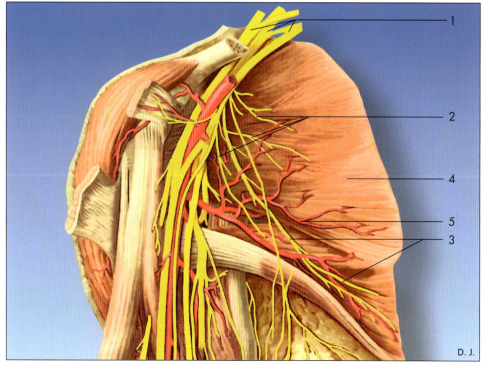

Fig. 11.1 Anatomy (anterior view):
(1) cords of the brachial plexus,
(2) subscapular nerve,
(3) thoracodorsal nerve,
(4) subscapular muscle,
(5) circumflex scapular artery

Starting physiotherapy at an early stage is an essential part of the treatment. The main problem here is that due to severe pain, the treatment cannot be carried out adequately in a large number of patients. The use of nerve blocks and targeted injections into the trigger points in the affected muscles shortly before carrying out physiotherapy makes it possible to achieve pain-free and effective treatment.

Anatomy (Figs. 11.1 and 11.2)

The subscapular nerves consist of two or three nerves emerging from various parts of the brachial plexus for the subscapular, teres major, and latissimus dorsi muscles. The longest and most important of these is the thoracodorsal nerve, which runs along the axillary border of the scapula and supplies the latissimus dorsi muscle.

The superior subscapular nerve emerges from C5 and C6 (C7) and enters the subscapular muscle. The medial subscapular nerve (C5–6) arises from the posterior secondary trunks and supplies the lateral lower part of the subscapular muscle and teres major muscle.

The inferior subscapular nerve (thoracodorsal nerve) is the largest in this group. It arises from the posterior secondary branches or from the axillary nerve, or more rarely from the radial nerve, and passes along the lateral edge of the scapula to the latissimus dorsi muscle.

The subscapular muscle is one of the most important of what are known as the rotator cuff muscles (see Table 11.1, Fig. 11.2 and Chapter 10, Fig. 10.2).

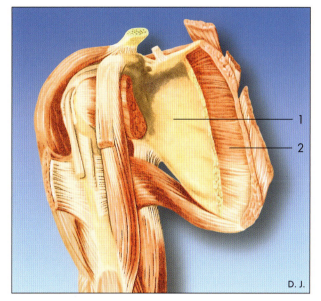

Fig. 11.2 Anatomy. (1) Subscapular fossa, (2) subscapular muscle

Anatomical insertions

The anatomical insertions of the subscapular muscle are medial to the interior surface of the scapula (Fig. 11.2) and lateral to the lesser tubercle on the anterior surface of the humerus.

Innervation and function

See Table 11.1.

Table 11.1 Rotator cuff muscle (dark blue) and neighboring muscles: innervation and function

Muscle	Innervation	Function
Supraspinatus	Suprascapular nerve (C5**; superior trunk*)	Abducts the upper arm and pulls the head of the upper arm into the glenoid cavity
Infraspinatus	Suprascapular nerve (C5, C6**; superior trunk*)	External rotation of the arm; stabilizes the head of the humerus in the glenoid cavity
Teres minor	Axillary nerve (C5, C6**; posterior fascicle*)	Almost identical to the infraspinatus muscle
Subscapularis	Subscapular nerves (C5, C6**; posterior fascicle*)	Internal rotation and adduction of the upper arm in the shoulder
Teres major	Inferior subscapular nerve (C5, C6**; posterior fascicle*)	Supports adduction, internal rotation and extension of the upper arm from a bent position
Deltoid	Axillary nerve (C5, C6**; posterior fascicle*)	Helps the supraspinatus muscle to abduct the upper arm in the shoulder
Latissimus dorsi	Thoracodorsal nerve (C6–C8**; posterior fascicle*)	Adduction and internal rotation of the arm; strong downward movement of the scapula
Coracobrachialis	Musculocutaneous nerve (C6, C7**; lateral fascicle*)	

* Brachial plexus.
** Spinal nerves

Chapter 11

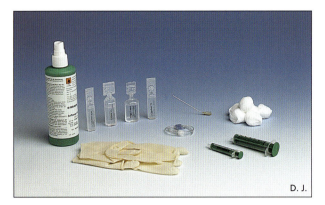

Fig. 11.3 Materials

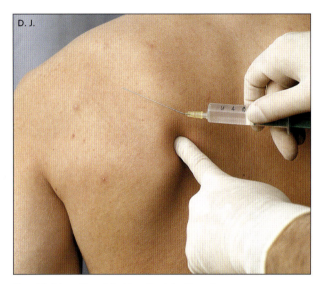

Fig. 11.4 Location. Marking the injection site (center of the medial border of the scapula)

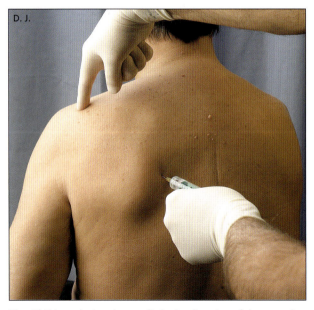

Fig. 11.5 Introducing the needle in the direction of the acromion

Symptoms

Activation of the trigger points and irritation of the neighboring nerves gives rise to pain with a classic distribution pattern. The pain involves the scapula, the posterior deltoid region, elbow and dorsum of the wrist.

Indications and contraindications
See Chapter 10, p. 125.

Procedure

Preparations
Check that the emergency equipment is complete and in working order; sterile precautions, intravenous access. Prior information for the patient is an absolute necessity.

Materials (Fig. 11.3)
Fine 25-mm long 26-G needle for local anesthesia, 70-mm long 20-G needle (with the needle shaft angled by about 20°), local anesthetic, disinfectant, swabs, 2 mL and 10 mL syringes.

Technique
Position
Sitting, with the neck comfortably tilted and the shoulders relaxed.

Location (Fig. 11.4)
- The patient's arm is pulled back, so that the contours of the scapula are easily recognized. The center of the medial border of the scapula is marked as the injection point.
- Acromion.

Skin prep, local anesthesia, drawing up the local anesthetic, testing the injection needle for patency.

> - Before the injection, the shaft of the injection needle should be bent by about 20°.
> - Targeted paresthesias are not elicited.
> - During the injection, observe the skin for possible subcutaneous spread of the local anesthetic.

Injection technique
- Introduce the 20° angled needle into the center of the medial border of the scapula, in the direction of the acromion (Figs. 11.5 and 11.6).
- The needle is introduced subscapularly parallel to the skin surface between the anterior surface of the

scapula (costal surface) and the posterior thoracic wall (ribs), into the subscapular fossa. If the needle meets the edge of the ribs, it is withdrawn as far as the subcutaneous tissue and reintroduced.

- At a depth of 4 cm, then 5 cm and finally 6 cm – depending on the anatomy – a total of 10–15 mL local anesthetic is then injected after prior aspiration (Fig. 11.5).

The signs of a successful injection are: spread extending into the shoulder joint, upper arm, and often as far as the wrist, corresponding to the radiation pattern of the trigger points of the subscapular muscle (Fig. 11.7) [15].

Dosage
Diagnostic
5 mL local anesthetic – e.g. 1% prilocaine or 1% mepivacaine.

Therapeutic
10–15 mL local anesthetic– e.g. 0.5–0.75% ropivacaine, 0.25–0.5% bupivacaine (0.25–0.5% levobupivacaine). In acute pain, the addition of 40 mg triamcinolone has proved useful.
In our experience, this block is superior to blocking the suprascapular nerve. A combination of the two techniques is possible and often desirable (Table 11.2).

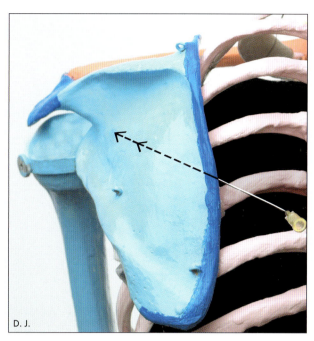

Fig. 11.6 Introducing the needle in the direction of the acromion (skeletal model)

Block series
In all indications, a series of six to eight blocks is useful if an improvement trend is seen after the first and second treatments.

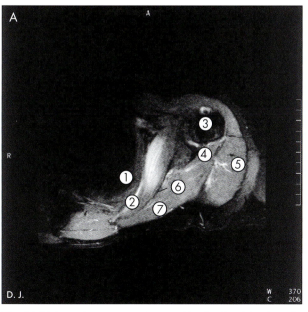 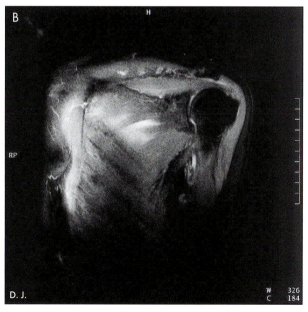

Fig. 11.7 Magnetic resonance images 10 min after injection of 10 mL ropivacaine, without radiographic contrast medium, into the subscapular fossa. **a** Axial (cross-section). **b** Paracoronal.
(1) Thorax wall, (2) subscapular muscle and subscapular fossa, (3) head of the humerus, (4) teres minor muscle, (5) deltoid muscle, (6) scapula, (7) infraspinatus muscle

Table 11.2 Shoulder–arm region: blocking techniques in pain therapy
Comparison of interscalene block of the brachial plexus, blocks of the subscapular and suprascapular nerves and blocks of the stellate ganglion

		Indications		
Surgical	Postoperative pain therapy	Acute and chronic pain conditions Target area		Mobilization of the shoulder
		Shoulder	Shoulder–arm	
Interscalene* +++++ Dosage: 20–25 mL 0.75% ropivacaine or 0.5% bupivacaine (0.5% levobupivacaine)	Interscalene** +++++ 20–25 mL 0.375–0.5% ropivacaine or 0.25% bupivacaine (0.25% levobupivacaine)	Subscapular nerves +++++ 10–15 mL 0.5–0.75% ropivacaine or 0.25% bupivacaine (0.25% levobupivacaine)	Interscalene +++++ 10–15 mL 0.375–0.5% ropivacaine or 0.25% bupivacaine (0.25% levobupivacaine)	Interscalene +++++ 20–25 mL 0.375–0.5% ropivacaine or 0.25% bupivacaine (0.25% levobupivacaine)
	Subscapular nerves** ++ 15 mL 0.5–0.75% ropivacaine or 0.25–0.375% bupivacaine (0.25–0.375% levo-bupivacaine)	Interscalene +++ 10–15 mL 0.375–0.5% ropivacaine or 0.25% bupivacaine (0.25% levobupivacaine)	Stellate ganglion ++ 10–15 mL 0.375% ropivacaine or 0.25% bupivacaine (0.25% levobupivacaine)	Subscapular nerves*** ++ 10–15 mL 0.5–0.75% ropivacaine or 0.25% bupivacaine (0.25% levobupivacaine)

+++++ Best method.
++++ Very suitable method.
+++ Suitable method.
++ Method suitable with some qualifications.
+ Less suitable method.
* Usually in combination with basic general anesthesia. This provides excellent pain relief.
** In severe pain, a combination of the two techniques is possible.
*** Usually in combination with a suprascapular nerve block: 8–10 mL 0.5–0.75% ropivacaine or 0.25% bupivacaine (0.25% levobupiva-caine).

Side effects

If the dosage is too high, transient weakness may occur in the shoulder and upper arm. Outpatients should be informed about this. A partial block of the intercostal nerves is possible due to spread of the local anesthetic, and is often desirable.

Complications

- There is a potential risk of pneumothorax (unlikely if the correct technique is observed).
- Intravascular injection.

12 Rotator cuff muscles
Injection techniques in the myofascial trigger points

Subscapular muscle

See Chapter 11.

Supraspinatus muscle

Anatomical insertions
The anatomical insertions are medial to the supraspinous fossa and lateral to the greater tubercle of the humerus (Fig. 12.1).

Innervation and function
See Chapter 11, Table 11.1.

Myotatic unit
This covers the middle part of the deltoid muscle and the upper part of the trapezius muscle, as synergists for abduction.

Trigger points
The two trigger points (TrPs) in the supraspinatus muscle are located deep in the supraspinous fossa of the scapulae, underneath the relatively thick part of the trapezius muscle. The medial TrP lies directly above the spine of the scapula, lateral to the medial border of the scapula. The lateral TrP can be palpated medial to the acromion. A third TrP may be located in the tendon of the muscle at its lateral insertion on the joint capsule and the greater tuberosity (Fig. 12.1) [15].

Symptoms
Pain in the middle deltoid region, sometimes radiating to the upper and lower arm, particularly in the area of the lateral epicondyle.

Procedure

Materials
Sterile precautions, 23-G needle 30 mm long, 2-mL and 5-mL syringes, local anesthetic.

Injection technique
The lower arm of the seated patient is placed behind the back at waist level ("hand behind the back"; Fig. 12.2). After palpation, injection into the medial TrP is carried out in the direction of the suprascapular notch (Fig. 12.3). After careful aspiration, injection of the local anesthetic follows. The lateral TrP is sought directly medial to the acromion. The muscle's insertion point at the greater tubercle of the humerus requires perpendicular puncture until bone contact is made (Fig. 12.4).

Dosage
1–2 mL local anesthetic – e.g. 0.2–0.375% ropivacaine.

Complications
Pneumothorax must be regarded as a potential complication when injecting into the medial TrP of the supraspinatus muscle.

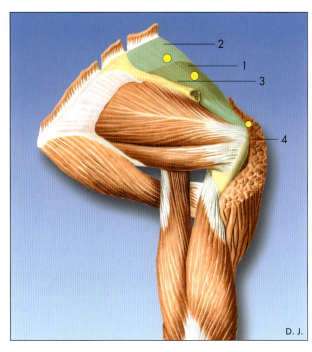

Fig. 12.1 Supraspinatus muscle. Anatomic insertions and myofascial trigger points (yellow circles); *adapted from Travell and Simons [15]*. (1) Infraspinatus muscle, (2) supraspinous fascia, (3) spine of the scapula, (4) greater tuberosity of the humerus

Chapter 12

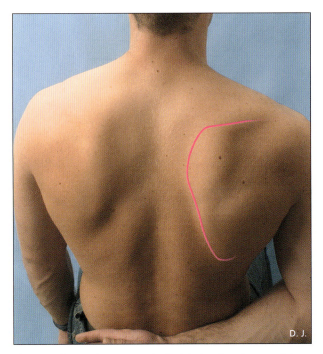

Fig. 12.2 Supraspinatus muscle. Positioning for trigger point injection ("hand behind the back" position)

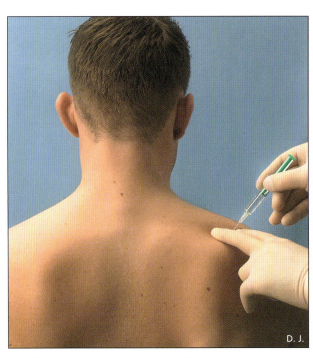

Fig. 12.3 Supraspinatus muscle. Injection into the medial trigger point in the direction of the suprascapular notch

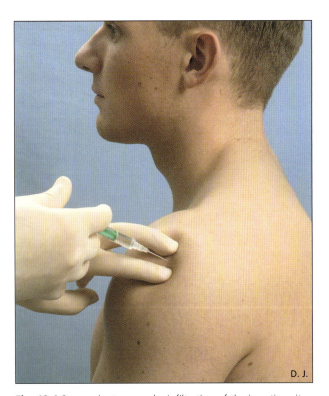

Fig. 12.4 Supraspinatus muscle. Infiltration of the insertion site at the greater tubercle of the humerus

Infraspinatus muscle

Anatomic insertions
The anatomic insertions are located medial to the infraspinous fossa of the scapula and lateral to the greater tuberosity of the humerus (Fig. 12.5).

Innervation and function
See Chapter 11, Table 11.1.

Myotatic unit
With the exception of external rotation of the arm, the infraspinatus muscle acts synergistically with the teres minor muscle (with almost identical function) and the posterior part of the deltoid muscle.

Trigger points
Two active trigger points (medial and lateral) can be located approximately 2 cm below the spine of the scapula, and sometimes there is also another possible trigger point slightly caudally (Figs. 12.5, 12.7) [15].

Symptoms
The symptoms consist of referred pain when sleeping in the lateral position and an inability to reach the rear trouser pockets or bra fastener, or to comb the hair or brush the teeth.

Procedure

Materials
Sterile precautions, 23-G needle 30 mm long, 2-mL and 5-mL syringes, local anesthetic.

Injection technique
The patient lies on the side that is not being treated. The arm is bent to 90° and the elbow is laid on a cushion. The contour of the scapula has to be clearly defined.
After careful disinfection and palpation of the trigger point (TrP), the needle is slowly introduced in the direction of the TrP. During injection into the medial TrP, the left middle finger is pressed against the caudal edge of the spine of the scapula. During injection into the lateral TrP, the left ring finger presses against the caudal edge of the spine of the scapula (Fig. 12.6).

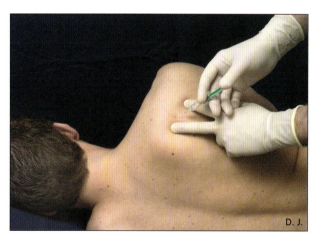

Fig. 12.6 Infraspinatus muscle. Injection into the medial trigger point in the direction of the caudal edge of the spine of the scapula

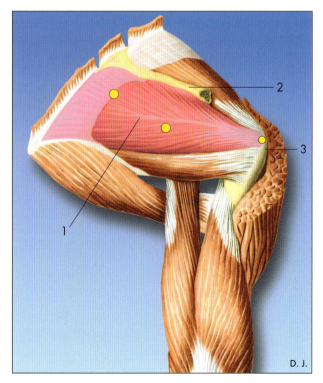

Fig. 12.5 Infraspinatus muscle. Anatomic insertions and myofascial trigger points (yellow circles); *adapted from Travell and Simons [15]*. (1) Infraspinatus muscle, (2) spine of the scapula, (3) greater tuberosity of the humerus

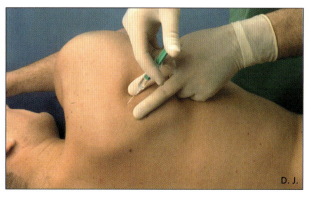

Fig. 12.7 Infraspinatus muscle. Injection into the caudal trigger point

Chapter 12

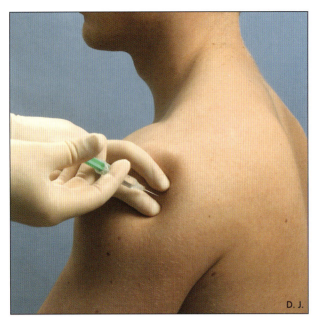

Fig. 12.8 Infraspinatus muscle. Infiltration of the insertion site on the greater tuberosity of the humerus

The puncture has to be carried out sensitively, as the scapula bones (part of the infraspinous fossa) sometimes offer very little resistance (resembling a fibrous membrane, so that there is a risk of pneumothorax). The insertion site of the muscle into the greater tuberosity of the humerus requires a perpendicular position to be maintained until bone contact is made (Fig. 12.8).

Dosage
1–2 mL local anesthetic – e.g. 0.2–0.375% ropivacaine.

Complications
- Pneumothorax is a potential complication [15].
- Infection.

Teres minor muscle

Anatomic insertions
The muscle's anatomic insertions are located directly alongside and caudal to those of the infraspinatus muscle (Fig. 12.9).

Innervation and function
See Chapter 11, Table 11.1.

Myotatic unit
The teres minor muscle acts synergistically with the infraspinatus muscle.

Trigger points
The teres minor muscle is one of the most rarely affected muscles in the rotator cuff (only involved in 7% of cases). The trigger point usually lies in the center of the muscle (Fig. 12.9) [15]. The teres minor muscle is located above the teres major muscle.

Symptoms
Pain in the posterior deltoid area.

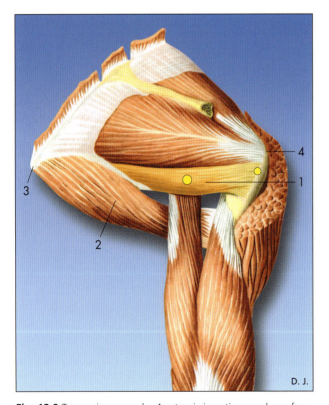

Fig. 12.9 Teres minor muscle. Anatomic insertions and myofascial trigger points (yellow circles); *adapted from Travell and Simons [15]*. (1) Teres minor muscle, (2) teres major muscle, (3) inferior angle of the scapula, (4) greater tuberosity of the humerus

Rotator cuff muscles. Injection techniques in the myofascial trigger points

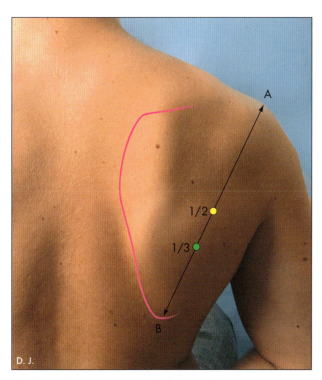

Fig. 12.10 Teres minor muscle (yellow) and teres major muscle (green). Landmarks for TrP injection. **A:** Acromion, **B**: inferior angle of the scapula

Procedure

Materials
Sterile precautions, 23-G needle 30 mm long, 2-mL and 5-mL syringes, local anesthetic.

Injection technique
The arm is bent to 90°. The contour of the scapula has to be clearly defined (Fig. 12.10).
The TrPs are sought between the teres major and infraspinatus muscles, near the lateral edge of the scapula. The index and middle finger fix the TrP. The 30-mm needle is directed toward the scapula (Fig. 12.11). The insertion site of the muscle on the greater tuberosity of the humerus requires a perpendicular needle direction until bone contact is made (Fig. 12.12).

Dosage
2 mL local anesthetic – e.g. 0.2–0.375% ropivacaine.

Complications
Pneumothorax is a potential complication.

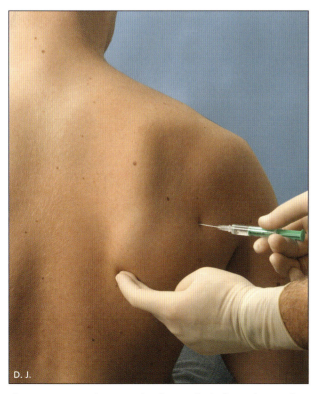

Fig. 12.11 Teres minor muscle. The needle is directed toward the scapula

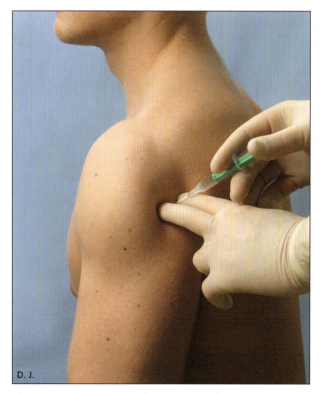

Fig. 12.12 Teres minor muscle. Injection at the insertion point of the greater tuberosity of the humerus

13 Shoulder region
Intra-articular injections

Intra-articular injection into the shoulder joint

Indications
Synovial inflammatory conditions (capsulitis), severe resting pain, humeroscapular periarthritis, after shoulder bruising, rheumatoid arthritis. The anatomy of the shoulder joint is shown in Fig. 13.1a, b.

Strictly aseptic conditions are necessary when carrying out intra-articular injections.

Materials
25-G needle 30–40 mm long, 2-mL and 5-mL syringes, sterile swabs, disinfectant, sterile gloves, sterile drape.

Injection techniques
Ventral access route
Landmarks (Fig. 13.1a, b)
- Coracoid process
- Head of the humerus
- Clavicle

Technique
The patient is seated with the supinated arm hanging freely, and the articular cavity is palpated directly medial to the head of the humerus. The needle is introduced underneath the clavicle, directly lateral to the coracoid process toward the outside and back. The path to the joint is very short with this approach (Fig. 13.2).

Dosage
2 mL local anesthetic – e.g. 0.5–0.75% ropivacaine or 0.25% bupivacaine mixed with 40 mg methylprednisolone.

Dorsal access route
Landmarks (Fig. 13.1a, b)
- Spine of the scapula
- Lateral corner of the acromion
- Coracoid process

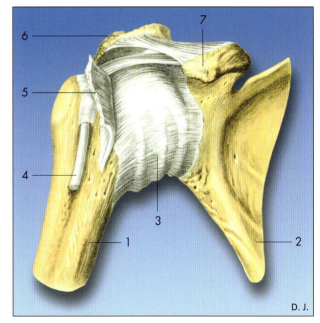

Fig. 13.1a Anatomy of the shoulder joint.
(1) Humerus, (2) scapula, (3) articular capsule, (4) tendon of the biceps brachii muscle, (5) subscapular muscle, (6) acromion, (7) coracoid process

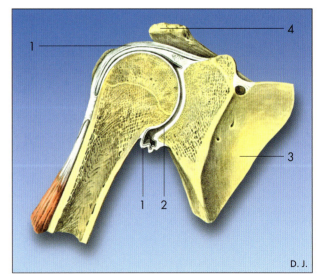

Fig. 13.1b Shoulder joint. Articular cavity and articular capsule.
(1) Articular capsule, (2) articular cavity, (3) scapula, (4) acromion

Shoulder region. Intra-articular injections

Technique
The patient is seated, with the upper arm slightly abducted and rotated inward, and the lateral corner of the acromion is palpated. The injection is made directly underneath this point and the needle is advanced between the posterior edge of the deltoid muscle and the tendon of the infraspinatus muscle (the muscle's dorsolateral tendon) in the direction of the coracoid process (Fig. 13.3). The articular cavity is reached after approximately 3–4 cm. After injection into the joint, a further 1 mL is distributed circumarticularly as the needle is withdrawn.

Dosage
2 mL local anesthetic – e.g. 0.5–0.75% ropivacaine or 0.25% bupivacaine mixed with 40 mg methylprednisolone.

> **Intra-articular injection into the acriomioclavicular joint**

Indications
Shoulder pain radiating to behind the ear, restricted mobility in the shoulder joint.

Landmarks
- Lateral edge of the clavicle
- Acromion
- Acromioclavicular ligament (Fig. 13.4)

> The acromioclavicular joint has a very small volume, so that only a small amount of the injection solution is needed.

Injection technique
The patient is seated, and the articular cavity between the lateral end of the clavicle and the acromion is palpated. The needle is advanced perpendicularly from above through the acromioclavicular ligament to a maximum depth of 1 cm. Provided there is no resistance, a small amount of the injection solution is injected (Fig. 13.5).

Dosage
0.5–1 mL local anesthetic – e.g. 0.5–0.75% ropivacaine or 0.25% bupivacaine mixed with 40 mg methylprednisolone or triamcinolone.

Side effects
Some 25% of patients report a transient increase in pain after an intra-articular injection in the shoulder joint. The patient should be advised of this potential side effect.

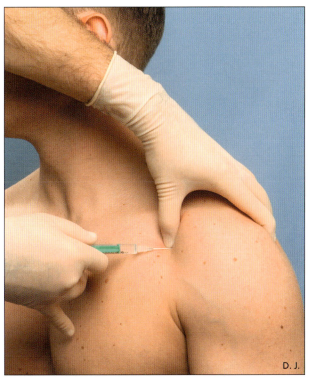

Fig. 13.2 Intra-articular injection into the shoulder joint from the ventral access route

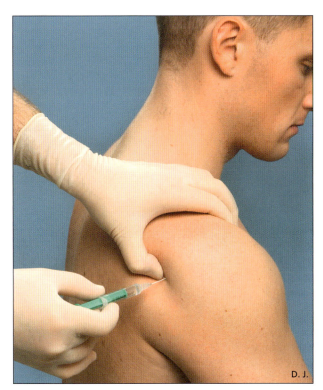

Fig. 13.3 Intra-articular injection into the shoulder joint from the dorsal access route

Complications
- Infection
- Hematoma (prophylactic compression should be carried out after the injection).

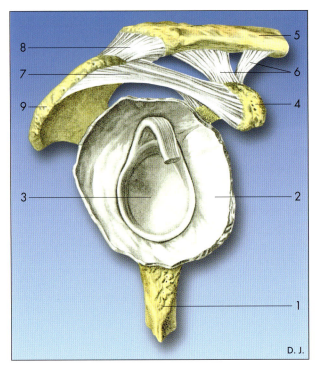

Fig. 13.4 Anatomy of the acromioclavicular joint and neighboring structures. (1) Scapula, (2) articular capsule, (3) glenoid cavity, (4) coracoid process, (5) clavicle, (6) coracoclavicular ligament, (7) coracoacromial ligament, (8) acromioclavicular joint, (9) acromion

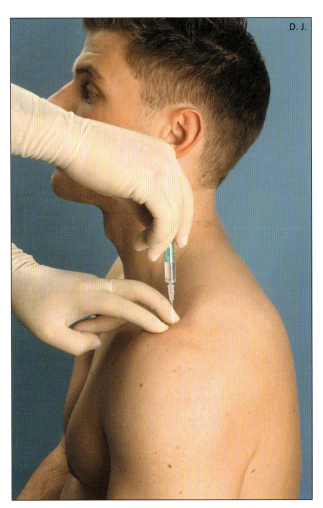

Fig. 13.5 Intra-articular injection into the acromioclavicular joint

Elbow and hand region

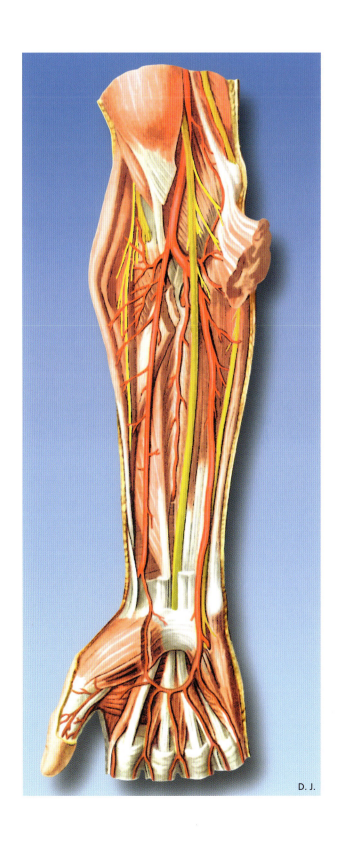

14 Peripheral nerve blocks in the elbow region

Anatomy (Fig. 14.1)

Ulnar nerve
The ulnar nerve originates from the medial cord of the brachial plexus (C8–T1, C7). The nerve runs on the medial side of the lower third of the upper arm, in the groove of the ulnar nerve on the posterior side of the medial epicondyle of the humerus.
The nerve is easily palpated at this location. In the forearm, it runs between the humeral and ulnar head of the flexor carpi ulnaris muscle on the medial side of the forearm.

Median nerve
The median nerve originates from the medial and lateral cords of the brachial plexus (C5, C6–C8, T1). At the elbow, it lies medial to the brachial artery, courses along the medial surface of the brachialis muscle downwards in the elbow, where it can be found behind the bicipital aponeurosis and in front of the insertion of the brachialis muscle and elbow joint.

Radial nerve and lateral antebrachial cutaneous nerve (musculocutaneous nerve)
These two nerves innervate the radial half of the forearm and the back of the hand, and have a close anatomical relationship.
The radial nerve (C5–C8, T1) is the longest branch of the brachial plexus, and represents a direct continuation of the posterior cord. It runs in the middle of the upper arm in the groove of the radial nerve along the dorsal side of the humerus. Before the lateral epicondyle of the humerus and the elbow joint capsule, it then enters the fissure between the brachioradialis muscle and the biceps muscle. At the level of the head of the radius, it divides into the deep branch (anterior interosseous nerve, mainly motor) and the superficial branch (mainly sensory). The latter follows the course of the radial artery.

Lateral antebrachial cutaneous nerve
The musculocutaneous nerve (C4, C5–C7) arises from the lateral cord of the brachial plexus. At the level of the elbow joint, it passes between the biceps muscle and the brachioradialis muscle to the brachial fascia,

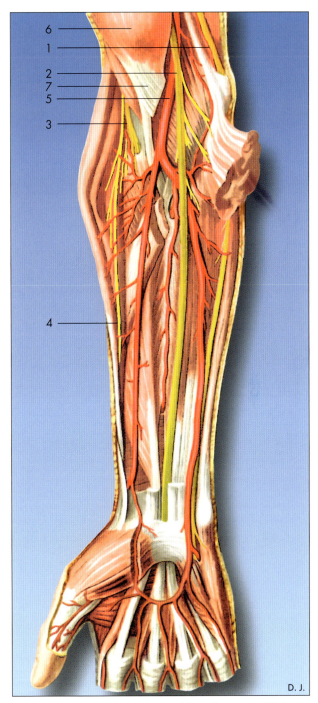

Fig. 14.1 Anatomy. (1) Ulnar nerve, (2) median nerve, (3) deep branch of the radial nerve (anterior interosseous nerve), (4) superficial branch of the radial nerve, (5) brachial artery, (6) biceps brachii muscle, (7) bicipital aponeurosis

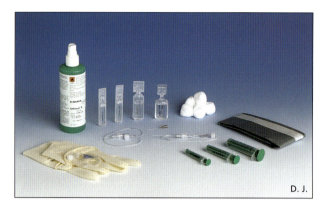

Fig. 14.2 Materials

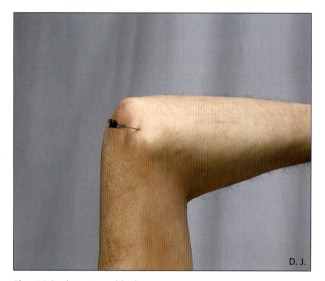

Fig. 14.3 Ulnar nerve block

which it penetrates, becoming the lateral antebrachial cutaneous nerve.

Indications

Surgical
- Minor interventions in the innervated area.
- Supplementation of incomplete anesthesia of the brachial plexus.

> Care must be taken to avoid nerve injury, since paresthesias do not occur as a warning signal (see p. 110).

Diagnostic
Differential diagnosis of painful conditions in the upper extremity.

Therapeutic
None.

Contraindications

Relative
- Local neuritis
- Carpal tunnel syndrome (median nerve)

> Distal blocks of the peripheral nerves of the arm are associated with a high incidence of nerve injury (particularly to the ulnar nerve). It is therefore advisable not to use these injections on a routine basis.
> During the injection, intraneural positioning of the needle must be excluded.

Procedure

Preparations
Check that the emergency equipment is complete and in working order; sterile precautions, intravenous access.

Materials (Fig. 14.2)
35–50 mm long atraumatic 25-G needle (15°), with injection lead ("immobile needle") – e.g. Stimuplex D® (B. Braun Melsungen) or 24-G Plexufix needles, 25–50 mm long, local anesthetic, disinfectant, swabs, drape, syringes: 2, 5, and 10 mL.

Technique

Ulnar nerve (Fig. 14.3)
Positioning
Supine, with the arm rotated outward and the elbow bent to 90°.

Location
The medial epicondyle of the humerus and olecranon are palpated. The ulnar nerve runs in the groove of the ulnar nerve at a depth of 0.5–1 cm, and can usually be palpated.
Skin prep, local anesthesia, covering with a sterile drape, drawing up the local anesthetic, checking the patency of the needle and functioning of the nerve stimulator, attaching electrodes.

Injection
After definite localization of the groove of the ulnar nerve, the needle should be introduced through infiltrated skin ca. 1–2 cm above this point at an angle of 90° to the long axis of the humerus.
After paresthesias have been elicited and intraneural positioning of the needle has been excluded, withdraw

the needle slightly and carry out a fan-shaped injection after aspiration.

Median nerve (Fig. 14.4)
Positioning
Supine, elbow joint extended.

Location
The intercondylar line is marked. Palpation of the brachial artery.

Injection technique
After palpation of the brachial artery, the needle is introduced through infiltrated skin, on the ulnar side of the artery. At a depth of 0.5–1 cm, paresthesias are elicited. After aspiration and exclusion of intraneural positioning of the needle, a fan-shaped injection is carried out.

Radial nerve and lateral antebrachial cutaneous nerve (musculocutaneous nerve) (Fig. 14.4)
These two nerves are closely related to one another anatomically, so that both can be blocked using this technique.

Positioning
Supine, elbow joint extended.

Location
Lateral humeral epicondyle, biceps tendon, brachioradial muscle.

Injection technique
At the level of the intercondylar line, the fissure between the brachioradialis muscle and the biceps tendon is palpated. The needle is introduced through infiltrated skin about 2 cm lateral to the biceps tendon, in a proximal and lateral direction towards the lateral epicondyle.
After paresthesias have been elicited, intraneural positioning has been excluded, and aspiration has been carried out, 5–8 mL of a local anesthetic are injected. After withdrawal of the needle, fan-shaped infiltration of 5 mL local anesthetic is carried out as far as the subcutaneous tissue.
If no paresthesias can be elicited, the needle is introduced as far as the lateral surface of the lateral humeral epicondyle, and after bone contact the first dose of 3–4 mL of the local anesthetic is injected. The needle is then withdrawn to a subcutaneous level and, after altering the direction slightly medially, the procedure is repeated two or three times. On each occasion, 2–3 mL of local anesthetic is injected. Finally, when withdrawing the needle, a fan-shaped infiltration of 5 mL local

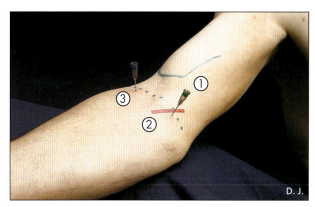

Fig. 14.4 Median nerve and radial nerve blocks.
(1) Median nerve, (2) brachial artery, (3) radial nerve

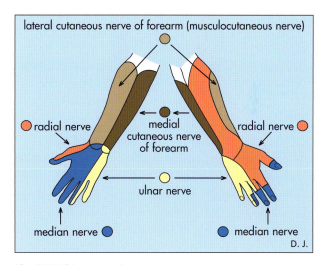

Fig. 14.5 Skin innervation

anesthetic as far as the subcutaneous tissue is carried out.

Dosage
Ulnar nerve: 2–5 mL local anesthetic.
Median nerve: 5 mL local anesthetic.
Radial nerve (and lateral antebrachial cutaneous nerve): 10–15 mL local anesthetic.

- 0.75% ropivacaine
- 0.5% bupivacaine
- 1% prilocaine
- 1% mepivacaine
- 1% lidocaine

Skin innervation
Fig. 14.5.

Complications
Neuritis after nerve puncture (particularly in the ulnar nerve).

15 Peripheral nerve blocks in the wrist region

Anatomy

Ulnar nerve (Fig. 15.1)
In the medial distal third of the forearm, about 5 cm proximal to the wrist, the ulnar nerve divides into a sensory branch – the dorsal branch; and a mixed branch – the palmar branch. The latter runs along the tendon of the flexor carpi ulnaris muscle in a distal direction. The ulnar artery lies directly radially, alongside the nerve.

Median nerve (Fig. 15.1)
The median nerve lies between the tendons of the palmaris longus muscle and the flexor carpi radialis muscle. It runs in the direction of the long axis of the radius.

Radial nerve (Fig. 15.2)
The superficial branch of the radial nerve runs – together with the radial artery, initially – in the forearm along the medial side of the brachioradialis muscle in the direction of the wrist. About 7–8 cm proximal to the wrist, it crosses under the tendon of the brachioradialis muscle and reaches the extensor side of the forearm. At the level of the wrist, the radial nerve divides into several peripheral branches.

Indications
Surgical
- Minor surgical interventions in the innervated area.
- Supplementation of an incomplete block of the brachial plexus.

Care must be taken to avoid nerve injury, since paresthesias do not occur here as a warning signal (see Chapter 9, brachial plexus, p. 110).

Diagnostic
- Differential diagnosis of painful conditions in the hand.

Therapeutic
- None.

Contraindications
Relative
- Neuritis.

Procedure

Preparations
Check that the emergency equipment is complete and in working order; sterile precautions, intravenous access.

Materials (Fig. 15.3)
35-mm long, atraumatic 25-G needle (15°), with injection lead – e.g. Stimuplex D® (B. Braun Melsungen; exception: circular block of the radial nerve; fine 25-G needles, 25 mm long).
Local anesthetic, disinfectant, swabs, drape, syringes: 2, 5, and 10 mL.

Technique
Skin prep, local anesthesia, drawing up the local anesthetic, checking patency of the injection needle and functioning of the nerve stimulator, attaching electrodes.

Ulnar nerve (Fig. 15.4)
Positioning
Supine, with wrist slightly flexed.

Location
Styloid process of ulna, ulnar artery, flexor carpi ulnaris muscle.

Injection technique
Palmar branch: proximal to the styloid process of the ulna, the ulnar artery and tendon of the flexor carpi ulnaris muscle are palpated. The needle is introduced perpendicularly between the tendon and the artery, in the direction of the pisiform bone. After paresthesias have been elicited (1–2 cm), the needle is minimally withdrawn. After excluding intraneural positioning of the needle and aspiration, the needle is fixed and the local anesthetic is injected.
If no paresthesias can be elicited, the needle is advanced until bone contact is made, and 1 mL of local anesthetic is injected.
During withdrawal of the needle, fan-shaped infiltration is then carried out. A further 3–5 mL of the local anesthetic is used for this.
Dorsal branch: fan-shaped infiltration medial to the tendon of the flexor carpi ulnaris muscle, in the direction of the styloid process of the ulna.

Median nerve (Fig. 15.4)
Positioning
Supine, with the elbow extended. The forearm musculature is tensed by making a fist, so that the muscular tendons become easily visible.

Location
Styloid process of the ulna, tendons of the palmaris longus and flexor carpi radialis muscles.

Injection technique
The needle is introduced perpendicularly at the level of the proximal crease of the wrist, in between the tendons of the palmaris longus and flexor carpi radialis muscle. After paresthesias have been elicited (0.5–1 cm), the needle is minimally withdrawn, an intraneural location is excluded, and after aspiration the local anesthetic is injected.

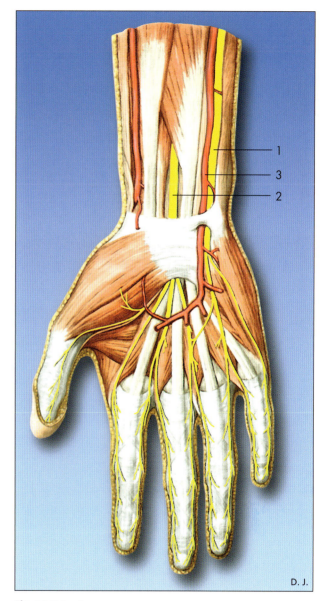

Fig. 15.1 Anatomy.
(1) Ulnar nerve, (2) median nerve, (3) ulnar artery

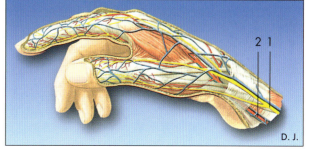

Fig. 15.2 Anatomy.
(1) Radial nerve (superficial branch), (2) radial artery

Chapter 15

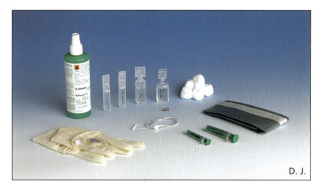

Fig. 15.3 Materials

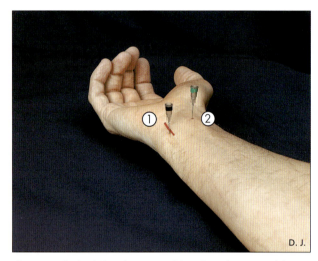

Fig. 15.4 Block of the ulnar nerve (1) and median nerve (2)

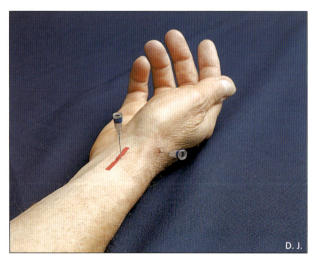

Fig. 15.5 Radial nerve block

Radial nerve (Fig. 15.5)
Positioning
Supine, with hand supinated.

Location
Level of the styloid process of the ulna, radial artery.

Injection technique
The needle is introduced through a skin spot perpendicular to the skin surface and lateral to the radial artery (0.5–1 cm). After paresthesias have been elicited, the needle is minimally withdrawn, an intraneural position is excluded, and after prior aspiration, the local anesthetic is injected. Supplementation of the block can be provided by subcutaneous infiltration of the peripheral branches and circularly between the radial artery on the ventral side and the tendons of the extensor pollicis longus and brevis muscles on the dorsal side. It is helpful for the patient to extend the thumb.

Dosage
Ulnar nerve: 3–5 mL local anesthetic.
Median nerve: 3–5 mL local anesthetic.
Radial nerve: 5–8 mL local anesthetic.

- 0.75% ropivacaine
- 0.5% bupivacaine
- 1% prilocaine
- 1% mepivacaine
- 1% lidocaine

Complications
Neuritis after puncture of a nerve.

16 Elbow and wrist
Infiltration of the myofascial trigger points and intra-articuar injections

Elbow

Area of the lateral epicondyle

Hand extensors

The **extensor carpi radialis brevis and longus muscles** (origin: distal lateral border of the humerus and lateral epicondyle of the humerus; insertion: base of metacarpal bones II and III; function: dorsal flexion and radial abduction in the wrist; innervation: radial nerve, C6, C7) and the **extensor carpi ulnaris muscle** (origin: lateral epicondyle of the humerus and antebrachial fascia; insertion: base of metacarpal bone V; function: dorsal flexion and ulnar abduction in the wrist; innervation: radial nerve, C7, C8) extend the hand at the wrist (Fig. 16.1).

The **extensor carpi radialis brevis and longus muscles** and the **extensor digitorum muscle** are the main muscles that cause "weak grip." The active trigger points (TrPs) in this "extensor muscle group" are located immediately next to each other in the proximal forearm, slightly distal to the lateral epicondyle of the humerus (Fig. 16.1).

Symptoms
The pain first appears in the lateral epicondyle and spreads to the back of the hand in the region of the articular facet of the radial head (Fig. 16.1). This type of pain is often referred to as "tennis elbow" (see also supinator muscle).

Procedure

Materials
Sterile precautions, 22-G needle 30 mm long, 2-mL and 5-mL syringes, swabs, local anesthetic.

Injection technique
The patient lies supine, with the arm on a cushion. As all of the hand extensors are located fairly superficially, their TrPs can be precisely located by palpation. The location and injection technique for the TrPs is illustrated in Fig. 16.2 (extensor carpi radialis brevis and longus muscles) and Fig. 16.3 (extensor carpi ulnaris muscle).

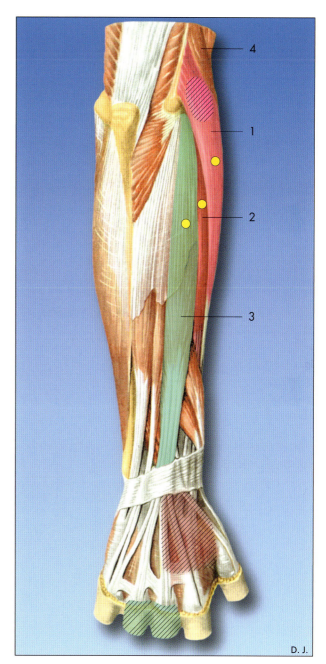

Fig. 16.1 Area of the lateral epicondyle of the humerus. (1) Extensor carpi radialis longus muscle, (2) extensor carpi radialis brevis muscle, (3) extensor digitorum muscle, (4) brachioradialis muscle. Myofascial trigger points (yellow circles) and referred pain (hatched red = extensor carpi radialis longus and brevis muscle; green = extensor digitorum muscle). *Adapted from Travell and Simons [3]*

Chapter 16

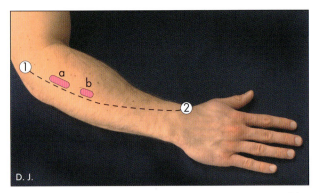

Fig. 16.2a The extensor carpi radialis longus (a) and brevis (b) muscles. Locating the injection site. Connecting line between (1) the lateral epicondyle of the humerus and (2) the styloid process of the radius

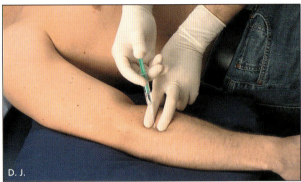

Fig. 16.2b The extensor carpi radialis longus muscle. Injection

Dosage
1 mL local anesthetic per TrP – e.g. 0.5% ropivacaine, 1% prilocaine.

Finger extensors (extensor digitorum muscle, extensor indicis muscle)

Pain referred from the **extensor digitorum muscle** (origin: lateral epicondyle of the humerus, antebrachial fascia; insertion: dorsal aponeurosis of fingers II–V; function: extension in the first joints of fingers II–V and middle and end joints, supports ulnar abduction in the wrist; innervation: deep nerve of the radial nerve, C7, C8) is projected along the forearm downward toward the back of the hand and often to the fingers (middle finger and ring finger; Fig. 16.1).

Symptoms
Patients report elbow pain or arthritis-like pain in the fingers (middle and ring finger).

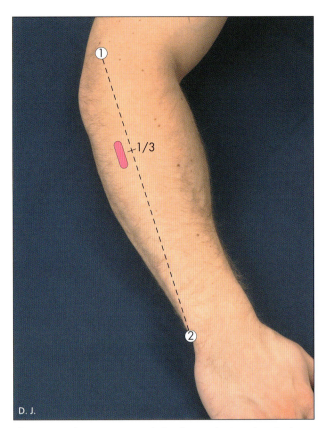

Fig. 16.3a The extensor carpi ulnaris muscle. Locating the injection site. Connecting line between (1) the lateral epicondyle of the humerus and (2) the styloid process of the ulna

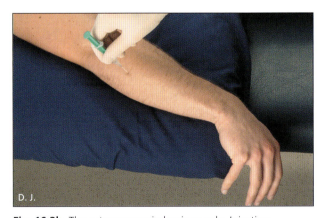

Fig. 16.3b The extensor carpi ulnaris muscle. Injection

Procedure

Materials
Sterile precautions, 22-G needle 30 mm long, 2-mL and 5-mL syringes, swabs, local anesthetic.

Elbow and wrist, Infiltration of the myofascial trigger points and intra-articular injections

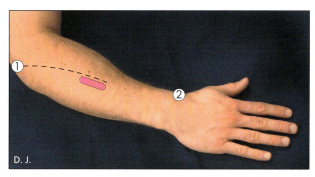

Fig. 16.4a The extensor digitorum muscle. Locating the injection site. (1) Lateral epicondyle of the humerus, (2) styloid process of the radius

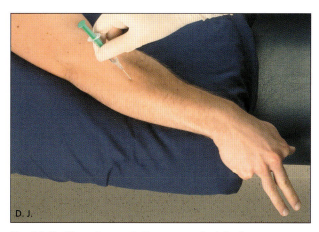

Fig. 16.4b The extensor digitorum muscle. Injection

Injection technique
The arm lies on a cushion, with the hand and fingers relaxed (this stretches the finger extensors slightly). The injection is carried out at a depth of ca. 2 cm. The deeper-lying TrP in the supinator muscle is sometimes reached (Fig. 16.4).

Dosage
1–2 mL local anesthetic per TrP – e.g. 0.5% ropivacaine, 1% prilocaine.

Supinator muscle ("tennis elbow")

"Tennis elbow" or lateral epicondylitis very often has a myofascial origin and can be traced back to the formation of trigger points in the supinator muscle (see hand extensors, above).
The origin of the supinator muscle is on the lateral epicondyle of the humerus, the radial collateral ligaments and annular ligaments and the ulna. Its insertion is located in the upper third of the lateral surface of the radius. Its function is supination of the forearm and its innervation is from the radial nerve (C5–C7; Fig. 16.5).

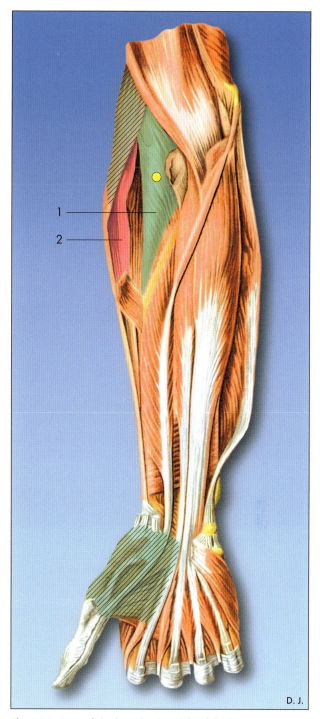

Fig. 16.5 Area of the lateral epicondyle of the humerus. (1) Supinator muscle, (2) extensor carpi radialis longus muscle. Myofascial trigger points (yellow circles) and referred pain (hatched green = lateral epicondyle of the humerus and thumb region). *Adapted from Travell and Simons [3]*

Symptoms
Stabbing elbow pain (lateral epicondyle) radiating as far as the thumb (Fig. 16.5). Almost all patients with pain in the area of the lateral epicondyle have an active TrP in the supinator muscle.

151

Chapter 16

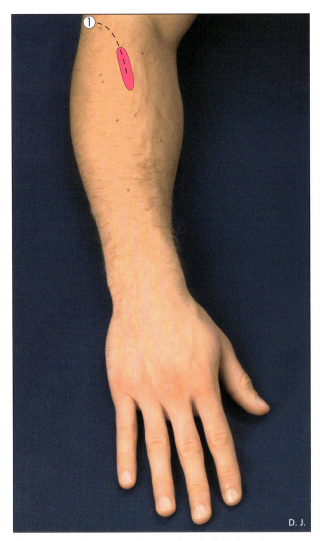

Fig. 16.6a Supinator muscle. Locating the injection site. (1) Lateral epicondyle of the humerus. Muscle groove between the extensor carpi radialis muscle and the extensor digitorum muscle

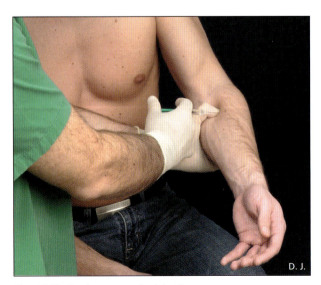

Fig. 16.6b Supinator muscle. Injection

Procedure

Materials
Sterile precautions, 23-G needle 30 mm long, 2-mL and 5-mL syringes, swabs, local anesthetic.

Injection technique
The needle is introduced directly lateral to the insertion of the biceps tendon (with the brachioradialis muscle pushed to the side) and advanced until bone contact is made with the radius. The needle is withdrawn slightly and the local anesthetic is then injected (Fig. 16.6). The extensor carpi radialis brevis muscle is usually penetrated as this is done.

Dosage
1 mL local anesthetic per TrP – e.g. 0.5% ropivacaine or 1% prilocaine (which may be mixed with 40 mg methylprednisolone if needed).

Area of the medial epicondyle ("golfer's elbow")

The area of the medial epicondyle, with its muscular components (pronator teres muscle, flexor carpi radialis and ulnaris muscles, and palmaris longus muscle) is often affected in golfers.

Palmaris longus muscle (Dupuytren's contracture)

The **anatomical insertions** of this muscle are located on the medial epicondyle of the humerus and on the palmar fascia, between the flexor carpi radialis muscle and the flexor carpi ulnaris muscle (Fig. 16.7). The **innervation** is from the median nerve.

Symptoms
The referred pain focuses on the wrist in the form of a superficial, needle-pricking pain. Experience shows that patients with Dupuytren's contracture often have one or more active trigger points (TrPs) in the fibers of the palmaris longus muscle (Fig. 16.7).

Procedure

Materials
Sterile precautions, 23-G needle 30 mm long, 2-mL and 5-mL syringes, swabs, local anesthetic.

Injection technique

The patient lies supine, with the affected elbow extended (Fig. 16.8a). After palpation of the TrP, the needle is introduced perpendicularly (Fig. 16.8b), the TrP is located and the local anesthetic is injected.

Dosage

1 mL local anesthetic per TrP – e.g. 0.5% ropivacaine or 1% prilocaine.

Pronator teres muscle

The pronator teres muscle is responsible for pronation of the forearm and flexion of the elbow. Its origin is on the medial epicondyle of the humerus, the antebrachial fascia and the coronoid process of the ulna, and its insertion is on the dorsal surface of the middle third of the radius. The innervation is from the median nerve (C6 and C7; Fig. 16.7).

Procedure

Materials
Sterile precautions, 22-G needle 30 mm long, 2-mL and 5-mL syringes, swabs, local anesthetic.

Injection technique

The patient lies supine, with the affected elbow extended (Fig. 16.8a). The injection technique is illustrated in Fig. 16.9. The flexor carpi radialis muscle is often also involved.

Dosage

1 mL local anesthetic per TrP – e.g. 0.5% ropivacaine or 1% prilocaine.

Hand and finger flexors in the forearm: flexor carpi radialis and ulnaris muscles

The **anatomic insertions** of the hand and finger flexors are located on the medial epicondyle and the distal phalanges of all of the fingers (Fig. 16.7). **The flexor carpi radialis muscle** is responsible for palmar flexion and radial abduction in the wrist, for pronation and elbow flexion, and the **flexor carpi ulnaris muscle** is responsible for palmar flexion and ulnar abduction in the wrist.

The **innervation** of the flexor carpi radialis muscle is from the median nerve (C6–C8), while that of the flexor carpi ulnaris muscle is from the ulnar nerve (C8, T1).

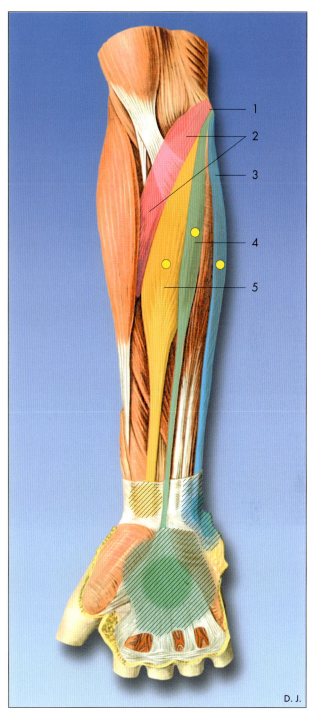

Fig. 16.7 Area of (1) the medial condyle of the humerus. (2) Pronator teres muscle, (3) flexor carpi ulnaris muscle, (4) palmaris longus muscle, (5) flexor carpi radialis muscle. Myofascial trigger points (yellow circles) and referred pain (hatched, yellow = flexor carpi radialis muscle, blue = flexor carpi ulnaris muscle, green = palmaris longus muscle). *Adapted from Travell and Simons [3]*

Chapter 16

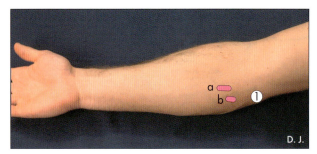

Fig. 16.8a Pronator teres muscle (a), palmaris longus muscle (b). Medial epicondyle of the humerus (1). Locating the injection sites

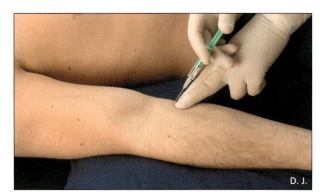

Fig. 16.8b Palmaris longus muscle. Injection

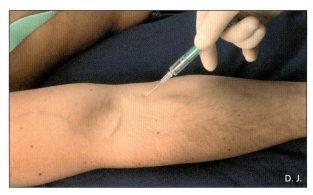

Fig. 16.9 Pronator teres muscle. Injection

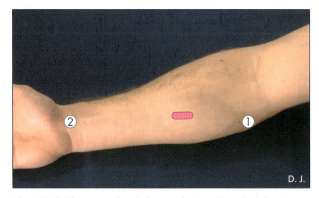

Fig. 16.10 Flexor carpi radialis muscle. Locating the injection site. (1) Medial epicondyle of the humerus, (2) muscle tendon

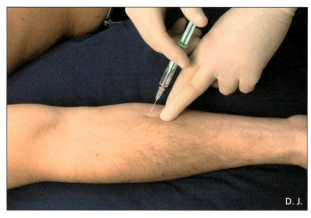

Fig. 16.11 Flexor carpi radialis muscle. Injection

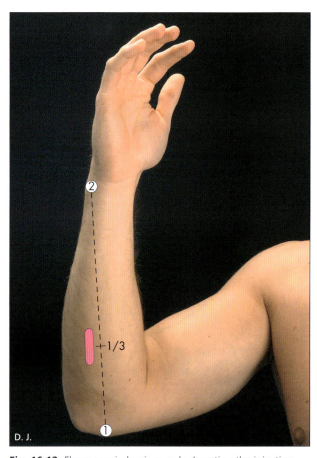

Fig. 16.12 Flexor carpi ulnaris muscle. Locating the injection site. (1) Medial epicondyle of the humerus, (2) styloid process of the ulna

Symptoms
Pain in the radial part of the palmar wrist fold (flexor carpi radialis muscle) or radiating to the ulnar side of the palmar surface of the hand (flexor carpi ulnaris muscle; Fig. 16.7).

Procedure

Materials
Sterile precautions, 23-G needle 30 mm long, 2-mL and 5-mL syringes, swabs, local anesthetic.

Injection technique
Flexor carpi radialis muscle: the patient lies in the supine position, with the affected elbow extended. After location and palpation (Fig. 16.10), the needle is introduced perpendicularly until bone contact is made. It is then withdrawn as far as the subcutaneous tissue and the injection is carried out (Fig. 16.11). To infiltrate an active TrP in **the flexor carpi ulnaris muscle** (the most superficial muscle), the patient's arm is bent, the TrP is located using extensive palpation (Fig. 16.12), and infiltration is carried out with direct tactile guidance (Fig. 16.13).

Dosage
1 mL local anesthetic per TrP – e.g. 0.5% ropivacaine or 1% prilocaine.

Intra-articular injection into the elbow joint

The **anatomy** of the elbow joint is shown in Fig. 16.14.

Indications
Pain on movement of the elbow joint, difficulty and pain in extending and bending the distal phalanx.

Procedure

Materials
Sterile precautions, 22-G needle 30 mm long, 2-mL and 5-mL syringes, swabs, local anesthetic (corticosteroids).

Injection technique

> As strict as possible aseptic conditions!

The patient places the forearm on the table, so that the upper arm and forearm form an angle of 90°. The needle is introduced from the dorsal direction, between the lateral epicondyle and the olecranon into the olecranon fossa in a mediopalmar direction (lateral to the tendon of the triceps muscle; Fig. 16.15). The articular cavity is reached after ca. 1 cm.

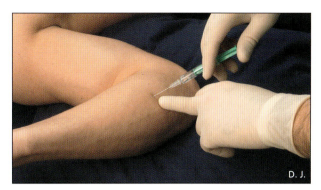

Fig. 16.13 Flexor carpi ulnaris. Injection

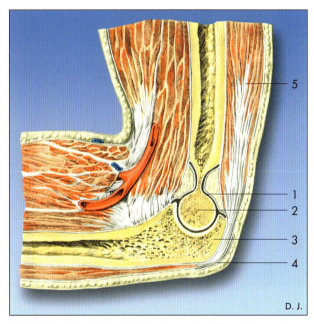

Fig. 16.14 Elbow joint. (1) Articular cavity, (2) trochlea of the humerus, (3) olecranon, (4) subcutaneous olecranon bursa, (5) triceps brachii muscle

Dosage
1–2 mL local anesthetic – e.g. 0.5–0.75% ropivacaine (which may be mixed with 40 mg methylprednisolone if needed).

Complications
Infection (prophylaxis: as strict as possible aseptic conditions), hematoma (prophylactic compression should be carried out after the injection).

Chapter 16

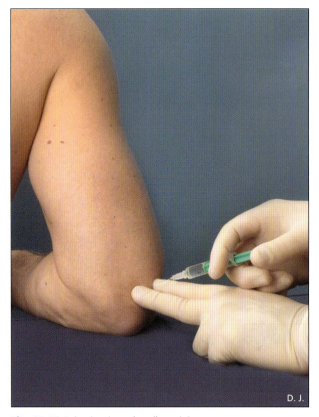

Fig. 16.15 Injection into the elbow joint

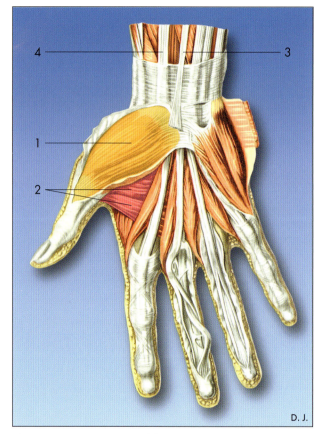

Fig. 16.16 Wrist. Anatomy: (1) opponens pollicis muscle, (2) adductor pollicis muscle, (3) palmaris longus muscle, (4) flexor carpi radialis muscle

Wrist

Adductor pollicis and opponens pollicis muscles ("Weeder's Thumb")

An active trigger point (TrP) in the **adductor pollicis muscle** causes severe pain along the radial side of the thumb and in the hand at the base of the thumb distal to the fold of the wrist. Pain from TrPs in this muscle is referred to the palmar surface of most of the thumb and wrist (Fig. 16.16). The adductor pollicis muscle adducts the carpometacarpal joint and metacarpophalangeal joint. Its innervation is from the ulnar nerve (C8, T1). The function of the **opponens pollicis muscle** (Fig. 16.16) is opposition at the carometacarpal joint of the thumb (flexion, abduction and slight rotation). Its innervation is from the median nerve (C7, C8, T1).

Symptoms
Pain, poorly controlled movements, and absence of fine movement in the thumb.

Procedure

Materials
Sterile precautions, 22-G needle 30 mm long, , swabs, local anesthetic.

Injection technique
Adductor pollicis muscle: the thumb is abducted and the located trigger points are infiltrated from the dorsal direction, in the area of the fold (Fig. 16.17).
With the thumb abducted, the TrP of the **opponens pollicis muscle** is reached in the upper thenar area and in the direction of the metacarpal bone (Fig. 16.18). The injection may be painful.

Infiltration therapy in carpal tunnel syndrome

The most frequent peripheral nerve compression syndrome is carpal tunnel syndrome. Predisposing factors include obesity, chronic polyarthritis, diabetes mellitus, gout and dysproteinemia. The feature common to all of these conditions is that they increase the content of the carpal tunnel. This compresses the median nerve (Fig.

Elbow and wrist, Infiltration of the myofascial trigger points and intra-articuar injections

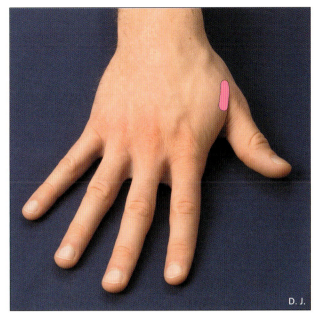

Fig. 16.17a Adductor pollicis muscle. Locating the injection site

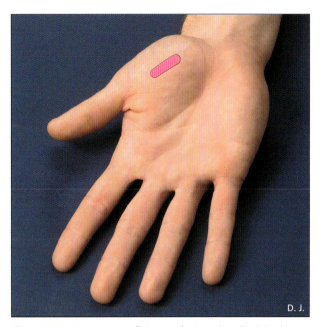

Fig. 16.18a Opponens pollicis muscle. Locating the injection site

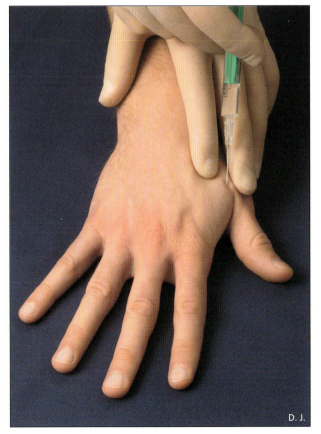

Fig. 16.17b Adductor pollicis muscle. Injection

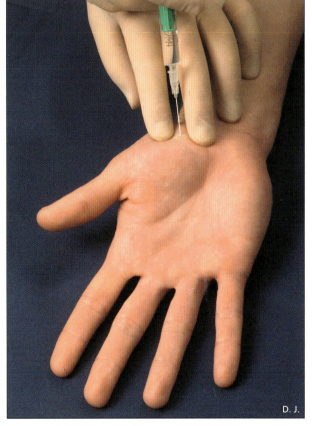

Fig. 16.18b Opponens pollicis muscle. Injection

157

16.16; see also Chapter 15, Fig. 15.1). Typically, carpal tunnel syndrome is associated with sensory and later with motor disturbances. Patients wake in the morning or at night with a feeling that their hands have "gone to sleep." The symptoms are provoked by pressure on the flexor retinaculum.

Procedure

Materials
Sterile precautions, **very short-beveled needle** – e.g. 24-G Plexufix 25 mm long (see Chapter 9, brachial plexus, Fig. 9.6a), swabs, local anesthetic, corticosteroid.

Injection technique
The needle is introduced at the level of the proximal wrist crease between the tendons of the **palmaris longus muscle** and the **flexor carpi radialis muscle** (Fig. 16.19). At a depth of 0.5–1 cm, paresthesias (median nerve) are often elicited. The needle is then withdrawn minimally, an intraneural position is excluded, and after aspiration the local anesthetic is injected.

Dosage
2 mL local anesthetic – e.g. 0.5–0.75% ropivacaine mixed with 40 mg methylprednisolone.

Complications
Infection, intravascular injection, neuritis after nerve puncture (prophylaxis: using short-beveled needles).

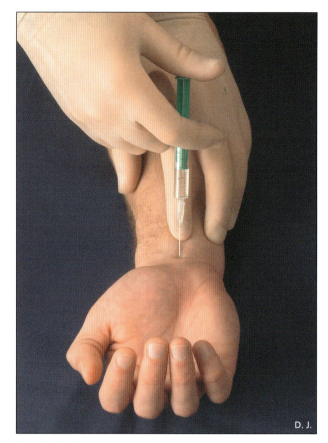

Fig. 16.19 Carpal tunnel syndrome. Injection

17 Intravenous regional anesthesia (IVRA)

The injection of local anesthetics into a vein in an exsanguinated extremity was first described by August Bier in 1908. It caused anesthesia and a motor block.

Indications
Outpatient surgical procedures with a maximum length of 1 hour in the forearm or hand (standard application) and in the lower leg and foot (more rarely; Figs. 17.1–17.3).

Specific contraindications
- Patient refusal
- Local infection in the area to be anesthetized
- Local nerve damage
- Peripheral vascular diseases
- Severe decompensated hypovolemia, shock
- Certain cardiovascular diseases
- Hypertonia, bradycardia, second-degree AV block, any history of a tendency to syncope
- Musculoskeletal diseases

Procedure

This block should only be carried out when full anesthetic facilities are available. Full prior information for the patient is mandatory.

Preparations
Check that the appropriate emergency equipment is present and in working order. Sterile precautions. Two intravenous access points (in the healthy extremity as well as the one being operated on), BP and ECG monitoring, pulse oximetry, anesthesia machine. Patient preparation is the same as for general anesthesia.

Materials (Fig. 17.4)
20-mL and 50-mL syringes, saline, cotton-wool padding, pneumatic tourniquet (double-lumen), Esmarch bandage, local anesthetic, disinfectant, pneumatic tourniquet device (e.g. VBM Medizintechnik Ltd., Sulz am Neckar, Germany; Fig. 17.5).

Patient positioning
Supine, with the extremity free.

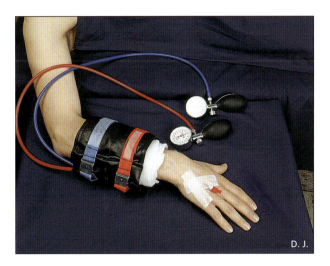

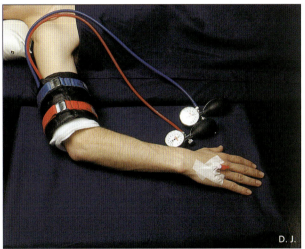

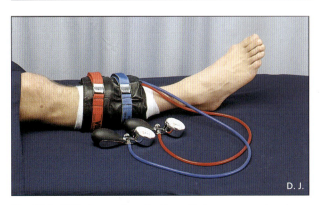

Fig. 17.1–17.3 Areas of application of intravenous regional anesthesia

Chapter 17

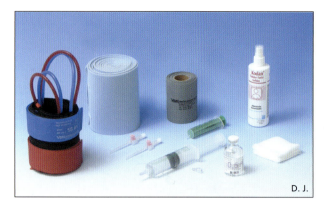

Fig. 17.4 Materials

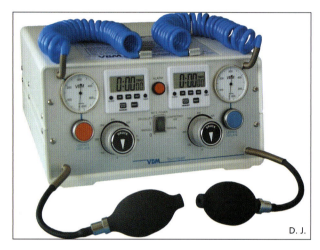

Fig. 17.5 Pneumatic tourniquet device (VBM Medizintechnik Ltd., Sulz am Neckar, Germany)

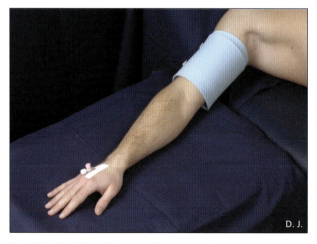

Fig. 17.6 Padding of the tourniquet area, intravenous access

Technical procedure
1. Insert two intravenous catheters – one in a healthy extremity and the other as distally as possible in the extremity being operated on.
2. Place the extremity being operated on in a free position and put soft padding under the tourniquet to help prevent nerve injury (Fig. 17.6).
3. Position the double-lumen tourniquet.
4. Elevate and massage the limb for a few minutes, then wrap it completely with an Esmarch bandage (Fig. 17.7).
5. Inflate the proximal cuff: the pressure in the cuff has to be ca. 80–100 mmHg higher than the patient's systolic blood pressure. The pressure that should be used depends on the thickness of the muscles being compressed. A pulse oximeter is used to document changes in, and cessation of, the pulse ("pulse occlusion pressure"), and the disappearance of the pulse in the radial artery. The "pulse occlusion pressure" can be used to determine the optimal pressure in the proximal cuff (Fig. 17.8).
6. Remove the bandage and place the extremity in a horizontal position.
7. Slowly inject the local anesthetic (20 mL/min; Fig. 17.9).
8. Perform stroking massage of the extremity (this improves the spread of the local anesthetic) and remove the catheters.
9. Good analgesia and muscle relaxation develop after ca. 5–10 min.
10. Inflation of the distal cuff, which is now in the analgesic area, so that the cuff is better tolerated. Deflate the proximal cuff. After the anesthetic effect has been tested, the operation can begin.

- Minimum tourniquet time is 15–20 min after injection of the local anesthetic. The tourniquet must not be released during this period (risk of toxic reactions!).
- Tourniquet pressure must be monitored continuously.
- After completion of the procedure: intermittent deflation over a period of 10 min, with complete inflation in between (Fig. 17.10).

Intravenous regional anesthesia (IVRA)

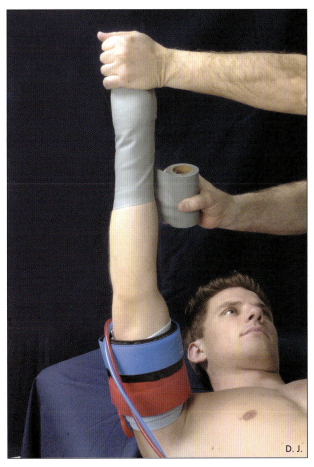
Fig. 17.7 Wrapping with an Esmarch bandage

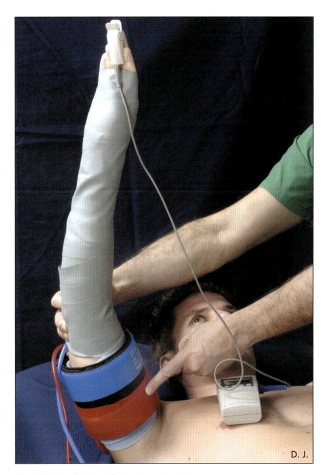
Fig. 17.8 Inflation of the tourniquet

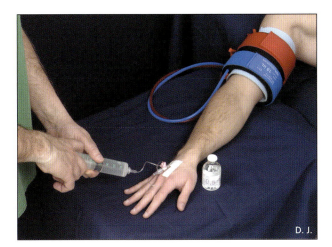
Fig. 17.9 Injection of the local anesthetic

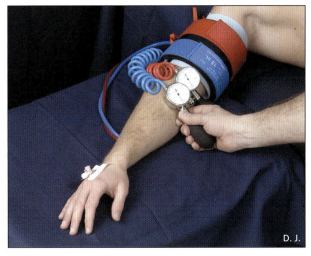
Fig. 17.10 Intermittent deflation of the cuff over a period of 10 min

Dosage

> Only local anesthetics that contain no vasoconstrictors may be used!

40–50 mL local anesthetic, e.g.
- Prilocaine 0.5%, 3–4 (5) mg/kg body weight [6,7]. Amongst the amide local anesthetics, prilocaine provides the best ratio between anesthetic potency and toxicity, and should be regarded as the agent of choice for intravenous regional anesthesia (see Chapter 1, p. 12).
- Mepivacaine 0.5% or lidocaine 0.5%, 1.5–3 mg/kg b.w. [6].

Additions to local anesthetic agents
- Clonidine 1 µg/kg or ketamine 0.1 mg/kg b.w. [3]
- Fentanyl (0.1–0.2 mg) [1]
- Morphine (1–6 mg) [2]

Complications
- Systemic toxic reactions can occur if the local anesthetic enters the circulation due to release of the tourniquet cuff (see Chapter 1, Table 1.7 and Chapter 6, p. 66).
Prophylaxis: intermittent opening of the tourniquet, maintaining verbal contact with the patient, avoiding strong premedication.
- Toxic effects on the cardiovascular system only occur after very high doses of local anesthetic and become apparent as a drop in blood pressure, bradycardia, circulatory collapse and cardiac arrest. This type of complication rarely occurs in intravenous regional anesthesia.
- Nerve damage due to the cuff pressure.

Advantages
- Simple technique
- No specific anatomical expertise is needed
- Wide safety margins and very high success rate (>98%) [7]
- Fast onset of effect (5–10 min)
- Good muscle relaxation
- Controllable spread of the anesthesia (below the tourniquet cuff)
- Fast return of sensation
- No risk of infection

Disadvantages
- Tourniquet cuff is needed
- Limited operating time (<1 h)
- Procedures in the upper arm are not possible
- Tourniquet pain during the procedure
- Nerve damage due to the tourniquet cuff
- Does not provide a blood-free operating area
- Insufficient postoperative analgesia due to fast recovery from the anesthesia

Intravenous regional anesthesia

Name: _____ Date: _____
Diagnosis: _____
Premedication: ☐ No ☐ Yes _____

Purpose of block:	☐ Surgical
i.v. access:	☐ No. 1 ☐ No. 2
Monitoring:	☐ ECG ☐ Pulse oximetry
Ventilation facilities:	☐ Yes (equipment checked)
Emergency equipment *(drugs)*:	☐ Checked
Patient:	☐ Informed

Position: ☐ Supine ☐ Other
Location of the tourniquet cuff: ☐ Right ☐ Left
☐ Forearm ☐ Upper arm ☐ Lower leg ☐ Thigh
BP: _____ mmHg Pulse _____ min
Ischemia: _____ mmHg At _____
Local anesthetic: _____ mL _____ % _____
☐ Addition to LA: _____ mL _____ µg
Ischemia: From _____ To _____
Cuff release over: ☐ 5 min ☐ 10 min intermittently

Patient's remarks during injection: ☐ None
☐ Pain ☐ Paresthesias ☐ Warmth ☐ Cold
Objective block effect after: ☐ 5 min ☐ 10 min
 ☐ Temperature measurement right _____°C left_____°C
☐ Sensory ☐ Motor
Monitoring after block: ☐ < 1 h ☐ > 1 h
 Time of discharge _____

Complications and side effects: ☐ None
☐ BP reduction ☐ Bradycardia ☐ Cardiac arrhythmia
☐ Fatigue ☐ Tingling lips ☐ Tongue paresthesia
☐ Perioral numbness ☐ Metallic taste ☐ Anxiety
☐ Restlessness ☐ Trembling ☐ Other

Special notes:
_____
_____
_____
_____
_____
_____
_____
_____
_____

Record and checklist

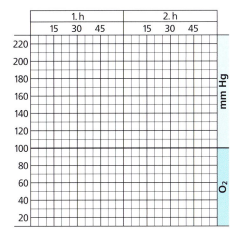

© Copyright ABW Wissenschaftsverlag 2004,
Jankovic, Regional nerve blocks and infiltration therapy, 3rd edition

18 Intravenous sympathetic block with guanethidine (Ismelin®)

Introduction

Guanethidine (1-[2-(perhydroazocin-1-yl)ethyl]guanidine monosulfate) is an inhibitor substance that acts at the postganglionic sympathetic efferents. Its pharmacological effect is based on depleting norepinephrine stores, with consequent block of the reuptake of the transmitter for several days. The substance, also used as an antihypertensive drug, is around 6800 times more effective than procaine for intravenous sympathetic block (microsympathectomy), and has been described as the "local anesthetic for the sympathetic nervous system" [5].

Other sympathetic blocking drugs have been used, such as reserpine or brotylium. There is controversy surrounding the need for guanethidine and whether it produces any useful effect.

Figures 17.1–17.3 (see Chapter 17, p. 159) show the most frequent areas of application for i.v. regional anesthesia.

Intravenous sympathetic block with guanethidine

Indications
Intravenous sympathetic block is a good alternative to stellate ganglion or plexus blocks when these are contraindicated or regional anesthesia cannot be used in patients receiving anticoagulant treatment.

Diagnostic
- Complex regional pain syndrome (CRPS)

Therapeutic
- Complex regional pain syndrome (CRPS) type I (sympathetic reflex dystrophy) and type II (causalgia)
- Perfusion disturbances in the extremities with burning pain, accompanied by hyperesthesia, hyperpathia, sensitivity to cold
- Post-sympathectomy syndrome
- Raynaud's disease
- Ischemic ulcers
- Diabetic angioneuropathy
- Post-traumatic neuralgia [9]

Specific contraindications
Infected extremity.

Procedure

This block should only be carried out when full anesthetic facilities are available.

Preparations
Check that the emergency equipment is complete and in working order. Sterile precautions. Two intravenous access points (healthy extremity and extremity being treated), BP and ECG monitoring, pulse oximetry, anesthetic machine.

Materials
5-mL syringe, 10-mL syringe, 20-mL syringe, 50-mL perfusion syringe, saline, cotton-wool cushioning, tourniquet (two-lumen with color-indicated proximal and distal parts), intubation kit, emergency drugs ready to hand, disinfectant (Fig. 18.1).

Skin prep
In all blocks.

Patient positioning
Supine, with the extremity free.

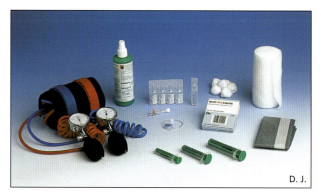

Fig. 18.1 Materials

Intravenous sympathetic block with guanethidine (Ismelin®)

Technical procedure

1. Place two plastic indwelling catheters, the first in a healthy extremity, and the second as distally as possible in the extremity being treated.
2. Place the extremity being treated in a free position and protect the tourniquet area for prophylaxis against nerve injury (Fig. 18.2).
3. Place the double-lumen cuff, with colored markers at the proximal and distal ends (Fig. 18.3).
4. Raise the extremity for ca. 5 min and massage it (Fig. 18.4).
5. Inflate the proximal cuff. The pressure must be ca. 100 mmHg higher than the patient's systolic blood pressure (Fig. 18.5). The change in the pulse wave amplitude is documented using a pulse oximeter.
6. Place the extremity horizontally and inject 5 mL local anesthetic – e.g. 1% prilocaine – through the plastic indwelling catheter (Fig. 18.6). Administration of the local anesthetic serves to reduce both pressure pain and pain after guanethidine administration to a tolerable level.
7. The distal cuff is then inflated. Here again, the pressure must be ca. 100 mmHg higher than the patient's systolic blood pressure. The distal cuff now lies in the anesthetized area, and the cuff pressure is better tolerated. Release the proximal cuff. Inject the guanethidine and allow it ca. 20 min to bind (Figs. 18.7 and 18.8).
8. To improve the distribution of the sympatholytic agent, the extremity must be moved about and constantly massaged during this period (Fig. 18.9).
9. After ca. 20 min, inflate the proximal cuff once again (ca. 100 mmHg above the patient's systolic pressure; Fig. 18.10).
10. After a further 10 min, slowly deflate the distal and proximal cuffs alternately, step by step (Fig. 18.11). This reduces reperfusion of the still unbound guanethidine to a minimum, and prevents systemic sympatholysis with a fall in blood pressure and bradycardia. At the end of the block, the patient must be monitored for one hour.

> The tourniquet should be applied as far distally as possible. This allows an optimal dose–effect ratio. During the block, the pressure in the block cuff must be constantly checked.
> Since accidental intravenous spread of the local anesthetic and/or the guanethidine can never be excluded, the patient must be carefully and constantly monitored.

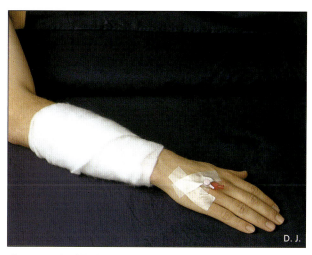

Fig. 18.2 The block area is wrapped

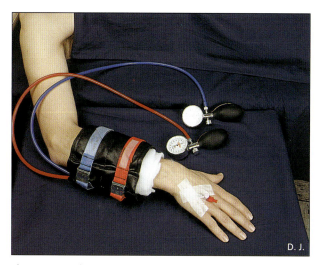

Fig. 18.3 Applying the cuff

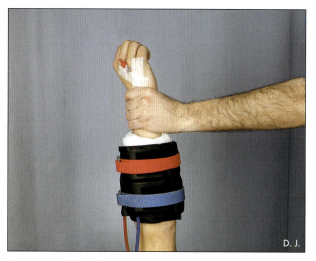

Fig. 18.4 Raising the extremity

Chapter 18

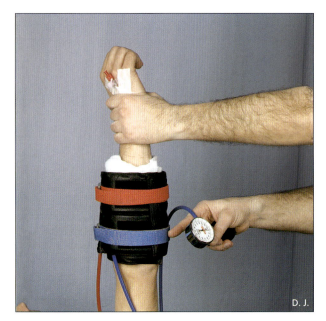

Fig. 18.5 Inflating the proximal section

Effects of the block

Two frequently occurring effects of the block are vasodilation (increased skin temperature and pulse wave) and inhibition of sweat gland function.

In particular, measurement of skin temperature before and after the block and comparison with the contralateral side is a reliable criterion for a successful block. Usually, the extremity being treated feels warmest on the first day after the block.

> During informed consent, the patient should be informed that fatigue, and rarely general weakness, may occur on the day of treatment or the following day. Complete elimination of the guanethidine takes up to 3 weeks.

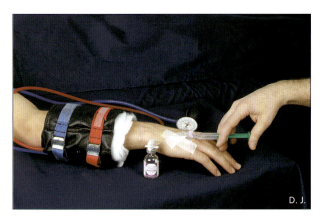

Fig. 18.6 Injecting 5 mL 1% prilocaine

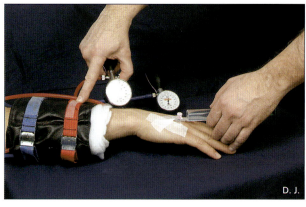

Fig. 18.7 The distal part of the cuff is inflated, and the proximal part is released

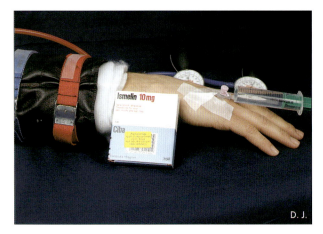

Fig. 18.8 The guanethidine is injected

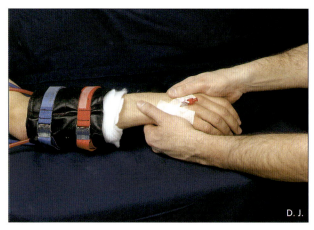

Fig. 18.9 The extremity must be constantly moved and massaged to ensure good distribution of the sympatholytic agent

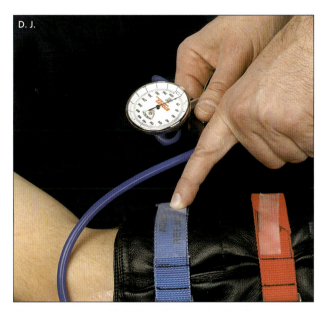

Fig. 18.10 Repeated inflation of the proximal cuff section

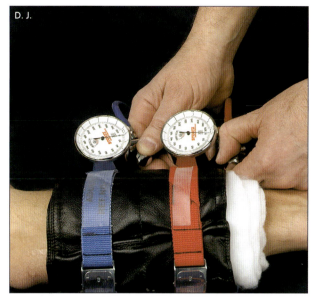

Fig. 18.11 The distal and proximal cuff sections are slowly and alternately released

Dosage
Diagnostic
5–10 mg guanethidine in 20 mL sodium chloride solution.

> No prophylactic administration of local anesthetic.

Therapeutic
Prophylactic administration of 5 mL of a local anesthetic – e.g. 1% prilocaine.
Forearm: 10–15 mg guanethidine in 20 mL sodium chloride solution.
Upper arm: 15–20 mg guanethidine in 30 mL sodium chloride solution.
Lower leg: 20-25 mg guanethidine in 50 mL sodium chloride solution.

Block series
An initial series of two or three therapeutic blocks can be carried out at intervals of 3–5 days. Thereafter, and only if there is clear evidence of effectiveness, periodic repetition is possible.

Side effects
Injection pain, tourniquet pain (prophylactic administration of a local anesthetic in therapeutic blocks, possibly with mild sedation), hypotension.

Complications
When the details of the technical procedure and dosage are precisely observed, no complications are expected.

Record and checklist

Intravenous sympathetic block
Block no. ☐ Right ☐ Left

Name: _____ Date: _____
Diagnosis: _____
Premedication: ☐ No ☐ Yes _____

Purpose of block:	☐ Diagnostic	☐ Therapeutic
i.v. access:	☐ No. 1	☐ No. 2
Monitoring:	☐ ECG	☐ Pulse oximetry
Ventilation facilities:	☐ Yes (equipment checked)	
Emergency equipment (drugs):	☐ Checked	
Patient:	☐ Informed	

Position: ☐ Supine
Location of the tourniquet cuff:
☐ Forearm ☐ Upper arm ☐ Lower leg ☐ Thigh
Local anesthetic: ☐ No ☐ Yes _____ mL _____ % _____
Injection mixture: Guanethidine _____ mg
                   NaCl 0,9 % _____ mL
Ischemic time: From _____ To _____ ☐ 20 min ☐ 25 min ☐ 30 min
Cuff release over: ☐ 5 min ☐ 10 min intermittently

Patient's remarks during injection: ☐ None
☐ Pain ☐ Paresthesias ☐ Warmth ☐ Cold
Objective block effect after 15 min:
☐ Temperature measurement right _____ °C left _____ °C
☐ Sensory ☐ Motor
Monitoring after block: ☐ < 1 h ☐ > 1 h
          Time of discharge _____

Complications and side effects:
☐ BP reduction ☐ Bradycardia ☐ Fatigue
☐ Cardiac arrhythmia ☐ Other _____

Subjective effects of the block: Duration: _____
☐ None ☐ Increased pain
☐ Reduced pain ☐ Relief of pain

VISUAL ANALOG SCALE

0 10 20 30 40 50 60 70 80 90 100

Special notes:
_____
_____
_____
_____
_____
_____

Thorax, abdomen, lumbar spinal and sacral region

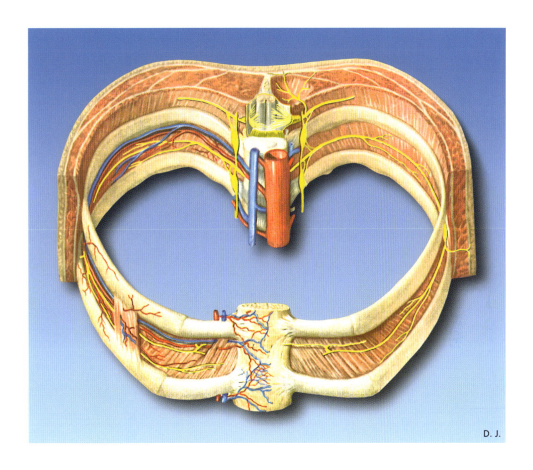

Thorax

19 Thoracic spinal nerve blocks

Anatomy

The thoracic spinal nerves form 12 pairs, which with the exception of the first two are narrow compared with the lower half of the cervical nerves. These spinal nerves emerge from the spinal cord with two roots – the receptor sensory dorsal root (posterior) and the effector motor ventral root (anterior) (Fig. 19.1). After leaving the dural sac, the two roots are surrounded by a dural sheath. The sensory root expands by taking up numerous nerve cells to form the **spinal ganglion**. Beyond the ganglion, the roots form a common mixed spinal nerve trunk, which divides into four branches after exiting through the intervertebral foramen:

- The **dorsal primary rami,**
- the **ventral primary rami,**
- the **meningeal branches**
  (which supply the spinal canal and the meninges), and
- The **white and gray communicating branches,** which anastomose with each neighboring ganglion of the sympathetic trunk and thus extend to the viscera and vessels, mediating and involving the sympathetic nervous system.
  They also carry sympathetic fibers to the spine.

The **dorsal rami of the thoracic nerves** pass between the two transverse processes to their area of distribution, and divide into the two typical branches, the medial and lateral branches; they give off muscular branches (back muscles) and cutaneous branches (spinous processes, posterior wall of the thorax, and lumbar region).

The **ventral rami of the thoracic nerves** are also termed **intercostal nerves,** and they are distributed segmentally (Fig. 19.2).

The 11 upper nerves are (relative to the thoracic ribs) genuinely intercostal, while the twelfth lies caudal to the twelfth rib and is known as the **subcostal nerve.** The six upper intercostal nerves run entirely in the in-

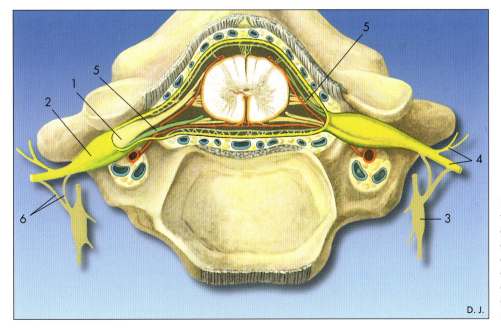

Fig. 19.1 Anatomy of the thoracic spinal nerves. (1) Spinal ganglion, (2) spinal nerve, (3) ganglion of the sympathetic trunk, (4) dorsal and ventral branch, (5) dorsal and ventral root, (6) white and gray communicating branches

tercostal spaces, as far as the edge of the sternum; the six lower ones reach the area of the linea alba. All of the intercostal nerves, with the exception of the twelfth, run in the relevant intercostal space in front of the superior costotransverse ligament and on the inner surface of the **external intercostal muscles.**

The **internal intercostal muscles** are absent from the spine far as the costal angle. Over this area, the intercostal nerves are only covered by the **endothoracic fascia** and **costal pleura.**

At the start of the internal intercostal muscles, the nerves lie between these muscles and the external intercostal muscles, and they are accompanied by the **intercostal vessels** (the **intercostal artery and vein**). They lie caudal to the vessels.

Special care needs to be taken during procedures, as due to the proximity of blood vessels to the nerves, toxic concentrations of local anesthetic can easily be reached.

Branches of the intercostal nerves
- **Muscular branches**
  It is advisable to distinguish between the six upper intercostal nerve pairs (which supply the subcostal muscle, serratus posterior superior muscle, and transversus thoracis muscle) and the lower five (which supply the subcostal muscle, serratus posterior inferior muscle, and transversus, obliquus, and rectus abdominis muscles).
- **Lateral cutaneous branches**
  For the skin and lateral sides of the thorax and abdomen. A small part of the first intercostal nerve (inferior trunk of the brachial plexus) supplies the skin of the axilla.
- **Anterior cutaneous branches**
  Supply the anterior side of the thorax.
- **Pleural and peritoneal branches**
  Supply the pleura and thoracic wall and the peritoneum of the lateral and anterior abdominal wall, as well as the pleural and peritoneal covering at the origin of the diaphragm.

Thoracic paravertebral somatic nerve block

Definition
A dorsal somatic block of the thoracic intercostal nerve below the transverse process, in its area of origin just after it exits from the intervertebral foramen and courses through the paravertebral space.

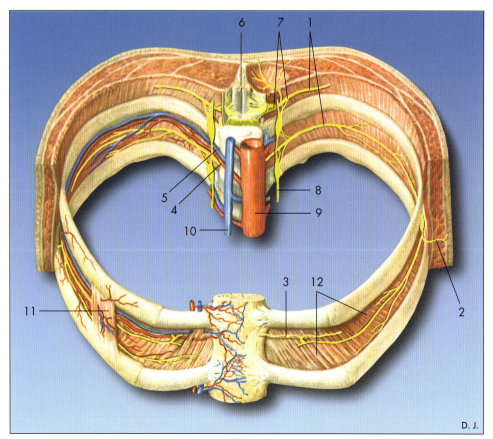

Fig. 19.2 Intercostal nerves. (1) Ventral branches (intercostal nerves), (2) lateral cutaneous branch, (3) anterior cutaneous branch, (4) posterior intercostal artery, (5) posterior intercostal vein, (6) spinal cord, (7) spinal nerve, (8) sympathetic trunk, (9) thoracic aorta, (10) azygos vein, (11) external intercostal muscles, (12) internal intercostal muscles

Indications

Surgical
- Inguinal herniorrhaphy (in combination with a lumbar paravertebral somatic block, T10–L2) [9, 14]. Large doses of local anesthetic will be required.

Diagnostic
- Differential diagnosis of somatic and autonomic pain.
- Differentiation and localization of intercostal neuralgia, causalgia, cardiac pain, etc.

Therapeutic
- A series of blocks in the appropriate dermatome is particularly useful in the acute phase of herpes zoster.
- Pain in the intercostal area (neuralgia, causalgia).
- Pain after fractured ribs or contusions of the chest wall.
- Postoperative pain after upper abdominal or thoracic operations (providing relief for coughing and deep breathing).

In most of the indications mentioned, an indwelling epidural catheter is preferred (see Chapters 41 and 42).

Block series
A series of six to eight blocks is recommended. When there is evidence of improvement in the symptoms, additional blocks can also be carried out.

Contraindications
Specific
- Anticoagulant treatment.
- Infections and skin diseases in the injection area.

Relative
- Slim patients.
- Chronic obstructive lung diseases.

Procedure

This block should only be carried out by experienced anesthetists, or under their supervision. A specific indication is required. Prior information for the patient is necessary.

Preparations
Check that the emergency equipment is complete and in working order; sterile precautions, intravenous access, ECG monitoring, pulse oximetry, intubation kit, ventilation facilities, emergency medication.

Materials (Fig. 19.3)
Fine 26-G needle, 25 mm long, for local anesthesia.
Atraumatic 24-G needle, 0.7 × 80 mm (15°) with injection lead (e.g. Stimuplex D®, B. Braun Melsungen) or 24-G spinal needle, 0.6 × 80 mm.
Syringes: 2, 5, and 10 mL.
Local anesthetic, disinfectant, swabs, sterile gloves and drape; flat, firm pillow.

Patient positioning
- **Prone position:** cushioned with a pillow under the lower thorax and upper abdomen. The patient's arms hang to the sides (Fig. 19.4).
  For blocks of the upper four thoracic nerves, it is recommended that the patient's head is positioned projecting over the end of the table, supported by an assistant (Fig. 19.10).
- Sitting: with the trunk leant forward (Fig. 19.13b).

Location
- Vertebra prominens (nuchal tubercle) (count down caudally).
- Iliac crest line of L4 (count up cranially).

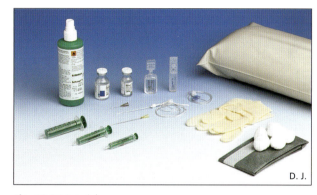

Fig. 19.3 Materials

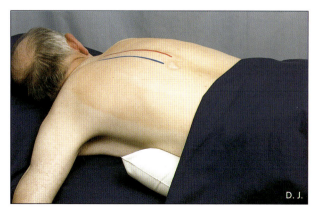

Fig. 19.4 Prone position

Chapter 19

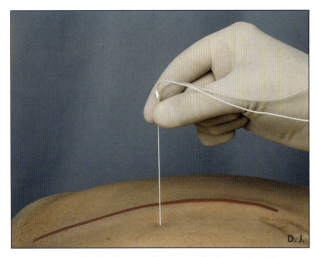

Fig. 19.5 Introducing the needle perpendicular to the skin surface

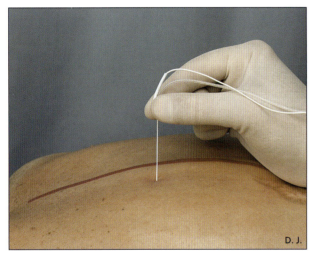

Fig. 19.6a Bone contact (transverse process)

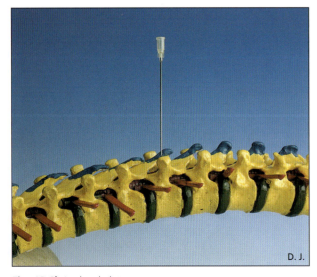

Fig. 19.6b In the skeleton

■ Upper edge of the transverse process selected.
A horizontal line is drawn on the segment above the level being blocked. The injection point is located ca. 3.5–4 cm (two fingerbreadths) paramedian to this.

Skin prep, local anesthesia, covering with a sterile drape, drawing up the local anesthetic, testing the patency of the injection needle.

During the injection, the following points must be observed without fail:
■ The person carrying out the injection must stand on the side being blocked.
■ The injection point must not be located more than 4 cm lateral to the midline (rib contact, risk of pneumothorax!)
■ There is a risk of perforating the dural cuff if the injection is made too far medially (epidural or subarachnoid injection).
■ The transverse process is ca. 0.6–0.7 cm thick.
■ If there is no bone contact after 2.5–5 cm (depending on the anatomy), the direction of the needle must be corrected (the transverse process has been missed; risk of pleural puncture).
■ If the patient coughs, it indicates pleural irritation. The procedure should be halted.
■ Eliciting paresthesias is not obligatory.
■ The injection should be carried out on an incremental basis, with frequent aspiration (blood, CSF?).

Injection technique
■ The injection needle is introduced perpendicular to the skin surface (Fig. 19.5) until bone contact is made (transverse process) (Fig. 19.6).
Depending on the anatomy, bone contact is made at a depth of 2.5–5 cm. The needle depth is marked.

Thoracic spinal nerve blocks

- The needle is withdrawn to lie subcutaneously, and introduced at an angle of 15–20° in a caudal or cranial direction, past the transverse process, up to 2 cm deeper (Fig. 19.7).
  Eliciting paresthesias is helpful, and confirms the correct position of the needle, but it is not obligatory, since optimal effectiveness of the block can be achieved with local anesthetic spread.
- After aspiration at various levels (blood, CSF?), incremental injection of local anesthetic is carried out.

After a successful somatic paravertebral block of the thoracic nerves, the injected local anesthetic diffuses via the plethora of communicating branches that are present towards the neighboring sympathetic chain, which is almost always blocked as well.

Dosage

Surgical
5 mL local anesthetic per segment (T10–L2) – e.g. 0.75 % ropivacaine or 0.5 % bupivacaine with the addition of epinephrine 1 : 400 000 [9] or 0.5 % levobupivacaine.

Diagnostic
5 mL local anesthetic per segment – e.g. 0.5% prilocaine, 0.5% mepivacaine, 0.5% lidocaine.

Therapeutic
5–10 mL local anesthetic per segment – e.g. 0.375% ropivacaine, 0.25–0.375% bupivacaine (0.25–0.375% levobupivacaine). In acute conditions (e.g. herpes zoster in the innervated area), 2–4 mg dexamethasone can be added.

Complications

- Pneumothorax (Fig. 19.8):
  This is a rare complication if the technique is carried out correctly. It is usually a small pneumothorax with spontaneous resorption. If there is any suspicion, however, a chest radiograph should be taken after 4–6 hours.
- Epidural or subarachnoid injection (avoid injecting too medially!) (see Chapter 36 and Chapter 41).
- Intravascular injection with toxic reactions (see Chapter 6, p. 65).
- Hypotension due to accompanying sympathetic block (e.g. with larger volumes of the local anesthetic).

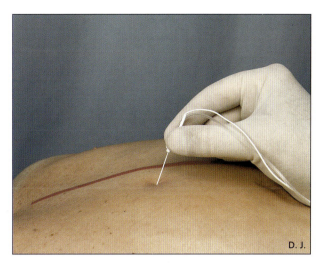

Fig. 19.7a The needle is withdrawn to lie subcutaneously and then introduced 2 cm deeper past the transverse process

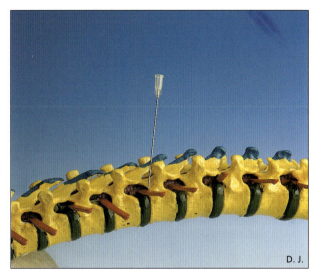

Fig. 19.7b In the skeleton

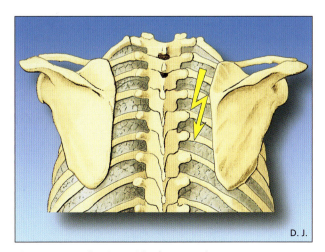

Fig. 19.8 Complications: risk of pneumothorax

Record and checklist

Thoracic paravertebral nerve block

Block no. ☐ Right ☐ Left

Name: _____ Date: _____
Diagnosis: _____
Premedication: ☐ No ☐ Yes
Neurological abnormalities: ☐ No ☐ Yes _____

Purpose of block: ☐ Diagnostic ☐ Therapeutic ☐ Surgical
Needle: G _____ Length _____ cm
i.v. access: ☐ Yes
Monitoring: ☐ ECG ☐ Pulse oximetry
Ventilation facilities: ☐ Yes (equipment checked)
Emergency equipment (drugs): ☐ Checked
Patient: ☐ Informed

Position: ☐ Prone ☐ Sitting
Injection level: ☐ T _____ _____ _____
Injection:
Local anesthetic: _____ mL _____ %
(in incremental doses)
Addition to LA: ☐ Yes _____ µg/mg ☐ No

Patient's remarks during injection:
☐ None ☐ Paresthesias ☐ Warmth ☐ Pain
Nerve area: _____
Objective block effect after 15 min:
☐ Cold test ☐ Temperature measurement right _____°C left _____°C
Segments affected: T _____
Monitoring after block: ☐ < 1 h ☐ > 1 h
Time of discharge _____

Complications:
☐ None ☐ Intravascular injection ☐ Subarachnoid/epidural
☐ Pneumothorax ☐ Other

Subjective effects of the block: Duration: _____
☐ None ☐ Increased pain
☐ Reduced pain ☐ Relief of pain

VISUAL ANALOG SCALE

0   10   20   30   40   50   60   70   80   90   100

Special notes:
_____
_____
_____
_____
_____

© Copyright ABW Wissenschaftsverlag 2004,
Jankovic, Regional nerve blocks and infiltration therapy, 3rd edition

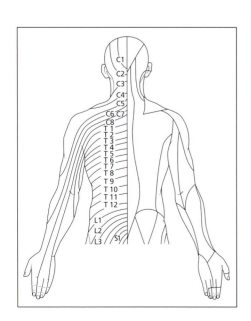

Blocks of the intercostal nerves

Definition
Block of one or more intercostal nerves at various points in their course, most often paravertebrally in the area of the costal angle, or dorsomedially in the area of the posterior axillary line; more rarely in the area of the anterior axillary line, or parasternally.

Indications
Surgical
- Superficial surgery in the innervation area.
- Insertion of a chest drain.

Diagnostic
- Differential diagnosis of somatic and autonomic pain conditions.

Therapeutic
- Pain in the intercostal area (neuralgia and causalgia).
- Pain after rib fractures or contusions of the thoracic wall, pleuritic pain.
- Acute phase of herpes zoster (in combination with a somatic paravertebral block).
- Postoperative pain therapy after upper abdominal and thoracic surgery, to relieve muscular spasms and wound pain (to allow coughing and deep breathing).

In most of the indications mentioned, an epidural catheter procedure is preferable (see Chapters 41 and 42).

Contraindications
Specific
- Anticoagulant treatment.
- Infections and skin diseases in the injection area.

Relative
- Slim patients.
- Chronic obstructive lung disease.

Procedure

Preparations
Check that the emergency equipment is complete and in working order; sterile precautions, intravenous access, ECG monitoring, pulse oximetry, endotracheal anesthesia set, ventilation facilities, emergency medication.

Materials (Fig. 19.9)
Fine 26-G needle, 25 mm long, for local anesthesia. Atraumatic 25-G needle, 0.5 × 35 mm (15°) with injection lead (e.g. Stimuplex D®, B. Braun Melsungen) or 24-G Plexufix needle, 0.55 × 25 mm. Syringes: 2, 5, and 10 mL.
Local anesthetic, disinfectant, swabs, sterile gloves and drape; flat, firm pillow (prone position).

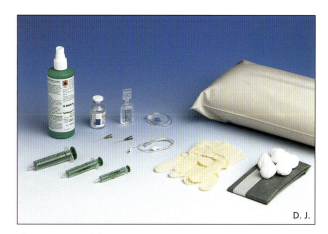

Fig. 19.9 Materials

Chapter 19

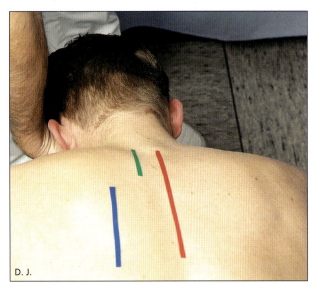

Fig. 19.10 Block of the first four intercostal nerves is carried out paravertebrally (green line)

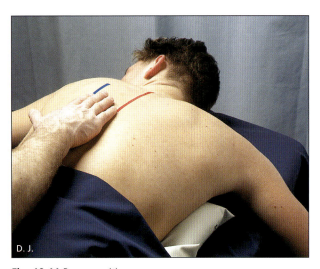

Fig. 19.11 Prone position

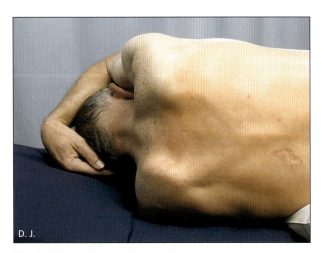

Fig. 19.12 Lateral recumbent position

The first four intercostal nerves are blocked paravertebrally, ca. 3.5–4 cm (ca. two fingerbreadths) lateral to the spinous processes (Fig. 19.10).

Intercostal block in the area of the costal angle

Patient positioning
- **Prone position:** with a pillow under the mid-abdomen, between the arch of the ribs and the iliac crest line, with the patient's arms hanging (Fig. 19.11). This position is particularly preferred with bilateral blocks.
- **Lateral recumbent:** more rarely, and with unilateral blocks (Fig. 19.12).
- **Supine:** (Fig. 19.13a).
- **Sitting:** e.g. in rib fractures (Fig. 19.13b).

Location
- Twelfth rib (count cranially).
- Costal angle (ca. 7–8 cm – four fingerbreadths – lateral to the midline and lateral to the musculature of the erector muscle of the spine) (Fig. 19.11).
- Caudal boundary of the rib being blocked (Fig. 19.14).

Skin prep, local anesthesia, covering with a sterile drape, drawing up the local anesthetic, checking the patency of the injection needle.

During the injection, the following points must be observed:
- The person carrying out the injection must stand on the side being blocked.
- The intercostal nerve runs dorsocaudal to the vessels in the inferior costal groove.
- The rib is ca. 0.6–0.7 cm thick.
- Start with the lowest rib.
- The injection must only be carried out after definite idenitification of the rib being blocked.
- Targeted paresthesias are not elicited.
- If the patient coughs, it indicates pleural irritation. The procedure should be halted.
- Injection should be carried out on an incremental basis, with frequent aspiration.

Injection technique

- The index and middle fingers of the left hand palpate the rib being blocked, and press the skin around the contours of the ribs. The index finger locates the lower edge of the rib.
- A 3.5-cm long needle is advanced at an angle of 80° to the skin surface until bone contact (costal periosteum) is made (Fig. 19.15).
- The needle is withdrawn slightly, and the skin and needle are then simultaneously pushed caudally until the needle slides under the lower edge of the rib (Fig. 19.16a).
- After loss of bone contact, the needle must only be introduced 2–3 mm deeper (Fig. 19.16b).
- The hub of the needle is fixed between the thumb and index finger as this is done; the middle finger fixes the shaft and directs the needle. The side of the left hand (left hypothenar eminence) rests on the patient's back; initially it serves as a brake, and then during the injection it serves as fixation (Fig. 19.17).
- After aspiration at various levels, the local anesthetic is injected on an incremental basis.

> Due to overlap, at least three nerves have to be blocked in order to achieve a complete segmental block.

Effects of the block

Block of the skin, lateral and anterior thoracic wall, motor block of the intercostal muscles, as well as of the pleura and thoracic wall.

The six lower intercostal nerves reach the area of the linea alba, leading to motor block of the abdominal musculature and sensory block of the skin and abdomen, as well as of the peritoneum and lateral and anterior thoracic wall.

Dosage

3–5 mL local anesthetic per segment – e.g. 0.5–0.75% ropivacaine, 0.25–0.5% bupivacaine (0.25–0.5% levobupivacaine).

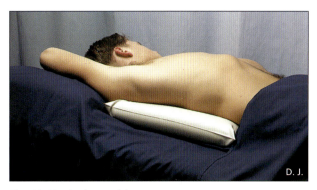

Fig. 19.13a Supine position

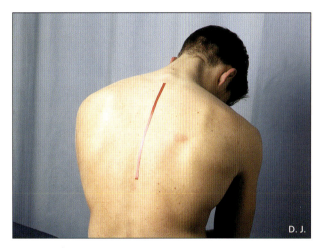

Fig. 19.13b Sitting

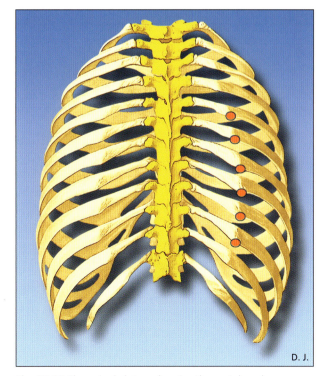

Fig. 19.14 Thoracic skeleton, showing the costal angles

Chapter 19

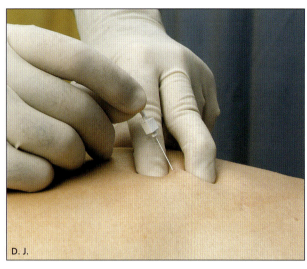

Fig. 19.15 The needle is advanced as far as the costal periosteum

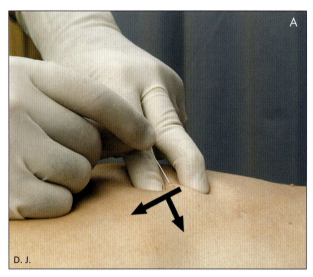

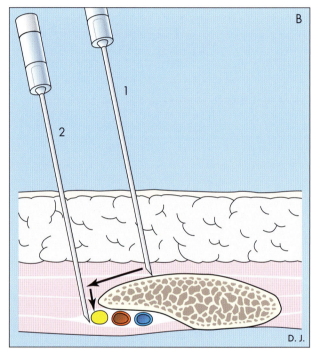

Fig. 19.16a, b The skin and the needle are simultaneously pushed caudally, and the needle is then introduced a further 2–3 mm

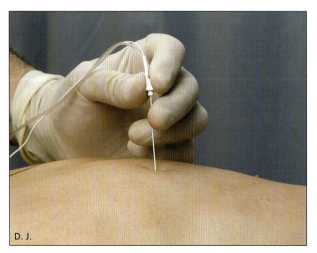

Fig. 19.17 Guiding the needle

As intercostal block is the procedure in which the highest blood levels of local anesthetic per milligram injected are achieved (due to very fast absorption), there is a risk of overdose.
The individual maximum dose must be carefully calculated, and must never be exceeded.

Dorsolateral intercostal block in the area of the posterior axillary line

This block is carried out ca. 2 cm dorsomedial to the posterior axillary line, with the patient in a supine position. Cushioning with a flat pillow under the back allows the relevant side of the chest to be raised at a slight angle. The patient's ipsilateral arm lies under the neck (Fig. 19.18).

This technique is suitable for blocking the lateral cutaneous branch of the intercostal nerve.

The materials and preparation, injection technique, dosage and complications are the same as those for the block of the costal angle described above.

More rarely, blocks of the intercostal nerves are carried out in the area of the anterior axillary line (distal third of the ribs and sternum), or parasternally (e.g. in sternum fractures).

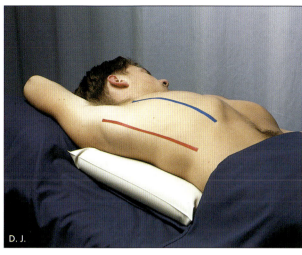

Fig. 19.18 Posterior axillary line (red), anterior axillary line (blue)

Complications
- Pneumothorax.
- Toxic reactions due to overdosage (see Chapter 1, p. 9 and Chapter 6, p. 66).
- Intravascular injection (see Chapter 6, p. 65).

Record and checklist

Intercostal nerve block

Block no. ☐ Right ☐ Left

Name: _____ Date: _____
Diagnosis: _____
Premedication: ☐ No ☐ Yes _____
Neurological abnormalities: ☐ No ☐ Yes _____

Purpose of block: ☐ *Diagnostic* ☐ *Therapeutic* ☐ *Surgical*
Needle: G _____ Length _____ cm
i.v. access: ☐ *No* ☐ *Yes*
Monitoring: ☐ *ECG* ☐ *Pulse oximetry*
Ventilation facilities: ☐ *Yes (equipment checked)*
Emergency equipment *(drugs)*: ☐ *Checked*
Patient: ☐ *Informed*

Position: ☐ *Prone* ☐ *Lateral recumbent* ☐ *Sitting* ☐ *Supine*
Access: ☐ *Costal angle* ☐ *Posterior axillary line* ☐ *Anterior axillary line* ☐ *Parasternal*
No. of nerves blocked: T _____ _____ _____ _____
Injection:
Local anesthetic: _____ mL _____ %
Addition to LA: ☐ *Yes* _____ µg/mg ☐ *No*

Patient's remarks during injection:
☐ *None* ☐ *Paresthesias* ☐ *Warmth* ☐ *Pain*
Nerve area: _____
Objective block effect after 15 min:
☐ *Cold test* ☐ *Temperature measurement right* _____°C *left* _____°C
Monitoring after block: ☐ *< 1 h* ☐ *> 1 h*
      Time of discharge _____

Complications:
☐ *None* ☐ *Intravascular injection* ☐ *Pneumothorax* ☐ *Toxic reaction*

Subjective effects of the block: Duration: _____
☐ *None* ☐ *Increased pain*
☐ *Reduced pain* ☐ *Relief of pain*

VISUAL ANALOG SCALE

|||||||||||||||||||||||||||||||||||||||||||||||||||
0   10   20   30   40   50   60   70   80   90   100

Special notes:
_____
_____
_____
_____
_____
_____

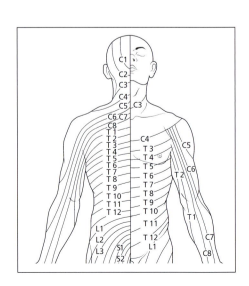

© Copyright ABW Wissenschaftsverlag 2004,
Jankovic, Regional nerve blocks and infiltration therapy, 3rd edition

Posterior branches of the thoracic spinal nerves

Anatomy
The posterior branches of the spinal nerve supply the skin of the back and the back musculature. Their area of distribution in the thoracic section stretches over the area between the spinous processes of the vertebrae and the costal angles (Fig. 19.19).

The posterior branches of the thoracic nerves each run between two transverse processes to their area of distribution, and divide shortly thereafter into a medial branch and a lateral branch. Together, these both supply the deep muscles of the back, but only one of each pair penetrates the subcutaneous tissue to become a cutaneous nerve.

Normally, the posterior branches of the eight upper thoracic nerves send off thick medial cutaneous branches, while the four lower ones send off thick lateral cutaneous branches.

The medial cutaneous branches pass through the trapezius muscle alongside the spinous processes of the vertebrae. The point of exit of the lateral cutaneous branches lies in the area of the musculotendinous line of the latissimus dorsi muscle.

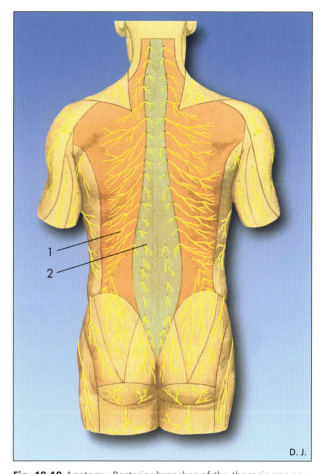

Fig. 19.19 Anatomy. Posterior branches of the thoracic nerves: (1) lateral cutaneous branches, (2) medial cutaneous branches

Indications
Therapeutic
- Muscular tension in the area of the trapezius muscle, serratus anterior and posterior muscles, rhomboideus muscle, levator scapulae muscle, splenius capitis muscle, and splenius cervicis muscle.
- Spasm of the deep paraspinal musculature.
- Shoulder pain, supplementing a block of the suprascapular and subscapular nerves (see Chapters 10 and 11).

Specific contraindications
None.

Procedure

Preparations
Check that the emergency equipment is complete and in working order. Sterile precautions.

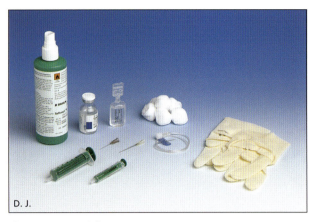

Fig. 19.20 Materials

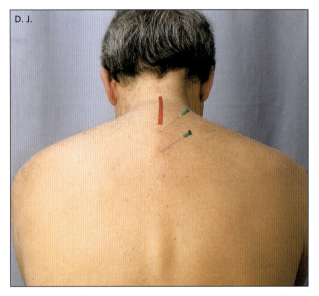

Fig. 19.21 Needle insertion into the intervertebral spaces of neighboring spinous processes

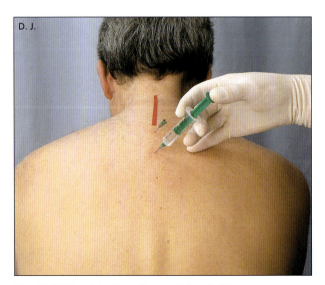

Fig. 19.22 Slow injection after careful aspiration

Materials (Fig. 19.20)
2-mL syringe, 5-mL syringe, fine 23-G needle (40 mm long), disinfectant.
Skin prep in all blocks.

Patient positioning
Sitting, with the head tilted forward slightly and the back muscles relaxed ("pharaoh posture").

Location
Spinous processes of the vertebral column in the C7–T1 and T2–T7 areas.

Injection technique
The intervertebral space between two neighboring spinous processes is palpated, and the needle is introduced at an angle of ca. 45° laterally, up to a depth of ca. 3–4 cm (Fig. 19.21).
After aspiration at various levels, the local anesthetic is injected slowly. When indicated, the neighboring segments can be anesthetized, starting at C7–T1 up to T7 and further along the spine (Fig. 19.22).

Effects of the block
Relaxation and pain relief in the area of the musculature of the nape of the neck and in the paraspinal musculature of the spine.
C7–T1: After the injection, a pleasant sensation of warmth develops, which radiates laterally to the shoulder and often cranially as far as the suboccipital area.
T2–T7: The lateral thoracic spread, with a sensation of warmth and slight itching, is about 20 cm.

Dosage
1–1.5 mL local anesthetic per segment – e.g. 0.5–0.75 ropivacaine, 0.25–0.5% bupivacaine (0.25–0.5% levobupivacaine). Up to 10–15 mL local anesthetic in total.

Side effects
No side effects are expected.

Spinal nerves (posterior branches)

Block no. ☐ Right ☐ Left ☐ Bilateral

Name: _____ Date: _____
Diagnosis: _____

Purpose of block:		☐ Diagnostic	☐ Therapeutic
Needle:	☐ 23 G	☐ 30 mm	☐ 40 mm
i. v. access:		☐ Yes	☐ No
Monitoring:		☐ ECG	☐ Pulse oximetry

Position: ☐ Sitting
Access: ☐ Median, angle ca. 45°; segment(s) _____
Local anesthetic: _____ mL _____ % per segment
Addition to injection solution: ☐ No ☐ Yes _____

Patient's remarks during injection:
☐ None ☐ Pain ☐ Paresthesias ☐ Warmth

Objective block effect after 15 min:
☐ Cold test ☐ Temperature measurement right ____°C left ____°C
Segments affected: _____ (numbness, warmth)
Monitoring after block: ☐ < 30 min ☐ > 30 min
Time of discharge _____

Complications:
☐ None ☐ Yes (which?) _____

Subjective effects of the block: Duration: _____
☐ None   ☐ Increased pain
☐ Reduced pain   ☐ Relief of pain

VISUAL ANALOG SCALE

|||||||||||||||||||||||||||||||||||||||||||||||||||||||||
0   10   20   30   40   50   60   70   80   90   100

Special notes:
_____
_____
_____
_____
_____
_____
_____
_____
_____
_____

© Copyright ABW Wissenschaftsverlag 2004,
Jankovic, Regional nerve blocks and infiltration therapy, 3rd edition

Record and checklist

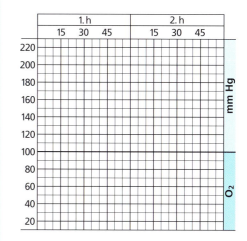

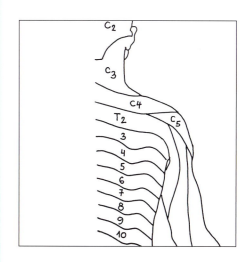

Lumbar spinal region

20 Lumbar paravertebral somatic nerve block

Definition
Dorsal somatic block of a lumbar nerve below the transverse process in its area of origin, just after it exits from the intervertebral foramen and runs through the paravertebral space.

Anatomy

Shortly after they exit from the intervertebral foramina, the spinal nerves divide into ventral branches (anterior) and dorsal branches (posterior). The smaller posterior branches turn dorsally and supply the skin and musculature of the back.
Together with the twelfth thoracic nerve, the longer ventral branches of the first four lumbar nerves form the lumbar plexus. The shorter muscular branches supply the psoas muscle and quadratus lumborum muscle (see pp. 218f). The lumbar plexus is connected to the lumbar part of the sympathetic chain via two or three long communicating branches.

Indications
Surgical
- Inguinal herniorrhaphy (in combination with a thoracic paravertebral somatic block, T10–L2) [9, 14]. High doses of local anesthetic are usually required.

Diagnostic
- Differentiation and localization of painful conditions in the lower abdominal quadrants, back, and lower extremities.

Therapeutic
- Pain in the lumbar, inguinal, and thigh region.
- Acute phase of herpes zoster in the appropriate dermatome.

Block series
A series of six to eight blocks is recommended. When there is evidence of improvement, additional blocks can be carried out.

Contraindications
Specific
- Anticoagulant treatment.
- Infections and skin diseases in the injection area.

Procedure

This block should only be carried out by experienced anesthetists, or under their supervision. Prior information for the patient is mandatory.

Preparations
Check that the emergency equipment is complete and in working order; sterile precautions, intravenous access, ECG monitoring, pulse oximetry, intubation kit, ventilation facilities, emergency medication.

Materials (Fig. 20.1)
Fine 26-G needle, 25 mm long, for local anesthesia.
Atraumatic 24-G needle, 0.7 × 80 mm (0.7 × 120 mm) (15°) with injection lead (e.g. Stimuplex D®, B. Braun Melsungen) or 24-G spinal needle, 0.6 × 80 mm, or 21-G spinal needle, 0.8 × 120 mm.
Syringes: 2, 5, and 10 mL.
Local anesthetics, disinfectant, swabs, sterile gloves, drape, flat, firm pillow.

Patient positioning
- Prone position: cushioned with a pillow in the mid-abdomen, to eliminate lumbar lordosis. The patient's arms should be dangling. It is also possible to carry out the injection with the patient in a sitting or lateral position.

Location
- Iliac crest line L4 (count cranially).
- Upper edge of the selected spinous process.

> Each of the lumbar somatic nerves leaves the intervertebral foramina slightly caudal and ventral to the transverse process.
> The upper edge of each spinous process in the lumbar region lies more or less on the same horizontal line as its own transverse process. After palpation of the upper edge of the spinous process, a horizontal line is drawn laterally. The injection point is located ca. 2.5–4 cm paramedian.

Skin prep, local anesthesia, covering with a sterile drape, drawing up the local anesthetic, checking the patency of the injection needle.

During the injection, the following points must be observed without fail:
- The person carrying out the injection must stand on the side being blocked.
- There is a risk of perforating the dural cuff if the injection is made too far medially (epidural or subarachnoid injection).
- The transverse process is ca. 0.6–0.7 cm thick.
- If there is no bone contact after 3.5–5 cm (depending on the anatomy), the direction of the needle must be corrected (the needle is located between two transverse processes).
- Producing paresthesias is not obligatory.
- The injection should be carried out incrementally, with frequent aspiration (blood, CSF?).
- Motor weakness in the leg must always be expected. Patients should be warned of this.

Injection technique
- The injection needle is introduced perpendicular to the skin surface (Fig. 20.2) until bone contact is made (transverse process).

Depending on the anatomy, bone contact is made at a depth of ca. 3–5 cm. The depth of the needle is marked (Fig. 20.3).

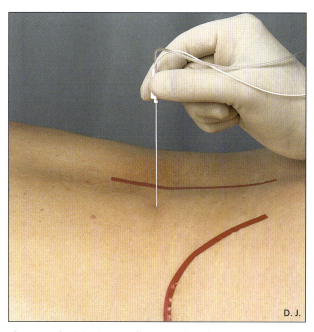

Fig. 20.2 The injection needle is introduced perpendicular to the skin surface

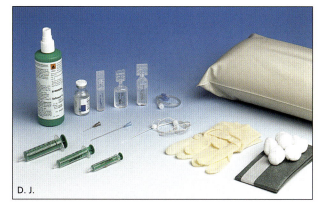

Fig. 20.1 Materials

Chapter 20

- The needle is then withdrawn to lie subcutaneously, and introduced at an angle of ca. 15–20° caudally (or cranially), past the transverse process, for a further 2–2.5 cm deeper (Fig. 20.4).
Eliciting paresthesias is helpful, and confirms the correct positioning of the needle, but it is not obligatory, since the optimal effect of the block can be achieved by spread of the local anesthetic.
- After aspiration at various levels (blood, CSF?), the local anesthetic is injected on an incremental basis.

> After a successful somatic paravertebral block in the lumbar region, the injected local anesthetic diffuses through the plethora of communicating branches that are present (particularly in the first and second lumbar nerves, but more rarely in the third) towards the neighboring sympathetic chain, which is almost always blocked as well.

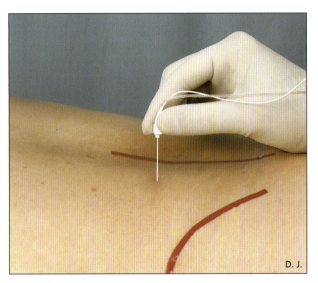

Fig. 20.3a Bone contact with the transverse process. Visual marking of the depth

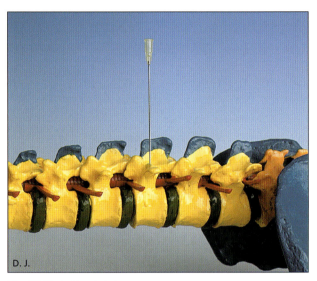

Fig. 20.3b In the skeleton

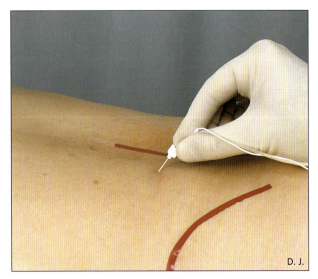

Fig. 20.4a Withdraw, and then introduce the needle past the transverse process

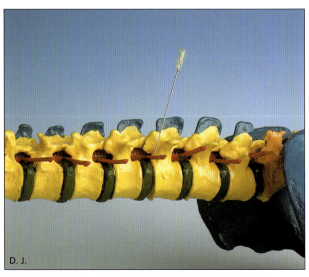

Fig. 20.4b In the skeleton

Dosage

Surgical
5 mL local anesthetic per segment (T10–L2) – e.g. 0.75% ropivacaine, 0.5% bupivacaine with 1 : 400000 epinephrine [9] (0.5% levobupivacaine).

Diagnostic
5 mL local anesthetic per segment – e.g. 0.5% prilocaine, 0.5% mepivacaine, 0.5% lidocaine.

Therapeutic
5–10 mL local anesthetic per segment – e.g. 0.5% ropivacaine, 0.25–0.375% bupivacaine (0.25–0.375% levobupivacaine). In acute conditions (e.g. herpes zoster), 2–4 mg dexamethasone can be added.

Important notes for outpatients
See Chapter 26, p. 224.

Complications
- Epidural or subarachnoid injection (avoid injecting too medially! See Chapters 36 and 41).
- Intravascular injection with toxic reactions (see Chapter 1, p. 9 and Chapter 6, p. 66).
- Intra-abdominal and retroperitoneal injection, or injection into the peritoneum (severe complications are not expected).
- Hypotension due to accompanying sympathetic block (e.g. with larger volumes of local anesthetic or too deep an injection).

Record and checklist

Lumbar paravertebral nerve block
Block no. ☐ Right ☐ Left

Name: _____ Date: _____
Diagnosis: _____
Premedication: ☐ No ☐ Yes _____
Neurological abnormalities: ☐ No ☐ Yes _____

Purpose of block: ☐ *Diagnostic* ☐ *Therapeutic* ☐ *Surgical*
Needle: G _____ Length _____ cm
i.v. access: ☐ *Yes*
Monitoring: ☐ *ECG* ☐ *Pulse oximetry*
Ventilation facilities: ☐ *Yes (equipment checked)*
Emergency equipment *(drugs)*: ☐ *Checked*
Patient: ☐ *Informed (what to do after block)*

Position: ☐ *Prone*
Injection level ☐ L _____ _____ _____
Injection:
Local anesthetic: _____ mL ____ %
(in incremental doses)
Addition to LA: ☐ *Yes* _____ µg/mg _____ ☐ *No*

Patient's remarks during injection:
☐ *None* ☐ *Paresthesias* ☐ *Warmth* ☐ *Pain*
Nerve area: _____
Objective block effect after 15 min:
☐ *Cold test* ☐ *Temperature measurement right* ____ °C *left* ____ °C
Segments affected: L _____
Monitoring after block: ☐ *< 1 h* ☐ *> 1 h*
Time of discharge: _____ *Motor / sensory status checked*

Complications:
☐ *None* ☐ *Intravascular injection* ☐ *Subarachnoid/epidural* ☐ *Other*

Subjective effects of the block: *Duration:* _____
☐ *None* ☐ *Increased pain*
☐ *Reduced pain* ☐ *Relief of pain*

VISUAL ANALOG SCALE
0 10 20 30 40 50 60 70 80 90 100

Special notes:
_____
_____
_____
_____
_____
_____

© Copyright ABW Wissenschaftsverlag 2004,
Jankovic, Regional nerve blocks and infiltration therapy, 3rd edition

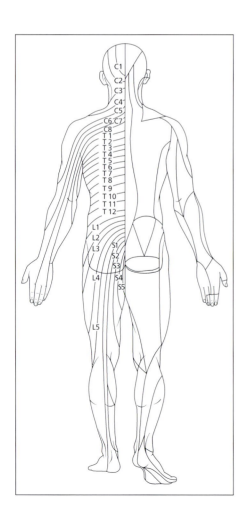

21 Lumbar sympathetic block

Definition
Injection of a local anesthetic or neurolytic in the sympathetic ganglia of the lumbar sympathetic trunk.

Anatomy (Figs. 21.1, 21.2)

From the T12 ganglion, the sympathetic trunk passes into the abdominal cavity. The abdominal part of the trunk reaches the anterolateral surface of the lumbar vertebrae, lying directly medial to the origin of the psoas, to the right behind the inferior vena cava and cisterna chyli and to the left beside the aorta. The lumbar part of the sympathetic trunk usually contains only four lumbar ganglia (due to fusion of the twelfth thoracic and first lumbar ganglion), with a spindle shape or oval shape. The final ganglion is usually the largest.
The average length of the ganglia is ca. 3–5 mm (more rarely, up to 10–15 mm). The psoas muscle and its fascia separate the sympathetic nerve trunk from the lumbar somatic spinal nerves.
The sympathetic trunks give off and receive communicating and visceral branches, as well as vascular, muscular, osseous and articular branches.
White communicating branches only reach the lumbar sympathetic ganglia from the two cranial spinal nerves, as well as from the three lumbar spinal nerves. They carry preganglionic fibers and visceral afferents. Gray communicating branches are given off from the corresponding ganglia to all the lumbar spinal nerves. They contain vasomotor, sudomotor and pilomotor fibers, which are distributed with the lumbar spinal nerves. From the lumbar part of the sympathetic chain, some branches run to the renal plexus, but most pass to the abdominal aortic plexus and the hypogastric plexus. Most of the sympathetic nerve fibers responsible for the lower extremity pass through the L2 (dominant) and L3 ganglia.

Indications
Diagnostic and prognostic
- Differentiation between various forms of vasospastic disease in the area of the lower extremities.
- Prognostic block to establish an indication for surgical sympathectomy or a neurolytic block.
- Checking (confirmation) of a surgical sympathectomy.

Therapeutic
- Pain caused by perfusion disturbances in vasospastic diseases in the region of the lower extremities, in the form of arterial or venous dysfunction or a combination of the two.
- Intermittent claudication.
- Embolism and thrombosis.
- Thrombophlebitis and post-phlebitic edema.
- Post-reconstructive vascular procedures.
- After frostbite or trauma.
- Complex regional pain syndrome (CRPS) types I and II.
- Phantom limb pain.
- Erythromelalgia.
- Acrocyanosis.
- Phlegmasia alba dolens (milk leg).
- Persistent infection of the leg.
- Poorly healing ulcers.
- Neuropathy after radiotherapy.
- Hyperhidrosis of the lower body.
- Acute phase of herpes zoster.
- Visceral pain (e.g. renal colic).

Block series
A series of six to eight blocks is recommended. When there is evidence of improvement in the symptoms, additional blocks can also be carried out.

Contraindications
- Anticoagulant treatment.
- Infections and skin diseases in the injection area.
- Addition of vasopressors in patients with peripheral circulatory disturbances.

Procedure

This block should only be carried out by experienced anesthetists, or under their supervision. Full information should be given to the patient.

Preparations
Check that the emergency equipment is complete and in working order; sterile precautions, intravenous access, ECG monitoring, pulse oximetry, intubation kit, ventilation facilities, emergency medication.

Materials (Fig. 21.3)
Fine 26-G needle, 25 mm long, for local anesthesia. Atraumatic 22-G needle, 0.7 × 120 mm (15°) with injection lead (e.g. Stimuplex D®, B. Braun Melsungen) or spinal needle, 0.7 (0.9) × 120 mm (150 mm), 20–22 G (e.g. Spinocan, B. Braun Melsungen).
Syringes: 2, 5 and 10 mL.
Disinfectant, swabs, compresses, sterile gloves and drape, flat, firm pillow.

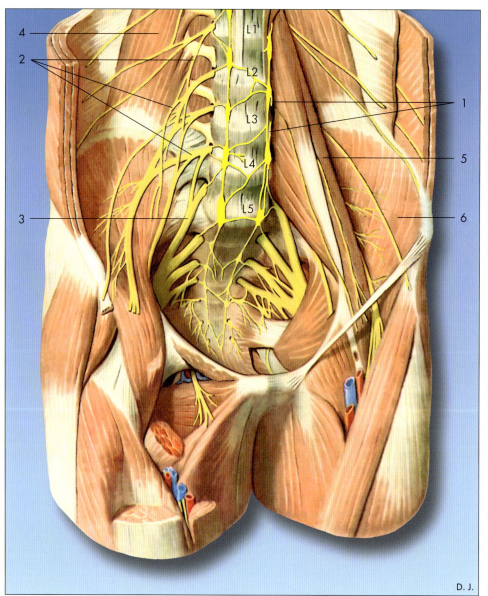

Fig. 21.1 Anatomy (anterior view):
(1) sympathetic trunk with communicating branches,
(2) lumbar plexus,
(3) lumbosacral trunk,
(4) quadratus lumborum muscle,
(5) psoas major muscle,
(6) iliac muscle

Lumbar sympathetic block

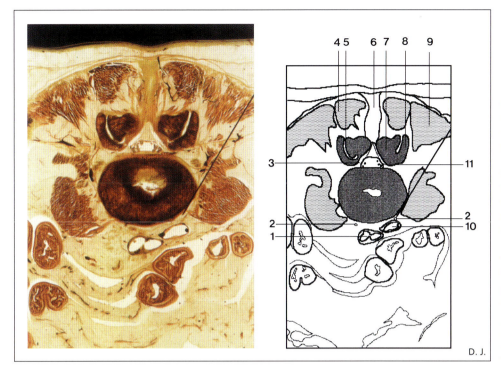

Fig. 21.2a Lumbar sympathetic block (anatomy and diagram). (1) Aorta, (2) sympathic ganglion, (3) epidural space, (4) medial tract of back muscles, (5) intervertebral joint, (6) interspinal ligament, (7) superior articular process of L3, (8) inferior articular process of L4, (9) lateral tract of back muscles, (10) vena cava, (11) filum terminale

[From: Grönemeyer and Seibel, *Interventionelle Computertomographie. Lehrbuch and Atlas zur interventionellen Operationstechnik and Schmerztherapie* (Vienna/Berlin: Ueberreutter Wissenschaft), 1989.]

Patient positioning

- Prone position: support with a pillow in the mid-abdomen (to eliminate lumbar lordosis). The patient's arms should be dangling.
  The patient should breathe with the mouth open, to reduce tension in the back muscles.
  This position is preferable, particularly when the block is carried out under radiographic control using an image intensifier.
- Lateral decubitus: the flank is supported with a pillow. The side being blocked should be uppermost.

Landmarks (Fig. 21.4)
- L4 iliac crest line.
- L2: a parallel line is drawn ca. four fingerbreadths (7 cm) from the midline. The intersection point between this line and the twelfth rib is at the level of L2.
- Mid-point of each spinous process of the relevant lumbar vertebra.

Disinfection, generous local anesthetic infiltration of the injection channel, covering with a sterile drape, drawing up the local anesthetic, testing the patency of the injection needle.

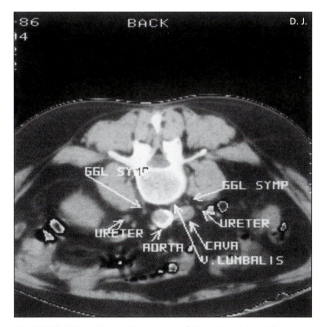

Fig. 21.2b CT section in the center of the L4 vertebra. The sympathetic ganglia are well delineated in the fatty tissue on each side. Neighboring structures, such as the vessels and ureters, can also be precisely differentiated

[From: Grönemeyer and Seibel, *Interventionelle Computertomographie. Lehrbuch and Atlas zur interventionellen Operationstechnik and Schmerztherapie* (Vienna/Berlin: Ueberreutter Wissenschaft), 1989.]

Chapter 21

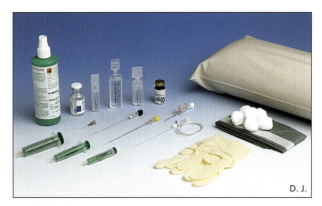

Fig. 21.3 Materials

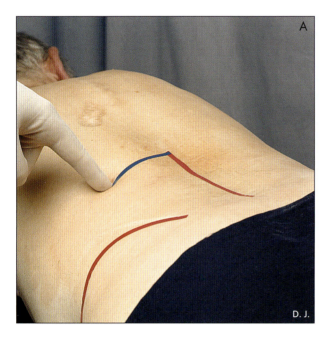

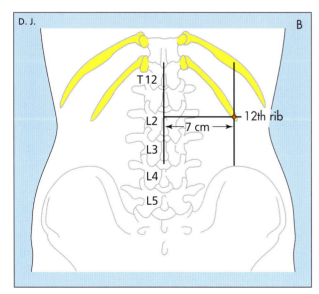

Fig. 21.4a, b Localization

During the injection, the following points must be observed:
- In clinical routine, a sympathetic block is started at the L2 segment; block of segment L4 follows.
- The person carrying out the injection must stand on the side being blocked.
- Usually, the injection point should not be located more than 8 cm lateral to the midline (risk of renal puncture) and no more than 5 cm medial to it (the lateral side of the vertebra is more difficult to reach).
- Paresthesias occur relatively frequently during introduction of the needle and indicate irritation of the lumbar somatic nerves.
- Inadvertent block of the lumbar somatic nerves can lead to motor weakness of the contralateral leg. The patient should be warned of this.
- There is a risk of perforating the dural cuff if the injection is made too far medially (epidural or subarachnoid injection).
- Aspirate frequently and inject incrementally.
- No neurolytics should be administered without precise confirmation of the needle position using radiographic control with an image intensifier.

Injection technique

- The injection needle is introduced in the direction of the intended vertebra, ca. four fingerbreadths (7 cm) lateral to the midline and at an angle of ca. 30–40° to the skin surface and slightly cranially (Fig. 21.5).
- Locating the transverse process at a depth of ca. 3-5 cm is helpful. The depth of the transverse process is marked (Fig. 21.6).
- The needle is withdrawn to lie subcutaneously.
- The needle is then reintroduced slightly more steeply, with stepwise correction of the direction cranially or caudally (to avoid the transverse process) and medially (to obtain contact with the vertebral periosteum).

After contact with the periosteum, the needle is rotated 180° so that the bevel is directed toward the vertebra and can slide off the bony edge. After sliding off, the needle is further advanced by 1–2 cm (Fig. 21.8).

> The lumbar sympathetic trunk lies about twice as deep as the distance between the skin and the transverse process (Fig. 21.7).
> The distance from the transverse process and the ganglia of the lumbar sympathetic trunk is ca. 3.8–5 cm and is relatively constant.
> The distance from the skin to the transverse process depends on the anatomy and is rather more variable.

Confirming the correct needle position
- Radiographic control.
- Loss-of-resistance technique with 0.9% saline or air.
  Perforation of the psoas fascia is similar to the sensation experienced when carrying out an epidural.
  A false loss of resistance can occur when the needle is positioned superficially between the psoas muscle and the quadratus lumborum muscle, leading to inadvertent block of the lumbar somatic nerves, with consequent numbness of the lower extremity during the period of effect of the local anesthetic.
  Injection of a neurolytic into this area without prior radiographic control of the position can have fatal consequences.
- After careful aspiration testing at all levels, resistance-free incremental injection of the local anesthetic is carried out.

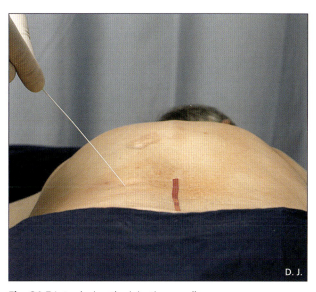

Fig. 21.5 Introducing the injection needle

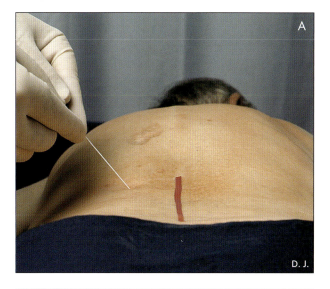

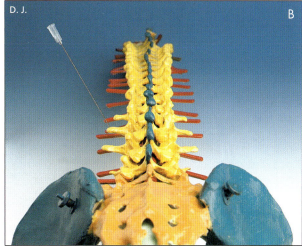

Fig. 21.6a, b Bone contact with the transverse process: in a patient **(a)** and in the skeleton **(b)**

Chapter 21

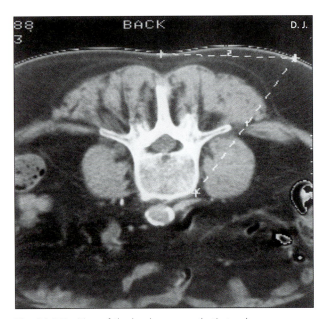

Fig. 21.7 Position of the lumbar sympathetic trunk

[From: Grönemeyer and Seibel, *Interventionelle Computertomographie. Lehrbuch and Atlas zur interventionellen Operationstechnik and Schmerztherapie* (Vienna/Berlin: Ueberreutter Wissenschaft), 1989.]

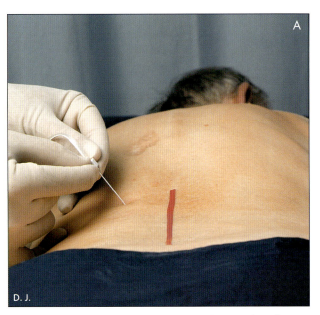

Fig. 21.8a After the needle has been withdrawn to lie subcutaneously, it is reintroduced at a steeper angle, followed by contact with the vertebral periosteum and rotation of the needle by 180°. The needle is then advanced 1–2 cm

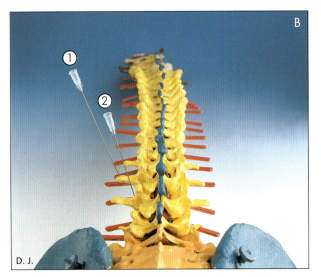
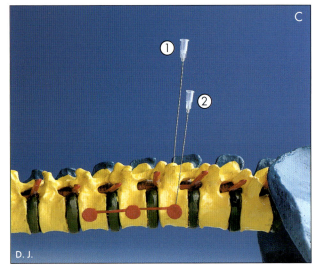

Fig. 21.8b, c In a skeleton (anterior and lateral views)

Neurolytic block

Injection of neurolytics – 45–95% ethanol, 7% phenol in water or 7–10% phenol in Conray (iothalamate meglumine) – at the lumbar sympathetic ganglia.
Prerequisite: the procedure must be carried out under radiographic guidance.
Usually, three needles are introduced at the level of L2, L3 and L4 and the neurolytic is only injected after definite confirmation of the correct needle position. After this, 1 mL of air is injected per needle, to clear any residual neurolytic from the needle.

Effects of the block
Signs of vascular dilation in the area of the ipsilateral leg are:
- Increase in skin temperature.
- Hyperthermia and anhidrosis.
- Loss of the sympathogalvanic reflex.
- Reduced pain or absence of pain.
- No signs of sensory or motor block (assuming that the lumbar somatic nerves have not been concomitantly anesthetized).

Dosage
Diagnostic
5 mL local anesthetic with contrast medium – e.g. 0.5 prilocaine, 0.5% mepivacaine, 0.5% lidocaine.

Therapeutic
20 mL local anesthetic (single-needle technique).
10 mL local anesthetic per needle (in the two-needle or three-needle technique) – e.g. 0.2–0.375% ropivacaine, 0.25% bupivacaine (0.25% levobupivacaine).

Neurolytics
3 mL per segment.

Side effects
- Transient motor weakness due to block of the lumbar somatic nerves. Paresthesias during the injection are a warning signal. This undesired effect is always liable to occur and is caused by superficial injection in the area of the lumbar somatic nerves or by spread after the administration of large volumes of a local anesthetic. It is therefore necessary to monitor the patient for at least 1 hour after the block (see Chapter 26, section on important notes for outpatients, p. 224).
- Fall in blood pressure due to sympathetic block.

Complications
Severe
- Intravascular injection (aorta, vena cava) with toxic reactions (see Chapter 6, p. 66).
- Epidural or subarachnoid injection (see Chapter 36 and Chapter 41).

Potential
- Retroperitoneal hemorrhage.
- Hemorrhage in the psoas area (with subsequent pain in the thigh and transient weakness in the quadriceps muscle).
- Renal injury accompanied by hematuria.
- Back pain.
- Perforation of an intervertebral disk.
- Ejaculation disturbances (in younger patients with bilateral block).

Complications of neurolytic block
- Injury to the lumbar somatic nerves (neuritis, 1%).
- Neuralgia in the genitofemoral nerve (5–10%).
- Ureteral stricture.

Chapter 21

Record and checklist

Lumbar sympathetic block

Block no. ☐ Right ☐ Left

Name: _____ Date: _____
Diagnosis: _____
Premedication: ☐ No ☐ Yes _____
Neurological abnormalities: ☐ No ☐ Yes _____

Purpose of block: ☐ Diagnostic ☐ Therapeutic
Needle: G _____ Length _____ cm
i.v. access: ☐ Yes
Monitoring: ☐ ECG ☐ Pulse oximetry
Ventilation facilities: ☐ Yes (equipment checked)
Emergency equipment *(drugs)*: ☐ Checked
Patient: ☐ Informed (what to do after block)

Position: ☐ Prone ☐ Lateral recumbent
Injection level ☐ L _____ _____ _____
Injection technique: ☐ X-ray image intensifier ☐ Loss of resistance ☐ CT-guided
Injection:
Local anesthetic: _____ mL _____ %
(in incremental doses)
Addition to LA: ☐ Yes _____ μg/mg ☐ No
Neurolytic: _____ mL _____ %
Addition: ☐ Yes ☐ No

Patient's remarks during injection:
☐ None ☐ Paresthesias ☐ Warmth ☐ Pain
Nerve area: _____
Objective block effect after 15 min:
☐ Cold test ☐ Temperature measurement right _____°C left _____°C
Segments affected: L _____
Monitoring after block: ☐ < 1 h ☐ > 1 h
Time of discharge: _____ *Motor / sensory status checked*

Complications:
☐ None ☐ Intravascular injection ☐ Subarachnoid/epidural
☐ Drop in BP ☐ Other

Subjective effects of the block: Duration: _____
☐ None ☐ Increased pain
☐ Reduced pain ☐ Relief of pain

VISUAL ANALOG SCALE

| 0 | 10 | 20 | 30 | 40 | 50 | 60 | 70 | 80 | 90 | 100 |

Special notes: _____

© Copyright ABW Wissenschaftsverlag 2004,
Jankovic, Regional nerve blocks and infiltration therapy, 3rd edition

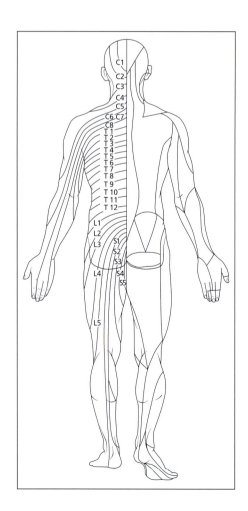

Abdomen

22 Celiac plexus block

Definition

Injection of a local anesthetic or neurolytic in the region of the celiac plexus.

Anatomy (Fig. 22.1)

The celiac plexus is the largest of the three large sympathetic plexuses (cardiac plexus – thorax; celiac plexus – abdomen; hypogastric plexus – pelvis).

It receives its primary innervation from the preganglionic splanchnic nerves (greater splanchnic nerve T5–10, lesser splanchnic nerve T10–11 and lowest splanchnic nerve T11–12), the postganglionic fibers of which, after synapsing in the celiac ganglion, radiate to the associated plexus and innervate most of the abdominal organs. This large network, with a diameter of about 50 mm, surrounds the origins of the celiac artery and superior mesenteric artery, extends laterally as far as the adrenal glands, upward as far as the aortic hiatus and downward as far as the root of the renal artery. It lies on the initial part of the abdominal aorta, at the level of the first lumbar vertebra, anterior to the medial crus of the diaphragm.

The most important roots of the celiac plexus are the splanchnic nerves, the abdominal branches of the vagus nerves and several branches of the last thoracic ganglion and two highest lumbar ganglia. Cranially, the celiac plexus is connected to the thoracic aortic plexus and caudally it continues into the abdominal aortic plexus. A paired celiac ganglion forms the basis for the celiac plexus. The left ganglion lies closer to the midline and partly on the aorta, while the right one (ventrolateral to the vena cava) lies slightly more to the side in the area of the fissure between the medial and lateral crura of the diaphragm. The two ganglia are connected to one another. With closer approximation and fusion, the double ganglion takes on a ring shape, which is also known as the solar ganglion (solar plexus).

The smaller superior mesenteric ganglion and aorticorenal ganglion are associated with the celiac ganglion.

The lesser splanchnic nerve usually enters the latter ganglion, while the greater splanchnic nerve passes to the posterior surface of the lateral part of the celiac ganglion. The phrenic ganglion is a third, unpaired, ganglion. The following, sometimes paired and sometimes unpaired, secondary (associated) plexuses emerge from the celiac plexus:
- Paired (phrenic plexus, suprarenal plexus, renal plexus and spermatic plexus).
- Unpaired (superior gastric plexus, hepatic plexus, splenic plexus and superior mesenteric plexus).

Indications

Diagnostic
- Differential diagnosis of pain in the abdominal region (visceral, epigastric or cardiac pain).

Prognostic
- In upper abdominal cancer pain, before a neurolytic block.

Therapeutic
- Relief of upper abdominal pain (pancreas, stomach).
- Treatment of the dumping syndrome.
- Injection of neurolytics as a palliative measure in malignant intra-abdominal disease (pancreas, stomach).

Contraindications
- Anticoagulant treatment.
- Infections and skin diseases in the injection area.
- Hypovolemia.
- General debility.
- Injection of a neurolytic without precise identification of the needle position (with guidance by CT or image intensifier).

Procedure

This block should be carried out by very experienced anesthetists. Full information for the patient is mandatory.

Chapter 22

Preparations
Check that the emergency equipment is complete and in working order; sterile precautions, intravenous access, ECG monitoring, pulse oximetry, intubation kit, ventilation facilities, emergency medication.

Materials (Fig. 22.2)
Fine 26-G needle for local anesthesia.
20–22-G spinal needle, 0.7 (0.9) × 120 mm (150 mm) (e.g. Spinocan, B. Braun Melsungen).
Syringes: 2, 10 and 10 mL.
Disinfectant, swabs, compresses, sterile gloves and drape, flat, firm pillow.

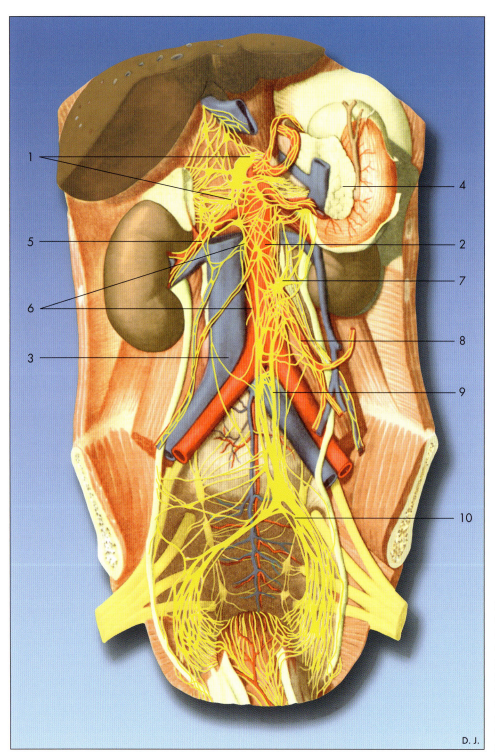

Fig. 22.1 Anatomy.
(1) Celiac plexus, (2) aorta, (3) inferior vena cava, (4) pancreas, (5) renal plexus, (6) abdominal aortic plexus, (7) inferior mesenteric ganglion, (8) inferior mesenteric plexus, (9) superior hypogastric plexus, (10) inferior hypogastric plexus

Celiac plexus block

Patient positioning
- Prone position: supported with a pillow in the mid-abdomen (to relieve lumbar lordosis). The patient's arms are dangling, with the head lying to the side. The patient breathes with the mouth open, to reduce tension in the back muscles. This position is preferable.
- Lateral decubitus position, with support under the flank. The side being blocked lies upward.

Location
- L4 iliac crest line (count the spinous processes cranially).
- L2: a parallel line is drawn about 7–8 cm lateral to the midline. The intersection between this line and the lower edge of the twelfth rib determines the level of the upper edge of L2 (see Chapter 21, Fig. 21.4b).
- T12–L1 is located in the midline and joined with dots to the lower edge of the twelfth rib. This produces a triangle, the equal sides of which provide basic guidance for the needle direction (Fig. 22.3).

Skin prep, generous local anesthetic infiltration of the injection channel, covering with a sterile drape, drawing up the local anesthetic, checking the patency of the injection needle.

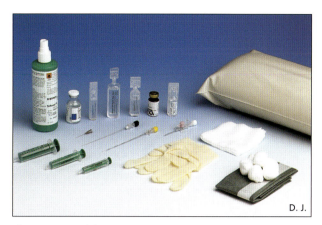

Fig. 22.2 Materials

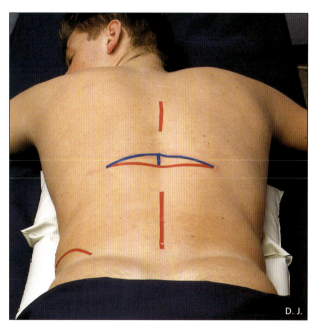

Fig. 22.3 Location

> During the injection, the following points must be observed:
> - In bilateral injections, it is advantageous to inject the left side first.
> - For a diagnostic block, a bilateral injection is unnecessary.
> - The operator performing the injection must stand on the side being blocked.
> - In most patients, the distance between the skin and the celiac plexus is about 9–11 cm.
> - Superficial bone contact (after 3–5 cm) indicates contact with the transverse process and requires correction.
> - Paresthesias during the introduction of the needle arise due to stimulation of the lumbar somatic nerves.
> - There is a risk of perforating the dural cuff (epidural or subarachnoid injection).
> - If the patient coughs, it indicates pleural irritation or injury. The procedure should be halted.
> - Aspirate frequently and inject on an incremental basis.
> - The method of choice when administering neurolytics is CT guided injection.

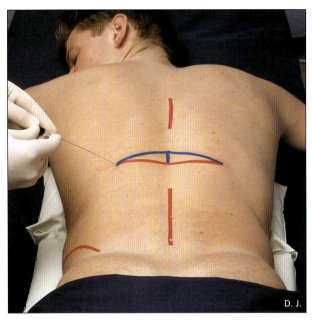

Fig. 22.4 Introducing the injection needle at an angle of about 45° to the skin surface

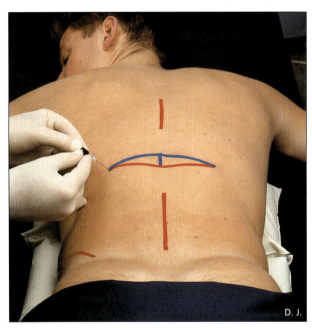

Fig. 22.5 Bone contact with the L1 vertebra. After visual marking of the depth, the needle is withdrawn back to the subcutis

Injection technique (dorsal, retrocrural)
- About 7–8 cm lateral to the midline (lower edge of the twelfth rib), at an angle of 45° to the skin surface and directed slightly cranially, the injection needle is advanced toward the L1 vertebra (Fig. 22.4). Bone contact is usually made at a depth of about 7–9 cm (Figs. 22.5, 22.7).
- The depth of the needle is marked visually.
- The needle is withdrawn to lie subcutaneously.
- The needle is then redirected at a steeper angle of 60° to the skin surface, so that it can just slide past the lateral edge of the L1 vertebra (Figs. 22.6, 22.7).
- The needle introduced on the left (the side of the aorta) can then be carefully advanced a further 1.5–2 cm deeper. After the needle is positioned in the periaortic space, pulsations are transmitted via the needle shaft to the fingertips.
  The needle introduced on the right side can be advanced in a similar fashion or slightly deeper (2–3 cm) (Figs. 22.7, 22.8).
- The end of the needle must be observed for spontaneous backflow of liquid (blood, CSF, urine?).
- Aspiration test at all four levels.
- Test dose of the local anesthetic.
- Resistance-free incremental injection of a local anesthetic.

> It is now the standard procedure to carry out this injection with guidance using a radiographic image intensifier or computed tomography (CT).

Neurolytic block
Unilateral or bilateral injection of neurolytics (50% ethanol) in the region of the celiac plexus.

Celiac plexus block

> The block should be carried out with CT guidance if possible, in order to reduce potential complications to a minimum and increase accuracy. Several access routes are possible (Figs. 22.8, 22.9).

A diagnostic block with local anesthetics is a prerequisite.
This measure can only achieve the desired result if the disease is not too far advanced and is not producing additional neuropathic pain (e.g. extension to the epigastric nerves, intercostal nerves or lumbar plexus) [5].

Effects of the block
- Hyperthermia in the upper abdominal region (vascular dilatation in the splanchnic region).
- Increased intestinal motility.
- Pain reduction.

Dosage
Diagnostic
20–30 mL local anesthetic – e.g. 0.5–1% prilocaine, 0.5–1% mepivacaine, 0.5–1% lidocaine.

Therapeutic
- Local anesthetics
  20–30 mL local anesthetic – e.g. 0.375–0.5% ropivacaine, 0.25–0.375% bupivacaine.
  A mixture with methylprednisolone is recommended in acute conditions.
- Neurolytics
  25–50 mL 50% ethanol in combination with 0.2% ropivacaine or 0.125% bupivacaine.
  Some authors recommended prior administration of 5 mL 2% lidocaine to relieve the pain of the ethanol injection.

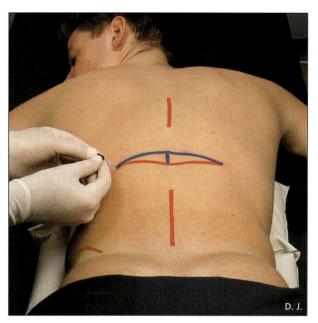

Fig. 22.6 Redirection of the needle at an angle of 60° to the skin surface

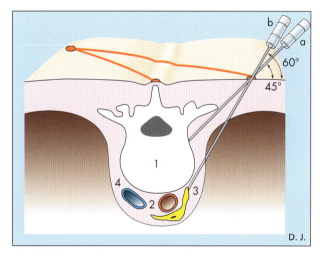

Fig. 22.7 Path of the needle to the celiac plexus. Diagram: (a) contact with the L1 vertebra, (b) introduction of the needle at a steeper angle of 60° to the skin surface. (1) L1 vertebra, (2) aorta, (3) celiac plexus, (4) inferior vena cava

Chapter 22

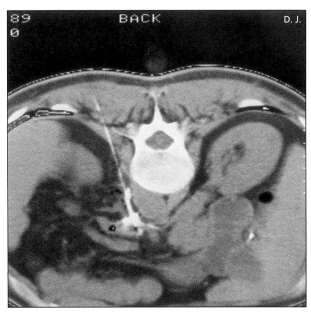

Fig. 22.8 Dorsal CT-guided celiac plexus injection. After injection of contrast medium, a good spread in the area of the celiac plexus can be seen

[From: Grönemeyer and Seibel, *Interventionelle Computertomographie. Lehrbuch and Atlas zur interventionellen Operationstechnik and Schmerztherapie* (Vienna/Berlin: Ueberreutter Wissenschaft), 1989.]

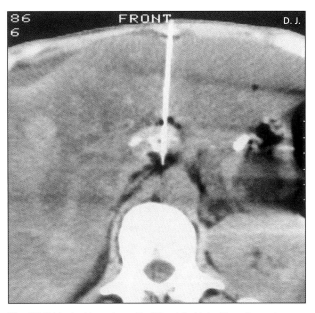

Fig. 22.9 Ventral transhepatic CT-guided injection. Several access routes are possible in celiac plexus injection. In this case, the injection was carried out using a ventral transhepatic approach. The tip of the needle lies directly alongside the celiac trunk. The alcohol spreads precisely within the celiac plexus

[From: Grönemeyer and Seibel, *Interventionelle Computertomographie. Lehrbuch and Atlas zur interventionellen Operationstechnik and Schmerztherapie* (Vienna/Berlin: Ueberreutter Wissenschaft), 1989.]

Side effects
Hypotension due to sympathetic block (caution in older patients).

Complications
Severe
- Intravascular injections (aorta, vena cava, celiac artery, renal artery) with toxic reactions (see Chapter 6, p. 66).
- Epidural or subarachnoid injection (see Chapter 36 and Chapter 41).
- Pneumothorax.

Potential
- Vascular injury (hemorrhage, retroperitoneal hematoma formation).
- Injection into kidneys and other intra-abdominal organs.
- Aortal pseudoaneurysm.
- Abscess or cyst formation.
- Intraosseous or psoas injection.

Complications of neurolytic block
- Paraplegia [3, 15].
- Monoparesis, with loss of sphincter function in the rectum and bladder.
- Sexual dysfunction.
- Diarrhea.
- Retroperitoneal fibrosis.
- Renal necrosis.
- Chemical peritonitis [2].
- Chemical pericarditis [12].

Celiac plexus block

Block no. ☐ Right ☐ Left

Name: _____ Date: _____
Diagnosis: _____
Premedication: ☐ No ☐ Yes _____
Neurological abnormalities: ☐ No ☐ Yes _____

Purpose of block: ☐ Diagnostic ☐ Therapeutic
Needle: G _____ Length _____ cm
i.v. access: ☐ Yes
Monitoring: ☐ ECG ☐ Pulse oximetry
Ventilation facilities: ☐ Yes (equipment checked)
Emergency equipment (drugs): ☐ Checked
Patient: ☐ Informed
Contraindications excluded: ☐

Position: ☐ Prone ☐ Lateral recumbent
Injection level: ☐ L1
Injection technique: ☐ Dorsal ☐ Ventral ☐ X-ray image intensifier guidance
 ☐ CT-guided
Injection:
Local anesthetic: _____ mL _____ %
(in incremental doses)
Addition to LA: ☐ Yes _____ ☐ No _____
Neurolytic: _____ mL _____ %
Addition: ☐ Yes ☐ No

Patient's remarks during injection:
☐ None ☐ Paresthesias ☐ Warmth ☐ Pain
Nerve area: _____
Objective block effect after 15 min:
☐ Cold test ☐ Temperature measurement before _____ °C after _____ °C
Monitoring after block: ☐ < 1 h ☐ > 1 h
 Time of discharge: _____

Complications:
☐ None ☐ Intravascular injection ☐ Subarachnoid/epidural
☐ Pneumothorax ☐ Drop in BP ☐ Nerve injury ☐ Other

Subjective effects of the block: Duration: _____
☐ None ☐ Increased pain
☐ Reduced pain ☐ Relief of pain

VISUAL ANALOG SCALE

| 0 | 10 | 20 | 30 | 40 | 50 | 60 | 70 | 80 | 90 | 100 |

Special notes:

© Copyright ABW Wissenschaftsverlag 2004,
Jankovic, Regional nerve blocks and infiltration therapy, 3rd edition

Record and checklist

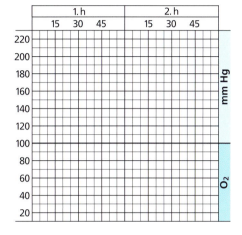

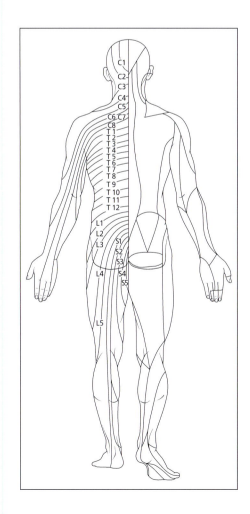

Lumbosacral region

23 Iliolumbosacral ligaments

Definition
Injection of a local anesthetic or a sclerosant solution along the ligamentous insertion points in the lumbosacral area.

Anatomy (Fig. 23.1)

The ligaments of the sacral and coccygeal region are very important, since they transfer the entire weight of the trunk via the hip bones to the lower extremities. This occurs through firm anchoring of the vertebrae, hip bones and sacrum.
The pelvic girdle only has one ligamentous connection of its own, the obturator membrane of the hip bone. **Ventrally**, the connection between the two hip bones is created by the pubic symphysis. **Dorsally**, there are connections with the trunk or spinal column – with the sacrum and coccyx, as well as the lumbar spine, via the sacroiliac joint and a number of ligaments.

The sacroiliac joint
The articular bones are the sacrum, hip bone and iliac bone. The joint capsule is under firm tension and posteriorly its place is taken by the interosseous sacroiliac joint.
The joint cavity is narrow and fissure-like. A number of ligaments are present as special features.
The **direct strengthening ligaments** are the anterior sacroiliac ligament **ventrally**, and **dorsally** the posterior sacroiliac ligament and the interosseous sacroiliac ligament.
The iliolumbar ligament, sacrospinous ligament and sacrotuberous ligament serve as **indirect strengthening ligaments.**
The **anterior sacroiliac ligaments** are usually not particularly thick and lie on the pelvic side of the joint capsule. They run from the pelvic fascia of the sacrum to the iliac bone.
The **posterior sacroiliac ligaments,** 1 cm thick, are anchored with their long fibers on the posterior superior iliac spine and the lateral parts of the third and fourth segments of the sacrum.

The **interosseous sacroiliac ligament** fills the deep cavity between the iliac tuberosity and the sacral tuberosity. The strongest ligament in this region, it is one of the body's thickest ligaments.
The **iliolumbar ligament** originates, with its strong bands, from the transverse processes of the fourth and fifth lumbar vertebrae, radiating over the iliac crest and the neighboring parts of the anterior and posterior surfaces of the iliac bone.
The **sacrotuberous ligament** is attached to the interior surface of the ischial tuberosity and originates from the lateral margin of the sacrum and coccyx. It extends up as far as the posterior and superior inferior iliac spine.
The **sacrospinous ligament** is shorter and thinner than the previous one and is connected to it. Its base is also attached to the lateral margin of the sacrum and coccyx, but its tip attaches to the ischial spine.
The sacrotuberous ligament and sacrospinous ligament form an essential part of the pelvic diaphragm.

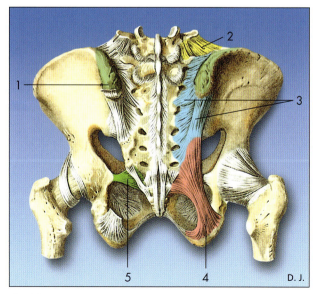

Fig. 23.1 Anatomy.
(1) Posterior superior iliac spine, (2) iliolumbar ligament, (3) dorsal sacroiliac ligament, (4) sacrotuberous ligament, (5) sacrospinous ligament

Iliolumbosacral ligaments

Indications

Diagnostic
- Differential diagnosis of various pain syndromes in the lumbosacral region.

Therapeutic
- Pain in iliolumbosacral ligamentous insufficiency.

Block series
A series of six to eight blocks is recommended. When there is evidence of improvement in the symptoms, additional blocks can also be carried out.

Contraindications
- Anticoagulant treatment.
- Infections and skin diseases in the injection area.

Procedure

Full information for the patient is mandatory.

Preparations
Check that the emergency equipment is complete and in working order; sterile precautions, intravenous access.

Materials (Fig. 23.2)
Fine 26-G needle, 25 mm long, for local anesthesia.
20–22-G needle, 70–80 mm long.
Syringes: 2 mL and 10 mL.
Local anesthetic, disinfectant, swabs, sterile gloves and flat, firm pillow.

Patient positioning
- Prone position: pillow under the mid-abdomen (to eliminate lumbar lordosis). The patient's arms are hanging.

Landmarks (Fig. 23.3)
- Iliac crest line of L4.
- The spinous process of the fifth lumbar vertebra is located about two fingerbreadths below the iliac crest line. The injection point is above the spinous process.

Injection targets (Fig. 23.4)
- Transverse process of the fifth lumbar vertebra.
- Dorsal cranial iliac spine.
- Lateral edge of the caudal part of the sacral bone.

Skin prep, local anesthesia, drawing up the local anesthetic, testing the patency of the injection needle.

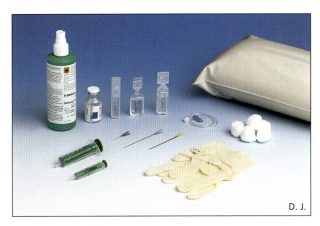

Fig. 23.2 Materials

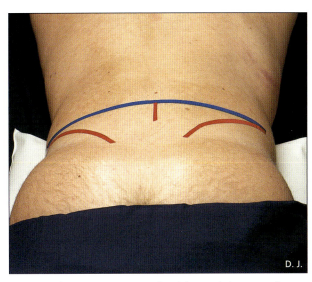

Fig. 23.3 The spinous process of L5 is located about two fingerbreadths below the iliac crest line

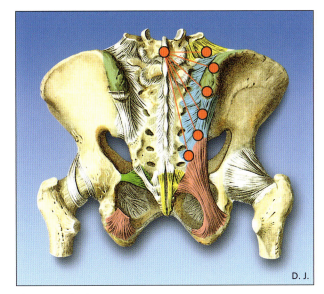

Fig. 23.4 Injection targets

Chapter 23

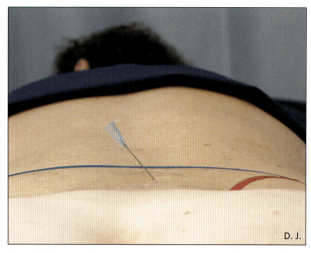

Fig. 23.5 Introducing the injection needle in the direction of the transverse process of L5 (45°)

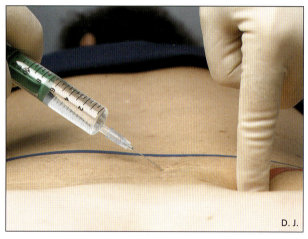

Fig. 23.6 The injection angle of ca. 30° in the direction of the iliac crest

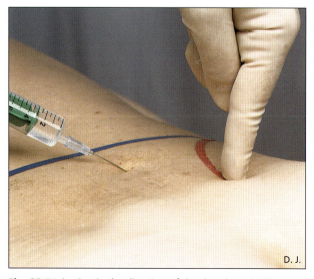

Fig. 23.7 Injection in the direction of the dorsal cranial iliac spine and then along the lower half of the sacrum

During the injection, the following points must be observed:
- The person carrying out the injection must stand on the opposite side to that being blocked.
- All insertions of the needle must be carried out from only one point.
- Elicit bone contact before injection.
- Aspirate before every injection.

Injection technique
Iliolumbar ligament
- The needle is introduced in the direction of the lateral part of the transverse process of the fifth lumbar vertebra, at an angle of 45° to the surface of the skin (Fig. 23.5).
- Bone contact is made after about 4–6 cm; the needle is then withdrawn by 1 mm and, after aspiration, 1–2 mL of local anesthetic is administered.
- The needle is then withdrawn to lie subcutaneously.
- The needle is then reintroduced at an angle of ca. 30° in the direction of the iliac crest, which is marked on the outside by the operator's index finger (Fig. 23.6).
  After bone contact, the needle is withdrawn by 1 mm and after aspiration, 1 mL of local anesthetic is injected.

If bone contact is not made at this depth, correct the angle of the needle, either craniolaterally or caudolaterally.

Sacroiliac, sacrotuberous and sacrospinous ligament
- The needle is withdrawn to lie subcutaneously.
- The needle is reintroduced at an angle of 30° in the direction of the dorsal cranial iliac spine, which is marked on the outside by the operator's index finger. After aspiration, 1 mL of local anesthetic is injected at two further points along the iliac spine.
- The needle is withdrawn to lie subcutaneously once more and then reintroduced two or three times at an angle of 20° along the lower half of the sacrum. The lateral edge is infiltrated with 1 mL local anesthetic at each level (Fig. 23.7).

Pain may increase during the injection.

Dosage
Diagnostic
10–15 mL local anesthetic – e.g. 0.5–1% prilocaine, 0.5–1% mepivacaine.

Therapeutic
- Unilateral block: 10 mL local anesthetic – e.g. 0.75 ropivacaine, 0.5% bupivacaine.
- Bilateral block: 15 mL local anesthetic – e.g. 0.5–0.75% ropivacaine, 0.25–0.5% bupivacaine, distributed on both sides.

In acute cases, 4 mg dexamethasone can be added with benefit.

Sclerosant solutions [4]
- 6 mL 40% glucose + 4 mL 1% mepivacaine (1 mL per injection site)
- Barbor solution with local anesthetic:
  Phenol crist. 2.0 vol%
  Glucose monohydrate 27.5 vol%
  Anhydrous glycerol 30.0 vol%
  Methylene blue 1.0 vol%
  Distilled water 39.5 vol%
  6 mL Barbor solution + 4 mL 0.5% bupivacaine = 10 mL (1 mL per injection site)

Repeated injection of sclerosant solution shows no benefit in comparison with a block series with a local anesthetic.

Complications
Block of a lumbar somatic nerve, with accompanying motor weakness during the local anesthetic effect (prophylaxis: no injection without bone contact).
Monitoring is obligatory after the block. The patient should be supported by a nurse when first standing up and should first use the leg on the unblocked side.
Complications are extremely rare and occur mainly due to poor technique.

24 Ganglion impar (Walther ganglion) block

Definition
Injection of a local anesthetic or neurolytic into the region of the most inferior (unpaired) ganglion of the sympathetic trunk, on the ventral side of the sacrococcygeal joint.

Anatomy

At the level of the pelvic inlet, the lumbar part of the sympathetic trunk becomes the sacral part of the sympathetic trunk. This lies behind the parietal peritoneum and the rectum in the parietal pelvic fascia and on the ventral surface of the sacrum immediately medial to the sacral foramina, with the vessels and nerves that course through them. The sacral part of the sympathetic trunk (Fig. 24.1) consists of three (but sometimes four or five) sacral ganglia, which have connections with the contralateral ganglia. From the two (or three) cranial ganglia emerge (two or three) **sacral splanchnic nerves,** with efferent (usually postganglionic) and afferent fibers to the **inferior hypogastric plexus.** The two sacral sympathetic trunks approach closer to each other caudally and join to form the ganglion impar (Walther ganglion), which is located in front of the coccyx (Fig. 24.2). White rami communicantes are absent, but gray rami communicantes with postganglionic sympathetic fibers course from each of the sacral ganglia to the corresponding spinal nerves in the sacrococcygeal region. Along with branches of the sacrococcygeal plexus, these fibers reach vessels, sweat glands, erector muscles of the hair, cross-striated muscles, bones and joints.

Indications
Diagnostic
- Differential diagnosis of pain in the anorectal and perineal region.

Prognostic
- In cancer pain, before a neurolytic block.

Therapeutic
- Pain conditions in the anorectal and perineal region.
- Injection of neurolytic agents as a palliative measure in malignant processes (rectum, cervix of the uterus, perineum, bladder, endometrium) [4–6].

Contraindications
- Anticoagulant treatment.
- Infections and skin diseases in the injection area.
- Advanced rectal carcinoma (causing blockage of the access route to the ganglion impar).

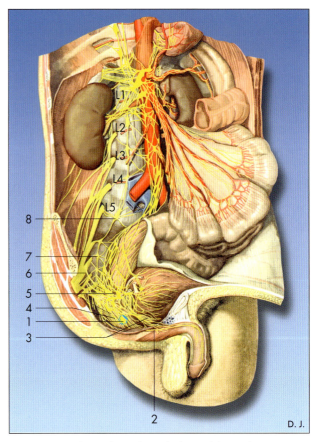

Fig. 24.1 Sacral ganglia and sacral plexus. (1) Ganglion impar, (2) pudendal nerve, (3) prostatic plexus, (4) rectal plexus, (5) ventral part of the inferior hypogastric plexus, (6) sacral plexus, (7) ganglion of the sympathetic trunk, (8) lumbosacral ganglion of the sympathetic trunk

Procedure

This block should be carried out by very experienced anesthetists. Full information for the patient is mandatory.

> Neurolytic agents should never be administered without precise localization of the needle position using radiographic guidance with an image intensifier. The method of choice is CT-guided injection.

Preparations
Check that the emergency equipment is complete and in working order; sterile precautions, intravenous access, ECG monitoring, pulse oximetry, intubation kit, ventilation facilities, emergency medication.

Materials
A fine 26-G needle for local anesthesia. A stable 70–80-mm long 20–22-G needle. The needle shaft curves in a sickle shape (Fig. 24.3), so that the needle can pass atraumatically to the ventral surface of the sacrococcygeal joint.

Patient positioning
Prone, or alternatively lateral recumbent (see Chapter 47 on caudal anesthesia, p. 361).

Localization
Palpation of the tip of the coccyx or sacrococcygeal joint.

Disinfection, generous local anesthetic infiltration of the needle channel, covering with a sterile drape, drawing up the local anesthetic. The patency of the previously bent injection needle should be checked.

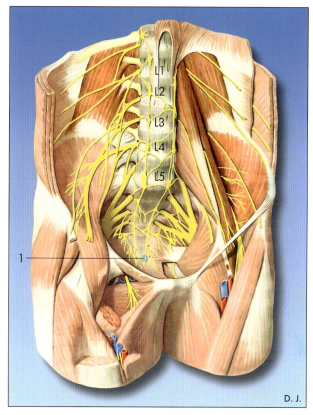

Fig. 24.2 Ganglion impar (Walther's ganglion). Ventral surface of the sacrococcygeal joint

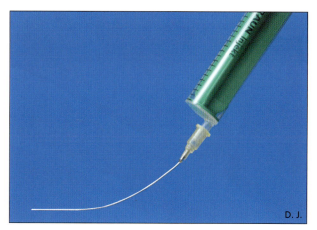

Fig. 24.3 70–80-mm long 20–22-G needle. The needle shaft is bent to form a sickle shape

Chapter 24

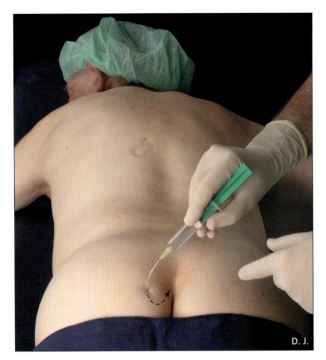

Fig. 24.4a Introduction of the sickle-shaped curved injection needle in a slightly cranial direction toward the ventral surface of the sacrococcygeal joint

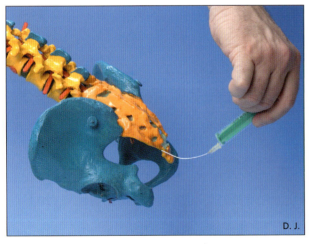

Fig. 24.4b In the skeleton

Injection technique
Approximately 3 cm laterally from the median sacral crest, thorough local anesthesia of the needle channel to a depth of ca. 3–4 cm is administered. After the onset of the local anesthetic effect, the sickle-shaped injection needle is introduced in a slightly cranial direction, toward the ventral surface of the sacrococcygeal joint (shown in Fig. 24.4a in a patient, Fig. 24.4b in the skeleton). After an intravascular position of the needle (aspiration of blood) has been excluded, as well as an intrarectal position (aspiration of air), and after aspiration, incremental injection of the local anesthetic is carried out.

Dosage
Diagnostic
5–10 mL local anesthetic – e.g. 1% prilocaine or 1% mepivacaine.

Therapeutic
- Local anesthetics:
  5–10 mL local anesthetic – e.g. ropivacaine 0.2–0.375% mixed with 40 mg triamcinolone.
- Neurolytics:
  4–6 mL 10% phenol [4–6].

Complications
- Intravascular injection (see Chapter 6, p. 65).
- Rectal perforation.
- Subperiosteal position (becomes evident due to high resistance and severe pain during the injection).
- Needle breakage (strong needles should be used).
- Infection (sterile precautions).

Ganglion impar block

Block no. ☐ Right ☐ Left

Name: _____ Date: _____
Diagnosis: _____
Premedication: ☐ No ☐ Yes _____
Neurological abnormalities: ☐ No ☐ Yes _____

Purpose of block: ☐ Diagnostic ☐ Therapeutic
Needle: G _____ Length _____ cm, curved
i.v. access: ☐ Yes
Monitoring: ☐ ECG ☐ Pulse oximetry
Ventilation facilities: ☐ Yes (equipment checked)
Emergency equipment *(drugs)*: ☐ Checked
Patient: ☐ Informed
Contraindications excluded: ☐

Position: ☐ Prone ☐ Lateral recumbent
Injection level: ☐ Sacrococcygeal joint
Injection technique: ☐ X-ray image intensifier guidance ☐ CT-guided
Injection:
Local anesthetic: _____ mL _____ %
(in incremental doses)
Addition to LA: ☐ Yes _____ ☐ No
Neurolytic: _____ mL _____ %

Patient's remarks during injection:
☐ None ☐ Paresthesias ☐ Warmth ☐ Pain
Nerve area: _____
Objective block effect after 15 min:
☐ Cold test ☐ Temperature measurement before _____ °C after _____ °C
Monitoring after block: ☐ < 1 h ☐ > 1 h
Time of discharge: _____

Complications:
☐ None ☐ Intravascular injection ☐ Subperiosteal position
☐ Rectal perforation ☐ Infection ☐ Coccygeal pain

Subjective effects of the block: Duration: _____
☐ None ☐ Increased pain
☐ Reduced pain ☐ Relief of pain

VISUAL ANALOG SCALE

|||||||||||
0   10   20   30   40   50   60   70   80   90   100

Special notes: _____

Record and checklist

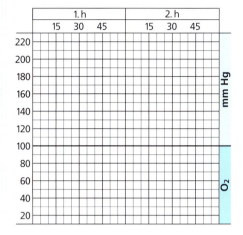

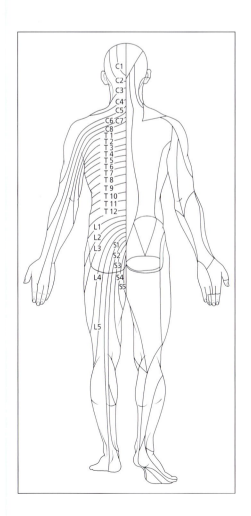

25 Infiltration of the piriform trigger points ("piriform syndrome")

Introduction

Activation of the trigger points in the piriform muscle ("double devil") and five other small external rotator muscles (the superior gemellus muscle, obturator internus muscle, inferior gemellus muscle, obturator externus muscle, and quadratus femoris muscle) and the resulting irritation of the neighboring nerves give rise to pain with a classic distribution pattern [14]. The name of the piriform muscle is derived from the Latin *pirum*, pear, and *forma*, shape. The muscle was named by the Flemish anatomist Adriaan van der Spieghel (Spigelius), who lived in the late sixteenth and early seventeenth centuries.

Anatomy

The piriform muscle, a thick, plump muscle, has its origin in the pelvis and anterior surface of the sacrum, between pelvic sacral foramina 1–4, and on the way to its insertion on the upper edge of the greater trochanter it passes through the greater sciatic foramen. This rigid opening is formed anteriorly and superiorly by the ilium, posteriorly by the sacrotuberal ligament, and inferiorly by the sacrospinal ligament (Fig. 25.1). The piriform muscle acts as an external rotator for the thigh and also supports abduction of the thigh. Its innervation is usually derived from the first and second sacral nerves. The neural structures in the greater sciatic foramen consist of: the superior gluteal nerve, sciatic nerve, pudendal nerve with the pudendal vessels, inferior gluteal nerve and the posterior cutaneous nerve of the thigh (Fig. 25.2). These nerves are jointly responsible for sensorimotor function of all the gluteal muscles, for sensorimotor function in the perineum, and for almost the whole of sensorimotor function in the posterior thigh and calf.

The most important blood vessels in this region are the superior gluteal artery and inferior gluteal artery.

Mechanism of pain

Numerous authors have recognized that contraction of the piriform muscle is capable of constricting the nerves and vessels that pass through the greater sciatic foramen.

The resulting inadequate blood supply to the muscle leads – due to accumulation of metabolic waste products that are normally disposed of by the circulating blood – to referred myofascial pain and often to blocking of the iliosacral joint.

Symptoms

Trigger points in the piriform muscle make a substantial contribution to complex myofascial pain syndromes in the area of the pelvis and hip. The piriform syndrome is often characterized by bizarre and initially apparently unconnected symptoms [11,14]. Patients report pain (and paresthesias) in the small of the back, groin, perineum, buttocks, hip, back of the thigh and calf, foot, and also in the rectum (during defecation) and in the area of the coccyx.

Some authors have suspected that contraction of the piriform muscle is an often overlooked cause of coccydynia [2, 13]. Edwards described the syndrome as "neuritis of the branches of the sciatic nerve" [11], while Te Poorten suspected involvement of the peroneal nerve [11].

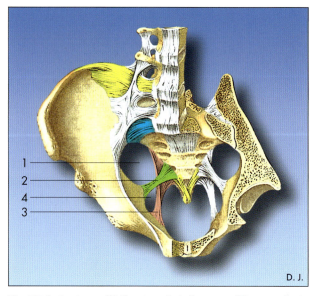

Fig. 25.1 Anatomy. (1) Greater sciatic foramen, (2) sacrospinal ligament, (3) sacrotuberal ligament, (4) lesser sciatic foramen

Swelling in the affected leg and disturbances of sexual function (dyspareunia in women and disturbances of potency in men) are very often present as accompanying symptoms.

Activation and provocation of trigger points in the piriform muscle can be initiated by the following factors: severe stress, trauma, prolonged immobility of the muscle, long car drives, chronic infections (pelvis, infectious sacroiliitis, arthritic hip), Morton's anomaly in the foot, asymmetry in the body, etc. [14].

Differential diagnoses include: "post-laminectomy syndrome," intervertebral disk prolapse, coccydynia, facet syndrome, spinal stenosis (bilateral pain), sacroiliitis, malignant neoplasms, local infections, etc.

Treatment of this syndrome includes: therapeutic injections of local anesthetics and corticosteroids [2–5, 8, 10], botulinum toxin injection [16], osteopathic manipulation [10, 11], intermittent cooling and stretching [14], corrective measures [10, 11, 14], self-stretching [14], transrectal or transvaginal massage of the muscle [13], and finally surgical decompression [2, 11, 14].

Procedure

Prior information for the patient is mandatory.

Preparations
See Chapter 28, sciatic nerve block, p. 231.

Materials
- Nerve stimulator (e.g. Stimuplex® HNS 11, B. Braun Melsungen).
- 22-G Stimuplex D® needle (15°), 80 mm long, with an injection lead – "immobile needle" (B. Braun Melsungen).
- 22-G spinal needle 80 mm long.
- 2-mL, 10-mL, and 20-mL syringes.
- Local anesthetics, disinfectant, swabs, compresses, sterile gloves and drape.

Technique

Positioning
Figure 25.3 (see Chapter 28, p. 231).

Landmarks
The important landmarks are the greater trochanter and posterior superior iliac spine. From the mid-point of the line connecting these, a line is drawn in a medial direction and the injection site is marked at 5 cm (Fig. 25.3).

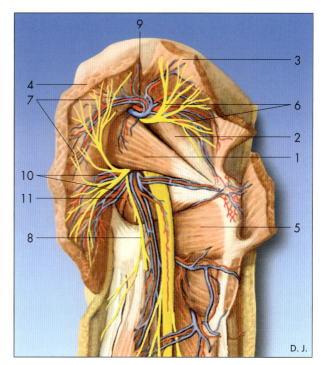

Fig. 25.2 Anatomy. (1) Piriform muscle and neighboring muscles, nerves, and vessels, (2) gluteus minimus muscle, (3) gluteus medius muscle, (4) gluteus maximus muscle, (5) quadratus femoris muscle, (6) superior gluteal nerve, (7) inferior gluteal nerve, (8) posterior cutaneous nerve of the thigh, (9) superior gluteal artery, (10) inferior gluteal artery and vein, (11) internal pudendal artery

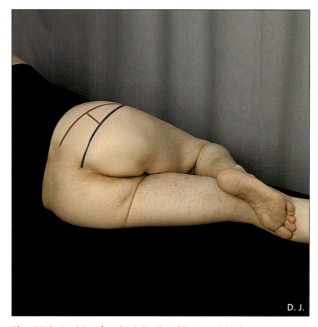

Fig. 25.3 Position for the injection (Sims position)

Injection technique
Transgluteal technique
The injection needle is introduced perpendicular to the skin (Fig. 25.4). Stimulation current starts at 1 mA at 2 Hz, with a stimulus duration of 0.1 ms. At a depth of ca. 6–8 cm, plantar flexion and dorsiflexion of the foot occurs in response to the stimulation of the tibial or perineal part of the sciatic nerve. The needle is then withdrawn slightly until the twitching completely disappears. After an aspiration test, injection of half of the planned amount of injection solution is carried out. The needle is then withdrawn to lie subcutaneously, and blindly advanced laterally in the direction of the greater trochanter in order to reach the muscle's lateral trigger point. After aspiration, the rest of the solution is then injected.

Pace transgluteal technique
The trigger points in the piriform muscle are located by transrectal palpation. The palpating index finger of the left hand serves as a guide for the 80-mm long 22-G spinal needle, which is introduced in a dorsal and transgluteal position [10, 13]. Fan-shaped infiltration into the belly of the muscle is carried out. This method is usually painful for the patient.

Dosage [2–6, 10]
5–10 mL local anesthetic – e.g. 0.5% ropivacaine or 0.5% lidocaine.
5–10 mL 0.2% ropivacaine or 0.08–0.25% bupivacaine.
Mixture with 20–40 mg long-acting corticosteroid (e.g. long-acting methylprednisolone) is also recommended. Experience shows that long-acting local anesthetics do not provide any substantial advantages over short-acting local anesthetics [2, 6, 14]. It should be pointed out to the patient that spreading of the local anesthetic (particularly with a long-acting agent) in the region of

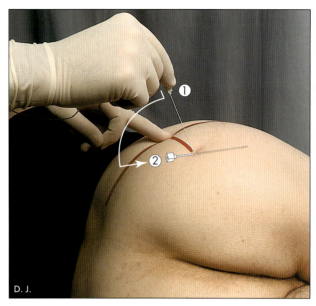

Fig. 25.4 Trigger point 1: the injection needle is introduced perpendicular to the surface of the skin. Trigger point 2: the needle is withdrawn and then advanced laterally in the direction of the greater trochanter

the sciatic nerve can lead to the leg suddenly giving away later (note the information required for outpatients; see Chapter 26, p. 224).

Complications
- See Chapter 28, p. 236.
- Nerve injury (see Chapter 26, p. 225). Injection of corticosteroid into the sciatic nerve must be avoided at all costs.
- Intravascular injection (see Chapter 6).
- CNS toxicity (see Chapters 1 and 6).
- Infection.
- Hematoma formation.
- Perforation of the rectum (transgluteal technique after intrarectal palpation of the trigger points).

Lower extremity

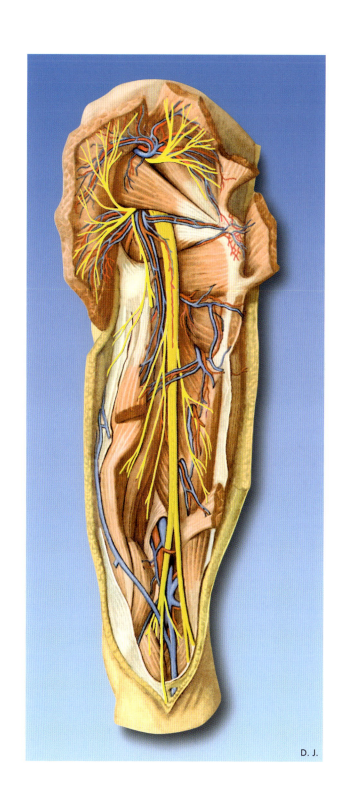

Anatomy of the lumbar plexus, sacral plexus and coccygeal plexus

These plexuses, closely related to one another, are formed by the ventral branches of the lumbar, sacral and coccygeal spinal nerves.

The **lumbar plexus** lies in front of the transverse processes of the lumbar vertebrae. It mainly arises from the ventral branches, the first three lumbar nerves, most of the fourth lumbar nerve and the twelfth thoracic nerve (subcostal nerve).

The most important branches of the plexus are located in a **fascial compartment** that is enclosed ("sandwiched") by the quadratus lumborum, psoas major and iliacus muscles.

The first lumbar nerve, which contains a branch from the twelfth thoracic nerve, divides into an upper branch (iliohypogastric nerve and ilioinguinal nerve) and a lower branch (genitofemoral nerve).

Most of the second, third and parts of the fourth lumbar nerves form ventral and dorsal branches, from which the femoral nerve and obturator nerve branch off. The lateral femoral cutaneous nerve is formed from fibers of the dorsal branches of L2/L3.

The caudal parts of the ventral branches of L4 and L5 combine to form the **lumbosacral trunk**. Together with the ventral branches of the first three sacral nerves and the upper part of the ventral branch of the fourth sacral nerve, the lumbosacral trunk forms the sacral plexus, the largest branch of which is the sciatic nerve. The lumbar plexus is also connected with the lumbar part of the sympathetic nervous system via two or three long communicating branches.

The thickness of the ventral branches of the lumbar nerves increases markedly from the first to the fifth nerve (L1 has a diameter of ca. 2.5 mm, L2 is already ca. 4 mm, L3 and L4 are ca. 6 mm and L5 is as large as 7 mm).

The **coccygeal plexus** arises from the lower part of the ventral branches of the fourth and fifth sacral nerves, as well as the coccygeal nerves.

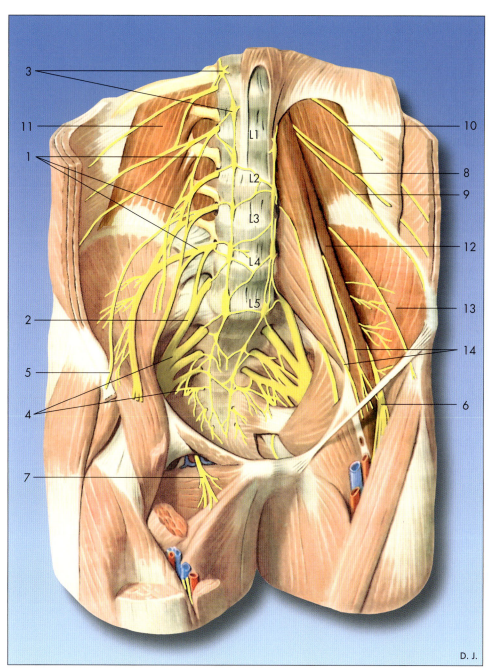

Anatomy: lumbar plexus, sacral plexus and coccygeal plexus.
(1) Lumbar plexus, (2) lumbosacral trunk, (3) sympathetic trunk, (4) sacral plexus, (5) lateral femoral cutaneous nerve, (6) femoral nerve, (7) obturator nerve, (8) iliohypogastric nerve, (9) ilioinguinal nerve, (10) subcostal nerve, (11) quadratus lumborum muscle, (12) psoas major muscle, (13) iliacus muscle, (14) genitofemoral nerve

Lumbar plexus blocks

26 Inguinal femoral paravascular block ("three-in-one" block)

Introduction

The concept underlying lumbar plexus blocks is that the course of the neural network from the transverse processes to the inguinal ligament lies within a perivascular and perineural space. Like the epidural space, this space limits the spread of the local anesthetic and conducts it to the various nerves.
Within the connective tissue and neural sheath, the concentration and volume of the local anesthetic determine the extent of the block's spread. Two techniques are described that belong to the standard methods for blocking the lumbar plexus:
- The caudal (ventral) psoas compartment block ("three in-one" inguinal femoral paravascular block).
- The cranial (dorsal) psoas compartment block.

Definition
The "three-in-one" block is an infero–antero approach to the femoral nerve, lateral femoral cutaneous nerve and obturator nerve. These three nerves (Fig. 26.1) are blocked with a single injection into the common connective tissue and neural sheath (Fig. 26.2) immediately below the inguinal ligament.
A volume of at least 35–40 mL of local anesthetic is necessary to block all three nerves.
The success of the block depends directly on the amount of local anesthetic injected. To produce complete anesthesia in the leg, it should be combined with a sciatic nerve block (Figs. 26.7, 26.8).

Advantages
- Suitable for postoperative or post-traumatic analgesia and for therapeutic blocks.
- Suitable for patients in whom a unilateral block is desired – particularly in outpatient procedures.

Disadvantages
- Success is unpredictable.
- Larger amounts of local anesthetic are necessary (particularly if the sciatic nerve is also being blocked).
- The likelihood of systemic toxicity is increased.
- Longer onset times have to be expected (surgical indications).
- Despite larger amounts of local anesthetic, not all nerves in the plexus are blocked (e.g. the lateral femoral cutaneous nerve).
- For surgical procedures with ischemia or a tourniquet, neuraxial anesthesia is preferable.

Indications
Surgical
- Superficial surgical interventions in the innervated area:
  Wound care, skin grafts, muscle biopsies.
- Blocking of the obturator reflex in transurethral prostate resection.
- Analgesia for positioning for neuraxial block anesthesia in femoral neck fractures.
- Performing surgical interventions in the area of the lower extremity in ischemia or tourniquet, in combination with sciatic nerve block.
  Larger volumes of local anesthetic have to be used here (toxicity!).
- Outpatient procedures.

Therapeutic
- Postoperative pain therapy (e.g. after femoral neck, femoral shaft, tibial and patellar fractures, knee joint operations).
- Post-traumatic pain.
- Postoperative neurolysis or nerve reimplantations for better innervation.
- Early mobilization after hip or knee joint operations.
- Arterial occlusive disease and poor perfusion in the lower extremities.
- Complex regional pain syndrome (CRPS) types I and II.

- Postamputation pain.
- Edema in the leg after radiotherapy.
- Diabetic polyneuropathy.
- Knee joint arthritis.
- Elimination of adductor spasm in paraplegic patients.

Block series
A series of six to eight blocks is recommended. When there is evidence of improvement in the symptoms, additional blocks can also be carried out.

Prophylactic
- Postoperative analgesia.
- Prophylaxis against postamputation pain.
- Prophylaxis against complex regional pain syndrome (CRPS).

Contraindications
Specific
- Infections (e.g. osteomyelitis, pyoderma) or malignant diseases in the inguinal region.
- Local hematoma.
- Anticoagulant treatment.
- Distorted anatomy (due to prior surgical interventions or trauma to the inguinal and thigh region).

Relative
The decision should be taken after carefully weighing up the risks and benefits:
- Hemorrhagic diathesis.
- Stable central nervous system disorders.
- Local nerve injury (when it is difficult to determine whether the cause is surgical or anesthetic).
- Contralateral nerve paresis.
- Patients with a femoral bypass.

Procedure

This block should be carried out by experienced anesthetists, or under their supervision. Full information for the patient is mandatory.

Preparations
Check that the emergency equipment is complete and in working order. Sterile precautions, intravenous access, ECG monitoring, pulse oximetry, intubation kit, ventilation facilities, emergency medication.

Materials (Fig. 26.3)
Fine 26-G needle, 25 mm long, for local anesthesia.
Nerve stimulator (e.g. Stimuplex® HNS 11, B. Braun Melsungen).

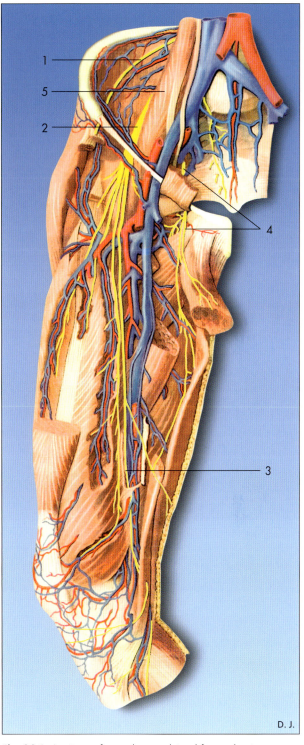

Fig. 26.1 Anatomy: femoral nerve, lateral femoral cutaneous nerve and obturator nerve.
(1) Lateral femoral cutaneous nerve, (2) femoral nerve, (3) saphenous nerve, (4) obturator nerve, (5) psoas major muscle

Chapter 26

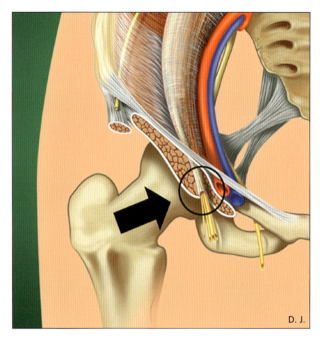

Fig. 26.2 Common connective tissue and neural sheath

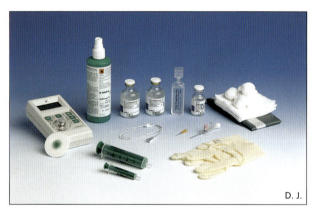

Fig. 26.3 Materials

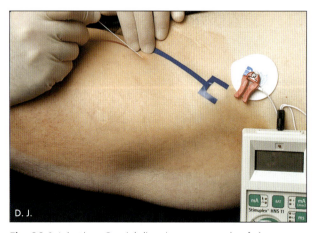

Fig. 26.4 Injection. Cranial direction, at an angle of about 30–40° to the skin surface

- Single-shot technique:
  50 (80)-mm long atraumatic 22-G needle (15°) with injection lead ("immobile needle" – e.g. Stimuplex D®, B. Braun Melsungen).
- Continuous technique:*
  Contiplex D® set: Contiplex® catheter 0.45 × 0.85 × 400 mm, with 18-G needle, 80 mm (15°), B. Braun Melsungen), or:
  Contiplex®–Tuohy set: 52 (102)-mm long 18-G Tuohy needle with Contiplex® catheter.

Syringes: 2 and 20 mL.
Local anesthetics, disinfectant, swabs, compresses, sterile gloves and drape.

Patient positioning
Supine, with the thigh slightly abducted. The patient's ipsilateral hand lies under the head. The person carrying out the injection must stand on the side being blocked.

Landmarks
The femoral artery is palpated 1–2 cm distal to the inguinal ligament. It is held between the spread index and middle finger. The injection point lies about 1–1.5 cm laterally.

Skin prep, subcutaneous local anesthesia, sterile drapes; draw up local anesthetic into 20-mL syringes, check patency of injection needles and functioning of nerve stimulator, attach electrodes.

Preliminary puncture with a large needle or stylet.

> The **quadriceps femoris muscle** and the **patella** must be observed throughout the procedure.

Injection technique
Single injection technique
- The injection is carried out in a cranial direction at an angle of about 30–40° to the skin surface, almost parallel to the course of the femoral artery. Stimultion current of 1–2 mA at 2 Hz is selected with a stimulus duration of 0.1 ms (Fig. 26.4).
- The needle is advanced until contractions of the **quadriceps femoris muscle** and **patellar movements** become visible ("dancing patella"). Contractions of the sartorius muscle alone suggest incorrect positioning and are inadequate (Fig. 26.5).

---

* If technical difficulties arise, the catheter and Tuohy needle must always be removed simultaneously. A catheter must never be removed through the Tuohy needle (as the catheter may shear!).

Inguinal femoral paravascular block ("three-in-one" block)

- Do **not** advance the needle further!
  The stimulation current is reduced to 0.3 mA. Slight twitching suggests that the stimulation needle is in the immediate vicinity of the nerve.
- Aspiration test.
- Test dose of 3 mL local anesthetic (e.g. 1% prilocaine). During the injection, the twitching slowly disappears.
- Incremental injection of a local anesthetic (injection–aspiration after each 3–4 mL).
- After the injection, **compression massage** of the injection area is carried out and then **flexing of the thigh** for about 1 min (Fig. 26.6).
- Careful cardiovascular monitoring.

> During the injection, distal compression should be applied with the finger to encourage proximal spread of the local anesthetic.

The distribution of the anesthetic is indicated in Figure 26.7.

Continuous technique
The site is located in the same way as described for the unilateral technique. The injection is carried out about 2–2.5 cm below the inguinal ligament and 1–1.5 cm lateral to the femoral artery and in a cranial direction at an angle of about 30–40°.
Using the Seldinger technique, the catheter is advanced at least 10 cm deep into the fascial compartment.
An aspiration test, administration of a test dose, fixation of the catheter and placement of a bacterial filter then follow. After aspirating again, the local anesthetic is given on an incremental basis.

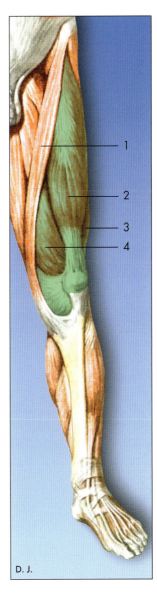

Fig. 26.5 Note the contractions of the quadriceps femoris muscle and patellar movements. (1) Sartorius muscle, (2) rectus femoris muscle, (3) vastus lateralis muscle, (4) vastus medialis muscle

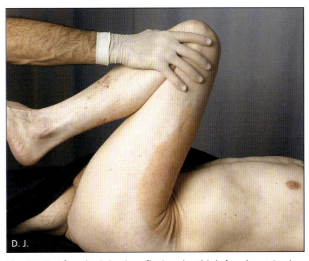

Fig. 26.6 After the injection: flexing the thigh for about 1 min

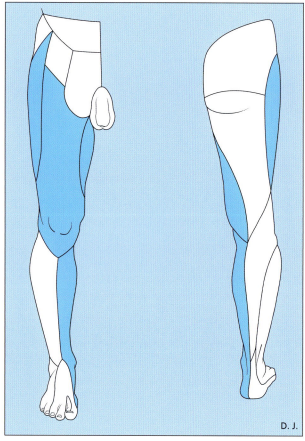

Fig. 26.7 The neural areas most frequently blocked after administration of a "three-in-one" block

Dosage

Surgical
40–50 mL local anesthetic – e.g. 0.5–0.75% ropivacaine, 0.5% bupivacaine (0.5% levobupivacaine), 1% prilocaine, 1% mepivacaine.
A combination of local anesthetics with longer-term and medium-term effect has proved particularly valuable for surgical indications – e.g. 1% prilocaine (20 mL) + 0.5–0.75% ropivacaine (20 mL) or 1% prilocaine (20 mL) + 0.25–0.5% bupivacaine (0.25–0.5% levobupivacaine; 20 mL).

Therapeutic
20 mL local anesthetic – e.g. 0.2–0.375% ropivacaine, 0.125–0.25% bupivacaine (0.125–0.25% levobupivacaine).

Important notes for outpatients
Long-lasting block can occur (even after administration of low-dose local anesthetics – e.g. 0.125% bupivacaine or 0.2% ropivacaine).
The blocked leg can give way even 10–18 hours after the injection.

The patient must therefore use walking aids during this period. The same rules apply to the treatment of post-amputation pain. During the period of effect of the local anesthetic, the patient should not wear a prosthesis.

> A record must be kept of patient information and consent.

Continuous technique
Test dose: 3–5 mL 1% prilocaine (1% mepivacaine).
Bolus administration: 30 mL 0.5–0.75% ropivacaine or 0.25–0.5% bupivacaine.
Maintenance dose:
Intermittent administration:
15–20 mL of local anesthetic every 4–6 hours (0.5–0.75% ropivacaine or 0.25–0.5% bupivacaine) after a prior test dose.
Reduction of the dose and/or adjustment of the interval, depending on the clinical picture.
Continuous infusion:
Infusion of the local anesthetic via the catheter should be started 30–60 minutes after the bolus dose. A test dose is obligatory.

Ropivacaine: 0.2–0.375%	**6–14 mL/h** (max. 37.5 mg/h)
Levobupivacaine: 0.125–0.25%	**8–15 mL/h**
Bupivacaine: 0.125%	**10–14 mL/h**
Bupivacaine: 0.25%	**8–10 mL/h**

If necessary, the infusion can be supplemented with bolus doses of 5–10 mL 0.5–0.75% ropivacaine (0.25–0.5% bupivacaine or 0.25% levobupivacaine).

> Individual adjustment of the dosage and period of treatment is essential.

Complications

- Nerve injuries
  Traumatic nerve injury is a rare complication of this technique. It can occur as a result of the use of sharp needles (due to nerve puncture), intraneural or microvascular injury (hematoma and its sequelae), prolonged ischemia, as well as toxic effects of intraneurally injected local anesthetic (see Chapter 9, p. n). Probable effects of intraneural injection include a transient neurological deficit (unexpectedly prolonged block, lasting up to 10 days) [6, 10].
- A suspicion of intraneural needle positioning arises if there is strong twitching even at low levels of stimulation current (e.g. 0.2 mA) and if there is no cessation of the twitching after administration of the test dose. The local anesthetic may also be difficult to inject.
  Correction of the needle position is essential.
  (On prophylaxis, see Chapter 9, p. 111).
- Intravascular injection (see Chapter 6, p. 65).
- CNS intoxication (see Chapter 6, p. 66 and Chapter 1, p. 9).
- Infection in the injection area (continuous techniques).
- Hematoma formation (note the obligatory prophylactic compression).

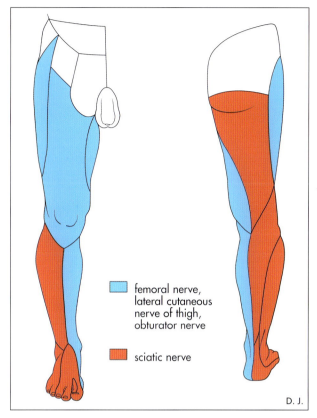

Fig. 26.8 Comparison of the innervation areas of the femoral nerve, lateral femoral cutaneous nerve and obturator nerve (blue) with the innervation area of the sciatic nerve (red)

27 Psoas compartment block (Cheyen approach)

Definition
The psoas compartment block represents a **cranial and dorsal paravertebral access route** to the lumbar plexus.
The concept is to block the closely juxtaposed branches of the lumbar plexus and parts of the sacral plexus by injecting local anesthetic through a high access route to the plexus (L4–L5).
When the quality of the block is good, the area of distribution is comparable with that of the "three-in-one" block (see Chapter 26, Fig. 26.7).
The following nerves are affected: lateral femoral cutaneous nerve, femoral nerve, genitofemoral nerve, obturator nerve, and parts of the sciatic and posterior femoral cutaneous nerve.
A combination of this block with block of the sciatic nerve is necessary to achieve complete anesthesia of the lower extremity (see Chapter 26, Figs. 26.7, 26.8).

Advantages
- Better block quality in comparison with the "three-in-one" block.
- Suitable for patients in whom a unilateral block is desired, particularly in outpatient procedures.
- The method is suitable for postoperative and post-traumatic analgesia and for therapeutic blocks.

Disadvantages
- Success of the block is unpredictable.
- Larger quantities of local anesthetic are needed (particularly if the sciatic nerve is also being anesthetized).
- There is an increased likelihood of systemic toxicity.
- There is a potential risk of intrathecal or epidural injection.
- Slower onset must be expected (surgical indications).
- For surgical procedures with ischemia or tourniquet, neuraxial anesthesia is preferable.

Indications
Surgical
- As a continuous or single-shot block for all surgical procedures in the region of the lower extremity, but in combination with a block of the sciatic nerve. A need for larger volumes of local anesthetics must be expected (toxicity!).
- Outpatient procedures.

Therapeutic
- Postoperative and post-traumatic pain therapy.
- Early mobilization after hip and knee operations.
- Arterial occlusive disease and poor perfusion of the lower extremities.
- Complex regional pain syndrome (CRPS), types I and II.
- Post-surgical neurolysis or nerve reimplantations for better innervation.
- Edema after radiotherapy.
- Postamputation pain.
- Diabetic polyneuropathy.
- Tumors and metastases in the hip joint and pelvis.

Block series
A series of six to eight blocks is recommended. When there is evidence of improvement in the symptoms, additional blocks can also be carried out.

Prophylactic
- Postoperative analgesia.
- Prophylaxis against postamputation pain.
- Prophylaxis against complex regional pain syndrome.

Contraindications
Specific
- Infection or hematoma in the injection area.
- Anticoagulant treatment.
- Lesion in the nerves to be stimulated distal to the injection site.

Relative
The decision should be taken after carefully weighing up the risks and benefits:
- Hemorrhagic diathesis.
- Stable systemic neurological diseases.
- Local nerve injury (when there is doubt whether the fault lies with the surgeon or anesthesiologist).
- Contralateral nerve paresis.

Procedure

This block should be carried out by experienced anesthetists, or under their supervision. Full information for the patient is mandatory.

Preparations
Check that the emergency equipment is complete and in working order. Sterile precautions, intravenous access, ECG monitoring, pulse oximetry, intubation kit, ventilation facilities, emergency medication.

Materials (Fig. 27.1)
Fine 26-G needle, 25 mm long, for local anesthesia.
- Electrostimulation technique:
  Nerve stimulator (e.g. Stimuplex® HNS 11, B. Braun Melsungen).
  120-mm long atraumatic 22-G needle (15°) with injection lead ("immobile needle" – e.g. Stimuplex D®, B. Braun Melsungen).
- Loss-of-resistance technique:
  120-mm (150-mm) long spinal needle, 20–22 G (e.g. Spinocan® 0.7–0.9 × 120 mm (150 mm), B. Braun Melsungen) and a smoothly moving 10-mL plastic or glass syringe.
- Continuous technique*:
  Contiplex®–Tuohy set: 1.3 × 102 (152) mm long 18-G Tuohy needle with Contiplex® catheter, or:
  18-G (15°) Contiplex D® needle (1.3 × 110 mm with Contiplex® catheter, B. Braun Melsungen).

Syringes: 2 and 20 mL.
Local anesthetics, disinfectant, swabs, compresses, sterile gloves and drape.

Patient positioning
Lateral decubitus or sitting, as in the position for neuraxial anesthesia; legs drawn up, with the leg being blocked on top.

Landmarks
The iliac crest and the midline of the spinous process are located. From the intersection between these (L4 spinous process), a line is drawn 3 cm caudally, and from the end of it another line is drawn 5 cm laterally as far as the medial edge of the iliac crest, and marked as the injection point (Fig. 27.2).

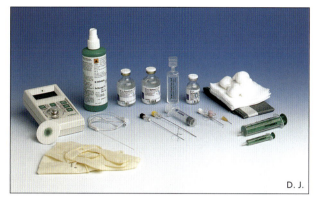
Fig. 27.1 Materials

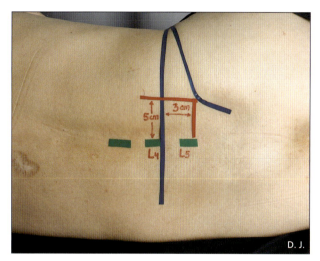
Fig. 27.2 Location

Skin prep, local anesthesia, sterile draping, drawing up the local anesthetic into 20-mL syringes, checking the patency of the injection needle and functioning of the nerve stimulator, attaching the electrodes.

Preliminary puncture with a large needle or stylet.

The quadriceps femoris muscle must be obsevred throughout the procedure (see Chapter 26, Fig. 26.5).

---
* If technical difficulties arise, the catheter and Tuohy puncture needle are always removed simultaneously. A catheter must never be withdrawn through a Tuohy puncture needle that remains in place (because of catheter shearing).

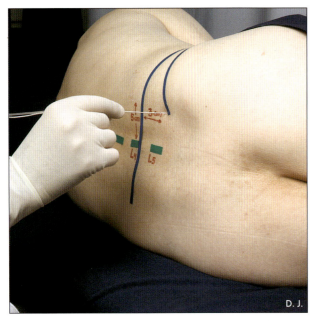

Fig. 27.3 The injection needle is introduced perpendicular to the skin surface until bone contact is made with the transverse process of L5

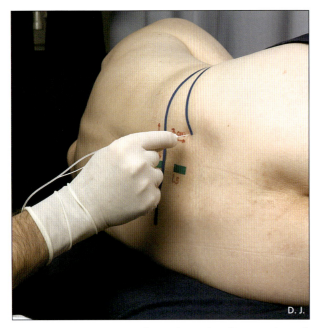

Fig. 27.4 The injection needle is advanced until contractions of the quadriceps femoris muscle become visible

Injection technique

Electrostimulation technique

- Introduce an electrostimulation needle perpendicular to the skin surface until bone contact is made with the transverse process of L5 (Figs. 27.3, 27.5). It is then withdrawn slightly and advanced further cranially, past the transverse process (Figs. 27.4, 27.5).
  Stimulation current of 1 mA at 2 Hz is selected with a stimulus duration of 0.1 ms.
- Advance the needle further until contractions of the **quadriceps femoris muscle** become visible.
- Reduce the stimulation current to 0.3 mA. If contractions of the muscle are still visible at this level of current, the needle is in the correct position.
- Aspiration test.
- Test dose of 3–5 mL of a local anesthetic.
- Incremental injection of a local anesthetic (injection–aspiration after each 3–4 mL).
- Careful cardiovascular monitoring.

Loss-of-resistance technique

- A 120-mm (150-mm) long 20–22-G spinal needle is introduced perpendicularly until bone contact is made with the transverse process of L5. After bone contact, the needle is withdrawn slightly, as in the paravertebral block, and then advanced in a cranial direction past the transverse process as far as the quadratus lumborum muscle.
- Removal of the trochar and aspiration.
- A 10-mL syringe filled with air or 0.9% saline is attached.
- The needle is slowly advanced with constant pressure on the plunger.
- After initial resistance from the surrounding muscle mass, perforation of the muscle fascia occurs and there is penetration into the fascial compartment between the quadratus lumborum muscle and the psoas major muscle, characterized by "loss of resistance." Experience shows that this occurs at a depth of about 12 ± 2 cm. Paresthesias are often, but not always, elicited.
- Once the psoas compartment has been reached, 10–20 mL of air is injected in order to dilate the space.
- Aspiration test.
- Test dose of 3–5 mL of a local anesthetic.
- Incremental injection of local anesthetic (injection–aspiration after each 3–4 mL).
- The patient must remain in the same position for about 5 min.
- Precise cardiovascular monitoring.

Continuous technique
The Contiplex® catheter is advanced through the previously placed 18-G Tuohy–Contiplex® needle (or alternatively a 110-mm long (15°) Contiplex® D needle) ca. 5 cm deep into the fascial compartment.

Dosage
Surgical
40–50 mL local anesthetic – e.g. 1% prilocaine (20–30 mL) + 0.5–0.75% ropivacaine (20 mL); 1% prilocaine (20–30 mL) + 0.25–0.5% bupivacaine (0.25–0.5% levobupivacaine; 20 mL).

Therapeutic
30 mL local anesthetic – e.g. 0.2–0.375% ropivacaine, 0.125–0.25% bupivacaine (0.125–0.25% levobupivacaine).

Important notes for outpatients
See Chapter 26, p. 224.

Continuous
See Chapter 26, p. 224.

Complications
- Nerve injury (extremely rare; see Chapter 26, p. 225).
- Intravascular injection (see Chapter 6, p. 65).
- CNS toxicity (see Chapter 6, p. 66 and Chapter 1, p. 9).
- Subarachnoid or epidural injection (see Chapter 36 and Chapter 41).
- Hematoma formation.
- Intra-abdominal injuries.
- Postinjection pain due to spasm in the lumbar paravertebral musculature.

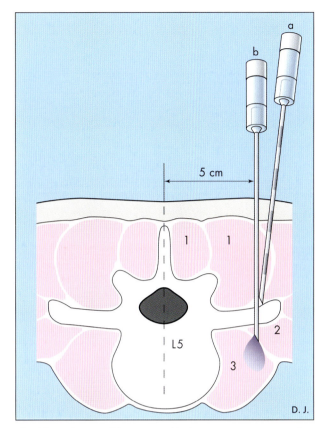

Fig. 27.5 Diagram: (a) contact with the transverse process of L5; (b) the needle is advanced past the transverse process until contractions of the quadriceps femoris muscle become visible. (1) Erector spinae muscle, (2) quadratus lumborum muscle, (3) psoas muscle

28 Sciatic nerve block

Definition

Block of the largest of the four nerves supplying the leg at the lower end of the lumbosacral plexus, after it exits from the greater sciatic foramen or infrapiriform foramen.

Anatomy (Fig. 28.1)

The **sciatic nerve** arises from the ventral branches of the spinal nerves from L4 to S3. Exiting from the pelvic cavity at the lower edge of the piriformis muscle (in about 2% of individuals, the nerve pierces the piriformis), its 16–20-mm thick trunk runs between the ischial tuberosity and the greater trochanter, turns downward over the gemelli, the obturator internus tendon and the quadratus femoris, which separate it from the hip joint, and leaves the buttock to enter the thigh beneath the lower border of the gluteus maximus.

Distal to this, the nerve lies on the posterior surface of the adductor magnus muscle, where it is covered by the flexor muscle originating from the ischial tuberosity and thus extends as far as the popliteal fossa. Here it lies slightly laterally and above the popliteal vein and artery, with thick popliteal fascia overlying it. At the proximal end of the popliteal fossa, the nerve usually divides into the thicker **tibial nerve**, which continues the trunk and the smaller **common peroneal (fibular) nerve**.

The sensory branches of the nerve innervate the dorsal thigh, the dorsolateral lower leg and lateral half of the foot, the hip and knee joint, as well as the femur.

Its **muscular branches** are responsible for supplying the biceps femoris, semimembranosus, semitendinosus and adductor magnus muscles.

Indications

Surgical
- Superficial procedures in the innervated area.
- Carrying out surgical procedures in the region of the lower extremity under tourniquet, but in combination with a block of the lumbar plexus ("three-in-one" block or dorsal psoas compartment block). A need for larger volumes of local anesthetics must be expected (toxicity!).

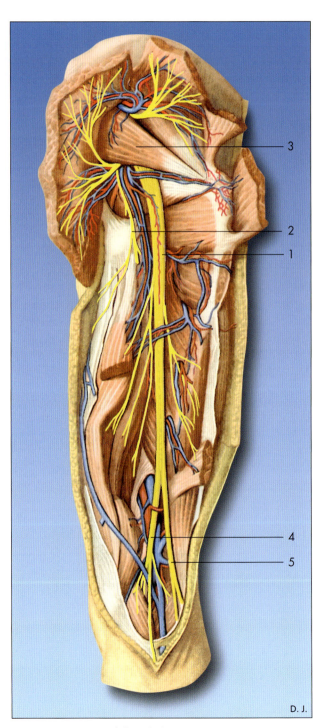

Fig. 28.1 Anatomy of the sciatic nerve.
(1) Sciatic nerve, (2) posterior femoral cutaneous nerve, (3) piriformis muscle, (4) tibial nerve, (5) common peroneal (fibular) nerve

Sciatic nerve block

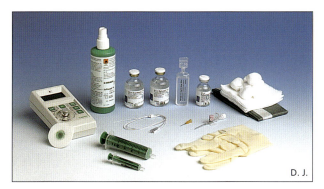

Fig. 28.2 Materials

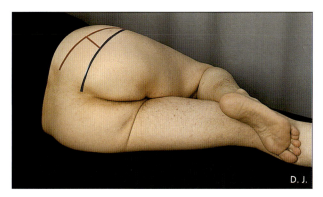

Fig. 28.3 Classic dorsal transgluteal technique (positioning)

Therapeutic
An isolated block of the sciatic nerve is rarely indicated. A combination with block of the lumbar plexus or femoral nerve is recommended (see Chapters 26, 27 and 29).

Block series
A series of six to eight blocks is recommended. When there is evidence of improvement in the symptoms, additional blocks can also be carried out.

Contraindications
Specific
- Infection or hematoma in the injection area.
- Anticoagulant treatment.
- Lesion in the nerves to be blocked distal to the injection site.

Relative
The decision should be taken after carefully weighing up the risks and benefits:
- Hemorrhagic diathesis.
- Stable central nervous system diseases.
- Local nerve injury.

Procedure

This block should be carried out by experienced anesthetists, or under their supervision. Full prior information for the patient is mandatory.

Preparations
Check that the emergency equipment is complete and in working order. Sterile precautions, intravenous access, ECG monitoring, pulse oximetry, intubation kit, ventilation facilities, emergency medication.

Materials (Fig. 28.2)
Nerve stimulator (e.g. Stimuplex HNS 11, B. Braun Melsungen).
- Single-shot technique:
  Fine 26-G needle, 25 mm long, for local anesthesia. 80-mm long (120–150 mm for ventral access), atraumatic 22-G needle (15°) with injection lead ("immobile needle") – e.g. Stimuplex D®, B. Braun Melsungen).
- Continuous technique:
  Contiplex®–Tuohy set: 102-mm long 18-G Tuohy needle with Contiplex® catheter.
  Contiplex D® set: 18-G Contiplex® needle (110 mm, 15°) with Contiplex® catheter.

Syringes: 2, 10 and 20 mL.
Local anesthetics, disinfectant, swabs, compresses, sterile gloves and drape.

Classic dorsal transgluteal technique (Labat technique)

Patient positioning (Fig. 28.3)
Lateral decubitus, with the leg being blocked on top (Sims position).
The upper leg is bent at the hip and knee joints and the upper knee lies on the table. The lower leg is straight.

Landmarks (Fig. 28.4)
The important landmarks are: the greater trochanter and posterior superior iliac spine (and/or sacral hiatus). The greater trochanter and posterior superior iliac spine are located. From the mid-point of the connecting line, a line is drawn medially and the injection point is marked at 5 cm (Labat line).
To check this, another line connecting the greater trochanter and the sacral hiatus is bisected (Winnie line). The two points should coincide.

Skin prep, local anesthesia, sterile draping, drawing up local anesthetic into a 20-mL syringe, checking patency of the injection needle and correct functioning of the nerve stimulator, attaching the electrodes.

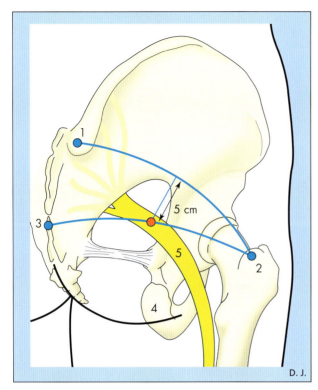

Fig. 28.4 Landmarks.
(1) Posterior superior iliac spine, (2) greater trochanter, (3) sacral hiatus, (4) ischial tuberosity, (5) sciatic nerve

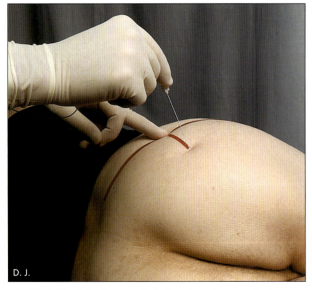

Fig. 28.5 The injection needle is introduced perpendicular to the skin surface

Preliminary puncture with a large needle or stylet.

During the procedure, the biceps femoris, semimembranosus and semitendinosus muscles and the foot must be observed (Fig. 28.6).

Injection technique
Electrostimulation
- The injection needle is introduced perpendicular to the skin surface (Fig. 28.5).
  Stimulation current of 1 mA at 2 Hz is selected with a stimulus duration of 0.1 ms.
- After about 1–4 cm, there should be direct stimulation of the **gluteus maximus muscle**.
- At a depth of about 5 cm, contractions of the **biceps femoris, semimembranosus and semitendinosus muscles** are produced (Fig. 28.6).
- After the needle is advanced further, at a depth of about 6–8 cm there is **plantar** and **dorsal flexion** of the foot as a response to the stimulus from the tibial or peroneal part of the sciatic nerve.
- Do **not** advance the needle any further.
- The stimulation current is reduced to 0.3 mA. Slight twitching suggests that the needle is positioned in the immediate vicinity of the nerve.
- Aspiration test.
- Test dose of 3 mL local anesthetic (e.g. 1% prilocaine). During the injection, the twitching should slowly disappear.
- Incremental injection of a local anesthetic (injection–aspiration after each 3–4 mL).
- Careful cardiovascular monitoring.

The area of anesthesia is shown in Figure 28.14.

Eliciting paresthesias
An atraumatic injection needle 80 mm long (rarely longer) is advanced using the technique described above until paresthesias are elicited that extend to the sole of the foot, or until bone contact is made, with subsequent correction of the needle direction. This technique is associated with a higher failure rate.

Problem situations
- Bone contact at a depth of 8 cm without visible twitching. The injection needle should be withdrawn and the direction should be altered laterally.
- Intraneural positioning:
  The following signs suggest intraneural positioning of the injection needle:
  – Strong twitching (even at a stimulant current of 0.2 mA).

- No disappearance of the twitching during injection of a test dose.
- High resistance and severe pain during the injection.

The injection must be stopped immediately and the needle must be withdrawn.

Continuous technique

The injection is carried out as in the single-shot technique.

An 18-G Tuohy needle 102 mm long or a Contiplex D® needle 110 mm long are usually used as stimulation needles. After correct stimulation and aspiration, a test dose is injected. The Contiplex® catheter is then advanced ca. 3 cm beyond the end of the container and the stimulation needle is slowly withdrawn while the thumb and index finger of the left hand simultaneously hold the catheter at the injection site. A bacterial filter is then placed and the catheter is fixed with a skin suture and dressing.

Anterior approach

Patient positioning
A supine position that is comfortable for the patient, with slight outward rotation of the leg being blocked.

Landmarks
Important landmarks are: the anterior superior iliac spine, pubic tubercle and greater trochanter. Two lines are drawn for orientation:
- A line connecting the anterior superior iliac spine with the pubic tubercle, which is marked into thirds.
- A second line parallel to the first, from the greater trochanter across the thigh.

A perpendicular line is drawn from the intersection of the medial and central third of the upper inguinal ligament line to the parallel line and marked as the injection point (Figs. 28.7, 28.8).

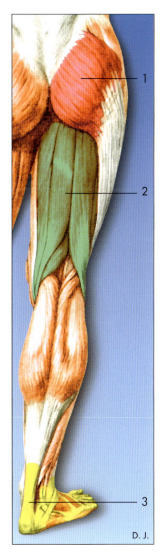

Fig. 28.6 Sequence of muscle contractions.
(1) Gluteus maximus muscle,
(2) semitendinosus muscle, semimembranosus muscle, biceps femoris muscle,
(3) plantar/dorsal flexion of the foot

Injection technique

A 22-G (15°) atraumatic injection needle 120–150 mm long, with an injection lead, is advanced perpendicular to the skin until bone contact is made with the femur. The needle is then withdrawn slightly and introduced about 5 cm deeper, past the medial border of the femur.

The correct needle position is confirmed when paresthesias or twitches are produced during electrostimulation. After aspiration and administration of a test dose, incremental injection of a local anesthetic is carried out.

233

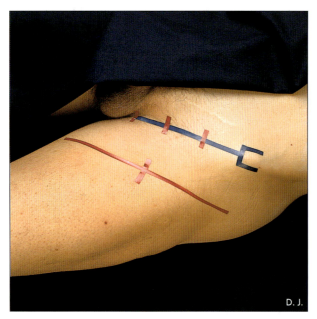

Fig. 28.7 Location (in patient)

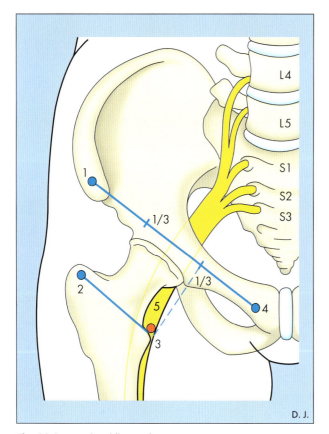

Fig. 28.8 Location (diagram).
(1) Anterior superior iliac spine, (2) greater trochanter, (3) injection site, (4) pubic tubercle, (5) sciatic nerve

Di Benedetto–Borghi subgluteal access route

Battista Borghi

The subgluteal block of the sciatic nerve has the advantage over the classic posterior transgluteal technique in that it is less stressful to the patient during the procedure, as the sciatic nerve has a more superficial course in the subgluteal region than in the gluteal region [4]. This access route also makes it easier to place and fix a catheter for postoperative analgesia.

Procedure

Patient positioning
Lateral decubitus, with the leg being blocked on top (Sims position; Fig. 28.3).

Landmarks
From the mid-point of a line connecting the greater trochanter and the ischial tuberosity, a second line is drawn to the upper edge of the popliteal fossa (known as the "sciatic line"). The injection site is located ca. 3–4 cm caudal to this (Fig. 28.9). If the patient is lying in the Sims position, for easier guidance one can palpate a groove along this line between the semitendinosus muscle and the biceps femoris muscle [4].

> In this technique, the distance between the skin and the sciatic nerve is shorter (4.7 cm) than in Labat's classic transgluteal access route (6.7 cm).

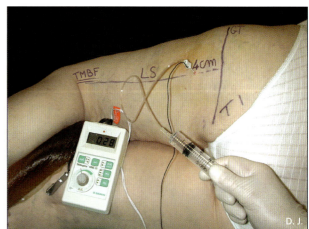

Fig. 28.9 Landmarks. GT = greater trochanter, TI = ischial tuberosity, LS = sciatic line, TMBF = tendon of the biceps femoris muscle

Preparations
Skin prep, local anesthesia, sterile draping, drawing up local anesthetic, checking the patency of the injection needle and correct functioning of the nerve stimulator, attaching the electrodes.

Injection
Preliminary puncture with a large needle or stylet.

> During the procedure, the biceps femoris, semimembranosus and semitendinosus muscles and the foot must be observed.

An injection needle ca. 50 (80) mm long is introduced perpendicular to the skin (Fig. 28.10). Stimulation current is applied at 1–1.5 mA at 2 Hz with a stimulus duration 0.1 ms. At a depth of ca. 4 cm, plantar flexion and dorsiflexion of the foot occur in response to the stimulation of the tibial or peroneal parts of the sciatic nerve. The needle should not be advanced any further. The stimulation current is reduced to 0.3 mA. Slight twitching indicates that the stimulation needle is located in the immediate vicinity of the nerve. After an aspiration test, a test dose (e.g. 3 mL 1% prilocaine) is injected and incremental injection of the local anesthetic follows.

Continuous subgluteal block of the sciatic nerve

After skin prep, an adhesive sterile transparent drape with a hole is applied.

Materials
Contiplex®–Tuohy set: 52 (102) mm long 18-G Tuohy needle with a Contiplex® catheter, or:
Contiplex D® set: 18-G Contiplex® needle 80–110 mm (15°) long with a Contiplex® catheter (B. Braun Melsungen).

Injection
The injection is carried out as in the single-shot technique. After injection of 5 mL 0.9% saline, the catheter is introduced through the already positioned needle. The catheter is advanced ca. 3–4 cm beyond the end of the needle or cannula (Fig. 28.11). After removal of the needle or cannula, fixing of the catheter and placement of a bacterial filter (Fig. 28.12), after careful aspiration and injection of a test dose, bolus administration of the local anesthetic is carried out (Fig. 28.13).

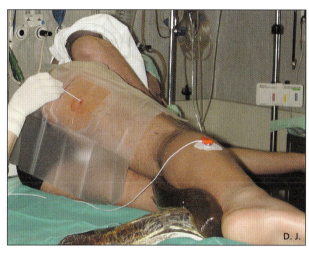

Fig. 28.10 Introducing the needle

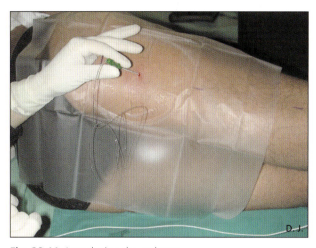

Fig. 28.11 Introducing the catheter

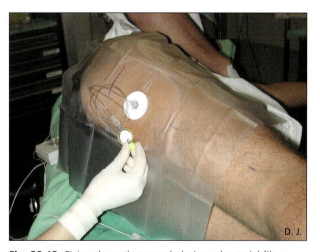

Fig. 28.12 Fixing the catheter and placing a bacterial filter

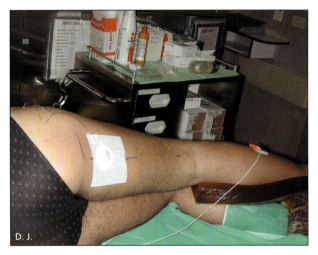

Fig. 28.13 Injecting the local anesthetic

Dosage
Surgical
30–40 mL local anesthetic – e.g. 0.5–0.75% ropivacaine, 0.5% bupivacaine (0.5% levobupivacaine), 1% prilocaine, 1% mepivacaine.
A combination of long-duration and medium-duration local anesthetics has proved particularly useful for surgical indications.

Continuous administration
0.2–0.375% ropivacaine,
5–15 mL/h (max. 37.5 mg/h)
Alternatively, as a bolus dose:
0.2–0.375% ropivacaine, 10–30 mL.

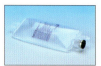

Subgluteal access
Patient-controlled analgesia (PCA) [4]: baseline rate of 4 mL/h 0.4% ropivacaine, 0.25% levobupivacaine, 0.25% bupivacaine.
Bolus dose of 2 mL.
Lockout time 10 min.

Therapeutic
10–20 mL local anesthetic – e.g. 0.2–0.375% ropivacaine, 0.125–0.25% bupivacaine.

Important notes for outpatients
See Chapter 26, p. 224)

Complications
Complications are rare, but possible:
- Nerve injury (see Chapter 9, p. 112 and Chapter 26, p. 225).
- Intravascular injection (see Chapter 6, p. 65).
- CNS toxicity (see Chapter 6, p. 66 and Chapter 1, p. 9).
- Infection in the area of the injection.
- Hematoma formation.

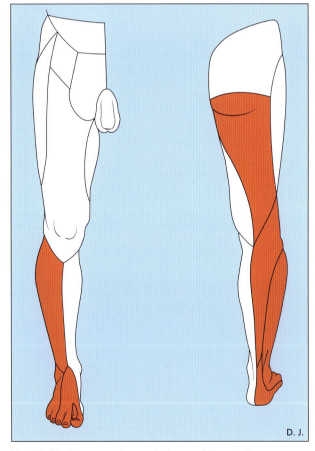

Fig. 28.14 Cutaneous innervated area of the sciatic nerve

Sciatic nerve block

Lumbosacral plexus and individual nerves in the plexus

Block no. ☐ Right ☐ Left

Name: _____ Date: _____
Diagnosis: _____
Premedication: ☐ No ☐ Yes
Neurological abnormalities: ☐ No ☐ Yes _____

Purpose of block: ☐ *Surgical* ☐ *Diagnostic* ☐ *Therapeutic*
Needle: G ___ Length ___ cm ☐ *15°* ☐ *30°* ☐ *Other*
i.v. access: ☐ *Yes*
Monitoring: ☐ *ECG* ☐ *Pulse oximetry*
Ventilation facilities: ☐ *Yes (equipment checked)*
Emergency equipment *(drugs)*: ☐ *Checked*
Patient: ☐ *Informed (behavior after block)*

Position: ☐ *Prone* ☐ *Lateral recumbent* ☐ *Sims-Position* ☐ *Sitting*
Injection: ☐ *Inguinal „3-in-one" block* ☐ *Dorsal psoas compartment block*
☐ *Sciatic nerve* ☐ *Femoral nerve* ☐ *Lateral cutaneous nerve of thigh*
☐ *Obturator nerve* ☐ *Ilioinguinal nerve / hypogastric nerve*
Location technique: ☐ *Electrostimulation* ☐ *Paresthesias* ☐ *Other*
Plexus (nerve): ☐ *Located* ☐ *Aspiration test* ☐ *Test dose*
Injection:
Local anesthetic: _____ mL ____ %
(in incremental doses)
☐ *Inguinal „3-in-one" block* ___ mL ☐ *Dorsal psoas compartmt. block* ___ mL
☐ *Sciatic nerve* ___ mL ☐ *Femoral nerve* ___ mL ☐ *Lateral cutaneous nerve of thigh* ___ mL ☐ *Obturator nerve* ___ mL ☐ *Ilioinguinal nerve/hypogastric nerve* ___ mL
☐ Addition to LA _____ µg/mg

Patient's remarks during injection:
☐ None ☐ Paresthesias ☐ Warmth ☐ Pain (intraneural position?)
Nerve area: _____
Objective block effect after 15 min:
☐ Cold test ☐ Temperature measurement before ___°C after ___°C
☐ Sensory ☐ Motor
Monitoring after block: ☐ < 1 h ☐ > 1 h
Time of discharge _____ ☐ Sensorimotor function checked

Complications:
☐ None ☐ Intravascular injection ☐ Signs of intoxication
☐ Hematoma ☐ Neurological complications ☐ Other

Subjective effects of the block: Duration: _____
☐ None ☐ Increased pain ☐ Reduced pain ☐ Relief of pain

VISUAL ANALOG SCALE

|||||||||||
0 10 20 30 40 50 60 70 80 90 100

Special notes:

Record and checklist

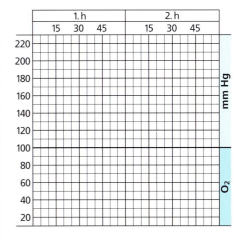

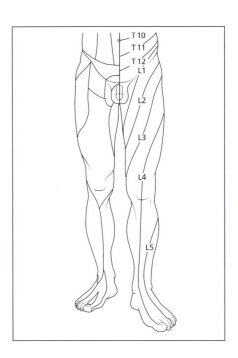

Blocking individual nerves in the lumbar plexus

29 Femoral nerve

Definition
Block of the largest nerve emerging from the lumbar plexus below the inguinal ligament.

Anatomy (Fig. 29.1)

The nerve, which is about 12 mm wide, arises from the ventral branches of the spinal nerves from **L2–L4**, runs through the psoas major muscle and the iliacus muscle and reaches the thigh behind the inguinal ligament. Above the inguinal ligament, the femoral nerve is located in a fascial compartment, which is surrounded by the iliac fascia laterally, the psoas fascia medially and the transversalis fascia ventrally. After passing the inguinal ligament, the nerve continues dorsolateral to the iliopsoas fascia, ventral to the inguinal ligament and fascia lata and medial to the iliopectineal fascia. Four to five centimeters below the inguinal ligament, the nerve divides into an anterior, mainly sensory, branch and a posterior, mainly motor one.

Its largest sensory branch is the saphenous nerve, which separates from it in the femoral triangle. The femoral nerve provides the sensory supply to the upper thigh and shares in the innervation of the hip and knee joints as well as of the femur. Its sensory end branch, the saphenous nerve, innervates the medioventral lower leg and the medial half of the foot. Its muscular branches supply the pectineus, sartorius and quadriceps femoris muscles (see Chapter 26, Fig. 26.1).

Indications
See Chapter 26, p. 220.

Surgical
- Superficial surgical procedures in the area of innervation, usually in combination with block of the neighboring lumbar plexus nerves or the sciatic nerve.

Therapeutic
Excellent results can be achieved with combined block of the femoral nerve and sciatic nerve (block series), particularly in:
- Postamputation pain.
- Complex regional pain syndrome (CRPS), types 1 and 2 (see case report, p. 240).
- In addition: in perfusion problems of the lower extremity, arterial occlusive disease (caution in patients with a femoral bypass), polyneuropathies, arthrosis of the knee joint, etc.

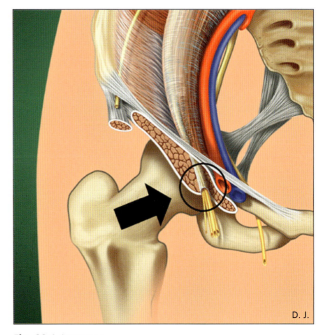

Fig. 29.1 Anatomy

Contraindications
See Chapter 26, p. 221.

Procedure

Full prior information for the patient is mandatory.

Preparations
See Chapter 26, p. 221.

Materials (Fig. 29.2)
Fine 26-G needle 25 mm long, for local anesthesia.
Atraumatic 23–25-G needle (15°), 40 mm long, with injection lead ("immobile needle" – e.g. Stimuplex D®, B. Braun Melsungen).
Syringes: 2, 10 and 20 mL.
Local anesthetics, disinfectant, swabs, compresses, sterile gloves and drape.

Patient positioning
Supine, with the thigh slightly abducted, with the ipsilateral hand under the head.

Landmarks
The femoral artery is palpated 1–2 cm distal to the inguinal ligament. It is held between the spread index finger and middle finger. The injection site is located about 1–1.5 cm lateral to this. The person performing the injection stands on the side being injected.

Skin prep, subcutaneous local anesthesia, covering with a sterile drape, drawing up the local anesthetic into a 10-mL or 20-mL syringe, checking the patency of the injection needle and correct functioning of the nerve stimulator, attaching the electrodes.

Injection technique
After a **preliminary puncture**, the injection needle is introduced perpendicular to the skin surface, with the femoral artery being pushed in a medial direction by the palpating finger (Fig. 29.3). The femoral nerve is located at a depth of ca. 2–3 cm. Producing paresthesias is helpful, but not obligatory.
After aspiration and administration of a test dose, incremental injection of a local anesthetic is carried out. If no paresthesias are produced, some of the local anesthetic is injected lateral to the artery in a fan-shaped fashion. The onset of effect is slow. A successful block is indicated if the patient is unable to extend the leg (Fig. 29.4).
It is helpful to use a nerve stimulator, as this allows a more targeted location of the nerve.
The distribution of anesthesia is shown in Fig. 29.5.

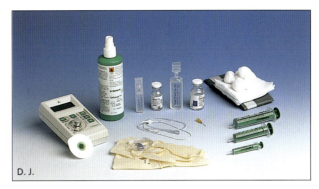

Fig. 29.2 Materials

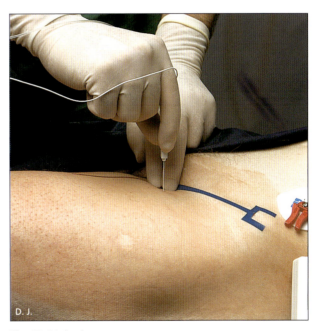

Fig. 29.3 Injection

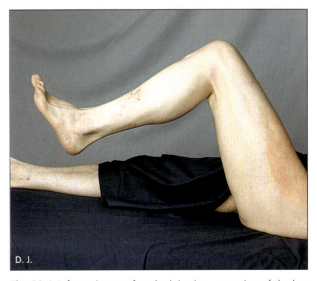

Fig. 29.4 A few minutes after the injection, extension of the leg is no longer possible

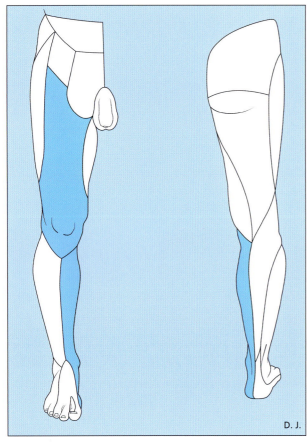

Fig. 29.5 Cutaneous innervation area of the femoral nerve

Dosage

Surgical
30 mL local anesthetic – e.g. 0.75% ropivacaine, 0.5% bupivacaine (0.5% levobupivacaine), 1% prilocaine, 1% mepivacaine.

Therapeutic
Single block of the femoral nerve:
10–15 mL local anesthetic – e.g. 0.2% ropivacaine, 0.125–0.25% bupivacaine (0.125–0.25% levobupivacaine).
In combination with a sciatic nerve block:
Femoral nerve: 5–8 mL local anesthetic.
Sciatic nerve: 8–10 mL local anesthetic – e.g. 0.2–0.375% ropivacaine, 0.125–0.25% bupivacaine (0.125–0.25% levobupivacaine).

Important notes for outpatients
See Chapter 26, p. 224.

Complications
See Chapter 26, p. 225.

Example case
Patient W.W. aged 54, with a four-month history.
The following symptoms developed after an Achilles tendon strain:
Livid soft-tissue swelling in the area of the left foot and ankle joint, with sensitivity to touch and severe pain, resistant to treatment.
Radiography showed osteoporosis, with thinning of cortical bone.
Investigations indicated a diagnosis of Sudeck's atrophy (CRPS).
Prior treatment with calcitonin, cortisone, NSAIDs and opioids had not led to any relief of the symptoms.

Start of treatment, 4 August 1994 (Fig. 29.6)
A series of blocks [19] of the femoral nerve and sciatic nerve with 0.5% bupivacaine, each 25 mL (femoral nerve 15 mL, sciatic nerve 10 mL).

End of treatment, 24 October 1994 (Fig. 29.7)
Complete resolution of the symptoms.

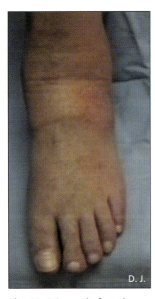

Fig. 29.6 Status before the start of treatment

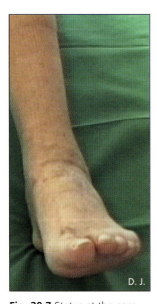

Fig. 29.7 Status at the completion of treatment

30 Lateral femoral cutaneous nerve

Definition
Block of this sensory nerve as it emerges from the lumbar plexus below the lateral inguinal ligament.

Anatomy (Fig. 30.1)

The lateral cutaneous femoral nerve arises from the ventral branches of the L2 and L3 spinal nerves, passing lateral to the psoas muscle and then to the iliacus muscle. Covered by the iliac fascia, it then runs to the region of the anterior superior iliac spine. It passes under the inguinal ligament and under the deep circumflex iliac artery, and enters the thigh, where it lies under the superficial sheet of the fascia and divides into a thicker descending branch and a smaller posterior branch, which penetrate the fascia separately. The posterior branch runs posteriorly over the tensor fascia lata muscle and reaches the gluteal region. The anterior branch runs 3–5 cm below the inguinal ligament, then downwards along the anterior surface of the vastus lateralis muscle as far as the lateral knee area, where it sends off lateral branches (see Chapter 26, Fig. 26.1).

Indications

Surgical
- Mainly for relief of tourniquet pain in combination with block of the neighboring nerves from the lumbar plexus and of the sciatic nerve.

Diagnostic
- Differentiation of various neuralgias in the thigh region.

Therapeutic (block series)
- Meralgia paraesthetica.

Contraindications
Infection at the injection site.

Procedure

Full prior information for the patient is mandatory.

Preparations
See Chapter. 26, p. 221.

Materials (Fig. 30.2)
Fine 26-G needle 25 mm long, for local anesthesia.
40 mm long, atraumatic 25-G needle (15°) with injection lead ("immobile needle" – e.g. Stimuplex D®, B. Braun Melsungen).

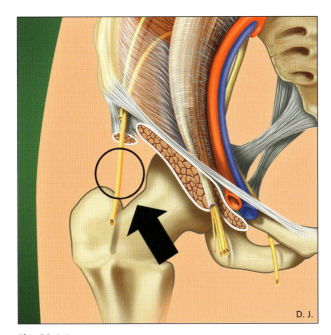

Fig. 30.1 Anatomy

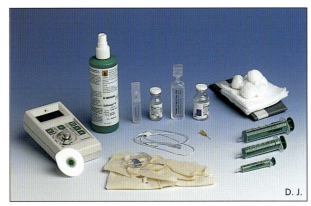

Fig. 30.2 Materials

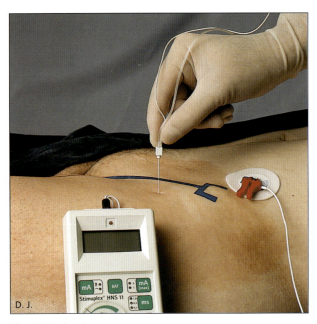

Fig. 30.3 Injection

Syringes: 2, 5, and 10 mL.
Local anesthetic, disinfectant, swabs, sterile gloves, drape.

Patient positioning
Supine, with the ipsilateral hand under the head.

Landmarks
The anterior superior iliac spine is palpated. The injection point lies about 2.5 cm medial and 2.5 cm caudal to it. The person carrying out the injection stands on the side being injected.

Skin prep, subcutaneous local anesthesia, drawing up the local anesthetic, checking the patency of the injection needle and correct functioning of the nerve stimulator if used, attaching the electrodes.

Injection technique (Fig. 30.3)
The injection needle is introduced slowly and perpendicularly in the direction of the fascia lata, penetration of which is recognized by loss of resistance or "fascial clicks."
Paresthesias are not elicited. Fan-shaped injection of the local anesthetic is carried out medially and laterally, subfascially as far as the ilium and also subcutaneously when withdrawing the needle.
When the electrostimulation technique is used, stimulation of the sensory nerve fibers is produced with a stimulus duration of 0.1 ms. Cooperation on the part of the patient is a prerequisite for this technique.

The distribution of the block is shown in Fig. 30.4.

Dosage

Surgical
10–15 mL local anesthetic – e.g. 0.5–0.75% ropivacaine, 0.5% bupivacaine (0.5% levobupivacaine), 1% prilocaine, 1% mepivacaine.

Therapeutic (block series)
5–10 mL local anesthetic – e.g. 0.2% ropivacaine, 0.125–0.25% bupivacaine (0.125–0.25% levobupivacaine).

Complications
No specific complications.

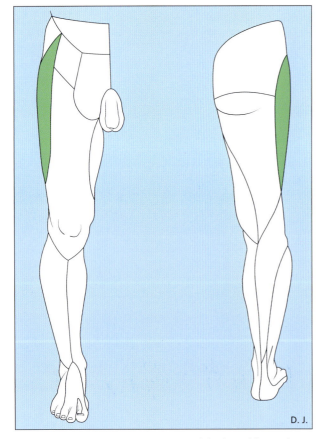

Fig. 30.4 Cutaneous innervation area of the lateral femoral cutaneous nerve

31 Obturator nerve

Definition
Block of the nerve emerging from the lumbar plexus in the obturator canal.

Anatomy (Fig. 31.1)

The obturator nerve arises from the ventral branches of the **L2–L4** spinal nerves.
The trunk runs downwards along the medial edge of the psoas muscle, passing behind the common iliac vessels to reach the pelvis and the obturator canal. Within the canal, it divides into its two end branches – the anterior and posterior branches. It provides the motor supply for the obturator externus muscle and the adductors of the thigh, sends off branches to the hip and knee joints and to the femur, and provides the sensory supply for a highly variable cutaneous area on the inside of the thigh and lower leg.

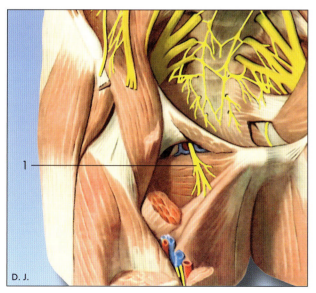

Fig. 31.1 Anatomy. (1) Obturator nerve

Indications
Surgical
- For procedures in the knee joint and above the knee joint, as well as in urological surgery, particularly for resections of bladder tumors in combination with blocks of neighboring nerves from the lumbar plexus and of the sciatic nerve.

Diagnostic
- Localization of hip joint pain.

Therapeutic
- Hip joint pain and elimination of adductor spasm.

Contraindications
Infection in the injection area.

Procedure

Full prior information for the patient is mandatory.

Preparations
See Chapter. 26, p. 221.

Materials (Fig. 31.2)
Fine 26-G needle, 2.5 cm long, for local anesthesia.
50 (80) mm long, atraumatic 22-G needle (15°) with injection lead ("immobile needle" – e.g. Stimuplex D®, B. Braun Melsungen), or an 80-mm long, 22-G spinal needle.
Nerve stimulator (e.g. Stimuplex® HNS 11, B. Braun Melsungen).
Syringes: 2, 10 and 20 mL.
Local anesthetics, disinfectant, swabs, sterile gloves and drape.

Chapter 31

Patient positioning
Supine, with slight abduction of the leg being blocked. The patient's ipsilateral hand is under the head.

Landmarks
Anterior superior iliac spine, pubic tubercle. The pubic tubercle is located. The injection site lies about 1.5 cm lateral and 1.5 cm caudal to it.

Skin prep, local anesthesia, drawing up local anesthetic, checking patency of injection needle and correct functioning of the nerve stimulator, attaching electrodes.

> The genitalia must be protected during skin prep.

Injection technique
- The injection needle is introduced perpendicular to the skin. At a depth of about 1.5–4 cm (depending on the anatomy), **bone contact** is made with the upper part of the inferior branch of the pubic bone. This depth is marked (Fig. 31.3a, b).
- The needle is then withdrawn and advanced in a **lateral** and slightly **caudal** direction, close beneath the upper part of the pubic bone (Fig. 31.4a, b).
- Entry into the **obturator canal** takes place after the needle has been advanced about 2–3 cm deeper than the position marked after bone contact with the lower part of the pubic bone. Paresthesias are not produced.
- When a nerve stimulator is being used, correct needle positioning is indicated when slight adductor twitches become visible after reduction of the stimulation current from 1 mA to 0.3 mA.
- Aspiration test.
- Injection of a local anesthetic is carried out on an incremental basis and in a fan shape (injection–aspiration).
- Success of the block depends directly on the amount of local anesthetic injected. A successful block is characterized by restricted adduction in the thigh.

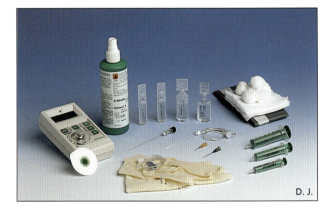

Fig. 31.2 Materials

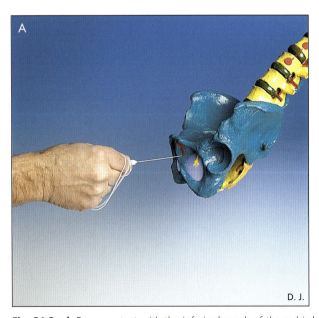
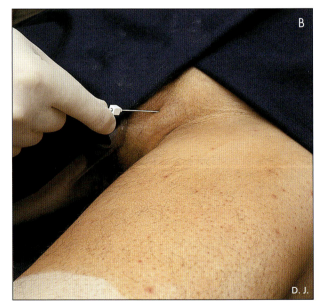

Fig. 31.3a, b Bone contact with the inferior branch of the pubic bone. **a** In the skeleton, **b** in the patient

Obturator nerve

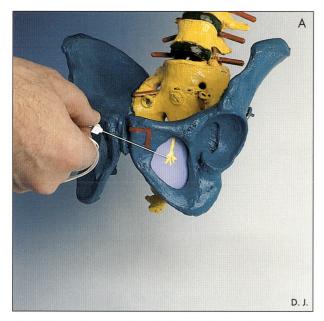 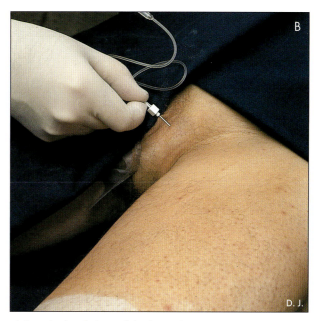

Fig. 31.4a, b Advancing the injection needle laterally and slightly caudally. **a** In the skeleton, **b** in the patient

Disadvantage
This technique is not easy to perform and the success rate is variable.

The distribution of anesthesia (very variable) is shown in Fig. 31.5.

Dosage
10–15 mL local anesthetic – e.g. 0.375–0.5% ropivacaine, 0.25–0.5% bupivacaine (0.25–0.5% levobupivacaine), 1% prilocaine, 1% mepivacaine.

Complications
Complications are very rare, but possible:
- Intravascular injection (the injection area is very well vascularized; see Chapter 6, p. 65).
- Hematoma formation.
- Puncture of or injury to the vagina or bladder.

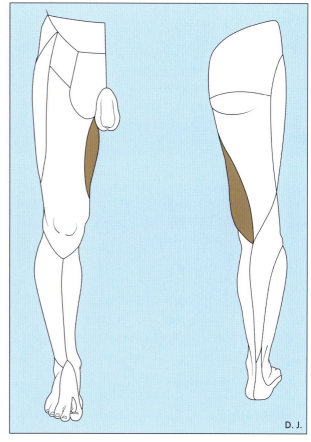

Fig. 31.5 Cutaneous innervation area of the obturator nerve

32 Ilioinguinal and iliohypogastric nerves

Definition
Block of these two neighboring nerves originating from the upper part of the lumbar plexus.

Anatomy (Fig. 32.1)

The **ilioinguinal and iliohypogastric nerves** arise from the upper branch of the first lumbar nerve in the lumbar plexus; the **genitofemoral nerve** is formed from the lower branch of the first lumbar nerve and from a small branch of the second lumbar nerve. These three nerves run parallel to the intercostal nerves, and participate in the innervation of the transversus and obliquus abdominis muscles.

The **ilioinguinal nerve** penetrates the internal oblique muscle at the level of the anterior superior iliac spine, and runs between this and the external oblique muscle in the direction of the inguinal ligament and the canal around the skin of the mons pubis, the scrotum (or labia majora in women) and the adjoining part of the femoral triangle.

The lateral cutaneous branch of the **iliohypogastric nerve** innervates the skin of the anterolateral part of the gluteal region, and ends in its anterior branch above the pubic bone.

The **genitofemoral nerve** passes through the psoas major muscle and divides into a genital branch and a femoral branch.

Indications
Surgical
- As an important part of field block in the inguinal region when carrying out herniorrhaphy.

Therapeutic
- Scar pain after herniorrhaphy.
- Post-herpetic neuralgia.

Contraindications
None.

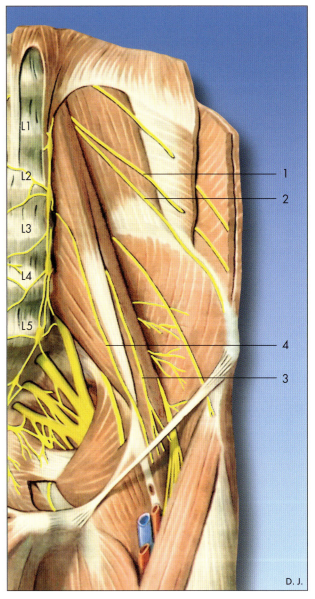

Fig. 32.1 Anatomy.
(1) Iliohypogastric nerve, (2) ilioinguinal nerve, (3) genitofemoral nerve (femoral branch), (4) genitofemoral nerve (genital branch)

Ilioinguinal and iliohypogastric nerves

Procedure

Full prior information for the patient is mandatory.

Preparations
See Chapter. 26, p. 221.

Materials (Fig. 32.2)
40–50 mm long injection needle, 23–25 G. When a nerve stimulator is used, a 35–50 mm long atraumatic 22-G needle (15°) with an injection lead (e.g. Stimuplex D, B. Braun Melsungen).
Syringes: 2, 5, and 10 mL.
Local anesthetics, antiseptic, swabs, sterile gloves and drape.

Patient positioning
Supine, with the ipsilateral hand under the head.

Landmarks
A line is drawn connecting the anterior superior iliac spine and the umbilicus.
The injection site is located about 3 cm medial to the iliac spine on this line (Fig. 32.3).

Skin prep, subcutaneous local anesthesia, covering with a sterile drape, drawing up the local anesthetic.

Injection technique
- The injection needle is introduced perpendicular and then slightly laterally until bone contact is made with the wing of the ilium. It is then withdrawn slightly, and after aspiration ca. 5 mL of the local anesthetic is injected.
- The needle is then withdrawn to lie subcutaneously, and the direction is altered medially along the connecting line until there is penetration of the fascia of the external oblique muscle and internal and transverse oblique muscles.
- After aspiration, fan-shaped injection of 10 mL of local anesthetic.

The cutaneous innervation of the ilioinguinal region is shown in Fig. 32.4.

Dosage

10–15 mL local anesthetic – e.g. 0.75% ropivacaine, 0.5% bupivacaine (0.5% levobupivacaine), 1% prilocaine, 1% mepivacaine.

Complications

None.

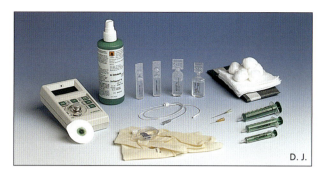

Fig. 32.2 Materials

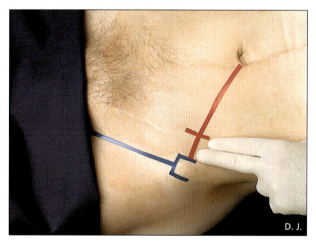

Fig. 32.3 Location

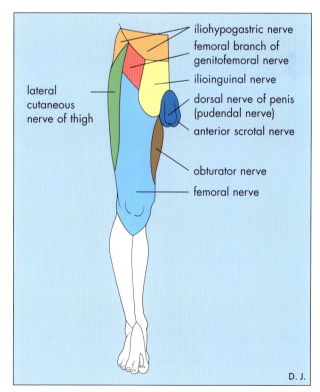

Fig. 32.4 Cutaneous innervation areas in the ilioinguinal region

33 Blocking peripheral nerves in the knee joint region

Anatomy

In the distal part of the thigh, the **sciatic nerve** divides into the **tibial nerve,** which runs medially and straight, and a lateral branch, the **common peroneal (fibular) nerve.** A third nerve in the area of the knee joint, the **saphenous nerve,** is the largest and thickest branch of the **femoral nerve.**

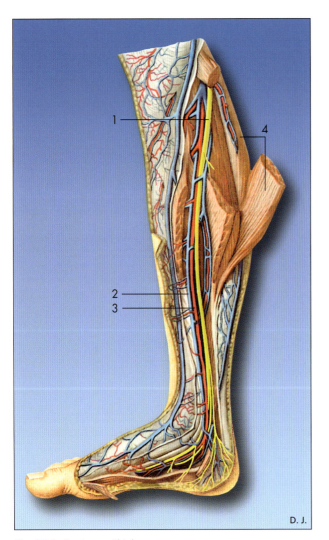

Fig. 33.1 Anatomy: tibial nerve.
(1) Tibial nerve, (2) posterior tibial vein, (3) posterior tibial artery, (4) gastrocnemius muscle

Sciatic nerve area

Tibial nerve (Figs. 33.1, 33.3)
Almost twice as thick as the common peroneal nerve, the tibial nerve is the continuation of the sciatic nerve, running down through the middle of the popliteal fossa and lying posterior and slightly lateral to the popliteal vessels.
It then passes between the two heads of the gastrocnemius muscle to the upper edge of the soleus muscle. Between the posterior tibial muscle and the soleus muscle, it runs distally together with the posterior tibial artery through the calf musculature, as far as the midpoint between the medial malleolus and the calcaneus, to the medial side of the foot joint.
It divides into its two end branches, the medial and lateral plantar nerves, behind the medial malleolus. These pass under the flexor retinaculum to the sole of the foot and provide it with its sensory innervation. While in proximity to the common peroneal nerve as part of the sciatic nerve, it gives off branches to the obturator internus muscle, gemelli muscles, quadratus femoris muscle, semitendinosus muscle, semimembranosus muscle, adductor magnus muscle and long head of the biceps.

Common peroneal (fibular) nerve (Figs. 33.2, 33.3)
After separating from the tibial nerve, the common peroneal nerve runs along the medial edge of the biceps femoris muscle over the lateral head of the gastrocnemius muscle to the lateral angle of the popliteal fossa. At the neck of the fibula, it passes to the lateral surface of the bone. Before entering the peroneus longus muscle, which originates here, it divides into the mainly sensory superficial peroneal nerve and the mainly motor deep peroneal nerve.
Up to the point at which it divides, its small branches supply the short head of the biceps femoris muscle, the lateral and posterior parts of the joint capsule and the tibiofibular joint, and it gives off the lateral sural cutaneous nerve. The anterior branch of this runs subcutaneously to the lateral surface of the lower leg as far as the lateral malleolus, and its posterior branch runs subfascially and then subcutaneously until it unites with the medial sural cutaneous nerve from the tibial nerve.

Area supplied by the femoral nerve

Saphenous nerve (Fig. 33.4)

The wholly sensory saphenous nerve is the longest branch of the femoral nerve (see Chapter 26, Fig. 26.1). It forms the continuation of the posterior trunk, and in the thigh it lies initially on the lateral surface and, further down, on the anterior surface of the femoral artery. Along with the femoral vessels, it enters the adductor canal and penetrates its anterior wall and, covered by the sartorius muscle, runs between the vastus medialis muscle and adductor magnus muscle to the medial side of the knee. Here, at the tendon of the sartorius muscle, it passes to lie below the skin and runs up to the great saphenous vein, then down subcutaneously alongside this vein in the lower leg. Its terminal nerves supply the skin on the medial edge of the foot and medial malleolus. One branch connects with the superficial peroneal nerve in the ankle. Apart from a branch to the knee joint, it also gives off the infrapatellar branch to the skin on the medial side of the knee as far as the anterior surface of the patella, and the medial crural cutaneous nerves, which supply the skin over the medial surface of the tibia and the medial calf skin.

Indications

Surgical

- Procedures on the lower leg (including those performed under tourniquet) using combined blocks of all three nerves, or superficial procedures in the region of the individual nerves, without using a tourniquet.
- Particularly suitable for outpatient procedures.
- Postoperative pain therapy.
- Supplementation of incomplete epidural anesthesia or incomplete block of the sciatic or femoral nerves.

Care must be taken to avoid nerve injury, as paresthesias are not available as a warning signal (see Chapter 9, section on axillary block, and Chapter 26).

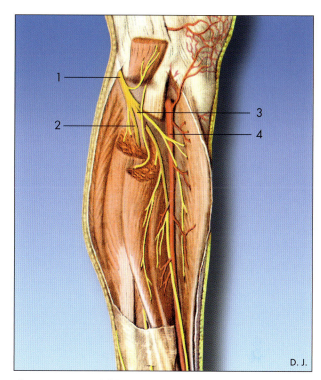

Fig. 33.2 Peroneal (fibular) nerve.
(1) Common peroneal (fibular) nerve, (2) superficial peroneal (fibular) nerve, (3) deep peroneal (fibular) nerve, (4) anterior tibial artery

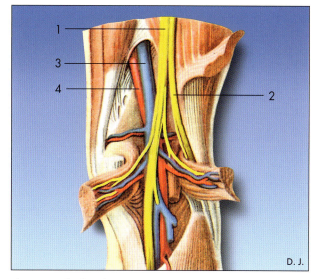

Fig. 33.3 Tibial and common peroneal (fibular) nerve in the popliteal area.
(1) Tibial nerve, (2) common peroneal (fibular) nerve, (3) popliteal vein, (4) popliteal artery

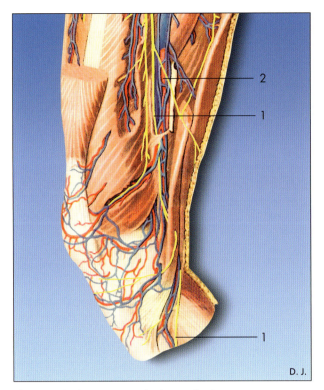

Fig. 33.4 Saphenous nerve in the popliteal area.
(1) Saphenous nerve, (2) femoral artery

Contraindications
- Lesions of the nerves being blocked distal to the injection site.
- Anticoagulant therapy.
- Infection in the injection area.

Procedure

Full prior information for the patient is mandatory.

Preparations
Check that the emergency equipment is complete and in working order. Sterile precautions, intravenous access, ECG monitoring, pulse oximetry, intubation kit, ventilation facilities, emergency medication.

Materials (Fig. 33.5)
- Single-shot technique:
  Atraumatic 22-G needle 40–55 cm long with injection lead ("immobile needle" – e.g. Stimuplex D®, B. Braun Melsungen) to block the peroneal and tibial nerves, 25-G needle 40 mm long to block the saphenous nerve.

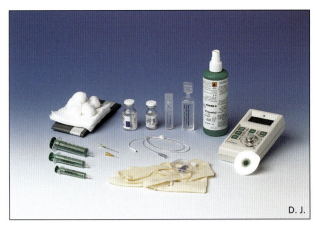

Fig. 33.5 Materials

- Continuous technique for postoperative analgesia: Contiplex D® set: 18-G Contiplex D® needle 55 (80) mm long (15°) with Contiplex® catheter, or: Contiplex®–Tuohy set: 18-G Tuohy needle 52 (102) mm long with Contiplex® catheter.

Syringes: 2, 10 and 20 mL.
Local anesthetics, disinfectant, swabs, compresses, sterile gloves and drape.

Simultaneous block of the tibial and common peroneal (fibular) nerve in the popliteal area (distal sciatic nerve block)

Popliteal fossa (Fig. 33.6)
The **caudal** boundary of the popliteal fossa is determined medially and laterally by the gastrocnemius muscle, **craniomedially** by the semimembranosus and semitendinosus muscles and **craniolaterally** by the biceps femoris muscle. The two nerves lie superficially and are located at a depth of about 1.5–2 cm.

Patient positioning
Prone, with the treated leg stretched out. The person carrying out the injection stands on the side being injected.

Landmarks
The popliteal fossa is divided into a medial and a lateral triangle, the base of which is represented by the intercondylar line between the lateral and medial epicondyles. The midpoint of the base is marked, and from there a line is drawn 5 cm proximally and then 1 cm laterally. This point determines the injection site (Fig. 33.7).

Skin prep, local anesthesia, covering with a sterile drape, drawing up the local anesthetic, checking the patency of the injection needle and the functioning of the nerve stimulator, attaching electrodes.

Injection technique (Fig. 33.7)
The injection needle is advanced at an angle of 45–60° and in an anterosuperior direction. After paresthesias have been produced at a depth of about 1.5–2 cm, incremental injection of a local anesthetic is carried out after aspiration.
When a nerve stimulator is used, either plantar flexion (as a motor response from the tibial nerve) or plantar dorsiflexion (common peroneal nerve) are sought.
After removal of the needle, better distribution of the local anesthetic is encouraged with pressure compression (3–5 min) and simultaneous massaging of the injection area. This also serves for hematoma prophylaxis.

Continuous technique
The injection is carried out as in the single-shot technique. After correct stimulation and aspiration, a test dose is injected. The Contiplex® catheter is then advanced ca. 2–3 cm beyond the end of the needle or cannula and the stimulation needle is slowly withdrawn while the thumb and index finger of the left hand simultaneously hold the catheter at the injection site.
A bacterial filter is then placed and the catheter is fixed with a skin suture and dressing.

Dosage
▪ Single-shot technique:
35–40 mL local anesthetic – e.g. 0.5–0.75% ropivacaine, 0.5% bupivacaine (0.5% levobupivacaine), 1% prilocaine, 1% mepivacaine.
A combination of long-duration and medium-duration local anesthetics has proved particularly suitable for surgical indications.
▪ Continuous technique:
0.2–0.375% ropivacaine,
5–15 mL/h (max. 37.5 mg/h), or alternatively for **bolus administration**: 10–20 mL 0.2–0.375% ropivacaine.
▪ Patient-controlled analgesia (PCA):
Baseline rate of **4–5 mL/h** 0.375% ropivacaine (max. 37.5 mg/h).
Bolus dose of **2–3 mL** 0.375% ropivacaine.
Lockout period of **10 min**.

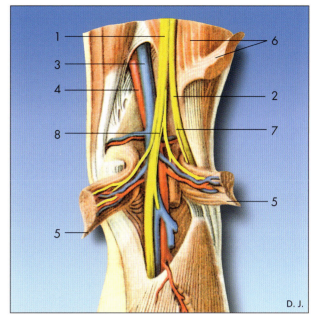

Fig. 33.6 Popliteal fossa.
(1) Tibial nerve, (2) common peroneal (fibular) nerve, (3) popliteal vein, (4) popliteal artery, (5) gastrocnemius muscle, (6) biceps femoris muscle, (7) lateral sural cutaneous nerve, (8) medial sural cutaneous nerve

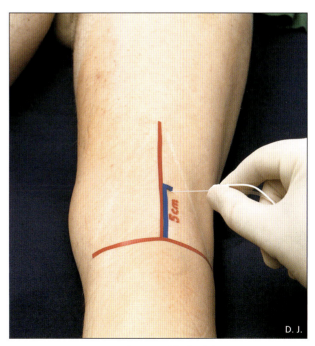

Fig. 33.7 Injection. Simultaneous block of the common peroneal (fibular) nerve and tibial nerve

Complications

Complications are extremely rare, but possible:
- Neuritis and dysesthesia.
- Intravascular injection.
- Hematoma formation.

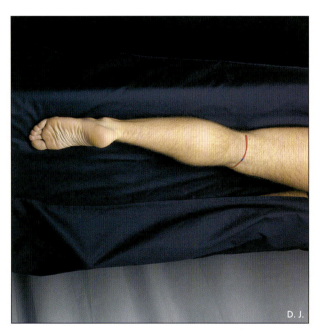

Fig. 33.8 Tibial nerve

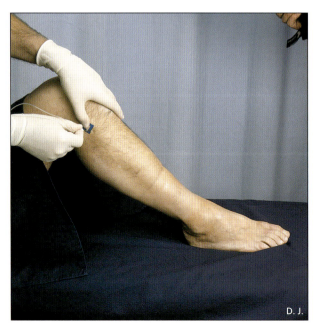

Fig. 33.9 Common peroneal (fibular) nerve

Tibial nerve block

Patient positioning
Prone, with the treated leg stretched out. The person carrying out the injection stands on the side being injected.

Landmarks
Popliteal fossa. The center of the connecting line between the lateral and medial epicondyles determines the injection point.

Injection technique (Fig. 33.8)
The injection needle is introduced perpendicular to the skin until paresthesias are produced. This normally occurs at a depth of about 1.5–3 cm. When a nerve stimulator is used, plantar flexion is noted as a motor response. After aspiration at two levels, incremental injection of local anesthetic is carried out.

Dosage
5–10 mL of local anesthetic – e.g. 0.75% ropivacaine, 0.5% bupivacaine (0.5% levobupivacaine), 1% prilocaine, 1% mepivacaine.

Complications
See the section on simultaneous block of the tibial and common peroneal (fibular) nerves in the popliteal area, above.

Block of the common peroneal (fibular) nerve

Patient positioning
Supine, with the treated leg positioned at a slight angle. The person carrying out the injection stands on the side being injected.

Landmarks
Head of the fibula, tendon of the biceps femoris muscle. The head of the fibula is palpated. The injection point lies about 2 cm below the head of the fibula.

Injection technique (Fig. 33.9)
The injection needle is advanced perpendicularly until paresthesias are produced at a depth of about 1 cm. When a nerve stimulator is used, plantar dorsiflexion is noted as a motor response. After aspiration at two levels, incremental injection of the local anesthetic is carried out behind the head of the fibula.

Dosage
5–10 mL of local anesthetic – e.g. 0.75% ropivacaine, 0.5% bupivacaine (0.5% levobupivacaine), 1% prilocaine, 1% mepivacaine.

Blocking peripheral nerves in the knee joint region

Complications
See the section on simultaneous block of the tibial and common peroneal (fibular) nerves in the popliteal area, p. 252.

Saphenous nerve block

Patient positioning
Supine, with the treated leg positioned at a slight angle.

Landmarks
Medial condyle of the tibia, tibial tuberosity, gastrocnemius muscle.

Injection technique (Fig. 33.10)
The medial condyle of the tibia is palpated. Distal to this, a continuous subcutaneous infiltration of the following areas is carried out: medial condyle, tibial tuberosity and gastrocnemius muscle.

Dosage
5–10 mL of local anesthetic – e.g. 0.75% ropivacaine, 0.5% bupivacaine (0.5% levobupivacaine), 1% prilocaine, 1% mepivacaine.

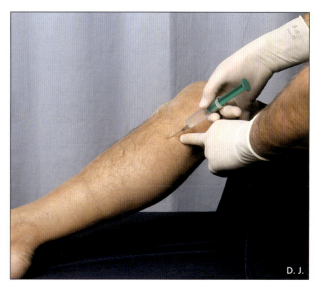

Fig. 33.10 Saphenous nerve

Complications
No specific complications.

The areas of cutaneous innervation of the individual nerves discussed in this Chapter are illustrated in Fig. 33.11.

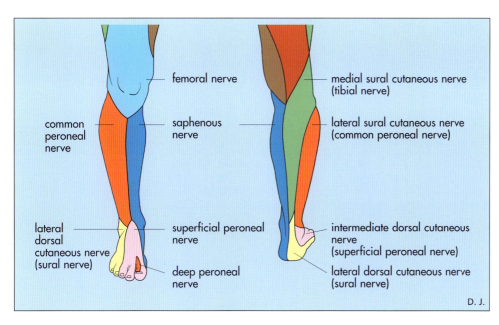

Fig. 33.11 Cutaneous innervation areas in the lower leg

34 Blocking peripheral nerves in the ankle joint region

Definition
Individual or combined infiltration anesthesia of the following nerves in the ankle joint region:
- Tibial nerve
- Superficial and deep peroneal (fibular) nerves.
- Sural nerve.
- Saphenous nerve.

Anatomy

Tibial nerve (Fig. 34.1)
The tibial nerve reaches the distal lower leg posterior to the medial malleolus. It gives off medial calcaneal branches to the heel and divides into its two end branches, the medial and lateral plantar nerves, which pass to the sole of the foot and provide it with its sensory supply.

Superficial peroneal (fibular) nerve
(Figs. 34.2, 34.3)
This nerve runs through the peroneus longus muscle, extends between the peroneus longus and brevis muscles, and penetrates the crural fascia in the distal third of the lower leg. Subcutaneously, or still at the subfascial level, it divides into the thicker medial dorsal cutaneous nerve and the smaller intermediate dorsal cutaneous nerve, providing the sensory supply for the skin on the back of the foot and the toes.

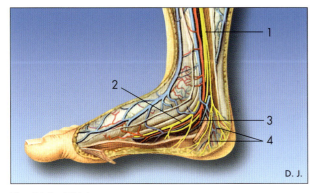

Fig. 34.1a Tibial nerve.
(1) Tibial nerve, (2) medial plantar nerve, (3) lateral plantar nerve, (4) calcaneal branches

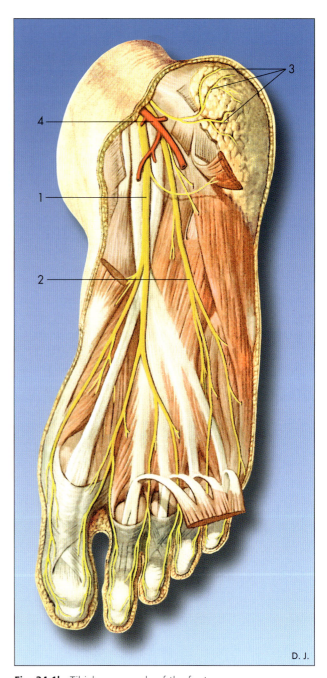

Fig. 34.1b Tibial nerve – sole of the foot.
(1) Medial plantar nerve, (2) lateral plantar nerve, (3) medial calcaneal branches, (4) posterior tibial artery

Blocking peripheral nerves in the ankle joint region

Deep peroneal (fibular) nerve (Figs. 34.2, 34.3)
This nerve runs between the tibialis anterior muscle and the extensor hallucis longus muscle in the direction of the ankle, where it divides into a medial and a lateral end branch. The medial end branch continues in same direction as the nerve trunk, and passes with the dorsalis pedis artery to the first interosseous space, crossing under the tendon of the extensor hallucis brevis muscle to the distal end of the interosseous space. Here it joins with a strand of the superficial peroneal nerve and divides into the end branches for the facing sides of the dorsal surfaces of the first and second toes. The lateral end branch turns laterally and supplies the extensor digitorum brevis muscle, sending off three interosseous nerves.

Sural nerve (Figs. 34.2, 34.3)
The medial sural cutaneous nerve arises in the proximal part of the popliteal fossa, runs down between the two heads of the gastrocnemius muscle, and joins the peroneal communicating branch to form the sural nerve. Accompanied by the small saphenous vein, the sural nerve runs behind the lateral malleolus and passes as the lateral dorsal cutaneous nerve along the lateral side of the foot, where it gives off a connecting branch to the intermediate dorsal cutaneous nerve and ends as the dorsalis digiti minimi nerve on the lateral edge of the dorsum of the small toe.

Behind the lateral malleolus it sends off branches (the lateral calcaneal branches) to the skin there and at the heel. The branches for the lateral side of the ankle, for the anterior capsular wall, and for the tarsal sinus originate proximal to the malleolus.

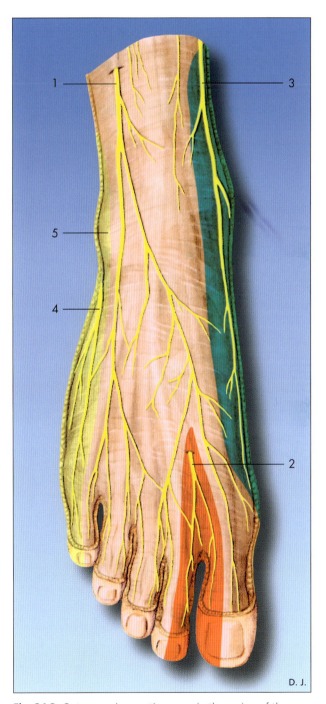

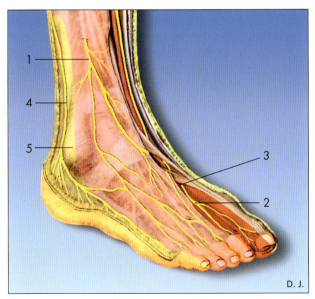

Fig. 34.2 Common, superficial, and deep peroneal (fibular) nerve, and sural nerve. Cutaneous innervation areas of the back of the foot (lateral).
(1) Superficial peroneal (fibular) nerve, (2) deep peroneal (fibular) nerve, (3) dorsalis pedis artery, (4) sural nerve, (5) lateral malleolus

Fig. 34.3 Cutaneous innervation areas in the region of the back of the foot (from the front).
(1) Superficial peroneal (fibular) nerve, (2) deep peroneal fibular) nerve, (3) saphenous nerve, (4) lateral dorsal cutaneous nerve (sural nerve), (5) lateral malleolus

Saphenous nerve (Fig. 34.3)

The saphenous nerve courses along the medial side of the lower leg and anterior to the medial malleolus, and sends off branches to the skin of the medial side of the foot. It usually ends in the metatarsal area, without reaching the big toe.

Indications
- Surgical procedures in the foot area.
- Outpatient surgery.
- Postoperative pain therapy.
- Supplementing incomplete epidural anesthesia or an incomplete sciatic nerve or femoral nerve block.

> Care must be taken to avoid nerve injury, as paresthesias are not available as a warning sign here (see Chapter 9, p. 111).

Contraindications
- Anticoagulant therapy.
- Infections in the injection area.

Procedure

Full prior information for the patient is mandatory.

Preparations
Check that the emergency equipment is complete and in working order; sterile precautions.

Materials (Fig. 34.4)
25-G needle 30 mm long.
Syringes: 2, 5, 10 mL.
Local anesthetics, disinfectant, swabs, sterile gloves, drape.

Skin prep, subcutaneous local anesthesia, drawing up the local anesthetic.

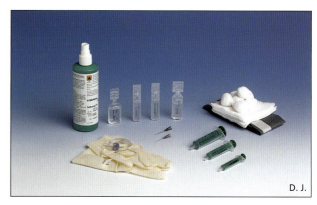

Fig. 34.4 Materials

Posterior tibial nerve

Patient positioning
Prone, with a pillow under the ankle (or the patient may be seated).

Landmarks
Medial malleolus, posterior tibial artery.

Injection technique (Figs. 34.5, 34.7)
Lateral to the palpated pulse of the posterior tibial artery, a fine 25-G needle, 30 mm long, is introduced at a right angle to the posterior side of the tibia and just posterior to the posterior tibial artery.
After paresthesias are elicited and after a negative aspiration test, 5 mL of local anesthetic is injected. If paresthesias cannot be elicited, then after reaching the posterior tibia the needle is withdrawn for about 1 cm, and 5–10 mL of local anesthetic is injected.
Another technique is to carry out perpendicular puncture of the skin at the level of the medial malleolus, dorsal and then ventral to the posterior tibial artery, and to distribute the total dose of local anesthetic in two equal halves on each side [8].

Deep peroneal nerve

Patient positioning
Supine, or sitting.

Landmarks
Dorsalis pedis artery, proximal back of the foot.

Injection technique (Fig. 34.6)
A fine 25-G injection needle, 30 mm long, is introduced perpendicular to the skin surface; 5 mL of the local anesthetic is injected on each side, first lateral to the artery and then medial to it [8].

Sural nerve and superficial peroneal nerve

Patient positioning
Supine, or sitting.

Landmarks
Lateral malleolus.

Injection technique (Fig. 34.8)
About 10 cm above the lateral malleolus, parallel to the upper ankle, fan-shaped subcutaneous infiltration of the Achilles tendon is carried out as far as the edge of the tibia, using about 10 mL of local anesthetic.

Saphenous nerve

Patient positioning
Supine, or sitting.

Landmarks
Medial malleolus.

Injection technique (Fig. 34.5)
About 10 cm above the medial malleolus, 5–10 mL of local anesthetic is injected subcutaneously around the long saphenous vein and, in a fan-shaped fashion, in a mediolateral direction.

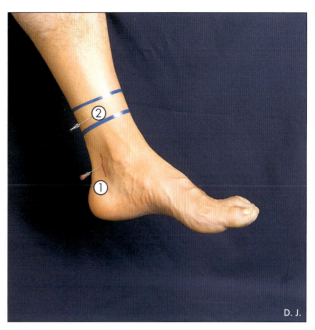

Fig. 34.5 Posterior tibial nerve (1) (red needle) and posterior tibial artery (red), (2) saphenous nerve (black needle)

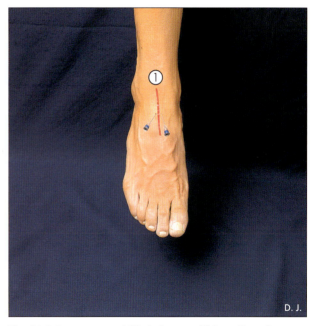

Fig. 34.6 Deep peroneal (fibular) nerve. (1) Dorsalis pedis artery

Chapter 34

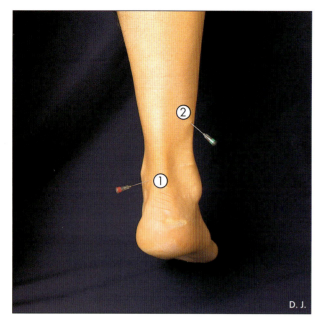

Fig. 34.7 Posterior tibial nerve (1) (red needle) and (2) sural nerve (green needle)

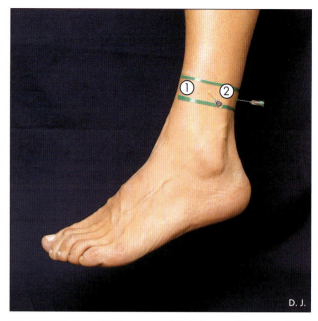

Fig. 34.8 (1) Superficial peroneal (fibular) nerve (blue needle) and (2) sural nerve (green needle)

The cutaneous innervation areas of the individual nerves are shown in Fig. 34.9.

Dosage
Tibial nerve and deep peroneal nerve
5–10 mL of local anesthetic.

Sural nerve, superficial peroneal nerve, saphenous nerve
10 (15)–20 mL of local anesthetic (subcutaneous fan-shaped infiltration).

Local anesthetics
0.5–0.75% ropivacaine, 0.25–0.5% bupivacaine (0.25–0.5% levobupivacaine), 1% prilocaine, 1% mepivacaine.

Complications
No specific complications.

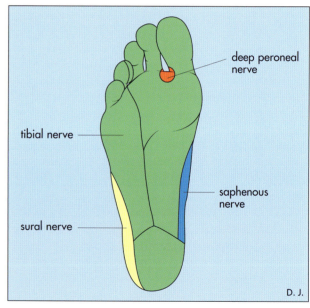

Fig. 34.9 Cutaneous innervation areas in the region of the sole of the foot

Blocking peripheral nerves – knee and foot

Block no. ☐ Right ☐ Left

Name: _____ Date: _____
Diagnosis: _____
Premedication: ☐ No ☐ Yes
Neurological abnormalities: ☐ No ☐ Yes _____

Purpose of block: ☐ Surgical ☐ Diagnostic ☐ Therapeutic
Needle : G ____ Length ____ ☐ Short-beveled ☐ Other
i.v. access: ☐ Yes ☐ No
Monitoring: ☐ ECG ☐ Pulse oximetry
Ventilation facilities: ☐ Yes (equipment checked)
Emergency equipment (drugs): ☐ Checked
Patient: ☐ Informed (behavior after block)

Knee area:
☐ Tibial nerve/common peroneal (fibular) nerve (simultaneously)
☐ Superficial/deep peroneal (fibular) nerve ☐ Tibial nerve ☐ Saphenous nerve

Foot area:
☐ Posterior tibial nerve ☐ Deep peroneal nerve
☐ Sural nerve/superficial peroneal nerve ☐ Saphenous nerve

Position : ☐ Supine ☐ Prone ☐ Sitting
Location technique: ☐ Electrostimulation ☐ Paresthesias
Injection:
Local anesthetic: _____ mL ____ %
(in incremental doses)
☐ Addition to LA _____ µg/mg

Patient's remarks during injection:
☐ None ☐ Paresthesias ☐ Warmth ☐ Pain (intraneural position?)

Nerve area: _____
Objective block effect after 15 min:
☐ Cold test ☐ Temperature measurement before ____°C after ____°C
☐ Sensory ☐ Motor
Monitoring after block: ☐ < 30 min ☐ > 30 min

Complications:
☐ None ☐ Intravascular injection ☐ Signs of intoxication
☐ Hematoma ☐ Neurological complications ☐ Other

Subjective effects of the block: Duration: _____
☐ None ☐ Increased pain ☐ Reduced pain ☐ Relief of pain

VISUAL ANALOG SCALE

0 10 20 30 40 50 60 70 80 90 100

Special notes: _____

Record and checklist

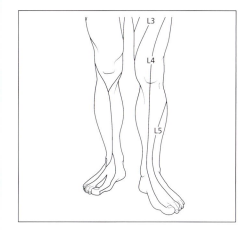

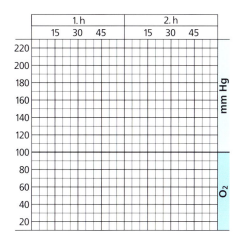

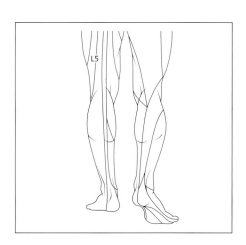

Neuraxial anesthesia

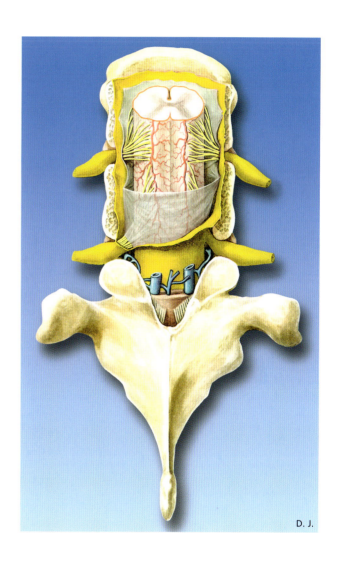

35 Neuraxial anatomy

Spine and sacrum

Spine

The spinal column consists of 33 vertebrae – seven cervical vertebrae; 12 thoracic vertebrae; five lumbar vertebrae; the sacrum, consisting of five fused sacral vertebrae; and the coccyx, consisting of four fused coccygeal segments (Fig. 35.1).
The average length of the spine in adult men is about 72 cm, while in women it is 7–10 cm shorter.

All of the vertebrae have the same basic shape, which is subject to certain variations in the individual sections of the spine. The basic shape consists of an anterior body (the body of the vertebra) and a dorsal arch (the vertebral arch), which consists of pedicles and laminae (Fig. 35.2).
The laminae of the vertebral arch join dorsally to form the spinous process. A transverse process branches off on each side of the vertebral arch, as well as a superior and an inferior articular process.
The vertebrae in the cervical region are smaller, but their size increases from cranial to caudal. The angle of

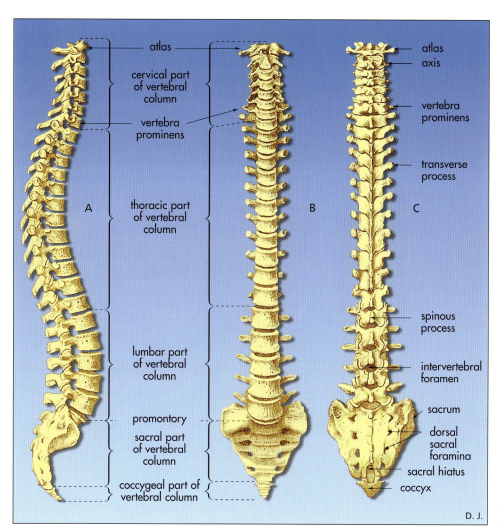

Fig. 35.1a–c Spine.
a Lateral, **b** Ventral, **c** Dorsal

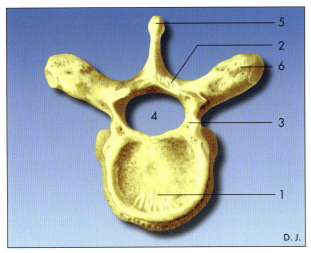

Fig. 35.2 Basic shape of a vertebra. (1) Vertebral body, (2) vertebral arch, (3) pedicle of the vertebral arch, (4) vertebral foramen, (5) spinous process, (6) transverse process

inclination of the spinous processes – important topographic signposts for neuraxial injections – varies at different levels of the spine.

The cervical spinous processes, the first two thoracic spinous processes and the lumbar spinous processes lie at the same level as their vertebrae. From T3 to L1, the spinous processes are angled caudally (particularly in the T4–T9 area) (Fig. 35.3a–c).

The vertebral canal (which provides excellent protection for the spinal cord) and the spinal cord, with its meningeal covering, extend throughout the whole length of the spine terminating in the cauda equina.

The spinal vessels and nerves emerge laterally through openings at the upper and lower margins of the roots of the arches of the adjoining vertebrae (the intervertebral foramina).

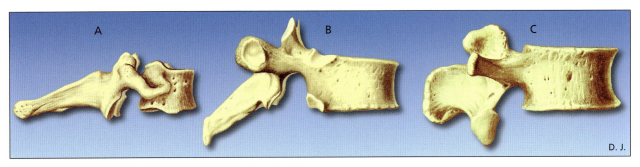

Fig. 35.3a–c Cervical, thoracic and lumbar spinous processes.
a C7 cervical vertebra (vertebra prominens, nuchal tubercle). **b** T8 thoracic vertebra. **c** L3 lumbar vertebra

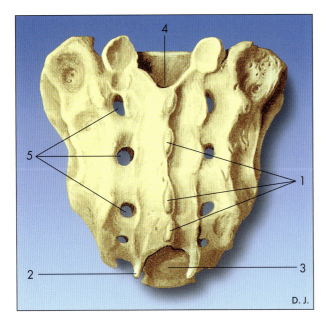

Fig. 35.4 Sacrum (dorsal view).
(1) Median sacral crest, (2) sacral horn, (3) sacral hiatus, (4) sacral canal, (5) posterior sacral foramina

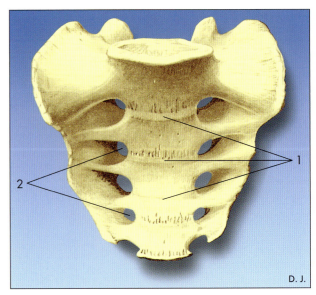

Fig. 35.5 Sacrum (ventral view).
(1) Transverse lines, (2) anterior pelvic sacral foramina

Sacrum

The sacrum is wedge-shaped and consists of five vertebrae fused together. It lies distal to the fifth lumbar vertebra and is connected distally, at its apex, to the coccyx.

Dorsally, the sacrum has a convex surface, in the middle of which the **median sacral crest** stands out (Fig. 35.4).

The crest is produced by the fusion of the rudimentary spinous processes of the upper third or fourth sacral vertebrae. Normally, the arch of the fifth and occasionally also of the fourth sacral vertebra is absent, so that there is a **sacral hiatus** at this point.

The hiatus is bounded by the sacral horn as a remnant of the caudal articular process, and it is used as a passage by the five small sacral nerves and by the coccygeal nerves.

Between the median sacral crest and the lateral sacral crest lie the four sacral openings (the posterior sacral foramina), through which the dorsal branches of the sacral spinal nerves emerge.

The anterior view shows a concave aspect. Alongside the transverse lines (fused vertebrae), there are large anterior openings (the anterior pelvic sacral foramina), through which the primary anterior parts of the sacral nerves emerge (Fig. 35.5).

Spinal ligaments

The vertebrae are supported from the axis to the cranial sacrum by intervertebral disks and by various ligaments (Fig. 35.6).

The intervertebral disks lie between neighboring vertebrae and function as fixed connecting elements and pressure-absorbing buffers. The disks are at their thinnest in the area of T3–T7 and thickest in the lumbar area.

The **anterior longitudinal ligament** is attached at the anterior edge of the vertebral bodies and intervertebral disks and is at its thickest in the thoracic area. The **posterior longitudinal ligament** is wider cranially than it is caudally and it lies behind the vertebral bodies in the medullary canal. The **supraspinous ligaments** extend as far as the sacrum along the tips of the spinous processes, with which they are connected, and continue cranially in the nuchal ligament and caudally in the **interspinous ligament.** They become thicker from cranial to caudal. The interspinous ligaments connect the roots and tips of the spinous processes.

The **intertransverse ligaments** serve to connect the transverse processes (Fig. 35.7).

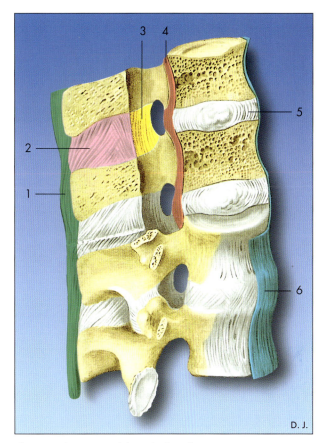

Fig. 35.6 Ligaments of the spinal cord.
(1) Supraspinous ligament, (2) interspinous ligament,
(3) ligamentum flavum, (4) posterior longitudinal ligament,
(5) intervertebral disk, (6) anterior longitudinal ligament

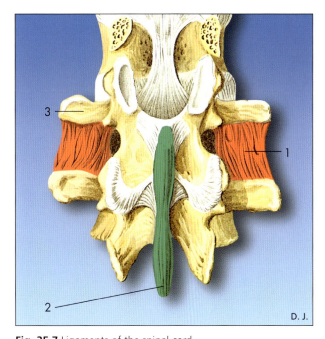

Fig. 35.7 Ligaments of the spinal cord.
(1) Intertransverse ligament, (2) supraspinous ligament,
(3) transverse process

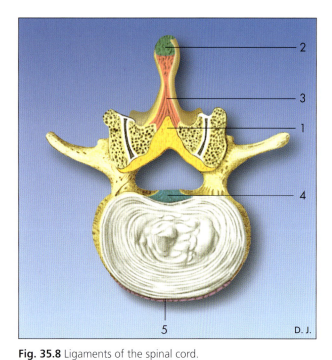

Fig. 35.8 Ligaments of the spinal cord.
(1) Ligamentum flavum, (2) supraspinous ligament,
(3) interspinous ligament, (4) posterior longitudinal ligament,
(5) anterior longitudinal ligament

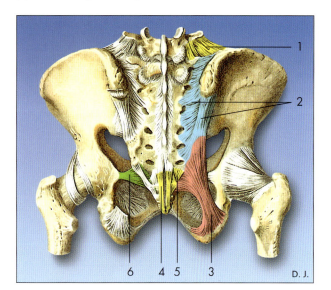

Fig. 35.9 Iliolumbosacral ligaments (dorsal view).
(1) Iliolumbar ligament, (2) dorsal sacroiliac ligament,
(3) sacrotuberous ligament, (4) superficial dorsal and deep dorsal sacrococcygeal ligaments, (5) lateral sacrococcygeal ligament,
(6) sacrospinous ligament

The **ligamentum flavum** largely consists of yellow, elastic fibers and it connects the neighboring laminae (Fig. 35.8).
It is at its thinnest in the midline (small fissure spaces exist for the veins running from the internal vertebral venous plexus to the external vertebral venous plexus), and its thickness increases laterally. The size and shape of the ligamentum flavum vary at the various levels of the spine. Caudally, for example, it is thicker than in the cranial direction.

Iliolumbosacral ligaments

The stability of the iliolumbosacral region is ensured by lumbosacral and sacroiliac connections that transfer the entire weight of the trunk via the hip bones to the lower extremities. These ligamentous connections serve to connect the vertebrae with one another and to stabilize the sacrum.
Clinically important ligaments: interspinous, supraspinous, iliolumbar, interosseous sacroiliac, sacrospinous and sacrotuberous ligaments (Figs. 35.9, 35.10).

Spinal cord

The spinal cord is about 46 cm long and is the caudal continuation of the medulla oblongata, which extends from the atlas to the conus medullaris (the lower edge of the first lumbar vertebra).
The **conus medullaris** continues in the threadlike median filum terminale as far as the posterior side of the coccyx (Fig. 35.11).
The dura mater and arachnoid, and consequently the subarachnoid space as well, extend downward as far as the level of the second sacral vertebra.

Meninges

The spinal cord is surrounded and protected by the meninges (the **dura mater, arachnoid mater** and **pia mater**) and by cerebrospinal fluid, epidural fatty tissue and veins (Fig. 35.12).
The **dura mater of the spinal cord,** a fibroelastic membrane, extends as far as the second sacral vertebra, where it ends in a blind sac. It encloses the anterior and posterior spinal nerve roots.

Neuraxial anatomy

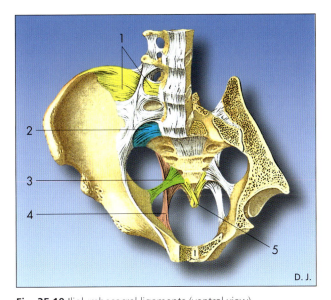

Fig. 35.10 Iliolumbosacral ligaments (ventral view).
(1) Iliolumbar ligament, (2) ventral sacroiliac ligament,
(3) sacrospinous ligament, (4) sacrotuberous ligament,
(5) ventral sacrococcygeal ligament

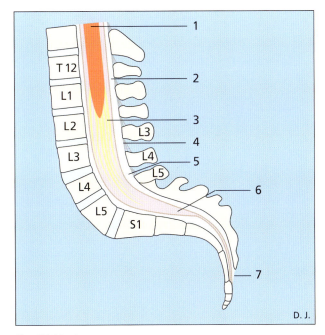

Fig. 35.11a Anatomy.
(1) Spinal cord, (2) dura mater, (3) cauda equina,
(4) ligamentum flavum, (5) epidural space, (6) subarachnoid space, (7) sacral hiatus

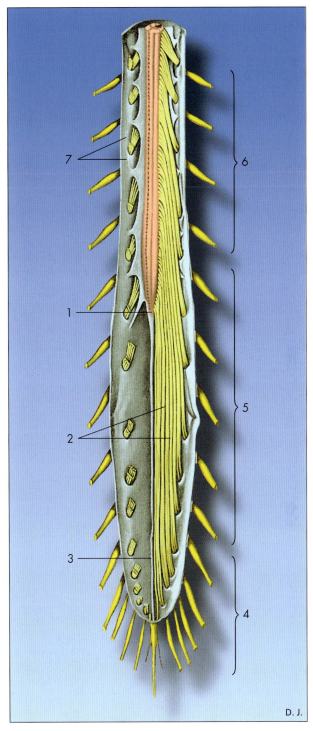

Fig. 35.11b Spinal cord (lower half).
(1) Conus medullaris, (2) cauda equina, (3) filum of spinal dura mater (filum terminale), (4) sacral nerves, (5) lumbar nerves, (6) thoracic nerves, (7) dura mater

Between the dura mater and the arachnoid, there is a space, the subdural space, in which a small amount of lymph-like fluid is located.

The **arachnoid mater,** a non-vascularized membrane, also ends at the level of the second sacral vertebra. Between the arachnoid mater and the pia mater lies the subarachnoid space, which is filled with cerebrospinal fluid.

The **spinal pia mater** is a thin, very well vascularized membrane that tightly encloses the spinal cord. Caudal to the medullary cone, it develops into the thin filum terminale, which descends medial to the cauda equina, penetrates the final part of the dural sac and arachnoid, and fuses with the connective tissue posterior to the first coccygeal segment.

The pia mater sends off 22 denticulate ligaments on each side, which attach to the dura mater and thus stabilize the spinal cord.

Spinal nerves

There are 31 pairs of spinal nerves in the human: eight cervical pairs, twelve thoracic pairs, five lumbar pairs, five sacral pairs and one coccygeal pair. These are connected to the spinal cord by a series of ventral and dorsal radicular filaments, which combine to form the nerve roots (Fig. 35.12).

The thicker **dorsal (posterior) root** is responsible for conducting afferent impulses (pain, temperature, touch, position). Each of the dorsal spinal nerve roots has a sensory **spinal ganglion** incorporated in it.

The **ventral (anterior) root** is responsible for conducting efferent impulses (muscles, glands). The nerve roots in the lower segments of the spinal cord descend

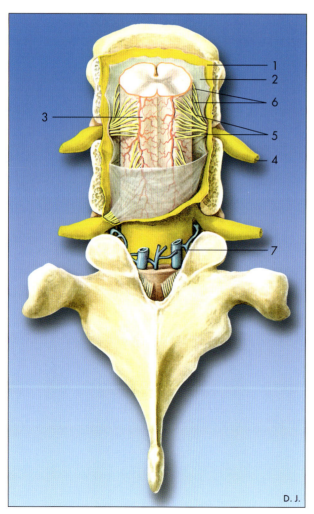

Fig. 35.12 Meninges.
(1) Dura mater, (2) arachnoid mater, (3) pia mater, (4) spinal nerve, (5) dorsal (posterior) root, (6) ventral (anterior) root, (7) internal vertebral venous plexus

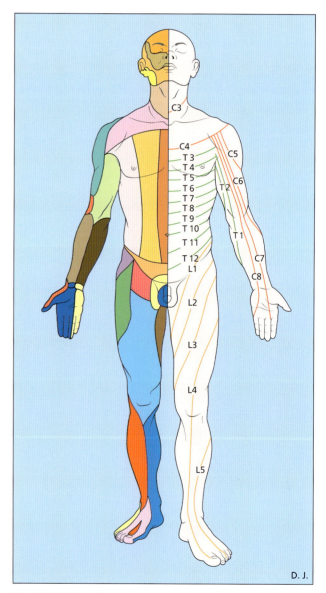

Fig. 35.13 Spinal dermatomes and the corresponding spinal-cord segments

Neuraxial anatomy

in the horsetail-like **cauda equina** to their exit openings.

After exiting from the subarachnoid space, the ventral and dorsal roots cross the epidural space.

In spinal anesthesia, the nerve roots are the principal targets for local anesthesia.

Spinal dermatomes

Via its branching spinal nerves, each segment of the spinal cord provides the sensory supply for a specific area of skin, known as the dermatome. These areas of skin, which often overlap, are very important for checking and verifying the spread of anesthesia (Figs. 35.13, 35.14).

Arteries of the spinal cord

The spinal cord is supplied by numerous radicular arteries, which form the **anterior spinal artery** and twin **posterior spinal arteries.**

The radicular arteries branch off from the cervical vertebral artery, the thoracic intercostal arteries and the abdominal lumbar arteries (Figs. 35.15, 35.16).

The **anterior spinal artery,** which arises from the fourth segment of the vertebral arteries, accompanies the spinal cord in the midline (anterior median fissure) along its entire course.

Via the central branches and small branches of the arterial pial network, the anterior spinal artery supplies the anterior two-thirds of the spinal cord.

The cervical and first two thoracic spinal cord segments receive blood from the radicular branches of subclavian artery branches.

In the mediothoracic spinal cord region (T3–T7), there is a radicular branch at the level of T4 or T5.

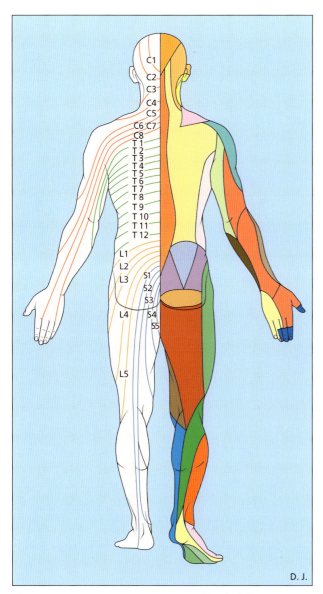

Fig. 35.14 Cutaneous innervation areas (detailed descriptions are given in the relevant chapters)

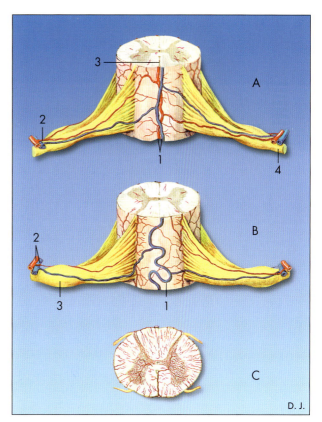

Fig. 35.15a–c Spinal cord.
a Ventral view: (1) anterior spinal artery and vein, (2) spinal branch, (3) anterior median fissure, (4) spinal nerve.
b Dorsal view: (1) posterior spinal vein, (2) dorsal branch of the posterior intercostal artery, (3) spinal ganglion.
c Cross-section

Chapter 35

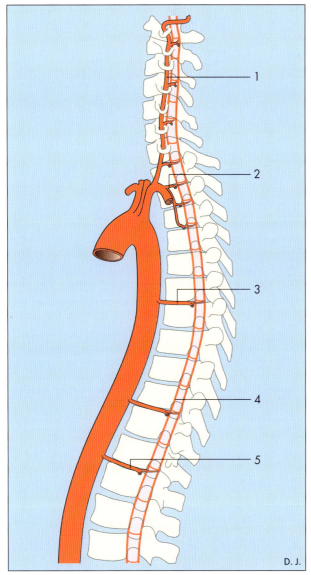

Fig. 35.16 Arteries of the spinal cord (side view).
(1) Vertebral artery, (2) deep cervical artery, (3) intercostal artery, (4) anterior and posterior spinal artery, (5) arteria radicularis magnus (artery of Adamkiewicz)

The thoracolumbar segment of the spinal cord (T8 to the medullary cone) draws its arterial supply mainly from the large-caliber arteria radicularis magnus (the artery of Adamkiewicz), which arises from an intercostal artery on the left side.

The cauda equina is supplied by branches of the lumbar, iliolumbar and lateral or median sacral arteries. These also supply the medullary cone.

The paired **posterior spinal arteries** arise from the fourth segment of the vertebral artery, receiving flow from 10–23 posterior radicular branches, and supply the dorsal third of the spinal cord.

Thin pial branches run from the spinal arteries, forming a network on the surface of the spinal cord known as the **arterial pial network**.

Veins of the spinal cord and vertebrae

The entire spinal canal is traversed by two venous plexuses, the **internal and external vertebral venous plexuses** (Figs. 35.17, 35.18).

Together, these form a ring around each vertebra, freely anastomosing with one another and receiving flow from the vertebrae, ligaments and spinal cord.

They are largely avalvular. Pressure changes in the thoracic or cerebrospinal fluid (CSF) spaces consequently affect the blood volume in the venous plexuses.

The plexuses are most strongly developed in the anterolateral area of the epidural space. They drain not only the spinal cord and its canal, but also part of the CSF.

Cerebrospinal fluid

The production of CSF is mainly achieved by active secretion and diffusion through the epithelial cells of the **choroid plexus,** but also to a small extent in the **subarachnoid space** and **perivascularly.**

The main tasks of the cerebrospinal fluid are:
- To function as a hemodynamic buffer and physical protection against forces affecting the spinal cord and brain.
- To substitute for the function of the lymphatic vessels, which are absent in the central nervous system.
- To allow metabolic exchange between blood and neural tissue.

There is a selective barrier between the blood and the CSF, the **blood–brain barrier,** which is formed by capillary endothelial cells and the choroid plexus. This barrier is clinically significant, as it is impermeable to many drugs.

The total quantity of the CSF in the adult is about 120–150 mL (with about 20–35 mL below the foramen ovale and about 15 mL below T5).

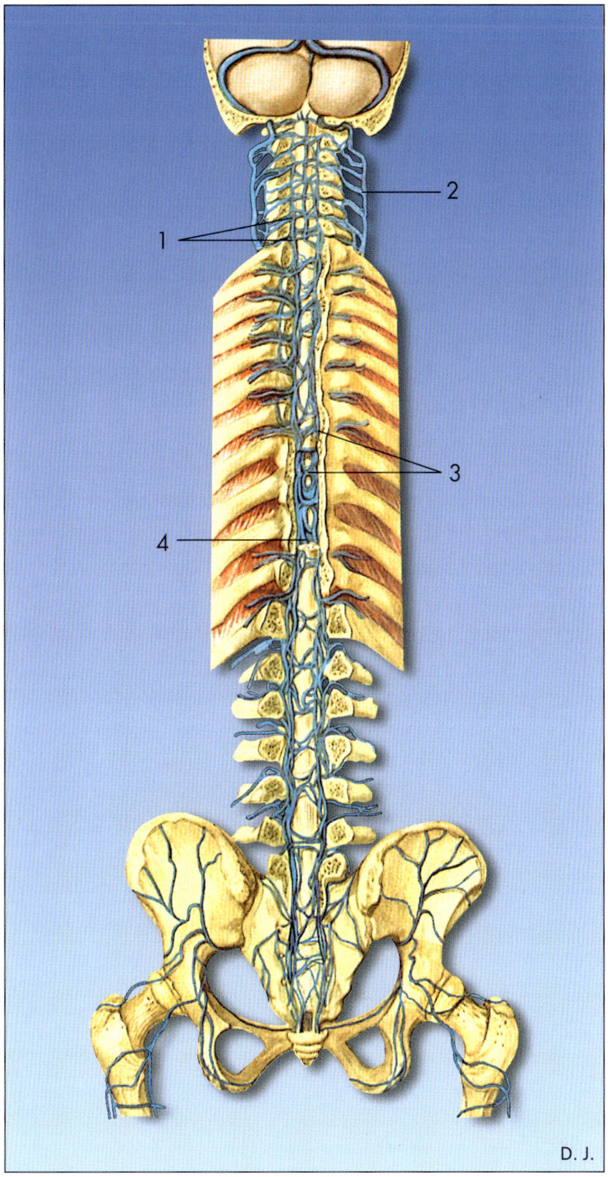

Approximately 400–450 mL of CSF is produced every day, and complete exchange of the fluid takes place every 10–12 hours.

Lumbar **CSF pressure** in a supine position is about 6–10 cmH$_2$O, while in a seated position it is about 20–25 cmH$_2$O.

The **specific gravity** of the CSF is 1.007 (1.003 to 1.009), and this must be taken into account in relation to the local anesthetic being used.

The **osmolarity** of CSF is comparable with that of the blood plasma (300 osmol/L), and the pH value is approximately the same as the physiological value.

Injected drugs mainly spread by diffusion, since CSF in the spinal canal circulates very little, if at all.

Resorption of CSF into the blood takes place via the **arachnoid granulations** and through the walls of the capillary vessels in the central nervous system and pia mater.

The liquid in the CSF sheaths of the cranial nerves and in the root pockets of the spinal nerves is an exception to the above rule. This liquid can enter the extradural lymphatic vessels directly.

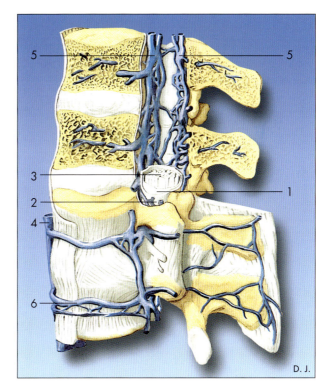

Fig. 35.17 Veins of the spinal cord.
(1) Vertebral veins, (2) deep cervical vein, (3) internal vertebral venous plexus, (4) spinal veins

Fig. 35.18 Veins of the spinal cord (lumbar region).
(1) Arachnoid, (2) dura mater, (3) cauda equina, (4) inferior vena cava, (5) internal vertebral venous plexus, (6) lumbar vein

Spinal anesthesia

36 Spinal anesthesia

Spinal anesthesia is one of the oldest, most valuable and most frequently used regional anesthesia techniques.

The injection of a local anesthetic into the subarachnoid space leads to temporary blocking of nerve conduction in the spinal nerve roots and paralysis of the autonomic, sensory and motor nerve fibers. Spinal anesthesia has the following characteristics:
- It is easy to perform.
- The onset is fast.
- Excellent anesthesia is produced.
- There is no systemic toxicity.

The application of spinal anesthesia depends on the following factors:
- The area of surgery.
- The type and expected duration of the procedure.
- The degree of muscle relaxation required.
- The presence of concomitant disease.
- The expected blood loss.

Indications
Surgical
Spinal anesthesia is particularly advantageous for all types of surgical procedures below the level of the umbilicus.
- Surgical procedures in the area of the lower extremities, hip joint and inguinal region.
- Vascular surgery.
- Prostate and bladder surgery.
- Gynecological and obstetric procedures.
- Surgery in the perineal and perianal region.
- Lumbar surgery – e.g. intervertebral disk operations [96].

Pain therapy
- Chemical intraspinal neurolysis with phenol in glycerol or alcohol (in advanced stages of malignant disease).

The use of spinal anesthesia has proved particularly valuable in:
- Patients with a full stomach.
- When tracheal intubation difficulties are expected.
- When there is a history of malignant hyperthermia, or a suspicion of malignant hyperthermia.
- Muscular disease.
- Cardiopulmonary disease.
- Metabolic disease.
- Renal and hepatic disease.
- Stable neurological diseases.
- After high spinal cord injury.
- Elderly patients.

Advantages
- Very good muscle relaxation.
- Very good postoperative analgesia.
- Increased bowel motility.
- Prophylaxis against thromboembolism caused by the sympathetic block.
- Suitable for outpatient procedures.
- Highly cost-effective, with easy and safe monitoring.

Disadvantages
- Unsuitable for upper abdominal procedures (high spinal anesthesia – e.g. T4–T6, is necessary).
- Lack of block of the vagus and phrenic nerves (leads to adverse effects such as nausea, vomiting, hiccup, pain and hypotension).

Contraindications
There are only a few contraindications to carrying out spinal anesthesia.

Specific
- Patient refusal
- Coagulation disorders, anticoagulant therapy.
- Sepsis

- Local infections at the injection site.
- Immune deficiency.
- Severe decompensated hypovolemia, shock.
- Specific cardiovascular diseases of myocardial, ischemic or valvular origin if the procedure being carried out requires sensory distribution of the anesthesia as far as T6.
- Acute cerebral or spinal cord diseases.
- Raised intracranial pressure.
- A history of hypersensitivity to local anesthetic agents, without a prior subcutaneous test dose.

Specific injection-related
- CSF mixed with blood (which does not clear even after repeated aspiration).
- No free CSF flow (even after rotating the needle at various levels and repeated attempts at aspiration).

Relative
These contraindications always require a risk–benefit assessment and are more medicolegal in nature.
- Severe spinal deformities, arthritis, osteoporosis, intervertebral disk prolapse or post intervertebral disk surgery. Following spinal fusion, spinal metastases.
- Spinal canal stenosis [84].
- Repetition of spinal anesthesia with hyperbaric solutions if the block originally carried out is ineffective [36, 60] (see Chapter 37 on neurological complications, p. 291). At least 10–15 minutes should be waited; attention should be given to possible mistakes with the initial injection procedure and a maximum of half of the original dose with no adjuncts should be administered.

Relative injection-related
- Further attempts after three unsuccessful injections.
- Inexperienced anesthetist without supervision.
- No anesthetic expertise.

> Head and back pain in the patient's history does not today represent a contraindication to spinal anesthesia, provided that small-caliber (>25 G) pencil-point injection needles are used and provided only one dural puncture is performed.

Procedure

Full prior information for the patient is mandatory.

Preparation and materials
- Check that the emergency equipment is complete and in working order (intubation kit, emergency drugs); sterile precautions, intravenous access, anesthetic machine.
- Start an intravenous infusion and ensure adequate volume loading (250–500 mL of a balanced electrolyte solution).
- Careful monitoring: ECG monitoring, BP, pulse oximetry.
- Skin prep.
- Local anesthetic.

The use of a ready-supplied spinal anesthesia kit – e.g. from B. Braun Melsungen, is recommended (Fig. 36.1).

Spinal needles (Fig. 36.2)
There are two possibilities here:
- **25–27 (29)-G spinal needles with conical tips** (pencil-point) – e.g. Pencan, Sprotte, Whitacre – in current standard use.
  When the dura is penetrated with these needles, the dural fibers are separated and then close together again. This means that the most troublesome complication – postdural puncture headache – hardly ever occurs when the dural puncture is carried out correctly.
- **Spinal needles with Quincke tip, 25–27 G**
  The needle bevel should be directed laterally during the puncture in order to pass through the dura in a

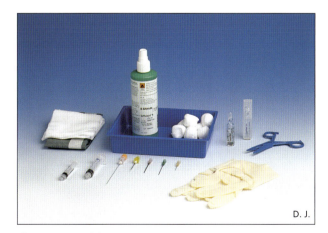

Fig. 36.1 Materials

Chapter 36

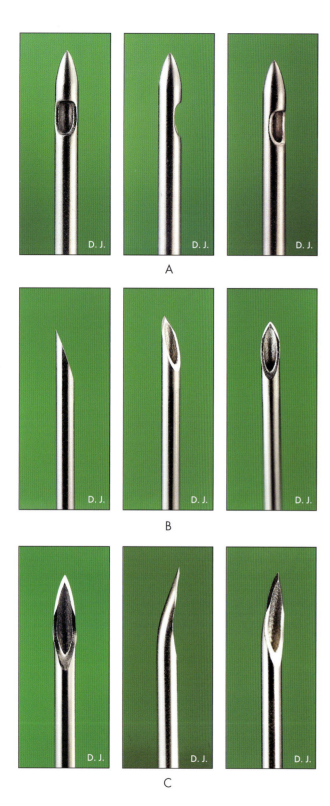

Fig. 36.2a–c Spinal needles.
a Pencan: pencil-point, 25 G
b Quincke: Spinocan Quincke tip, 27 G
c Atraucan: Atraucan Special Cut, 26 G

longitudinal direction. A 22-G needle is only used in exceptional cases – e.g. in older patients or when there are difficulties with positioning.

Patient positioning

Optimal patient positioning during puncture and during the fixation phase of the local anesthetic is a prerequisite for successful spinal anesthesia.

The following positions are possible:
- Lateral decubitus position.
- Sitting.
- Prone.

In all three positions, it is important to locate the **midline** and to follow it during the entire injection procedure. Lumbar lordosis must be minimised.

Lateral decubitus position
The assistant stands in front of the patient. If the anesthetist is right-handed, the patient is placed in the left lateral position. The patient is asked to adopt a "hunchback" position (legs flexed up against the abdomen and chin flexed down onto the chest) in order to bend the spine and allow optimal expansion of the intervertebral spaces.
It is important here for the spine to be parallel and for the intercristal line and the line connecting the two scapular tips to be perpendicular to the operating table (Fig. 36.3).

Advantages:
- More comfortable for the patient and thus particularly suitable for frail patients (risk of collapse).
- The reduction in blood pressure is less marked.
- When hyperbaric solutions are used, anesthesia concentrating on one side or unilateral anesthesia is possible.
- Can be used in pregnant patients (note the left lateral decubitus position).

Sitting
The patient is seated on the edge of the operating table and is supported by an assistant standing in front of him or her (Fig. 36.4).

Spinal anesthesia

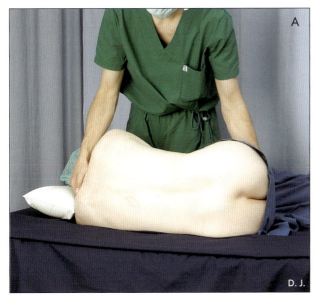
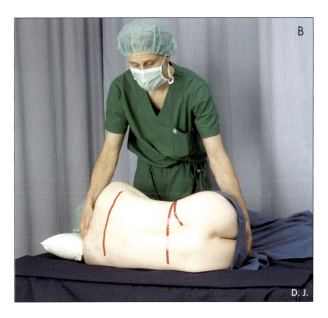

Fig. 36.3a, b Position: lateral decubitus

Advantages:
- When palpation of the spinous processes is difficult (e.g. in obese patients or those with spinal deformities), it is easier to locate the midline.
- The position is less painful for patients with fractures of the hip or lower extremities. Particularly in older patients with femoral neck fractures, we additionally administer 4–6 mg Hypnomidate (etomidate) before the injection, to make the short sitting phase easier.
- When anesthesia in the perineal or perianal region is required.
- The CSF flows more quickly.

Disadvantages:
- This position may lead to a hypotension (risk of collapse) and should be avoided in frail and heavily sedated patients, as well as in pregnant patients (aortocaval compression).
- An assistant is always required to support the patient.

Prone jackknife
This position is only used in the very rarely practiced hypobaric technique for spinal anesthesia (procedures in the rectum, perineum, sacrum, lower spine). An assistant and subsequent repositioning of the patient are not required (Fig. 36.5).

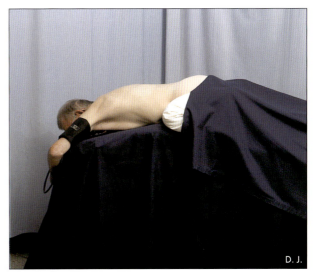

Fig. 36.4 Position: sitting

Fig. 36.5 Position: prone ("jackknife" position)

Chapter 36

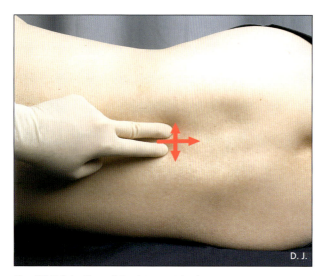

Fig. 36.6 Palpation of the intervertebral space

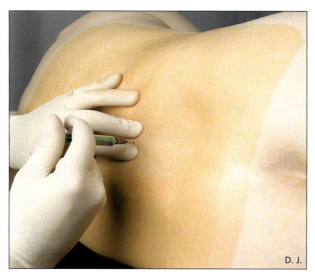

Fig. 36.7 Local anesthesia

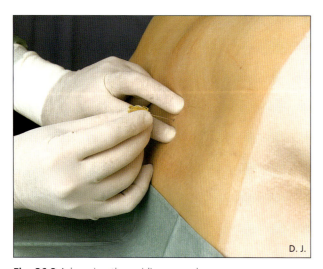

Fig. 36.8 Advancing the guiding cannula

Injection technique

Median approach (midline)
Landmarks
The injection is carried out in the midline below the L2 segment (conus medullaris), usually between the spinous processes of L2/3 or L3/4 (depending on the desired level of anesthesia).
The patient is asked to draw the legs tightly up to the abdomen and to place the chin on the chest. A line is drawn from one iliac crest to the other. This connection (Tuffier's line) crosses either the spinous process of L4 (50%) or the intervertebral space of segments L4/L5.
The intervertebral space is palpated, the **midline** is located as the most important signpost, and the injection site is marked with the thumbnail. As this is done, the palpating fingers move in a craniocaudal direction, or side to side (Fig. 36.6).

Strict asepsis
Thorough, repeated and wide skin prep and drying and covering of the injection site with a drape.

Local anesthesia
The skin and supraspinous and interspinous ligaments are anesthetized with 1–1.5 mL of a local anesthetic (e.g. 1% prilocaine).
The injection is carried out between the spread index and middle fingers of the left hand (Fig. 36.7).

Injection
Advancing the introducer
Without moving the spread index and middle finger of the **left** hand away from the intervertebral space, the introducer is grasped between the thumb and index finger of the **right** hand and advanced parallel to the operating table and slightly cranially (10°) far enough for it to lie firmly in the interspinous ligament (Fig. 36.8). It should be ensured that the **midline position** is maintained.
After this, the introducer is fixed with the thumb and index finger of the left hand, with the dorsum of the hand lying firmly on the patient's back.

Introducing the spinal needle, puncture of the subarachnoid space
The spinal needle, held between the thumb and index finger (or middle finger) of the right hand, is introduced through the interspinous ligament, ligamentum flavum, epidural space and dura/arachnoid as far as the subarachnoid space. The characteristic "dural click" occurs when the subarachnoid space is reached (Fig. 36.9).

Spinal anesthesia

When a Quincke needle is used, it should be ensured that the needle bevel is directed laterally, so that the dura is punctured in a longitudinal direction.

Removing the stylet
The following may occur here:
- *CSF flows freely*

  The injection needle is advanced 1 mm and fixed between the thumb and index finger of the left hand, which is supported on the patient's back. The desired amount of local anesthetic can now be injected (Fig. 36.10).

  With the single-injection technique, aspiration of CSF (0.1 mL) should be attempted immediately before and after injection of local anesthetic. The subarachnoid injection is made at the rate of 1 mL per 5 s.
- *Blood in the CSF*

  Slightly bloody CSF, which clears quickly (spontaneously, or after aspiration) usually occurs after penetration of an epidural vein on the way into the subarachnoid space. The local anesthetic can be injected.

  However, when pure blood flows, it indicates that the injection needle is positioned within a vein. A new attempt at puncture must be made in a different intervertebral space.
- *No CSF flow*

  Rotation of the needle to all four quadrants and careful aspiration. After replacing the trochar, the needle is advanced slightly.

  If no CSF flows in spite of all these measures, the needle should be removed and the procedure repeated with a different needle direction.

  Unexpectedly deep bone contact suggests that the posterior side of the vertebra or an intervertebral disk has been reached. CSF appears in most cases after the needle has been slightly withdrawn and aspiration has been repeated.
- *Paresthesias during puncture* (Fig. 36.11)

  These occur if the spinal needle touches a nerve root or the periosteum on its path. The needle direction needs to be altered.

  When paresthesias are produced at the **subarachnoid** level, the needle must be withdrawn slightly.

  When paresthesias occur **during the injection,** the needle must be repositioned before any further drug is injected.

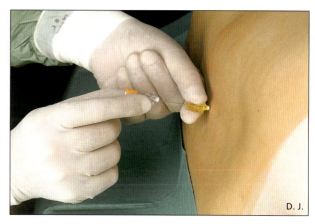

Fig. 36.9 Introducing the spinal needle. Puncture of the subarachnoid space

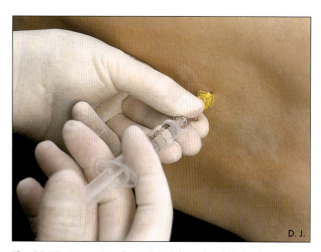

Fig. 36.10a Removing the stylet. Subarachnoid injection

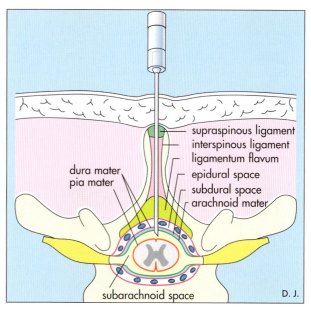

Fig. 36.10b Subarachnoid position of the needle (diagram)

> The local anesthetic must never be injected without evidence of CSF!
> The location and distribution of paresthesias arising during the puncture procedure must be recorded.

Experience shows that failure is usually due to the following causes:
- The needle has deviated from the midline.
- The needle is angled too cranially.

Alternative techniques

Paramedian approach
(Figs. 36.12, 36.14) (lateral, paraspinal)
In this technique, the supraspinous and interspinous ligaments are avoided, so that the ligamentum flavum is the primary target on the way to the subarachnoid space.

Procedure
This technique can be used in all the patient positions mentioned above. Flexion of the spine is not required. The caudal edge of the spinous process is marked. The injection site is located 1–1.5 cm lateral and caudal to this. The puncture is carried out in a craniomedial direction, at an angle of about 10–15°. The dura is reached after about 4–6 cm.
Most mistakes arise when the needle is angled too cranially.

This technique can be used in:
- Degenerative changes in the spine.
- Older patients with marked calcification of the supraspinous and interspinous ligaments.
- Obesity.
- Fractures or other pathological conditions in which pain makes it impossible to flex the spine.

Taylor's approach (Figs. 36.13, 36.14)
This lumbosacral approach is a paramedian injection via the intervertebral space of L5 and S1, the largest interlaminar space in the spinal region.

Procedure
Lateral decubitus position, or sitting. The injection site is located about 1 cm medial and about 1 cm caudal to the posterior superior iliac crest. The injection needle is advanced in a craniomedial direction and at an angle of about 55°. If it touches the periosteum (sacrum), the needle must be withdrawn and its direction must be corrected.

The rare indications for this access route include procedures in the perineal and perianal region.

Positioning of the patient after the injection

The level of the anesthetic spread is controlled by patient positioning measures and checked with cold tests at intervals of 2–5 minutes.

Hyperbaric spinal anesthesia
Lateral decubitus position
The patient remains on the side of surgery for 10–15 minutes if unilateral anesthesia is desired.
The patient is laid supine if bilateral anesthesia is required.

Sitting position
The patient is immediately laid down to allow the anesthetic to spread.
The patient remains sitting if sacral spread is desired.

Isobaric spinal anesthesia
Horizontal positioning is adequate; other positions have no significant influence on the spread of the anesthesia.

Hypobaric technique
Hypobaric spinal anesthesia is not suitable for everyday routine and is rarely used. It is mainly used for operations requiring a prone "jackknife" position, so that the patient does not need to be repositioned (Fig. 36.5).

Fixation phase
The phase immediately after injection of the local anesthetic is particularly critical and requires precise monitoring. The fixation phase lasts about 10–15 minutes.

Properties of local anesthetics in the subarachnoid space

Injecting a local anesthetic into the subarachnoid space blocks sensory and motor function. The main targets of local anesthesia are the posterior roots with the ganglia and anterior roots of the spinal nerves, the autonomic nerve fibers and mixed neural trunks.
The spread of the anesthesia should be checked at short intervals (2–5 min) and confirmed (with a cold spray) shortly before the start of the operation. The first sign of an effect on the spinal nerve roots is a subjective sensation of warmth in the feet. The further development of the block encompasses touch, deep pres-

Spinal anesthesia

sure, motor function, vibration sensitivity and positional sense.

Motor function is completely blocked at the site of the greatest concentration of the local anesthetic. **Sensory** block covers two to four segments and **sympathetic** block extends for a further two to four segments cranially. Subsidence of the block is marked by a return of motor function.

Elimination of local anesthetic that has been injected into the subarachnoid space takes place by subarachnoid vascular resorption (through the vessels of the pia mater and spinal cord), or epidurally [14].

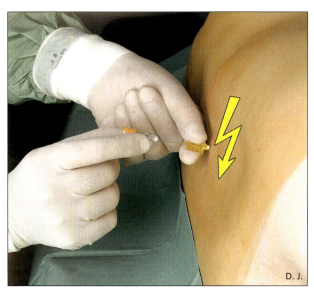

Fig. 36.11 Paresthesias during the injection

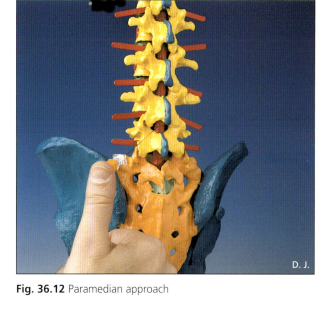

Fig. 36.12 Paramedian approach

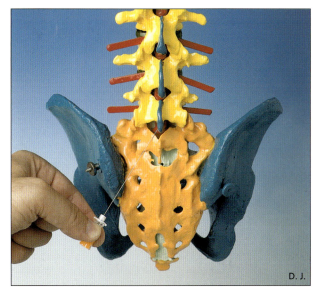

Fig. 36.13 Taylor's approach

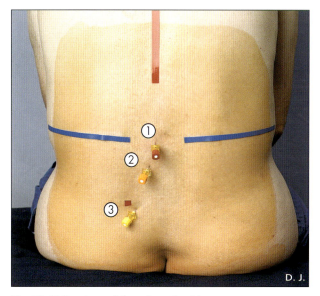

Fig. 36.14 Puncture of the subarachnoid space:
(1) median, (2) paramedian, (3) Taylor

Table 36.1 Dosage of hyperbaric local anesthetics*

Local anesthetic		0,5% bupivacaine 5–8% glucose		5% lidocaine 7.5% glucose		4% mepivacaine 9.5% glucose		1% tetracaine 5% glucose	
		mL	mg	mL	mg	mL	mg	mL	mg
Level of anesthesia									
T6	High	2.5–4.0	12.5–20.0	1.5–2.0	75–100	1.5–2.0	60–80	1.5–2.0	7.5–10.0
T10	Medium	2.0–2.5	10.0–12.5	1.0–1.5	50–75	1.0–1.5	40–60	1.0–1.5	5.0–7.5
L1	Deep	1.5	7.5	1.0–1.2	50–60	1.0–1.2	40–48	1.0–1.2	5.0–6.0
S1–S5	Saddle block	1.0	5.0	0.6–1.0	30–50	0.6–1.0	24–40	0.5–1.0	2.5–5.0
Onset of effect (min)		10–20		5–10		5–10		10–20	
Duration of effect (min)		Up to 160		Up to 60		Up to 60		Up to 150	
Prolongation of effect with vasopressors		No clinically significant effect with bupivacaine, lidocaine, or mepivacaine [24, 25, 91]						Up to ca. 180–240 min	

* Note the dose reduction (20–30 %) in obese patients and pregnant patients.

Local anesthetics

The following local anesthetics are the main ones used as hyperbaric and isobaric solutions:
- 0.5% **bupivacaine** and 0.5% **ropivacaine** as long-acting local anesthetics.
- 2–4% **mepivacaine** or 2% **prilocaine** or 2–5% **lidocaine** as medium-duration local anesthetics.

The local anesthetic of the ester group, 0.5–1% **tetracaine** (pantocaine), is mainly used in the USA.
Local anesthetics administered into the subarachnoid space reach body temperature in about 60 s.

Hyperbaric technique

This is the most frequently used and preferred technique for spinal anesthesia. Mixing a local anesthetic with glucose (5–10%) increases its baricity in comparison with CSF and the level of anesthesia can be determined by patient positioning (Table 36.1).

Isobaric technique

In the isobaric technique, the position of the patient does not have a significant effect on the spread of the anesthesia. With a slow injection, the local anesthetic remains in the vicinity of the injection site and with a fast injection or barbotage, higher levels of anesthesia can be achieved.
The most important parameter for the spread of the anesthesia is the volume of local anesthetic injected (Table 36.2).

Table 36.2 Dosage with isobaric local anesthetic*

Prilocaine	2%	3–4 ml (60–80 mg), duration of effect: 60–120 min
Mepivacaine	2%	3–5 ml (60–100 mg), duration of effect: 30–90 min
Lidocaine	2%	3–5 ml (60–100 mg), duration of effect: 30–90 min
Bupivacaine	0.5%	3–4 ml (15–20 mg), duration of effect: bis 160 min
Ropivacaine	0.5%	3–5 ml (15–25 mg), duration of effect: 120–180 min

* Note the dose reduction (20–30 %) in obese patients and pregnant patients.

Unilateral spinal anesthesia

Definition

Unilateral spinal anesthesia is always intended to block only the anterior and posterior roots on the side being operated on, while the contralateral side – and particularly its sympathetic fibers – remains unblocked. This leads to a reduced incidence of hypotension.

Indications

Surgical and orthopedic procedures on the lower extremities.

Advantages

- Reduction in the extent of the sympathetic block (by about 70%), since small volumes and slower injection of the local anesthetic mean that fewer spinal segments are involved [40, 95].

- Hemodynamic stability (hypotension is only observed in ca. 5% of patients) [20, 61].
- Faster recovery from anesthesia.
- Suitable for outpatient procedures.
- Greater acceptance by patients.

Disadvantages
- Strict unilateral anesthesia is only rarely achieved.
- The procedure requires considerable patience (time factor).

Contraindications
See p. 272.

Procedure

Preparations and materials
See p. 273.

Patient positioning
Lateral decubitus position, lying on the side that is to be operated on.

Injection technique
This is the same as for conventional spinal anesthesia. The opening of the pencil-point needle is rotated to the operating side, and the desired amount of local anesthetic is slowly injected [41].

Patient position after the injection
The patient remains lying on the side that is to be operated on for ca. 20 min.

Dosage
0.5% bupivacaine, hyperbaric	1.2–1.6 mL (6–8 mg)
Injection speed:	2.5 mL/min [77]
	1.2 mL/min [21, 22]

Complications
See Chapter 37.

Factors affecting the spread and duration of spinal anesthesia [66]

Spread
The following factors are very important:
- The dose and volume of local anesthetic solution injected.
- The speed of injection of the anesthetic solution.
- The position of the patient during and immediately after the injection.

Important factors are:
- The patient's age, weight and height.
- The anatomic configuration of the spinal column.
- The volume of cerebrospinal fluid.
- The level of the injection site.
- The speed and barbotage of the injection.
- The direction of the injection needle's beveled tip.
- Intra-abdominal pressure.
- The diameter of the needle.

Less important factors are:
- CSF pressure.
- The concentration of the local anesthetic.

Duration
- Type and dosage of the local anesthetic.
- Anesthetic level achieved.
- Patient's age.
- Vasopressor addition: only with tetracaine; no clinical significance with bupivacaine or lidocaine [24, 25, 91].

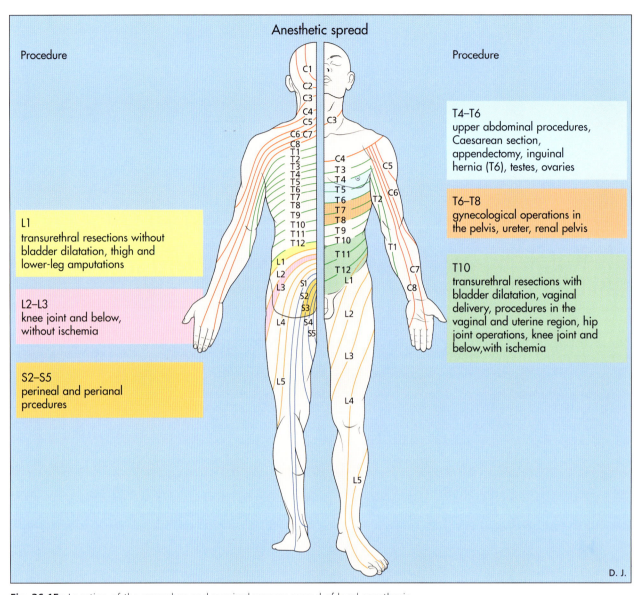

Fig. 36.15a Location of the procedure and required sensory spread of local anesthesia

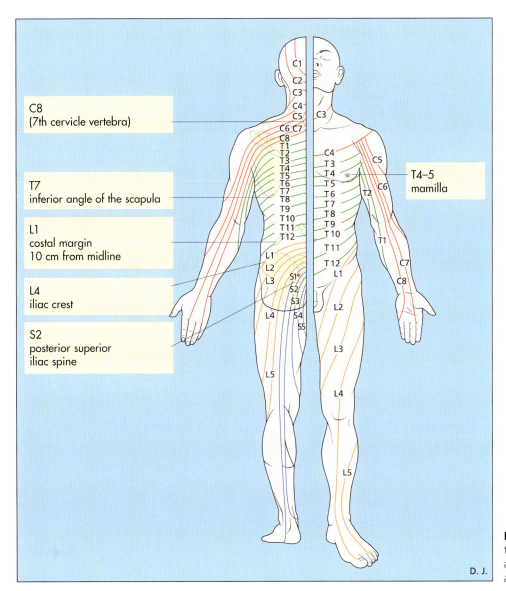

Fig. 36.15b Landmarks for testing the spread of a local anesthetic after neuraxial anesthesia

Chapter 36

Record and checklist

Spinal anesthesia

Name: _____ Date: _____
Diagnosis: _____
Premedication: ☐ No ☐ Yes
Neurological abnormalities: ☐ No ☐ Yes _____

Purpose of block: ☐ Surgical
Needle: ☐ Pencil-Point G _____ ☐ Quincke ☐ Other
i.v. access, infusion: ☐ Yes
Monitoring: ☐ ECG ☐ Pulse oximetry
Ventilation facilities: ☐ Yes (equipment checked)
Emergency equipment (drugs): ☐ Checked
Patient: ☐ Informed (behavior after block)

Position: ☐ Lateral recumbent ☐ Sitting
Access: ☐ Median ☐ Paramedian ☐ Taylor
Injection level: ☐ L3/4 ☐ Other
CSF: ☐ Clear ☐ Slightly bloody ☐ Bloody
Abnormalities: ☐ No ☐ Yes _____
Injection:
Local anesthetic: _____ % _____ mg
☐ Hyperbaric ☐ Isobaric
Addition to LA: _____ % _____ µg/mg

Patient's remarks during injection:
☐ None ☐ Pain ☐ Paresthesias ☐ Warmth
Duration and area: _____
Objective block effect after 15 min:
☐ Cold test ☐ Temperature measurement before ____°C after ____°C
☐ Sensory: L _____ T _____
☐ Motor

Complications:
☐ None ☐ Pain
☐ Radicular symptoms ☐ Vasovagal reactions
☐ BP drop ☐ Total spinal anesthesia
☐ Subdural spread ☐ Respiratory disturbance
☐ Drop in body temperature ☐ Muscle tremor
☐ Bladder emptying disturbances ☐ Back pain
☐ Postdural puncture headache ☐ Neurological complications

Special notes:
_____
_____
_____
_____
_____

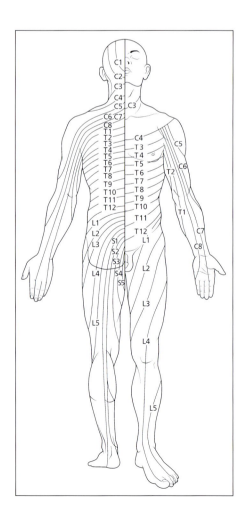

© Copyright ABW Wissenschaftsverlag 2004,
Jankovic, Regional nerve blocks and infiltration therapy, 3rd edition

37 Complications of spinal anesthesia

Complications during the injection

Collapse (vasovagal syncope)

This is a harmless complication, which often occurs in young, nervous and anxious patients during injections in the sitting position. It involves a "neurogenic," normovolemic shock state, which requires no treatment other than lying the patient supine.

Prophylaxis

Injection in lateral decubitus position, mild sedation.

Complications immediately after the injection and during the fixation phase

Hypotension

This is the most frequent complication of spinal anesthesia. It arises due to blockade of sympathetic fibers and is usually accompanied by bradycardia (preganglionic block of the sympathetic nerves to the heart, T1–4) and nausea.

Mechanism

Vasodilation, postarteriolar pooling of blood, reduction in the effective circulating blood volume and venous return to the heart [11, 14].
The higher the spread of the spinal anesthesia or sympathetic block, the greater the reduction in arterial blood pressure.
A drop in blood pressure is also possible after the fixation period of the local anesthetic and it is often exacerbated by acute blood loss, repositioning maneuvers or quick release of a pneumatic tourniquet.

Treatment

The aim is to increase venous return to the heart and to raise cardiac output, using the following physiological and pharmacological measures:
- Volume infusion.
- Oxygen administration.
- Raising the legs.
- Place the patient in a slight Trendelenburg position (10°). This does not produce significant spread of the anesthetic.
- Atropine when there is bradycardia.
- Small intravenous doses of a vasopressor may also be needed (e.g. ephedrine 10–20 mg).

Prophylaxis

- Before spinal anesthesia is administered, any deficits in intravascular volume should be corrected and an additional volume of at least 500 mL of a balanced electrolyte solution should be infused.
- Accurate assessment of the patient's degree of cardiovascular risk.
- In pregnant patients, as well as older or obese patients: reduced dose of the local anesthetic, opioid, or combination.

Prophylactic administration of a vasopressor is not recommended.

High and total spinal anesthesia

Causes

- Overdosage of the local anesthetic.
- Positioning error.
- Inadvertent spinal anesthesia when attempting epidural anesthesia (most frequent cause!)

The clinical picture has a dramatic course, characterized by restlessness, breathing difficulties, a severe drop in blood pressure and loss of consciousness. It is life-threatening and requires immediate treatment.

Therapy

- Immediate tracheal intubation (thiopental 1–2 mg/kg b.w. routinely ca. 150 mg i.v.); succinylcholine if appropriate, since the muscles of mastication are not affected [66].
- Ventilation with 100% oxygen.
- Raising the legs.
- Rapid volume administration.
- Atropine.
- Vasopressor.
- Dopamine infusion.
- Careful cardiovascular monitoring.

Subdural spread of the local anesthetic

Subdural injection can never be excluded with certainty. It may occur slightly more frequently after spinal anesthesia or myelography than after epidural anesthesia.

The subdural space is at its widest in the cervical region, particularly dorsolaterally. It does not end at the great foramen as does the epidural space, but continues cranially.

Warning signs

An unusually high sensory block, which develops very slowly (even after 20 minutes) and a much less marked motor block.

The clinical picture resembles that of total spinal anesthesia and is characterized by moderate hypotonia, breathing difficulties with retained consciousness and often involvement of the cranial and cervical nerves:

Trigeminal nerve: trigeminal nerve palsy, with accompanying paresthesias in the area supplied by the nerve and transient weakness of the muscles of mastication with simultaneous Horner's syndrome, has been observed after high epidural anesthesia or subdural spread [31, 45, 89, 92].

Horner's syndrome: Horner's syndrome is produced after neuraxial anesthesia with a high spread of the injected local anesthetic and block of very sensitive sympathetic nerve fibers in the areas of segments T4–C8 [54, 83]. Most often, Horner's syndrome is seen after high spinal or epidural anesthesia in obstetrics and when there is subdural spread of the local anesthetic [28, 34].

Relatively rapid resolution of the symptoms is characteristic.

Differential diagnosis

Total spinal anesthesia: dramatic course, blood pressure unrecordable, respiratory arrest, longer time required for symptoms to resolve.

Prophylaxis

- Individual dosage and dose reduction in older patients, pregnant patients, obese patients and those with diabetes mellitus or arteriosclerosis.
- Incremental injection in epidural anesthesia.

Respiratory disturbances

These only arise after spread of the local anesthetic above segment T8. They result from block of the intercostal nerves and accompanying paralysis of the intercostal muscles. Resting ventilation is largely unaffected, thanks to a compensatory increase in diaphragmatic movement.

Therapy

- Mild sedation.
- Oxygen administration.
- Reassure the patient.

Gastrointestinal tract disturbances

Due to blocking of sympathetic inhibition, disturbances of bowel tone and motility may occur, becoming manifest as nausea or, more rarely, as vomiting. These disturbances are very often associated with a drop in blood pressure and bradycardia.

Reduced body temperature

Particularly in cool surroundings and when there is intraoperative blood loss, sympathetic block and the associated vasodilatation can lead to a drop in body temperature.

Complications in the early postoperative phase

Urinary retention

This affects 14–56% of patients, mainly older ones, and results from autonomic dysfunction caused by block of the parasympathetic segments from S2 to S4, which recovers last after spinal anesthesia.

Clinical symptoms

Patients complain of severe lower abdominal and back pain; this is often accompanied by an increase in blood pressure.

Therapy

If physical measures, early mobilization or administration of carbachol (Miostat, Carbastat; i.m.) are not successful, urinary catheterization can lead to a rapid improvement in the symptoms.

Late complications

Late complications are usually caused by the technique of spinal anesthesia. They manifest as:
- Postdural puncture headache.
- Back pain.
- Neurological complications.

Postdural puncture headache (PDPH)

This is a very unpleasant complication after spinal anesthesia, diagnostic lumbar puncture, myelography or diagnostic or therapeutic sympathetic block [63]. It usually develops after 24–48 hours or even later.

Frequency

0.2–24% [14] up to 76.5% [31, 35, 101] after puncture with large-diameter needles.

Mechanism

PDPH is thought to represent a multistep phenomenon initiated by dural puncture and resultant CSF leakage. Two proposed mechanisms for PDPH pain have been discussed in the literature. The first theory proposes that a decrease in CSF pressure produces traction on structures within the cranium, resulting in the generation of pain. The second hypothesis suggests that decreased CSF pressure leads to intrathecal hypotension and painful vasodilatation of the intracranial blood vessels (known as the "intracranial vascular response" [17, 101]). Mainly when the patient is in a standing position, painful areas dilate (meninges, tentorium, vessels) and there is further pain transmission via the cerebral nerves and upper cervical nerves.

Etiology

Postdural puncture headache occurs most frequently in younger patients and women, particularly during pregnancy. Repeated dural perforation, puncture with large-diameter needles, and in particular accidental spinal anesthesia when attempting to carry out epidural anesthesia, are liable to lead to postdural puncture headache.

Location

Usually occipitofrontal (occipital: 25%, frontal: 22% or occipitofrontal: 25%) [13, 101].

Clinical symptoms

Position-dependent headache, which is more severe when sitting and standing, coughing or straining, with marked relief when lying down.

Associated symptoms

Pain in the nape of the neck, stiffness in the neck, nausea, vomiting, sensitivity to light, smells and noise, auditory disturbances, tinnitus, loss of appetite, depressive mood.

CSF hypotension syndrome and involvement of the cranial and cervical nerves

All of the cranial nerves, with the exception of the olfactory nerve, glossopharyngeal nerve and vagus nerve, can be affected by low CSF pressure. The abducent nerve and vestibulocochlear nerve are most frequently affected (Fig. 37.1).
- Abducent nerve:
  The long intracranial course of this nerve leads to traction and consequent irritation of the nerve when there are changes in intracranial pressure. The patient complains of double vision, with parallel horizontal images and difficulties in focusing on objects [7, 34, 97].
- Vestibulocochlear nerve
  When precise audiometric examinations are carried out, unilateral or bilateral hypacusis can be observed in 0.4–40% of patients with CSF hypotension syndrome [34]. The prognosis is good.

Differential diagnosis

- Migraine.
- Tension headache.
- Cervical myofascial pain, particularly in the sternocleidomastoid muscle, with what is known as "pseudospinal headache" [39].
- CNS infections (bacterial meningitis).
- Sinus thrombosis (in the second half of pregnancy or in the puerperium, frequently in preeclampsia).
- Pneumocephalus (after accidental dural perforation in attempted epidural anesthesia when using the loss-of-resistance technique with air [51]).

Therapy

When there is a diagnosis of postdural puncture headache, various treatment approaches are possible.

Noninvasive conservative therapy

This is used initially and includes traditional symptomatic measures such as:
- Bed rest (compulsory).
- Analgesics.
- Sedatives.
- Antiemetics.

The majority of patients experience marked improvement in the symptoms or complete recovery after 5–7 days with this form of treatment [101]. In ca. 80% of patients, the symptoms improve spontaneously within 2 weeks without any treatment ("tincture of time" [23]).

> Treatment measures recommended in the past, such as massive fluid intake or obligatory 24-hour bed rest after the injection, are unnecessary.

Caffeine sodium benzoate is often used as part of noninvasive conservative treatment, with considerable success (> 85%) [13, 17, 43, 52, 88, 89]. The substance leads to cerebral vasoconstriction and a reduction in cerebral blood flow [87].
Caffeine sodium benzoate can be administered orally or intramuscularly [17, 51]. The following infusion is used most frequently: 2 liters of liquid are administered over 2 hours, with the first liter containing 500 mg caffeine sodium benzoate. When there is residual pain, the treatment can be repeated after 4 hours [58].

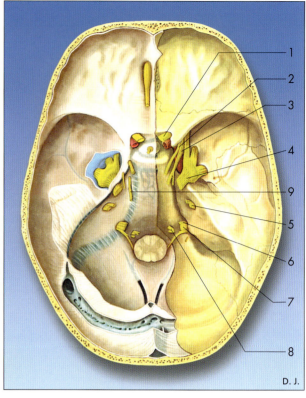

Fig. 37.1 Cranial nerves.
(1) Optic nerve, (2) oculomotor nerve, (3) trochlear nerve, (4) trigeminal nerve, (5) vestibulocochlear nerve, (6) glossopharyngeal nerve, (7) vagus nerve, (8) hypoglossal nerve, (9) abducent nerve

Mild CNS stimulation and dizziness have been observed as side effects.
Hypertonus, a history of epilepsy, and pre-eclampsia are contraindications.
This form of treatment is particularly indicated in immune-suppressed patients, when there is a risk of infection, when there are difficulties in performing epidural puncture ("blood patch") and in postdural puncture headache after thoracic or cervical injections. Other alternatives that have been reported in the area of noninvasive conservative treatment of postdural puncture headache include administering adrenocorticotropic hormone (ACTH) [6] or sumatriptan (a serotonin type Id receptor agonist) [18].

> None of the conservative treatment approaches removes the cause of postdural puncture headache; they merely bridge the period until the dural leak closes naturally.

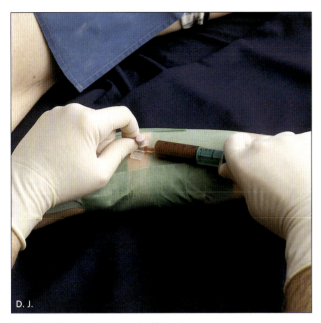

Fig. 37.2 Sterile withdrawal of blood

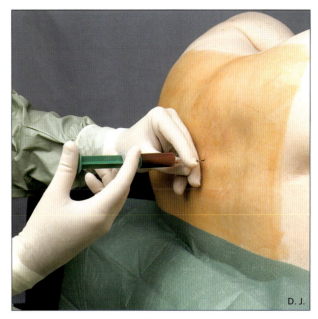

Fig. 37.3 Epidural injection of homologous blood

Invasive therapy

The method of choice in treatment-resistant postdural puncture headache is administration of a "blood patch" at the dural perforation site.

Prerequisites
- Correct diagnosis.
- Exclusion of all contraindications.
- Informing the patient.
- Experienced anesthetist.

> This procedure should never be carried out without a correct diagnosis!

Procedure

10–20 mL of blood, taken from the patient in sterile conditions (Fig. 37.2), is reinjected epidurally. The injection is carried out at the same level as the original spinal anesthesia procedure or one segment caudally (Fig. 37.3).

The injection is carried out slowly (1 mL in 3–4 s). After the injection, the patient lies supine for ca. 30–60 min. This procedure can be repeated after 24 hours. The patient is recommended to maintain bedrest for ca. 24 hours.

Using magnetic resonance imaging, Beards et al. [10] traced the spread of the extradurally injected homologous blood. The maximum compression effect on the dura was seen after an interval of 30 min–3 hours, encompassing four to five neighboring segments. After about 7 hours, this effect subsided.

Other authors [19] have observed a spread over six segments above and three segments below the puncture site after extradural injection of radioactively marked blood.

Extradurally injected blood also spreads in the subarachnoid space [90] and particularly in the subcutaneous fatty tissue in the region of the lumbar spine. It has been suggested that this is a possible cause of postinjection back pain.

Complications

Back pain (35.9%), pain in the nape of the neck (0.9%), increased temperature (5%) and dizziness are temporary phenomena and do not require treatment [14]. The treatment has a 95% success rate.

> Epidural injection of homologous blood is not normally painful. If injection pain occurs, the procedure should be stopped.

Potential complications
- Inadvertent subarachnoid injection.
- Hematoma formation, with compression of the spinal cord.
- Risk of infection.
- Persistent back pain.
- Radicular pain.
- Facial palsy [76].
- Nerve injury [13, 58].
- Cramps [93].

Alternative methods
- Epidural dextran patch [98, 101].
  Initially, a test dose of 20 mL Promit (dextran 1) is injected intravenously, to avoid potential allergic reactions.
  Then, at the level of the dural perforation site, a slow epidural injection of 20–25 mL dextran 40 is carried out. The viscosity and high molecular weight of dextran 40 lead to very slow resorption from the epidural space, so that a longer period of compression of the dural defect is achieved.
- Epidural patch with fibrin glue [32, 46, 48].
- Infusion of isotonic saline via an epidural catheter: 150–200 mL/day [8, 31, 53]. This method represents a temporary solution for the problem.
- Intrathecal injection of 10 mL saline 0.9% immediately after dural puncture, using an epidural needle.

Prophylaxis against postdural puncture headache

- Use thin pencil-point spinal needles: 25–29 G – e.g. Pencan, Sprotte, Whitacre.
- If needles with a Quincke tip are being used, the bevel should be positioned so as to be parallel to the mainly longitudinal dural fibers.
- Atraumatic technique: avoid multiple perforations of the dura.
- Experienced anesthetist.

> When these prerequisites are observed, spinal anesthesia can also be carried out in patients with a history of headache and in young patients.

Back pain

This complication is a frequent occurrence after spinal anesthesia (2–25%), but it is no more frequent than after general anesthesia. Diseases of the spine make this complication more likely.

Mechanism

- Tissue trauma after multiple attempts at puncture.
- Position-dependent pressure during surgery on bones, joints and ligaments in the lumbar region.

Treatment

Symptomatic.

Transient neurologic symptoms (TNS)
[3, 42, 79, 86, 99]

Definition

Transient occurrence of neurological symptoms, usually caused by spinal anesthesia (rarely after epidural techniques). Neurological findings are lacking (absence of motor, sensory, or sphincter disturbances). The symptoms develop within 24 hours, after complete disappearance of neuraxial anesthesia and 2–4 hours after the patient has been mobilized. In most cases, the symptoms resolve completely after a few hours or days, and at the latest after a week.

Clinical symptoms

Severe back pain, pain and dysesthesia in the area of the buttocks, radiating to the legs. These are bilateral symptoms. Muscle spasms are often present.

Etiology

The etiology of TNS is not known. Possible causes of this strange phenomenon that have been proposed include the following:

- Specific local anesthetic toxicity – primarily with hyperbaric lidocaine and mepivacaine (the frequency of the condition after spinal anesthesia has been administered with hyperbaric lidocaine is reported to be 0–40% in the literature).
- Extremely slow injection using narrow-lumen pencil-point spinal needles, creating "sacral pooling" of the local anesthetic.
- Intrathecal pethidine administration.
- Intraoperative patient positioning. In this case, the symptoms – particularly after procedures conducted with the patient in what is known as the "lithotomy" position (dorsosacral position; 30–36%) and after knee arthroscopy (18–22%) are seen much more frequently than in procedures conducted using a supine position during surgery (4–8%). Mechanical stretching of the spinal nerve roots probably promotes the development of TNS.
- Early mobilization after outpatient procedures.
- Injection trauma and obesity may also play a role.

It is regarded as proven that the following factors do not promote the development of TNS: sex, age, ethnic group, ASA physical status, weight, a history of back pain, type of injection needle used, position during the injection, and the addition of opioids such as fentanyl and sufentanil, or glucose.

What to do for suspected TNS

Neurological complications should be excluded on an urgent basis (epidural/spinal abscess, anterior spinal artery syndrome, cauda equina syndrome (CES). It is necessary to maintain constant verbal contact with the patient, particularly after outpatient procedures.

Treatment

The most effective form of treatment is symptomatic – particularly the administration of nonsteroidal anti-inflammatory drugs, muscle-relaxing agents and injections at the affected trigger points.

Prophylaxis

The only way of providing absolute protection against the development of TNS is to avoid administering neuraxial anesthesia. Caution is advisable when selecting the local anesthetic. Local anesthetics such as bupivacaine or prilocaine should be used at the lowest possible dosages and concentrations (e.g. 7.5–10 mg bupivacaine, possibly with the addition of fentanyl or sufentanil). Vasopressors should not be added. Particular caution is needed in outpatients undergoing operations in the lithotomy position or knee arthroscopy.

Neurological complications

See also Chapter 41, p. 325.
Neurological complications occur extremely rarely after spinal anesthesia.

> If there is the slightest suspicion, an immediate neurological consultation should be requested!

Etiology [62]

- Traumatic nerve lesions due to direct trauma by the needle or catheter, or due to intraneural injection of the local anesthetic.
- Toxic effects of the injected local anesthetic (see the section on cauda equina syndrome, below).
- Hemorrhage into the spinal canal, particularly in patients with coagulation disorders (subarachnoid or subdural hemorrhage, epidural hematoma).
- Vascular causes (thrombosis and spasm in the anterior spinal artery).
- Infection in the form of bacterial meningitis, which may be caused by inadequate asepsis or bacterial transmission via blood or lymph.
- Chemical irritation by substances used for skin prep at the puncture site.
- Introduction of foreign bodies.
- Exacerbation of latent neurological diseases (e.g. multiple sclerosis, tabes, tumor, viral infections).
- Injury due to poor surgical positioning.
- Psychogenic causes – e.g. as the initiating factor in paraplegic symptoms [27, 49].

Neurological complications can become manifest as arachnoiditis, myelitis, spinal or epidural abscess, cauda equina syndrome, or anterior spinal artery syndrome.

Cauda equina syndrome (CES)

Cauda equina syndrome is an extremely rare complication [33], which can occur after both intrathecal and epidural injections (single-shot or continuous techniques).

Clinical symptoms
Peripheral paralysis, often asymmetric, of both legs, "saddle-like" sensory disturbances of all types in the lumbar and sacral segments, pain, absence of spontaneous bladder or rectal emptying, impotence.

Diagnosis
MRI, CT and/or myelography [57, 78].

Nerves of the cauda equina
The nerves of the cauda equina, located in a poorly vascularized distal area of the dural sac, possess only a weak protective layer [57, 59, 60].

Consequently, they react particularly sensitively to:
- The effects of local anesthetics [60, 74], depending on the type, dose, baricity and duration of exposure, particularly when an epidural dose is inadvertently administered intrathecally.
  Harmful effects of various local anesthetics (chloroprocaine [80] and hexylcaine [98]) have been reported in the past. Since the 1990s, there have also been reports that hyperbaric lidocaine can damage the nerves of the cauda equina [85], particularly after intrathecal administration via microcatheters [60, 84, 85].
  Bupivacaine has proved to be safe, although there have also been individual reports of CES after intrathecal administration of hyperbaric solutions or after continuous epidural administration [60].
- Direct trauma caused by the needle or by a catheter, particularly microcatheters (see Chapter 38, p. 293).
- Chemical irritation due to bacterial contamination.

Risks
Repetition of spinal anesthesia with a hyperbaric solution when the original block is incomplete represents a potential risk (see Chapter 36, section on relative contraindications, p. 273). In patients with spinal canal stenosis, caution should be exercised due to potential accumulation or incorrect spread of the local anesthetic [36, 37, 60, 84].

Most important prophylactic measures [56]
- Always choose the lowest possible concentration of the local anesthetic and inject it on an incremental basis.
- Caution should be exercised when using hyperbaric solutions (5% lidocaine in particular should be avoided).
- Advance the spinal catheter a maximum of 2–3 cm beyond the needle tip (see Chapter 38, p. 293).

Anterior spinal artery syndrome

This syndrome can be caused by direct trauma to the vessel or by ischemia in the anterior two-thirds of the distal spinal cord [62].
Injury to the artery produces a clearly definable clinical syndrome: motor disturbances and loss of pain and temperature sensitivity below the level of the lesion, with preserved positional sense and vibration sensitivity [74].

38 Continuous spinal anesthesia (CSA)

Continuous spinal anesthesia requires placement of a catheter in the subarachnoid space. Continuous administration of a local anesthetic or opioid, or a combination of the two, is carried out via the catheter to produce adequate intraoperative and postoperative analgesia.

History of continuous spinal anesthesia
1907 H.P. Dean reported the first use of CSA via an intrathecal spinal needle during surgery.
1944 E. Tuohy: a urethral catheter was introduced through a 15-G needle (PDPH > 30%).
1964 D. Bizzari, J.G. Giuffrida: 27-G catheter through a 21-G needle.
1983 D.D. Peterson used standard epidural instruments (18-G Hustead needle with 20-G plastic catheter).
1989 Introduction of the microcatheter technique (by Boom in the USA), 28-G spinal microcatheter through a 22-G needle.
1992 Reports on cauda equina syndrome (14 per 50 000). The Food and Drug Administration (FDA) banned the use of the spinal microcatheter in the USA. Suspected causes:
 – Overdosage with hyperbaric 5% lidocaine or 1% tetracaine.
 – Extremely slow injection through the small diameter catheter, leading to "sacral pooling" of the local anesthetic.
 – Caudal migration of the spinal microcatheter.
1993 In Germany, the BGA confirmed the above causes, but the continued use of spinal microcatheters for CSA was allowed.
1994 Development of a new "over-the-needle" CSA macrocatheter system (analogous to indwelling venous cannulas): lower risk of PDPH.

CSA is characterized [9, 56, 66] by:
- Rapid onset.
- Lowest possible dose of the local anesthetic or opioid by careful titration.
- Low incidence of cardiovascular and respiratory complications.
- Allows anesthesia to be prolonged as long as required.
- Shorter recovery times.
- Postoperative pain therapy.

Advantages over "single-shot" spinal anesthesia
- Injection of a local anesthetic only after placing the patient in the surgical position, with a consequent reduction in cardiopulmonary risk.
- Better checking and control of the spread of anesthesia due to careful titration.
- Prolongation of anesthesia for as long as required.
- Precise control and short recovery time, due to injection of medium-duration local anesthetics.
- At the end of the operation, the transition to opioid administration for postoperative pain therapy is made easier.

Advantages over continuous epidural anesthesia
- Easier identification of the subarachnoid space, and thus higher success rates, particularly when there are anatomical difficulties.
- Easy preoperative confirmation of subarachnoid positioning of the catheter.
- Only about 10% of the usual epidural dose is needed, so that the risk of toxicity is very low.
- Faster onset.
- Reliable block.
- Shorter recovery time.
- Lower risk of catheter migration.

Advantages over combined spinal and epidural anesthesia (CSE)
- Easy preoperative confirmation of subarachnoid positioning of the catheter.
- Reliable implementation of the anesthesia and postoperative pain therapy using only a single technique ("all-in-one system").
- Continuity and better control with rapidly-acting subarachnoid top-ups.
- Test dose to check the catheter position is unnecessary.

Indications
- Long surgical procedures with subsequent postoperative pain therapy.
- Older patients and high-risk patients.
- Anatomical difficulties.
- Use in vascular surgery, orthopedics, urology, gynecology and obstetrics, and in postoperative pain therapy.

Contraindications
These are the same as the general contraindications for neuraxial anesthesia (see Chapter 36).

Procedure

Full prior information for the patient is mandatory.

> Continuous spinal anesthesia (CSA) should only be carried out by experienced anesthetists.

Preparations and materials
- Check that the emergency equipment is complete and in working order (intubation kit, emergency drugs).
- Strict asepsis.
- Intravenous access, anesthesia machine.
- Ensure adequate intravenous volume loading with a balanced electrolyte solution (250–500 mL).
- Careful monitoring: ECG monitoring, BP, pulse oximetry.

The use of a specific CSA set is recommended (Fig. 38.1).

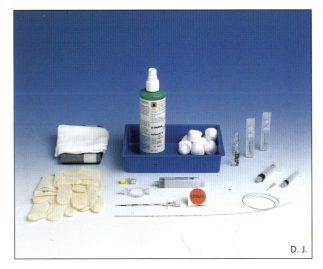

Fig. 38.1 Materials

Classic technique – through-the-needle system
Standard 18-G epidural Tuohy needle, with a 20-G epidural catheter (e.g Perifix®, B. Braun Melsungen) or a standard spinal needle (25–26 G), with a 32-G microcatheter or 22-G pencil-point spinal needle with a 28-G microcatheter.

Over-the-needle system (spinal needle lying in the catheter)
22-G or 24-G Spinocath, epidural guiding needle with a 30° beveled tip, smoothly moving; catheter connector, flat epidural filter (0.2 mm, antibacterial), B. Braun Melsungen.

Patient positioning
The lateral decubitus position is preferred, but the paramedian approach, which offers the best angle for catheter placement, is also often used.

Injection technique
Classic technique – through-the-needle system
- The needle bevel (Quincke, Tuohy or pencil-point) is first directed cranially. Shortly before the ligamentum flavum is reached, the needle is rotated 90° or directed laterally (Quincke, Tuohy), in order to puncture the dura after penetrating the ligamentum flavum. When the subarachnoid space has been reached, the bevel is rotated so as to face cranially.
- After removal of the stylet and free flow of CSF, the injection needle is advanced by 1–2 mm.
  The catheter is then carefully advanced into the subarachnoid space up to a maximum of 2–3 cm beyond the needle tip, to avoid neural irritation or vascular puncture.
- Once the catheter has been placed in the desired position, the needle is slowly withdrawn over the catheter.
- The catheter connector and bacterial filter are then attached, with the catheter being fixed in the same way as an epidural catheter.
- Careful aspiration of CSF (in microcatheters, aspiration can be very difficult or even impossible).

> If there are technical difficulties, the catheter and injection needle are always removed together. A catheter must never be withdrawn through the needle.

The patient is then placed in the position required for the operation, and the drugs for subarachnoid administration are prepared (diluted with 0.9% saline when appropriate).

Continuous spinal anesthesia (CSA)

Over-the-needle system
- Epidural puncture is carried out using the loss-of-resistance technique, with a needle that has a 30° bevel. This serves as the guiding needle for the Spinocath catheter system. The stylet is withdrawn (Fig. 38.2).
- The catheter and internal spinal needle are grasped with the thumb, index finger, and middle finger at the end of the needle, ensuring secure fixation of the spinal needle in the catheter for the dural puncture (Fig. 38.3).
- Dural puncture with the spinal needle and catheter tip (advance about 5 mm). The dural click and dilation of the hole in the dura by the catheter tip are usually easily felt.
- CSF appears at the end of the spinal needle (lateral eye of the spinal needle) within about 3–6 s (22 G) or 6–10 s (24 G).
- The catheter is grasped with one hand about 3 cm behind the guiding needle, and the pull-out wire is grasped at its end and stretched with the other hand (Fig. 38.4).
- Advance the catheter over the spinal needle 2–3 cm at most into the spinal space (technique analogous to indwelling venous catheters).
- Withdraw the spinal needle from the catheter completely with the withdrawal wire (Fig. 38.5).
- Remove the epidural guiding needle, fixing the spinal catheter in the usual way.
- The connector and flat filter are then attached.

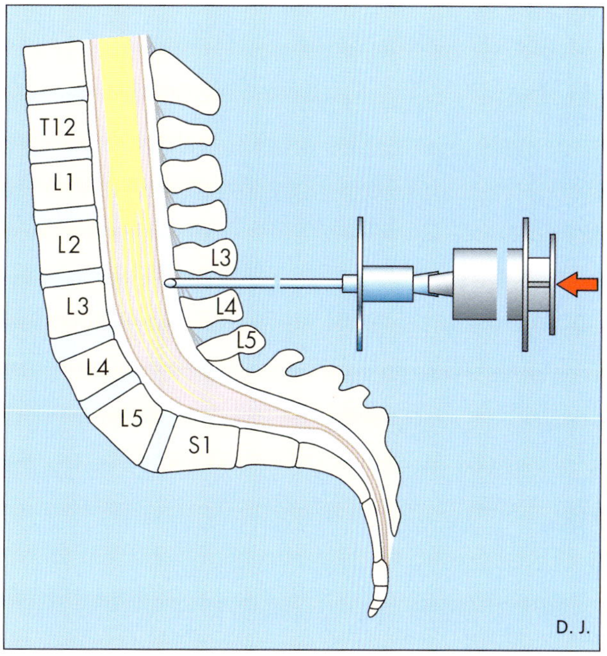

Advantages
Easy puncture, secure positioning, little trauma, gentle dilation with the cone-shaped catheter tip, immediate sealing, no initial CSF loss and thus a reduced risk of postdural puncture headache.

Problem situation with the two techniques
Intrathecal positioning of the catheter – cranial or caudal?

Dosage

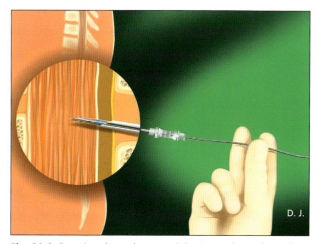

Fig. 38.2 Guiding needle. Epidural puncture using the loss-of-resistance technique

Fig. 38.3 Grasping the catheter and the internal spinal needle

> The lowest possible dose and concentration of local anesthetic or opioid must be selected. Always carry out injections in small, incremental doses (careful titration).

Surgical
Local anesthetic
0.5% bupivacaine (isobaric): 1–1.5 mL = 5–7.5 mg (± 0.2 mL) after careful titration.

0.5% bupivacaine (hyperbaric) for unilaterally accentuated anesthesia [71].

Combination
0.5% bupivacaine 2.5–5 mg and sufentanil 7.5–10 µg.
0.5% bupivacaine 2.5–5 mg and fentanyl 25 µg.

> Repeat doses should be 30–50% of the initial dose.

Chapter 38

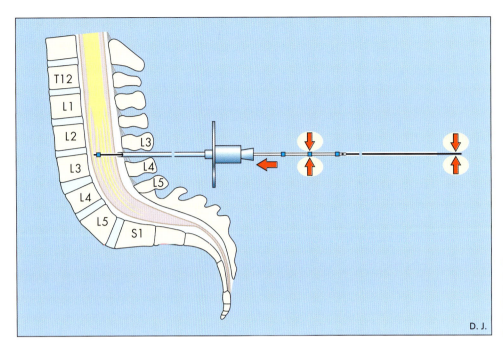

Fig. 38.4 Advance the catheter about 2–3 cm over the spinal needle (keeping the catheter stretched with the other hand on the pull-out wire as this is done)

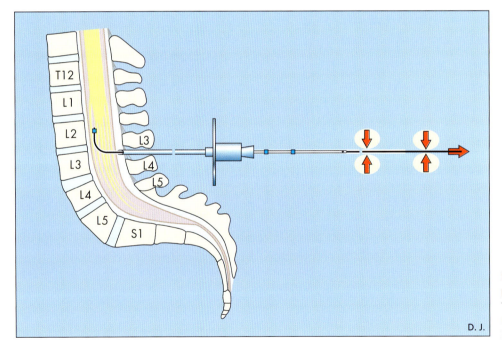

Fig. 38.5 Fix the catheter in position with one hand. Using the other hand, the spinal needle is withdrawn on the pull-out wire

Postoperative pain therapy [70]
Intermittent intrathecal administration:
0.25% bupivacaine (isobaric) – 1 mL every 4 h.
When there is inadequate analgesia, an additional injection of 0.5 mL 0.25% bupivacaine is given every 30 minutes (maximum dose 2.5 mL/4 h).

Continuous intrathecal infusion:
0.25% bupivacaine (isobaric) – 10 mL/24 h.
When there is inadequate analgesia, an additional injection of 1 mL 0.25% bupivacaine is administered initially; a maximum of 1 mL 0.5% bupivacaine can be given subsequently.

Disadvantages and complications
(see also Chapter 37)

Postdural puncture headache (PDPH)
The aim is to reduce the incidence of postdural puncture headache through the use of microcatheters (e.g a 32-G microcatheter through a 26-G injection needle or a 28-G catheter through a 22-G pencil-point injection needle) or the Spinocath catheter system. It is assumed that an inflammatory reaction occurs in the area of the puncture site, which allows sealing of the dural perforation site and thus reduces or prevents CSF loss [56]. The initial CSF loss after catheter placement is in theory avoided when the Spinocath system is used.

Cauda equina syndrome (CES)
The etiology of the cauda equina syndrome is probably multifactorial. The microcatheter technique and subarachnoid injection of hyperbaric lidocaine or tetracaine have been linked to the development of CES [37, 85].

The causes are thought to be high doses and sacral pooling of the injected local anesthetic, due to the high injection resistance in the microcatheter. It is still unclear whether the neurological damage is caused by direct toxic effects of the local anesthetic or by indirect ischemic effects in the cauda equina area, which has a poor blood supply [56, 59].
It should also be emphasized that the subarachnoid space is very sensitive to any accidental injection of unintended medications – in contrast to the epidural space, which is very robust and more "forgiving" [12].

Shearing of the catheter
This rare complication can occur during catheter placement and catheter removal (particularly with the microcatheter technique).

Prophylaxis
- When technical difficulties arise, never withdraw a spinal catheter through the needle.
- A catheter should always be removed with extreme care. The patient is placed in the lateral position, with the back flexed in order to stretch the ligamentum flavum [4].
- Never use force to pull the catheter, particularly against elastic resistance.
- If difficulties arise, wait until the patient is able to stand.
- Subsequent inspection of the catheter after removal to check that it is complete, and keeping a record of the removal, are obligatory.

Opioid side effects
See Chapter 50, additions to local anesthetics, section on opioids, p. 393.

Record and checklist

Continuous spinal anesthesia

Name: _____ Date: _____
Diagnosis: _____
Premedication: ☐ No   ☐ Yes _____
Neurological abnormalities: ☐ No   ☐ Yes _____

Purpose of block: ☐ Surgical   ☐ Therapeutic (postoperative)
Needle: ☐ G _____ Tip: _____ ☐ Spinal catheter G _____ (micro, macro) _____
i.v. access, infusion: ☐ Yes
Monitoring: ☐ ECG   ☐ Pulse oximetry
Ventilation facilities: ☐ Yes (equipment checked)
Emergency equipment (drugs):   ☐ Checked
Patient: ☐ Informed

Position: ☐ Lateral recumbent   ☐ Sitting
Access: ☐ Median   ☐ Paramedian
Injection level: ☐ L3/4   ☐ Other _____
Technique: ☐ Through-the-needle   ☐ Over-the-needle
Subarachnoid space: ☐ Identified
Catheter: ☐ Advanced 2–3 cm
Aspiration test: ☐ No   ☐ Yes
Bacterial filter: ☐ No   ☐ Yes
Abnormalities: ☐ No   ☐ Yes _____
Injection :
Local anesthetic (isobaric, hyperbaric): _____ mg _____ %
  (incremental)
☐ Opioid _____ (µg)   ☐ Other _____ µg/mg/mL
☐ Subsequent injection of _____ mL _____ %

Patient's remarks during injection:
☐ None   ☐ Pain   ☐ Paresthesias   ☐ Warmth
Duration and area: _____
Objective block effect after 15 min:
☐ Cold test   ☐ Temperature measurement before ____°C after ____°C
☐ Sensory: L _____ T _____
☐ Motor

Complications:
☐ None   ☐ Pain
☐ Radicular symptoms   ☐ Vasovagal reactions
☐ BP drop   ☐ Total spinal anesthesia
☐ Subdural spread   ☐ Respiratory disturbance
☐ Drop in body temperature   ☐ Muscle tremor
☐ Bladder emptying disturbances ☐ Back pain
☐ Postdural puncture headache   ☐ Neurological complications

Special notes:
_____
_____

© Copyright ABW Wissenschaftsverlag 2004,
Jankovic, Regional nerve blocks and infiltration therapy, 3rd edition

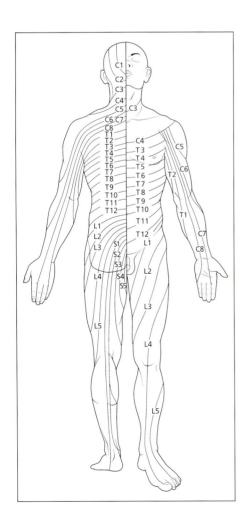

39 Continuous spinal anesthesia (CSA) in obstetrics

The first reports on the use of CSA in obstetrics were published in 1951. However, due to the high incidence of postdural puncture headache, use of the procedure was very limited until the 1980s. The development of improved equipment, as well as the introduction of opioids for subarachnoid and epidural applications (particularly lipid-soluble sufentanil, fentanyl and pethidine), encouraged the wider use of this method.
However, further experience is still needed before this valuable method can be used routinely in obstetric anesthesia [4].

Patient selection
Candidates for continuous epidural anesthesia in obstetrics are also suitable for continuous spinal anesthesia.

Advantages
- Easy identification of the subarachnoid space.
- Higher success rate.
- Lowest possible dosage of local anesthetic, opioids or a combination of the two and thus low incidence of cardiotoxic effects.
- Faster onset of anesthesia and analgesia.
- Bilateral spread.
- Particularly suitable in high-risk patients [1, 15, 55].

Procedure
Full prior information for the patient is mandatory.

Preparation and materials
- Check that the emergency equipment is complete and in working order (intubation kit, emergency drugs). Intravenous access, anesthetic machine.
- Strict asepsis.
- Ensure adequate intravenous volume loading with a balanced electrolyte solution (250–500 mL).
- Careful monitoring: ECG, BP, pulse oximetry.
- Antacid administration (see Chapter 43, p. 334).
- Prepare the drugs, diluting them with 0.9% saline when appropriate.

Patient positioning and injection
Puncture is carried out with the patient in the left lateral decubitus position, followed by placement of the spinal catheter, fixing of the catheter in position and placement of a bacterial filter.
Injection of a local anesthetic or opioid is always carried out on an incremental basis and at the lowest possible dosage, with careful monitoring (ECG, pulse oximetry; blood pressure monitoring: every 3 minutes during the first 30 minutes).

> In obstetrics, it is recommended that the spinal catheter should not be left in place for more than 24 hours (risk of an increased PDPH rate).

Dosages (Table 39.1) [4, 73]
In addition to local anesthetics (bupivacaine), opioids can also be administered intrathecally – particularly the lipid-soluble drugs sufentanil, fentanyl and pethidine.

> Injection of the local anesthetic should only be carried out once the patient is in an optimal position and with careful titration.

Local anesthetics for vaginal delivery
Initial dose: 1 mL 0.25% bupivacaine.
If this dose is inadequate, it can be supplemented with 0.5% bupivacaine, titrated with small boluses of 0.25 mL each [4].

Opioids for vaginal delivery
Sufentanil: 7.5–10 µg.
Fentanyl: 25 µg.
In contrast to fentanyl, sufentanil (10 µg) has a faster onset and is more effective [64].

Cesarean section
Local anesthetics:
0.5% bupivacaine (isobaric or hyperbaric), 2 mL increments = 10 mg (the maximum dose of 20 mg is rarely necessary) [4, 71].

Table 39.1 Vaginal delivery: dosage and duration of effect of subarachnoidally administered drugs [4, 73]

Drug	Dose	Onset of effect	Duration of effect	Notes
Sufentanil	10 µg	2–10 min	60–180 min	Better analgesia than with fentanyl
Fentanyl	25–50 µg	2–10 min	30–120 min	
Pethidine	10–20 mg	2–10 min	60–180 min	Has sedative effects (higher dosage), more frequent vomiting
Morphine*	0.2–2 mg	30–60 min	8–24 h	Respiratory depression
Bupivacaine	2.5–5 mg	15–20 min	30–60 min	Frequent tachyphylaxis

* Doses ≥ 2.5 mg are often accompanied by itching, nausea and vomiting.

Combination of opioids and local anesthetics
Initial dose: 1.5 ± 0.2 mL 0.5% bupivacaine, hyperbaric, with the addition of 10 µg sufentanil.
Sufentanil and pethidine are more effective than fentanyl. All three opioids can lead to a slight decrease in blood pressure (not greater than 15% of the baseline). The Apgar score in neonates remains normal [4].

Opioid side effects [4]
See Chapter 50, section on opioids, p. 393.

Other complications
When CSA is used in obstetrics, the same complications must be expected as described earlier for continuous spinal anesthesia (see Chapter 38, p. 297) and continuous epidural anesthesia in the obstetric field.
The occurrence of cauda equina syndrome after CSA in obstetrics has not yet been reported [4].
Various postpartum neuropathies (e.g. of the femoral nerve or obturator nerve), the duration of which is limited, must not be confused with cauda equina syndrome.

40 Chemical intraspinal neurolysis with phenol in glycerol

Chemical intraspinal neurolysis of the posterior spinal cord roots allows transient selective blocking of pain without any significant effect on cutaneous sensation or proprioception [47, 66, 69].

Neurolytic substances at appropriate concentrations (phenol in glycerol, alcohol and chlorocresol) are used to destroy the thin C fibers, A-delta fibers and A-gamma fibers, while only having a slight effect on the larger motor fibers [47] (Fig. 40.1).

At low doses of phenol, there is neither permanent motor weakness nor long-term loss of sensibility. Glycerol is used as the carrier substance for phenol. Phenol not only has destructive neurolytic effects, but also acts as a local anesthetic.

Indications
- Pain in the advanced stages of malignant disease (e.g. rectum, prostate, bladder, gynecological tumors). This method is particularly valuable for tumor-related pain in the rectal area.
- When opioids are ineffective in the terminal stages (method of choice in poor prognoses and poor general condition).
- When the patient declines neurosurgical pain-relieving procedures.
- Spastic paraplegia with no hope of functional recovery (spasticity, hyperreflexia and pain).

Contraindications
- The general contraindications for spinal anesthesia apply (see Chapter 36, p. 272f).
- No anesthetic expertise.

Procedure

Full prior information for the patient is mandatory.

Preparations and materials
- Check that the emergency equipment is complete and in working order (intubation kit, emergency drugs); sterile precautions, intravenous access, anesthetic machine.
- Commence intravenous infusion and ensure adequate volume loading (250–500 mL of a balanced electrolyte solution).
- Careful monitoring: ECG, BP control, pulse oximetry.
- Spinal needle with Quincke tip, 22 G (due to the high viscosity).
- 1-mL tuberculin syringe.
- 2-mL syringe with 1–2 mL 0.9% saline.
- Ampoule with 5% or 10% phenol in glycerol (Fig. 40.2).

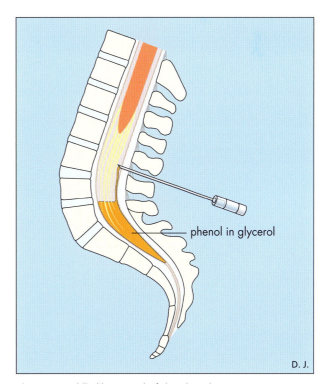

Fig. 40.1 Saddle-like spread of the phenol

Chapter 40

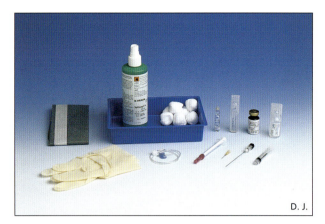

Fig. 40.2 Materials

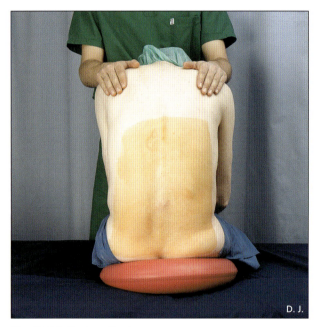

Fig. 40.3 Patient positioning

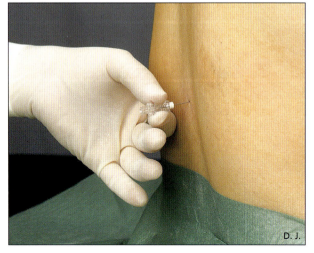

Fig. 40.4 Free CSF flow (proof) in all four quadrants

Warm the phenol ampoule to body temperature to reduce the viscosity [66] and then draw it up into the tuberculin syringe.

Prerequisites
Prerequisites for a neurolytic injection are:
- A prior prognostic spinal block with a local anesthetic (e.g. with hyperbaric 4% mepivacaine). This is the only way to identify the correct dose and avoid giving patients with central pain an injection that is not indicated.
- Very experienced anesthetist.
- No analgesics and no premedication on the day of the block, so that the effect of the neurolytic can be more easily assessed.

Positioning and injection technique
- The patient is placed in a sitting position, since the aim is to achieve saddle-block anesthesia. In cases of rectal carcinoma, sitting is almost impossible due to severe "fireball" pain in the anal region. A rubber ring is very helpful in such cases (Fig. 40.3).
- Puncture with a 22-G spinal needle in the region of the L5/S1 segment.
- Free CSF flow must be demonstrated in all four quadrants (rotate the needle and bevel) (Fig. 40.4). There is a risk of necrosis if phenol is inadvertently injected into neighboring tissues.
- Very slow injection of phenol (0.5 mL over 30 min) (Fig. 40.5). The correct dosage is based on the test block with local anesthetic. Normally, symptoms improve quickly after the administration of 0.1–0.2 mL phenol, so that the patient ceases to feel any pain while sitting. If this improvement does not occur, it is usually because the phenol concentration selected was too low.
  A 10% solution is preferred by the author.
- Constant checking of sensation by the assistant during the injection: pin-prick method (Fig. 40.6).
- After injecting the required amount of neurolytic (the authors recommend 0.5–0.6 mL per session), the spinal needle is cleared of residual phenol by the injection of 1 mL 0.9% saline and withdrawn (Fig. 40.7).
- The patient remains seated for the following 2–3 hours. After this, only 5% of the phenol is still bound to the glycerol and an optimal saddle block is achieved.

Chemical intraspinal neurolysis with phenol in glycerol

To minimize the risks and achieve better distribution of the phenol, spread the total dose of 1–1.2 mL over two successive days.

Observations after the block
- Transient numbness in the calf region often occurs on the day of the injection.
- The first injection rarely produces adequate pain reduction.
- A repeat block is possible when the pain recurs.
- The average duration of pain reduction is about two to three months, although in the author's experience the duration of effect is difficult to assess in advance. It can range from 1–2 days to 6 months.

Opioids should not be abruptly discontinued. Instead, they should if possible be reduced gradually.

Complications
Complications are rare and transient [69].

The sensory and motor supply to the urinary bladder and rectum originates in the lumbosacral segments. If the procedure is not carried out carefully, there is therefore a possibility of loss of sphincter function in the bladder and rectum. In the extensive literature over the last 40 years, the frequency of this complication is reported to be 3–5%.

The loss of function is transient and usually limited to 4–6 weeks, depending on the recovery period required by the nerve fibers affected by the neurolytic. The patient must be made aware of this potential complication.

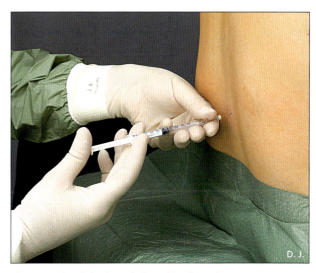

Fig. 40.5 Slow injection of phenol in glycerol

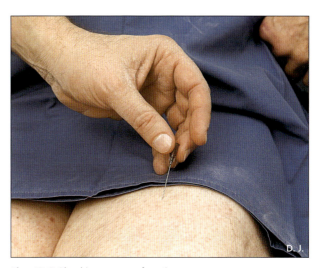

Fig. 40.6 Checking sensory function

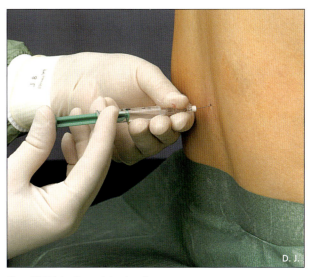

Fig. 40.7 Injection of 1 mL saline

Chapter 40

Record and checklist

Neurolysis with phenol in glycerol

Name: _____ Date: _____
Diagnosis: _____
Premedication: ☐ No ☐ Yes _____
Neurological abnormalities: ☐ No ☐ Yes _____

Purpose of block: ☐ Therapeutic
Needle: ☐ Quincke 22 G
i.v. access, infusion: ☐ Yes
Monitoring: ☐ ECG ☐ Pulse oximetry
Ventilation facilities: ☐ Yes (equipment checked)
Emergency equipment (drugs): ☐ Checked
Patient: ☐ Informed ☐ Consent
☐ Prognostic spinal anesthesia carried out

Position: ☐ Sitting
Access: ☐ Median
Injection level: ☐ L5–S1 ☐ Other _____
Free CSF flow: ☐ At all 4 levels
CSF: ☐ Clear ☐ Slightly bloody ☐ Bloody
Abnormalities: ☐ No ☐ Yes _____
Injection:
Phenol in glycerol: _____ mL ☐ 5 % _____ mL ☐ 10 %
Injection time: _____ min
☐ Sensory and motor function checked during injection

Patient's remarks:
☐ During the injection: _____
After phenol administraion:
Injection of 1 mL 0,9 % NaCl through the spinal neddle:
☐ Yes ☐ No

Complications:
☐ None ☐ Bladder emptying disturbances
☐ Bowel emptying disturbances ☐ Postdural puncture headache
☐ Back pain ☐ Neurological complications

Subjective effects of block:
☐ None ☐ Increased pain
☐ Reduced pain ☐ No pain

VISUAL ANALOG SCALE

|||||||||||||||||||||||||||||||||||||||||||||||||||||||||
0   10   20   30   40   50   60   70   80   90   100

Special notes:
_____
_____
_____

© Copyright ABW Wissenschaftsverlag 2004,
Jankovic, Regional nerve blocks and infiltration therapy, 3rd edition

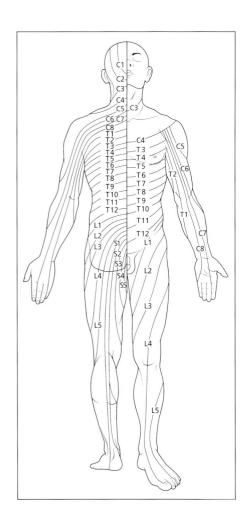

Epidural anesthesia

41 Lumbar epidural anesthesia

In epidural anesthesia, drugs are injected into the extradural space in order to interrupt conduction in the somatic and autonomic nerve fibers. In addition to local anesthetics, opioids, steroids and homologous blood, other substances can also be used, mainly as adjuvants – e.g. the alpha-2-adrenoceptor agonist clonidine, vasopressors, or ketamine.

Anatomy

The epidural space (cavum epidurale) lies between the widely separated laminae of the meninges: the thin periosteal lamina (lamina externa, endorrhachis), which covers the spinal cord; and the lamina interna – the spinal dura mater.

Laterally, the epidural space is bounded by periosteum and by the intervertebral foramina. Ventral and dorsally, it is enclosed by the anterior longitudinal ligament of the vertebrae and the ligamentum flavum (Fig. 41.1). In the cervical region, the ligamentum flavum is much thinner and not very elastic.

The ligamentum flavum is thickest in the midline in the lumbar region. The distance between the skin and the epidural space is about 4 cm in approximately 50% of patients and between 4 cm and 6 cm in 80%

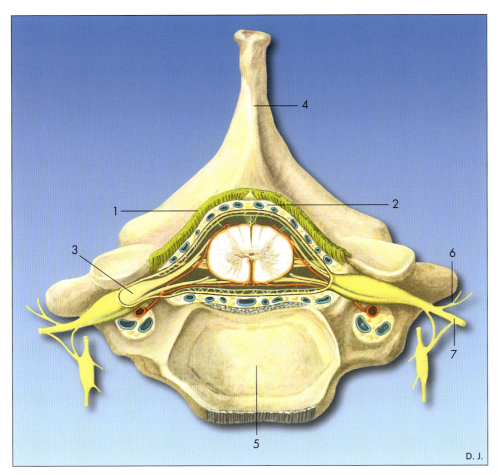

Fig. 41.1 Cross-section of the epidural space. (1) Ligamentum flavum, (2) epidural space with venous plexus, (3) spinal ganglion, (4) spinous process, (5) body of vertebra, (6) dorsal branch of spinal nerve, (7) ventral branch of spinal nerve

of patients. The range extends from less than 3 cm (in slim individuals) to more than 8 cm (in obese patients).

The distance between the ligamentum flavum and the dura mater varies from 2–3 mm in the cervical area to up to 5-6 mm in the mid-lumbar region [23].

The volume of the epidural space, with a capacity of about 118 mL (up to 150 mL), is not as large as that of the subarachnoid space [11]. The epidural space extends from the foramen magnum to the sacrococcygeal ligament. It is connected via the intervertebral foramina with the paravertebral space. It has an indirect transdural link to the CSF. The substantial epidural venous network is connected to the azygos vein and to the pelvic, abdominal and thoracic veins [11, 23].

In addition to fat and connective tissue, the epidural space contains lymph, the internal and external vertebral venous plexuses and the roots of the spinal nerves. The width of the epidural space is 4–7 mm in the lumbar region, 3–5 mm in the thoracic region and 3–4 mm in the cervical region (C7–T1). The dura mater is 0.3–0.7 mm thick in the lumbar region, 1 mm thick in the central thoracic region, and 1–1.5 mm thick in the cervical region. There is negative pressure in the epidural space in some 80–90% of patients. However, the negative pressure is not the same at all levels and it varies according to intrathoracic respiratory pressure variations, as well as to posture. The negative pressure increases in the sitting position, while in the supine position it is reduced. It is also reduced in pulmonary diseases (emphysema, asthma) and during heavy coughing or straining.

Indications

The use of epidural anesthesia has proved particularly valuable in the following groups of patients:
- Those with a full stomach.
- Those in whom tracheal intubation difficulties are expected.
- Those with a history or suspicion of malignant hyperthermia.
- Muscle disease.
- Cardiopulmonary disease.
- Metabolic disease.
- Renal and hepatic disease.
- Stable neurological diseases.
- Elderly patients.

Surgical indications
- Procedures in the area of the lower extremities, hip joints and inguinal region.
- Vascular surgery.
- Upper abdominal and thoracic procedures, in combination with general anesthesia.
- Urological procedures (prostate, bladder).
- Gynecological and obstetric procedures.
- Procedures in the perineal and perianal region.
- Interventional radiology.

Postoperative and post-traumatic pain therapy
Usually in combination with local anesthetics and opioids.

Therapeutic block with injection of depot corticoids
Caudal, lumbar or cervical.

Epidural injection of homologous blood or dextran, or fibrin glue patch in postdural puncture headache

Contraindications
Specific
- Patient refusal.
- Patients under general anesthesia.
- Coagulation disorders, anticoagulant therapy.
- Sepsis.
- Local infections at the injection site.
- Immune deficiency.
- Severe decompensated hypovolemia, shock.
- Specific cardiovascular diseases of myocardial, ischemic or valvular origin, if the procedure being carried out requires sensory spread up to or beyond T6.
- Acute diseases of the brain and spinal cord.
- Raised intracranial pressure.
- A history of hypersensitivity to local anesthetics, without a prior intradermal test dose.

Relative
These contraindications always require a risk–benefit analysis and are more medicolegal in nature:
- Chronic disorders of the brain and spinal cord.
- Severe spinal deformities, arthritis, osteoporosis, intervertebral disk prolapse or pain after intervertebral disk surgery.
- After spinal fusion, spinal metastases.

Injection-related
- Additional attempts after three unsuccessful punctures.
- Inexperienced anesthetist without supervision.
- No anesthetic expertise.

Lumbar epidural anesthesia

- Insertion should always be carried out below the level of L2 (conus medullaris). Insertion above the L2 segment must only be carried out by a technically highly skilled anesthetist and should have specific indications [13].
- Any severely radiating pain occurring during the insertion is a warning signal. The needle must not be advanced any further.
- Epidural insertion in patients under general anesthesia, particularly above the L2 segment, should generally be avoided, except in the hands of the most skilled anesthesiologists. One exception to this rule is epidural insertion in children, which must be left to experienced pediatric anesthesiologists [13, 54].

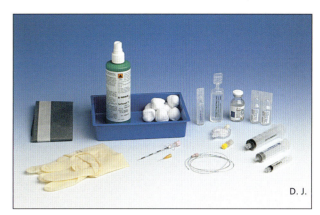

Fig. 41.2 Materials

Procedure

Full prior information for the patient is mandatory.

Preparations and materials
- Check that the emergency equipment is complete and in working order (intubation kit, emergency drugs); sterile precautions, intravenous access, anesthetic machine.
- Insert an intravenous cannula and give a volume load (250–500 mL of a balanced electrolyte solution).
- Precise monitoring: ECG, BP, pulse oximetry.

The use of purpose-designed kit for epidural anesthesia is recommended (e.g. from B. Braun Melsungen) (Fig. 41.2).
- Disinfectant.
- Local anesthetic.

Epidural needles
Tuohy, Hustead, Crawford, or Weiss (Fig. 41.3).

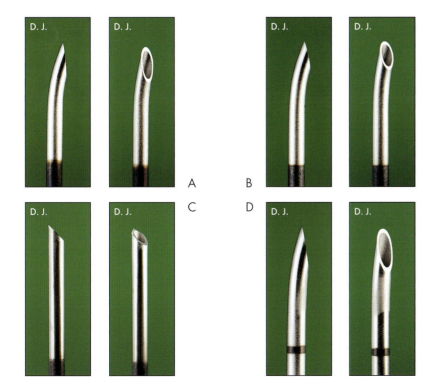

Fig. 41.3a–d Epidural needles.
a Tuohy, **b** Hustead, **c** Crawford, **d** Weiss

307

Single-shot technique

Patient positioning
Optimal positioning of the patient during the injection and fixation phase of the local anesthetic is the prerequisite for success. Lumbar epidural anesthesia can be carried out with the patient in the lateral decubitus position (preferred) or sitting.

> It is important with both positions to minimise lumbar lordosis and to identify the midline.

Injection technique

Median approach
Landmarks
The injection is carried out in the midline below the L2 segment (conus medullaris), usually between the spinous processes of L2/L3 or L3/L4. The intervertebral space is palpated and the midline is located to serve as the most important signpost. In the midline, the ligamentum flavum is at its thickest, the epidural space is widest and the blood vessels are at their smallest. The injection site is marked with the thumbnail (Fig. 41.4).

Strict asepsis
Thorough, repeated and wide skin prep, drying and covering of the injection site with a drape.

Local anesthesia
Local infiltration of the skin and supraspinous and interspinous ligaments is carried out between the spread index and middle fingers of the left hand, using 1–1.5 mL of a local anesthetic (e.g. 1% prilocaine) (Fig. 41.5).

Skin incision
Using a stylet or a large needle (Fig. 41.6).

Puncture of the supraspinous and interspinous ligaments and ligamentum flavum
Without moving the spread index and middle fingers of the left hand from the intervertebral space, an epidural needle is fixed between the thumb of the right hand (hub) and the index and middle finger (shaft) and advanced through the skin incision (Fig. 41.7). After passing the supraspinous ligament, which is about 1 cm thick, the needle, with its bevel directed laterally, is advanced a further 2–3 cm (depending on the anatomy), until it rests firmly in the interspinous ligament.

The trochar is removed and a low friction syringe is attached (Fig. 41.8).

> Care should be taken to ensure that the needle is kept in the midline.

Inadvertent deviation from the midline leads to the needle passing the supraspinous ligament, with a angled entry into the interspinous ligament with only brief resistance and a subsequent false loss of resistance. This type of puncture ends in the paravertebral musculature and is accompanied by local pain. The laminae and superior and inferior articular processes of the vertebrae may also be affected. As the articular processes are innervated, puncture trauma is accompanied by severe localized ipsilateral back pain, spasm of the paravertebral muscles and pain radiating into the leg. This type of pain is often confused with radicular pain.

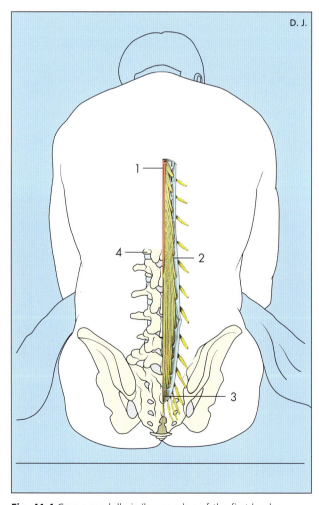

Fig. 41.4 Conus medullaris (lower edge of the first lumbar vertebra). (1) Conus medullaris, (2) cauda equina, (3) dural sac, (4) L1 segment

Lumbar epidural anesthesia

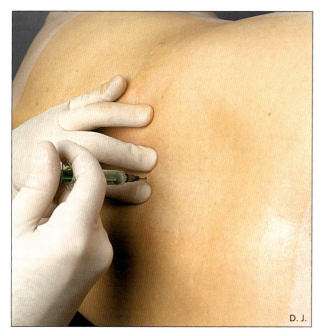

Fig. 41.5 Local anesthesia

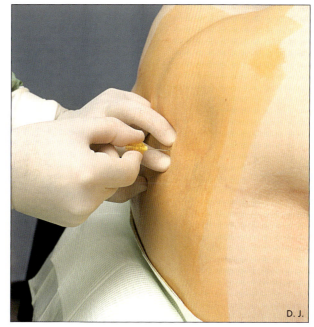

Fig. 41.6 Skin incision

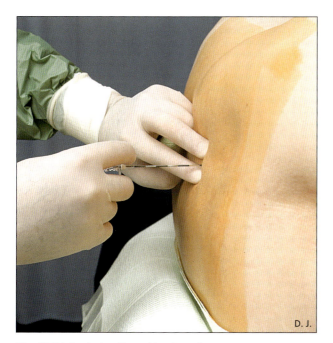

Fig. 41.7 Introducing the epidural needle

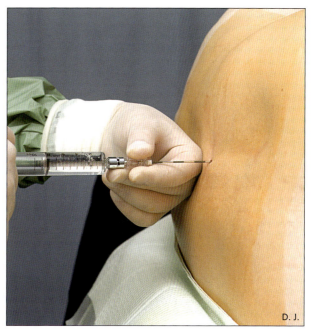

Fig. 41.8 Removing the stylet and attaching a low-friction syringe

After passing the interspinous ligament, the needle must be advanced carefully, millimeter by millimeter, in the direction of the ligamentum flavum.

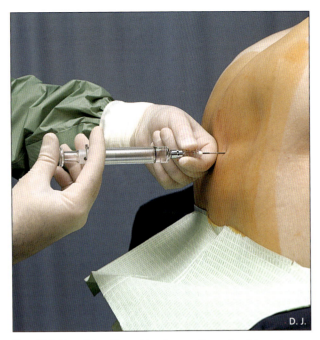

Fig. 41.9 Identifying the epidural space (loss of resistance)

Puncturing the epidural space
The thumb and index finger of the left hand, which is resting with the back of the hand firmly against the patient's back, secure the needle, advance it millimeter by millimeter and at the same exercise a braking function. The thumb of the right hand applies pressure on the syringe plunger. Loss of resistance indicates that the epidural space has been reached. The contents of the syringe are easily injected. Identification of the epidural space is carried out using the **loss-of-resistance technique** (Fig. 41.9).

The following variations on this technique can be applied:

Technique using saline or air
Saline: after the interspinous ligament has been reached, the stylet is removed and a low-friction syringe filled with a saline solution and with a small air bubble in it, serving as a visual indicator, is attached. When the ligamentum flavum is encountered, the air bubble is compressed by pressure on the syringe plunger (Fig. 41.10a); when the epidural space is reached, the bubble returns to its normal, larger shape (Fig. 41.10b).
Air: this technique is not suitable for inexperienced anesthetists or in insertions likely to be associated with technical difficulties [80, 82].

Advantage
When the epidural space has been reached, no fluid should emerge from the needle. Any CSF that emerges is therefore more easily identified.

Disadvantages
The loss of resistance is not as clear and the dura is not pushed aside from the needle tip in the same way as it is using the saline injection. Complications have been reported [6, 80, 88] – e.g. pneumocephalus, compression of the spinal cord and nerve roots by air collecting in the epidural space, air embolism, air collecting retroperitoneally, subcutaneous emphysema.

After air has been injected into the epidural space, irregular spread of the epidural anesthesia may occur, as the air bubbles act as a mechanical barrier. However, an even more important aspect is that when epidural anesthesia is combined with general anesthesia, the injected air may pose a danger to the patient. If nitrous oxide is used, it may diffuse quickly into the air bubbles and substantially expand them. Like large hematomas, large gas bubbles can compress the spinal cord and thereby cause transient or permanent neurological injury.

"Hanging drop" technique
After the interspinous ligament has been reached, a drop of saline is placed within the hub of the needle (Fig. 41.11a). After the ligamentum flavum has been passed and the epidural space has been reached, the drop is "sucked in" by the vacuum that is usually present during the inspiration phase (Fig. 41.11b).

Lumbar epidural anesthesia

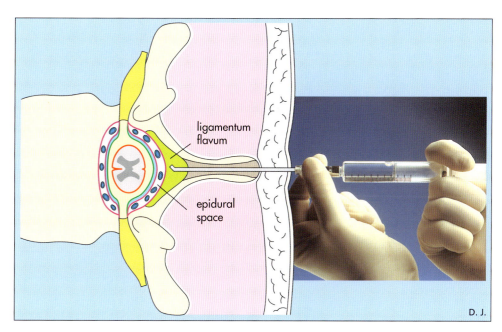

Fig. 41.10a Loss-of-resistance technique with saline. The air bubble is compressed by pressure on the syringe plunger

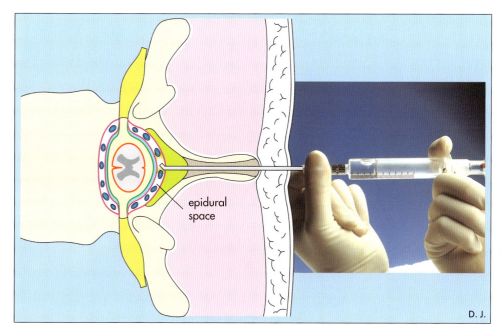

Fig. 41.10b Loss-of-resistance technique with saline. The epidural space has been reached. The air bubble has returned to its normal, loose shape

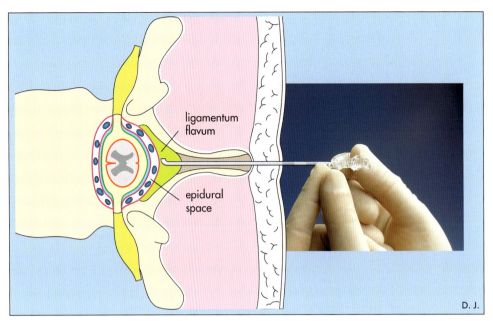

Fig. 41.11a "Hanging drop" technique. The epidural needle is positioned in the ligamentum flavum

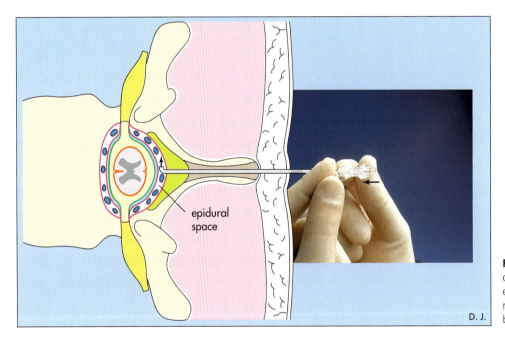

Fig. 41.11b "Hanging drop" technique. The epidural space has been reached. The drop is sucked back in

Lumbar epidural anesthesia

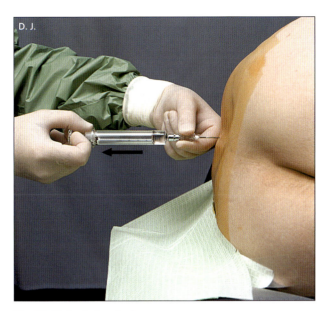

Fig. 41.12 Aspiration test

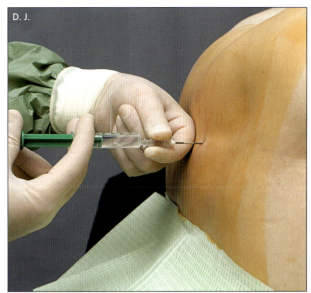

Fig. 41.13 Test dose

Aspiration and injection of a test dose
Careful aspiration is carried out (Fig. 41.12). The needle continues to be secured by the thumb and index finger of the left hand, resting with the back of the hand firmly against the patient's back.

After negative aspiration, a test dose of 3–4 mL of local anesthetic, usually with epinephrine added, can be injected. This allows easier detection of possible intravascular injection if tachycardia occurs (Fig. 41.13).

The test dose should be allowed 5 minutes to take effect. During this period, the needle should be rotated at 1-minute intervals (Fig. 41.14).

Five minutes after administration of the test dose, the spread of the anesthesia is checked to exclude inadvertent subarachnoid injection. The patient is asked whether there is a sensation of warmth or numbness in the lower extremities. The following points are important in this phase:
- Maintaining constant verbal contact with the patient.
- Careful cardiovascular monitoring.

If all is well, a local anesthetic can be injected.

The addition of epinephrine can lead to unreliable results in the following groups of patients [63]:
- Patients taking beta-blockers [42, 62].
- Patients under general anesthesia [29, 58, 95].
- Older patients [43].
- Pregnant patients [19].

Caution when adding epinephrine is required in:
- Pregnant patients (transient fetal bradycardia due to reduced uterine blood flow [57]).
- Older patients with coronary heart disease.
- Arteriosclerosis, hypertonia, diabetes.

Contraindications to the addition of epinephrine are:
- Glaucoma (with closed iridocorneal angle).
- Paroxysmal tachycardia, high-frequency absolute arrhythmia.

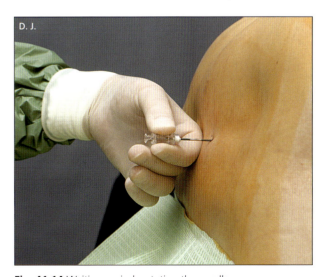

Fig. 41.14 Waiting period: rotating the needle

313

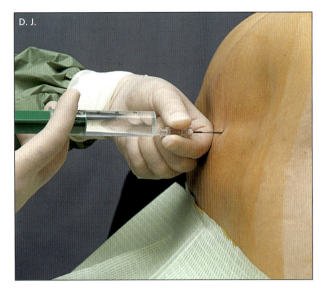

Fig. 41.15 Incremental injection of local anesthetic

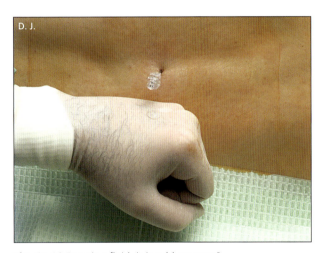

Fig. 41.16 Escaping fluid: is it cold or warm?

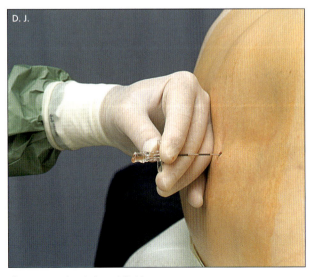

Fig. 41.17 Blood-tinged fluid

Injection of a local anesthetic (Fig. 41.15)
After aspiration has been repeated, incremental administration of a local anesthetic is carried out. In a "single-shot" injection, half of the planned dose is initially injected at a speed of <0.3–0.5 mL/s; the syringe is disconnected again, a check is made for any escaping fluid and only then is the remainder of the dose administered. After aspiration has been repeated shortly before the end of the injection, the needle is withdrawn and the patient is placed in the desired position.

> The hand securing the needle must remain constantly resting on the patient's back during puncture, aspiration, injection of the test dose, the test dose period and during injection of the local anesthetic.
> - Repeated aspiration.
> - Use of the smallest possible dose.
> - Always inject in incremental amounts (several test doses).
> - Verbal contact.
> - Careful checking of the spread of the anesthesia.
> - Careful cardiovascular monitoring.

Problem situations
Escaping fluid
After the epidural space has been identified or after administration of the test dose, a few drops of fluid may still drip from the positioned needle. This phenomenon often worries inexperienced anesthetists.
Procedure:
- During an attempt at aspiration, the viscosity of the fluid should be noted.
- The patient is asked to breathe in and out deeply. If the needle is positioned epidurally, there is synchronous movement of the fluid drop.
- A few drops of fluid can be tested on the back of the hand to check whether they are cold or warm: colder and slowly dripping fluid suggests saline, whereas warmer and quickly dripping fluid suggests CSF (Fig. 41.16).
- Test the glucose content of the fluid.

Escaping blood (Fig. 41.17)
The following steps are possible:
- Another attempt at insertion, one segment higher or lower.
- Administer general anesthesia.
- In all other indications – e.g. therapeutic blocks – it is advisable to abandon the procedure.

Escaping CSF
- The method of choice in surgical procedures is to carry out spinal anesthesia when the CSF is clear.
- Another attempt at insertion. It should be taken into account that an epidural dose of local anesthetic can spread intrathecally through the existing dural leak (larger puncture needles, 16–18 G) and can lead to total spinal anesthesia.
- Administer general anesthesia.
- In all other indications – e.g. therapeutic blocks – it is again advisable to abandon the procedure.
- Patients must be informed about the possibility of postdural puncture headache.

The following measures have proved valuable for reducing the risk of complications: aspiration, test dose of a local anesthetic containing epinephrine and incremental administration of the local anesthetic.

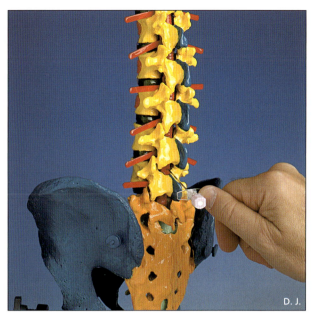
Fig. 41.18 Paramedian puncture

Paramedian (paraspinal) approach (Fig. 41.18)
This technique, which is independent of lumbar lordosis or the ability of the spine to flex, avoids puncture of the supraspinous ligament and the frequently ossified interspinous ligament. The puncture site is located in the selected intervertebral space, about 1.5–2 cm lateral from the upper edge of the lower spinous process.
Fan-shaped local anesthesia identifies the depth of the vertebral arches (laminae), which are marked (4–6 cm). The epidural needle (usually 18-G Crawford) is introduced in a craniomedial direction at an angle of about 15° to the sagittal level and about 35° to the skin surface, so that it passes the laminae and slides into the interlaminar fissure. The only ligament that needs to be penetrated on the way to the epidural space is the ligamentum flavum. Reaching this is characterized by a "leathery" resistance. The most important step in this technique is to identify the depth of the ligamentum flavum. The trochar is then removed from the puncture needle and identification of the epidural space is carried out in the same way as described for the single-shot technique.

Record and checklist

Lumbar epidural anesthesia

Name: _____ Date: _____
Diagnosis: _____
Premedication: ☐ No ☐ Yes _____
Neurological abnormalities: ☐ No ☐ Yes _____

Purpose of block: ☐ Surgical ☐ Therapeutic ☐ Diagnostic
Needle: ☐ Tuohy G ____ ☐ Other ____
i.v. access, infusion: ☐ Yes
Monitoring: ☐ ECG ☐ Pulse oximetry
Ventilation facilities: ☐ Yes (equipment checked)
Emergency equipment (drugs): ☐ Checked
Patient: ☐ Informed

Position: ☐ Lateral decubitus ☐ Sitting
Access: ☐ Median ☐ Paramedian
Injection level: ☐ L3/L4 ☐ Other _____
Injection technique: ☐ Loss of resistance ☐ Other _____
Epidural space: ☐ Identified
Aspiration test: ☐ Carried out
Test dose: _____ Epinephrine added: ☐ Yes ☐ No
Check on sensorimotor function after 5 min: ☐ Carried out
Abnormalities: ☐ No ☐ Yes _____
Injection:
☐ Local anesthetic: _____ mL _____ %
(incremental)
☐ Addition: _____ μg/mg

Patient's remarks during injection:
☐ None ☐ Pain ☐ Paresthesias ☐ Warmth
Duration and area: _____
Objective block effect after 20 min:
☐ Cold test ☐ Temperature measurement before _____ °C after _____ °C
☐ Sensory: L _____ T _____
☐ Motor

Complications:
☐ None ☐ Pain
☐ Radicular symptoms ☐ Vasovagal reactions
☐ BP drop ☐ Dural puncture
☐ Vascular puncture ☐ Intravascular injection
☐ Massive epidural anesthesia ☐ Total spinal anesthesia
☐ Subdural spread ☐ Respiratory disturbance
☐ Drop in body temperature ☐ Muscle tremor
☐ Bladder emptying disturbances ☐ Postdural puncture headache
☐ Back pain ☐ Neurological complications

Special notes: _____
_____

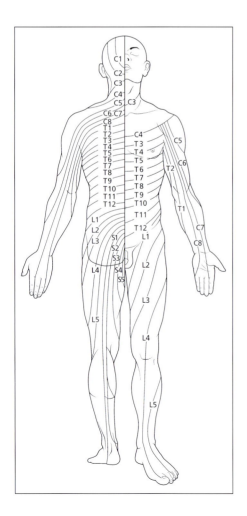

© Copyright ABW Wissenschaftsverlag 2004,
Jankovic, Regional nerve blocks and infiltration therapy, 3rd edition

Lumbar epidural anesthesia

Continuous epidural anesthesia*

Procedure

The identification of the epidural space is carried out in the same way as in the single-shot injection. After the epidural space has been reached and loss of resistance has been confirmed, the aspiration test is carried out. Before the catheter is introduced, the needle bevel should be directed cranially.

The thumb and index finger of the left hand secure the epidural needle, with the back of the hand lying firmly on the patient's back. The catheter is advanced cranially, using the thumb and index finger of the right hand, to a maximum of 3–4 cm (Fig. 41.19).

Advancing it further than this can lead to lateral deviation of the catheter, with accompanying paresthesias.

After placement of the catheter in the desired position, the needle is slowly withdrawn (Fig. 41.20a), while at the same time the thumb and index finger of the left hand secure the catheter at the injection site (Fig. 41.20b).

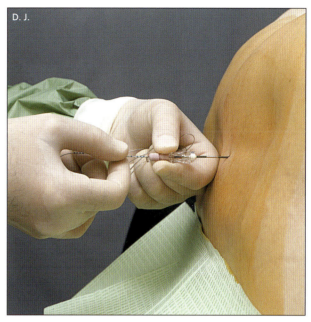

Fig. 41.19 Introducing the catheter

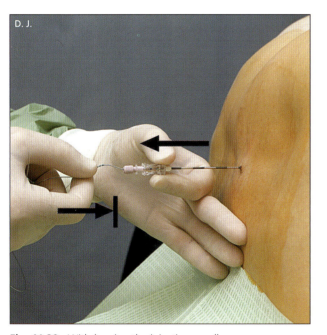

Fig. 41.20a Withdrawing the injection needle

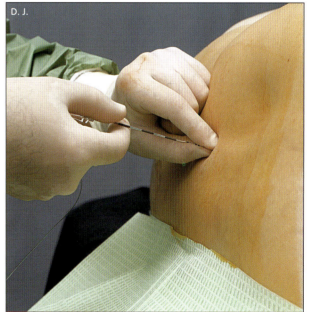

Fig. 41.20b The catheter is secured at the injection site with the thumb and index finger

---

* If technical difficulties are experienced, the catheter and puncture needle must always be removed simultaneously. The catheter must never be withdrawn through the positioned puncture needle.

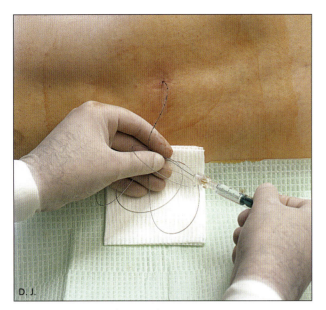

Fig. 41.21 Injection of 1 mL saline

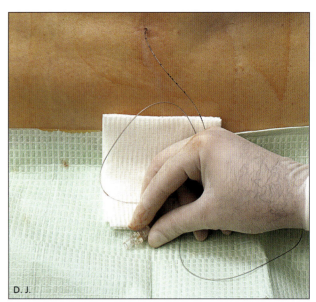

Fig. 41.22 The end of the catheter is placed below the injection site

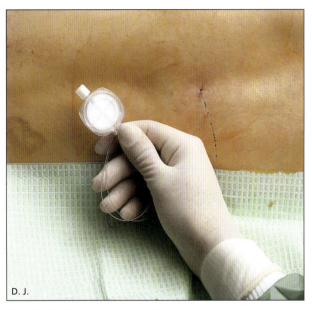

Fig. 41.23a Placing a bacterial filter

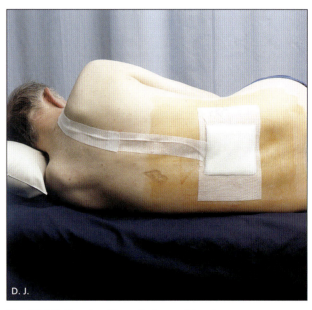

Fig. 41.23b Securing the catheter and dressing

An adapter is attached to the end of the catheter. The patency of the catheter is tested by injecting 1–2 mL saline (Fig. 41.21). After aspiration, the syringe is disconnected and the open end of the catheter is placed on a sterile drape below the puncture site. Attention must be given to any escaping fluid (CSF or blood) (Fig. 41.22).

A bacterial filter is then attached (Fig. 41.23a) and the catheter is secured with a skin suture and a dressing (Fig. 41.23b).

The patient is placed in the desired position and a test dose is administered, as with the single-shot injection. During the waiting period, it is important to maintain verbal contact with the patient and to check the spread of the anesthesia, to exclude the ever-present risk of inadvertent subarachnoid injection.

Lumbar epidural anesthesia

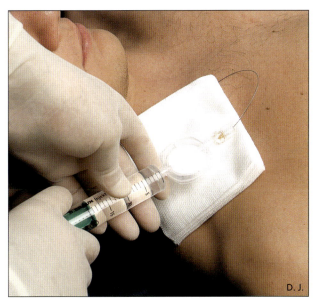

Fig. 41.24 After the test dose, incremental injection of local anesthetic

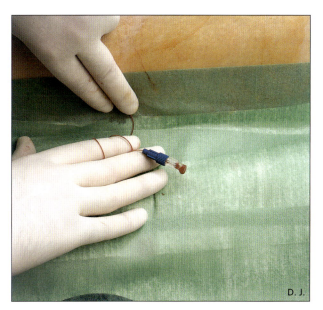

Fig. 41.25 Blood in the catheter

A subdural injection cannot always be excluded with absolute certainty, in spite of all precautions.
After 5 minutes, the remainder of the dose, adjusted for the individual patient, can be administered on an incremental basis (max. 5 mL each injection) until the desired level of anesthesia is reached (Fig. 41.24).

Problem situations
Blood in the catheter (Fig. 41.25).
The catheter is withdrawn 0.5–1 cm and rinsed with 2–3 mL saline. After waiting and subsequent aspiration, a test dose can be given if no further blood is observed. If blood is still present, the catheter must be withdrawn.

Escaping CSF
When subarachnoid positioning of the catheter is demonstrated, the following steps are possible:
- Inject a spinal dose and then remove the catheter.
- Carry on with continuous spinal anesthesia.
- Remove the catheter and administer general anesthesia.

The patient must be informed about the possibility of postdural puncture headache.

Monitoring an epidural catheter
Continuous pain therapy using an epidural catheter also requires continuous monitoring and checking of efficacy. This includes the following points in particular:
- Daily checking of the catheter position, so that intravascular or subarachnoid migration can be recognized early.
- Changing the bacterial filter and dressing every 2 days, with careful checking of the puncture site, to minimize the risk of bacterial colonization and associated infection.
- Continuous monitoring of efficacy and – if necessary – adjustment of the dose of local anesthetic, opioid, or other adjuvant substance.
- Records must be kept.

Chapter 41

Record and checklist

Lumbar catheter epidural anesthesia

Name: _____ Date: _____
Diagnosis: _____
Premedication: ☐ No   ☐ Yes _____
Neurological abnormalities: ☐ No   ☐ Yes _____

Purpose of block: ☐ Surgical   ☐ Therapeutic
Needle: ☐ Tuohy G ____   ☐ Other ____
i.v. access, infusion: ☐ Yes
Monitoring: ☐ ECG   ☐ Pulse oximetry
Ventilation facilities: ☐ Yes (equipment checked)
Emergency equipment (drugs):   ☐ Checked
Patient: ☐ Informed

Position: ☐ Lateral decubitus   ☐ Sitting
Access: ☐ Median   ☐ Paramedian
Injection level: ☐ L3/L4   ☐ Other _____
Injection technique: ☐ Loss of resistance ☐ Other _____
Epidural space: ☐ Identified
Catheter: ☐ Advanced 3–4 cm cranially
Aspiration test: ☐ Carried out
Catheter end: ☐ Placed deeper than the puncture site
Bacterial filter: ☐
Test dose: _____ Epinephrine added: ☐ Yes ☐ No
Check on sensorimotor function after 5 min: ☐ Carried out
Abnormalities: ☐ No   ☐ Yes _____
Injection:
☐ Local anesthetic: _____ mL ____ %
   (incremental)
☐ Addition: _____ µg/mg
☐ Subsequent injection (incremental): _____ mL ____ %

Patient's remarks during injection:
☐ None   ☐ Pain   ☐ Paresthesias   ☐ Warmth
Duration and area: _____
Objective block effect after 20 min:
☐ Cold test   ☐ Temperature measurement before _____ °C   after _____ °C
☐ Sensory: L _____ T _____   ☐ Motor

Complications:
☐ None ☐ Radicular symptoms ☐ BP drop ☐ Vascular puncture
☐ Massive epidural anesthesia ☐ Subdural spread ☐ Drop in body temperature
☐ Bladder emptying disturbances ☐ Back pain ☐ Pain ☐ Vasovagal reactions
☐ Dural puncture ☐ Intravascular injection ☐ Total spinal anesthesia
☐ Respiratory disturbance ☐ Muscle tremor ☐ Postdural puncture headache
☐ Neurological complications

Special notes: _____

© Copyright ABW Wissenschaftsverlag 2004,
  Jankovic, Regional nerve blocks and infiltration therapy, 3rd edition

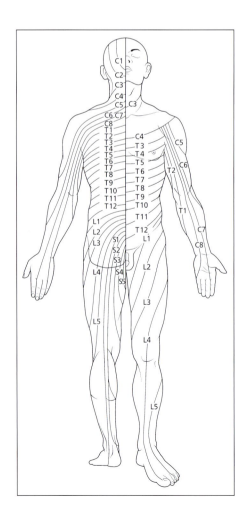

Effect of local anesthetics in the epidural space

Local anesthetic in the epidural space may take three routes.
- Resorption into the circulation via the epidural venous plexus.
- Transdural diffusion into the cerebrospinal fluid.
- Lateral spread through the intervertebral foramina and associated paravertebral block of the spinal nerves.

The targets of epidural injection of local anesthetic are the intradurally located roots of the spinal nerves, which are reached by diffusion through the dura. The spread of the injected local anesthetic is influenced by the following factors:
- Volume and concentration have the greatest influence.
- The speed of injection has a minimal influence on the quality of the anesthesia. Too fast an injection can lead to dangerous cerebrospinal and cardiotoxic complications.
- The positioning of the patient is much less important than in spinal anesthesia.
- Location of the injection and diameter of the nerve roots:
  In injections in the lumbar region, the local anesthetic tends to spread more cranially, so that (particularly when injecting lipophilic local anesthetics such as etidocaine) block of segments L5–S2 is markedly delayed and they are incompletely blocked – probably due to the larger diameter of the nerve roots (S1 about 3.8 mm, S2 about 3.4 mm).
  For the same reasons, the upper thoracic and lower cervical segments show resistance to the effect of local anesthetics.
- Injection level: the closer the injection site, the shorter is the latency.
- Anatomic relationships: Spinal deformities or operations near the spinal cord often lead to alterations of relationships in the epidural space and consequently affect the spread of local anesthetics.
- Height:
  Bromage's recommendation for patients aged between 20 and 40 has been widely accepted for clinical routine in the lumbar area [23].
  The dose of the local anesthetic (2% lidocaine) is between 1 mL and 1.6 mL per segment. For a patient height of 150 cm, ca. 1 mL per segment is used and for each further 5 cm of body height an additional 0.1 mL per segment is added: 150 cm = 1 mL, 160 cm = 1.2 mL, 170 cm = 1.4 mL, 180 cm = 1.6 mL, 190 cm = 1.8 mL of local anesthetic.

The dose of local anesthetic in the thoracic region and in various groups of patients (e.g. pregnant patients, obese patients, elderly patients, as well as in those with diabetes or arteriosclerosis) is reduced by 15–30%.

The time sequence of an epidural block is as follows:
- Sympathetic block with vasodilation.
- Block of temperature perception and deep pain.
- Loss of sensitivity to surface pain, pressure and touch.
- Block of motor functions.

Dosages

Surgical anesthesia

Medium-duration amide local anesthetics
(Table 41.1)

These local anesthetics are characterized by their low molecular weight, low lipophilia, moderate protein binding and high dissociation constant. At concentrations of 1.5–2%, they produce rapid and good analgesia and a low motor block.

Table 41.1 Medium-duration amide local anesthetics

Local anesthetic	Epidural dose	Onset of effect	Maximum dose	Duration of effect
1.5–2% lidocaine with epinephrine	15–30 ml	10–30 min	300 mg 500 mg	80–120 min 120–180 min
1.5–2% mepivacaine with epinephrine	15–30 ml	10–30 min	300 mg 500 mg	90–140 min 140–200 min
1.5–2% prilocaine with epinephrine	15–30 ml	12–16 min	400 mg 600 mg	ca. 100 min ca. 140 min

Long-duration amide local anesthetics (Table 41.2)

Table 41.2 Long-duration amide local anesthetics

Local anesthetic	Epidural dose	Onset of effect	Maximum dose	Duration of effect
0.75% ropivacaine	15–25 ml	10–20 min	250 mg (300)	180–300 min
1% ropivacaine	15–20 ml	10–20 min	250 mg (300)	240–360 min
0.5% levobupivacaine	15–20 ml	18–30 min	150 mg	160–210 min
0.5–0.75% bupivacaine	15–30 ml	18–30 min	150 mg	165–240 min
1% etidocaine	15–30 ml	10–15 min	300 mg	150–280 min

Incomplete epidural anesthesia

In incomplete epidural anesthesia (failure to spread to specific segments or inadequate motor block), it is recommended that an additional injection be carried out after a delay of about 30 minutes for safety. The additional injection into the epidural catheter should be half of the initial dose – e.g. 2% lidocaine with added epinephrine.

Diagnostic and therapeutic blocks

Medium-duration amide local anesthetics
(Table 41.3)

Table 41.3 Medium-duration amide local anesthetics

Block	Sympathetic	Sensory	Motor
Lidocaine	0.5%	1%	2%
Mepivacaine	0.5%	1%	2%
Prilocaine	0.5%	1%	2%

Long-duration amide local anesthetics (Table 41.4)

Table 41.4 Long-duration amide local anesthetics

Block	Sympathetic	Sensory	Motor
Ropivacaine	0.2%	0.375%	0.75–1%
Bupivacaine	0.125%	0.25%	0.5–0.75%
Levo-bupivacaine	0.125%	0.25%	0.5–0.75%

Postoperative or post-traumatic pain therapy

Continuous epidural infusion

- Local anesthetics
  - 0.2–0.3% ropivacaine
    Speed: **6–14 mL/h**
    (usually 10 mL/h, max. 37.5 mg/h).
  - 0.125% bupivacaine
    Speed: **8–18 mL/h (usually 10–14 mL/h).**
  - 0.25% bupivacaine
    Speed: **4–16 mL/h (usually 8–10 mL/h).**
  - 0.125–0.25% levobupivacaine
    Speed: **5–8 mL/h**
    (bolus 2–4 mL every 15 min).

> Individual adjustment of the dosage and duration of treatment is absolutely necessary.

- Opioids (see Chapter 50, section on opioids, p. n)
  Sufentanil: 30–50 µg
  Fentanyl: 50–100 µg
  Morphine: 2–5 mg

- Combination of local anesthetic and opioid
  Ropivacaine and sufentanil (fentanyl)
  Bolus injection:
  e.g. 15 mL 0.1% ropivacaine + 1–2 µg/mL sufentanil (10–20 µg)
  Continuous infusion starting after 30 min:
  0.1% ropivacaine + 0.2–0.3 µg/mL sufentanil.
  Speed: 6–10 mL/h.

  Or

  Bolus injection:
  15 mL 0.1% ropivacaine + 2 µg/mL fentanyl (30 µg).
  Continuous infusion starting after 30 min:
  0.1% ropivacaine + 2 µg/mL fentanyl.
  Speed: 10 mL/h.

  Bupivacaine and sufentanil (fentanyl)
  Bolus injection:
  e.g. 10 mL 0.25% bupivacaine + 1–2 µg/mL sufentanil (10–20 µg)
  Continuous infusion starting after 30 min:
  0.125–0.0625% bupivacaine + 0.2–0.3 µg/mL sufentanil.
  Speed: 6–10 mL/h.

  Or

  Bolus injection:
  e.g. 10 mL 0.25% bupivacaine + 50 µg/mL fentanyl.
  Continuous infusion starting after 30 min:
  0.125–0.0625% bupivacaine + 1–2 µg/mL fentanyl.
  Speed: 10 mL/h.

- Patient-controlled epidural analgesia (PCEA)
  Sufentanil and ropivacaine
  0.1% ropivacaine + 1 µg/mL sufentanil
  Speed: 5–10 mL/h
  Bolus injection: 5 mL
  Lockout time: 10–20 min.

  Fentanyl and ropivacaine
  0.1% ropivacaine + 2 µg/mL fentanyl
  Speed: 10 mL/h
  Bolus injection: 10 mL (max. 32 mL/h)
  Lockout time: 10–20 min.

- Epidural administration of clonidine (see Chapter 50, section on clonidine, p. 394)
  Bolus injection:
  5–10 µg/kg b.w.
  Epidural infusion:
  20–50 µg/h.

Chapter 41

Complications (Fig. 41.26)

Early complications

During injection or when introducing the catheter

- Collapse (vasovagal reaction).
- Dural perforation.
- Catheter shearing.
- Spinal cord injury.
- Trauma to a nerve root.

After identifying the epidural space and administering a test dose

- Subarachnoid injection.
- Intravascular injection.

During and after injection of the full dose of a local anesthetic, during the fixation phase

- Massive epidural anesthesia.
- Total spinal anesthesia.
- Subdural spread.
- Intravascular injection, with toxic reactions.

During the surgical procedure

- Drop in blood pressure.
- Respiratory disturbance.
- Drop in body temperature.
- Muscle tremor.

Complications in the early postoperative phase

- Difficulty with micturition.

Late complications

- Postdural puncture headache.
- Back pain.
- Neurological complications.

Complications that can develop at any time with an epidural catheter in position

- Dural perforation.
- Total spinal anesthesia.
- Subdural injection.
- Intravascular injection.
- Urinary retention.
- Infections.

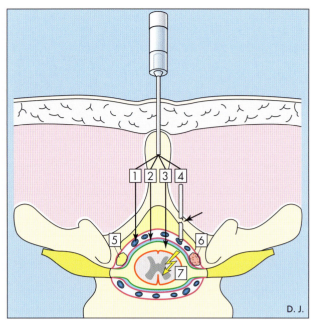

Fig. 41.26 Complications.
(1) Intravascular injection, (2) subdural injection, (3) subarachnoid injection, (4) catheter shearing, (5) epidural abscess, (6) epidural hematoma, (7) injury to the spinal cord and nerve roots

- Catheter shearing when removing the catheter.
- Neurological complications.

Inadvertent dural puncture

This is caused by poor technique. As epidural puncture needles have a large lumen (16–18 G), the probability of developing postdural puncture headache is very high (70–80%; see Chapter 37, p. 287).
Depending on whether or not the inadvertent dural puncture is noticed, various steps can be taken.

When dural puncture is noted:
- Administer a spinal dose and carry out spinal anesthesia.
- New attempt at insertion.
- Switch to general anesthesia.

When dural perforation is not noticed:
- Accidental subarachnoid injection of an epidural dose leads to total spinal anesthesia, with very serious sequelae (see Chapter 37, section on high and total anesthesia, p. 285).

The patient should be informed immediately and made aware of the possible complications.

Prophylaxis
- Stay in the midline during the insertion procedure.
- Always advance the needle millimeter by millimeter after passing the ligamentum flavum.
- Aspiration test.
- Test dose.
- At every additional injection into the positioned epidural catheter, observe the same safety measures as with the single-shot injection.
- Maintain constant verbal contact with the patient.
- Check the spread of anesthesia frequently.
- Careful monitoring.

Therapy
See Chapter 37, section on postdural puncture headache, p. 287.

Massive epidural anesthesia

Massive epidural anesthesia arises due to overdose of local anesthetic and its absorption at the injection site. The condition develops more slowly than with an intravascular injection and in extreme cases it can lead to generalized tonic–clonic seizures (see Chapter 6).

Subdural spread of local anesthetic

See Chapter 37, p. 286.

Intravascular injection

This can occur during the administration of a test dose, during a single-shot injection or during the injection of a local anesthetic through the catheter and it can lead to severe toxic reactions (see Chapter 6, p. 66 and Chapter 1, p. 9).

Prophylaxis
Before any single-shot injection or injection through the positioned catheter:
- Aspiration test.
- Test dose of a local anesthetic containing epinephrine.

Involvement of cranial and cervical nerves

High spread of an epidurally injected local anesthetic or a sudden increase in CSF pressure can lead to the following complications, which are mostly transient: hearing loss caused by transfer to the cochlear perilymph space; visual defects (in the most severe cases, retinal bleeding or even blindness); trigeminal nerve palsy, with weakness in the muscles of mastication; facial palsy (see Chapter 37, blood patch injection, p. 289); the development of Horner's syndrome.

Catheter shearing

Shearing of the catheter can occur both when it is being introduced and when it is being removed.

Prophylaxis
When placing the catheter:
When technical difficulties occur during insertion, the catheter and the spinal needle are always removed simultaneously. A catheter must never be withdrawn through the needle.

During catheter removal:
When the catheter is being removed, any elastic resistance should be noted. Force should never be used when pulling. If necessary, wait until the patient is able to stand up and pull the catheter during flexion or slight extension of the back.
After the catheter has been removed, it should be checked to ensure the tip has not broken off. A record must be kept.
If shearing occurs, the patient must be informed immediately. Neurological monitoring is obligatory, but surgery is very rarely indicated.

Transient neurological symptoms (TNS)

See Chapter 37, p. 290.

Neurological complications

Injury to the spinal cord and nerve roots
This is an extremely rare complication, since most insertions are carried out below the conus medullaris. Neurological injuries can occur in all forms of neuraxial regional anesthesia.

Prophylaxis
- Advance the puncture needle with the utmost care.
- Stop the procedure immediately if pain occurs
  - During insertion
  - While introducing the catheter
  - During the injection (intraneural placement)
- A catheter should be advanced at most 3–4 cm into the epidural space
- Puncture should be avoided at all costs in adult patients under general anesthesia, particularly above the L2 segment.

Bacterial meningitis

Strict asepsis is absolutely necessary when carrying out the block. A block is contraindicated when there is septic disease or infection in the area of the injection site.

Epidural abscess

The main cause of epidural abscess is *Staphylococcus aureus* [24]. The symptoms, which develop slowly (high fever, significant cervical or cervicothoracic and/or lumbar pain) require urgent investigation (erythrocyte sedimentation rate, blood culture, CSF measurement, myelography, CT, MRI). Immediate surgical treatment (laminectomy, drainage) within 12 hours is important to reduce complications.

Epidural abscesses are extremely rare and usually occur spontaneously. Earlier references to them in the literature involved continuous caudal blocks in which the necessary sterile conditions were ignored. However, numerous studies [1, 2, 12, 24, 40, 76, 92] report evidence of a connection between pre-existing sepsis and the development of abscesses after epidural anesthesia.

Systemic and local infections at the injection site are therefore an absolute contraindication to epidural anesthesia.

Epidural hematoma

This is an extremely rare but feared complication. It is characterized by rapid development of the classic symptoms, although these are not necessarily all evident in the reported occurrences in every patient affected: initial loss of consciousness, severe pain, substantial neurological disturbances, a lucid interval with normalization of the neurological status, headache and increasing clouding of consciousness, simultaneous pupillary dilatation, Cheyne–Stokes respiration, bradycardia, unconsciousness.

Any complaints by the patient regarding pain, fever, or radicular symptoms must be immediately investigated. Maintaining constant contact with the patient, particularly after an outpatient procedure, is mandatory. Immediate diagnostic clarification (myelography, CT, MRI) and immediate neurosurgical treatment within the first 12 hours are important for the prognosis.

The risk factors reported in the literature [44, 91, 101] include trauma, vascular disease, coagulation disturbances and anticoagulant treatment.

Cauda equina syndrome

See Chapter 37, p. 292.

42 Thoracic epidural anesthesia

Epidural injection or placement of a catheter for continuous epidural administration of a local anesthetic, opioid, or combination of the two in the region of the thoracic spine.

Advantages
- Excellent analgesia.
- The injection of local anesthetic takes place directly into the selected thoracic segment. This allows a lower dose per segment (e.g. 0.5–0.8 mL) and provides more targeted anesthesia of the surgical area – without affecting sensory or motor function in the pelvis or lower extremities, or bladder function.
- Better postoperative pulmonary function.
- Early mobilization.
- Improved blood flow to the area of surgery.
- Improved peristalsis.
- In addition, the risk of toxic reactions is lower.

Disadvantage
Potential traumatic puncture of the spinal cord. A specific and valid indication is therefore necessary.

Prerequisite
Very experienced, technically skilled anesthetist.

Anatomy (Figs. 42.1, 42.2)

The thoracic spinous processes form varying angles with their vertebral bodies. At the upper and lower boundaries of the thoracic spine with the cervical spine (C7, T1–3) and lumbar spine (T10–12, L1), the spinous processes are almost parallel to the sagittal plane. The angle of puncture when locating the epidural space is thus almost identical to that in the lumbar region. It should also be noted that in the region of the lower thoracic spine (T10–12, L1) the distance from the skin to the spinal canal is slightly less, due to the shorter spinous processes.

In the central area of the thoracic spine (T4–9), the spinous processes have a very caudal angle and the laminae of the vertebral bodies are slanted. The ligamentum flavum becomes thinner over its lumbar to cranial course and the epidural space becomes narrow-

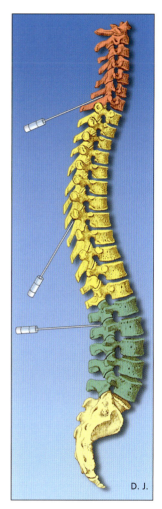

Fig. 42.1 Anatomy: cervical, thoracic and lumbar spine

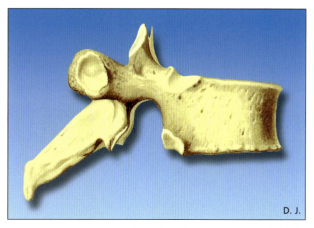

Fig. 42.2 Steep caudal angle of the spinous processes in T4–T9

er: 6 mm in the lumbar spine, 3–5 mm in the thoracic spine and 2–3 mm in the cervical spine. In the central thoracic area, the dura mater is ca. 1 mm thick.
These anatomic facts determine the puncture technique.

Indications

Surgical indications (Table 42.1)
- Upper abdominal, thoracic and thoraco-abdominal procedures in combination with general anesthesia, with subsequent continuation of continuous postoperative pain therapy with local anesthetics, opioids, or a combination of the two.

Table 42.1 Thoracic epidural anesthesia combined with basic general anesthesia

Surgical procedures and injection levels required

	Procedure	Injection level
Chest	Cardiac surgery	T2
	Pulmonary resection, esophagectomy	T4–6
Upper abdomen	Gastrectomy, liver and pancreatic surgery	T6
Lower abdomen	Bowel resection, gynecological tumor surgery	T10
Extraperitoneal and retroperitoneal procedures	Vascular surgery, retroperitoneal lymphadenectomy, renal surgery, prostatectomy	T8

Indications for pain therapy
- Fractures to a series of ribs.
- Post-herpetic neuralgia.
- Acute pancreatitis.
- Cancer pain.

Contraindications
- The contraindications are the same as those for lumbar epidural anesthesia (see Chapter 41, p. 306).
- Puncture is absolutely contraindicated in adult patients under general anesthesia.

Procedure

Full prior information for the patient is mandatory.

Preparation and materials
- Check that the emergency equipment is complete and in working order (intubation kit, emergency drugs); sterile precautions, intravenous access, anesthetic machine.
- Start an intravenous infusion and give a volume load (250–500 mL of a balanced electrolyte solution).
- Careful monitoring: ECG, BP, pulse oximetry.
- Skin prep.
- Local anesthetic.

Epidural needles
18-G Tuohy or Crawford (see Chapter 41, Fig. 41.3).

Access routes
Puncture of the epidural space is carried with on the same principles as for the lumbar region.

> Epidural puncture must be avoided at all costs in patients who are under general anesthesia.

The acute insertion angle in the T4–T9 region should be noted. Insertion can be carried out in the midline (median) or laterally (paramedian), with the patient sitting or in the lateral decubitus position. For a midline insertion, the cervicothoracic transition (C7, T1–3) or the lower thoracic region (T10–12) are suitable. A paramedian puncture can be used at all levels of the thoracic spine, particularly in the central area from T4 to T9.

Midline insertion in the sitting position
The sitting position is helpful, as it increases the negative pressure in the epidural space, particularly during inspiration.
The patient sits relaxed and leaning slightly forward, with the neck flexed and the arms crossed, supported by an assistant. The patient must be aware of the importance of sitting still during the puncture procedure.

Location, skin prep, local anesthesia, skin incision
After thorough skin prep (strict asepsis), a sterile drape is placed on the puncture area and the puncture site in the selected intervertebral space is anesthetized with 1.5–2 mL 1% prilocaine. During infiltration with a needle 3 cm long, the insertion angle is assessed. A skin incision with a stylet or lumen needle follows.

Puncture of the supraspinous and interspinous ligament and ligamentum flavum
An 18-G Tuohy needle with the bevel directed cranially, or a Crawford needle with a caudally directed bevel, is introduced at an angle of about 45° up to a depth of about 2.5 cm, until it is lying firmly in the interspinous ligament. The trochar is then removed.

Thoracic epidural anesthesia

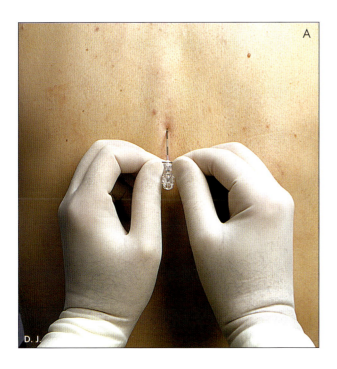
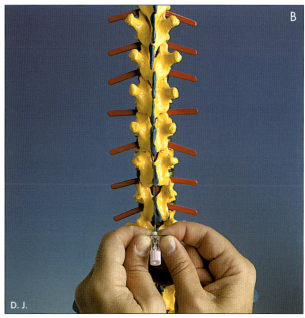

Fig. 42.3a, b Median puncture. "Hanging drop" technique

> Advancing the needle further after leaving the interspinous ligament must be carried out millimeter by millimeter and carefully, towards the ligamentum flavum

Puncturing the epidural space
Identification of the epidural space can be carried out using the loss-of-resistance technique or using the "hanging drop" technique with saline.

Loss-of-resistance technique (Fig. 42.4)
See Chapter 41, Fig. 41.10.

"Hanging drop" technique (Fig. 42.3; see Chapter 41, Fig. 41.11)
With this technique, high negative pressure in the thoracic epidural space during inspiration is helpful. After removal of the trochar from the puncture needle, a drop of the saline or local anesthetic is placed within the hub of the needle and the needle is advanced toward the ligamentum flavum.

The thumbs and index fingers of both hands secure the needle and advance it millimeter by millimeter, with both thumbs firmly supported on the patient's back fulfilling a braking function. The anesthetist's eyes are fixed on the "hanging drop." When the epidural space is reached, the drop is sucked in during the inspiration phase and a loss of resistance in the tissue is felt.

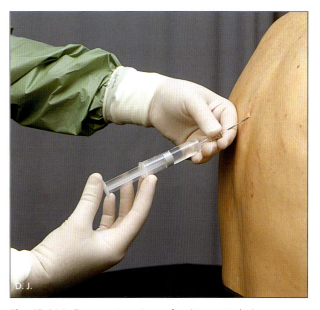

Fig. 42.4 Median puncture. Loss-of-resistance technique

Paramedian insertion
This access route circumvents the sharply angled spinous processes and the supraspinous and interspinous ligaments.
Local anesthesia is applied about 1.5 cm lateral to the caudal tip of the spinous process in the selected area.
This fan-shaped anesthesia allows the depth of the laminae to be measured and marked.

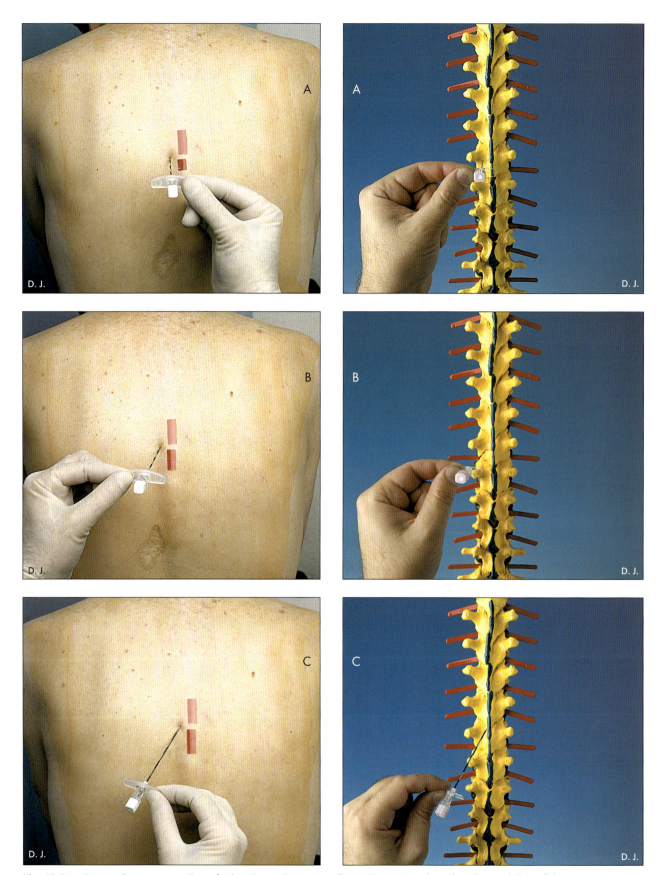

Fig. 42.5a–c Paramedian puncture. Steps for location. **a** Step 1: needle position 1.5 cm lateral to the caudal tip of the spinous process. **b** Step 2: angle of 15° to the sagittal plane. **c** Step 3: angle of 55–60° to the skin surface

The epidural needle is advanced alongside the spinous process at an angle of 15° to the sagittal plane and 55–60° to the skin surface or long axis of the spine (Fig. 42.5). After the ligamentum flavum has been passed, identification of the epidural space is carried out using the loss-of-resistance technique with saline.

Dosages

The dose of local anesthetic in the thoracic region is 15–30% lower than in the lumbar region, at about 0.5–0.8 mL per segment.

Local anesthetics

Ropivacaine

Incremental bolus injection: 0.75%, 5–15 mL (depending on the injection site).
Epidural infusion: 0.2%, 8–10 mL/h (max. 37.5 mg/h).

Bupivacaine

Incremental bolus injection: 0.25–0.5%, 4–6 mL (for 2–4 thoracic segments).
Epidural infusion: 0.125%, 5–10 mL/h.

Levobupivacaine

Incremental bolus injection: 0.25–0.5%, 4–6 mL (for 2–4 thoracic segments).
Epidural infusion: 0.125%, 5–10 mL/h.

Combination of local anesthetics and opioids

Ropivacaine and sufentanil

Bolus injection: Ropivacaine 0.5% (7–9 mL, puncture site T8–T9), (10–12 mL, puncture site T9–T11) + sufentanil 30 µg.
Epidural infusion: Ropivacaine 0.2% + sufentanil 0.5 µg/mL. Speed: 5–7 mL/h.

Bupivacaine and sufentanil

Bolus injection: Bupivacaine (0.25%), 5 mL + 1 µg/mL sufentanil.
Epidural infusion: Bupivacaine (0.125–0.0625%) + sufentanil 0.2–0.3 µg/mL. Speed: 6–10 mL/h.

Bupivacaine and fentanyl

Bolus injection: Bupivacaine (0.25–0.5%), 5 mL + 50 µg fentanyl.
Epidural infusion: Bupivacaine (0.125%) + 1–2 µg/mL fentanyl. Speed: 6–10 mL/h.

Administration of opioids via the epidural catheter – lumbar or thoracic?

Lipid-soluble opioids

The precise mechanism involved in the action of epidurally administered lipid-soluble opioids is a matter of controversy. According to a number of more recent investigations, the blocking of pain by lipid-soluble opioids after epidural administration is more the result of systemic uptake than a direct effect on spinal opioid receptors. The positioning of the epidural catheter would therefore be of secondary importance.

As some studies have reported [4, 48, 60, 74], opioid infusion via a lumbar epidural catheter has been used successfully for pain relief after thoracotomy.

The authors conclude that the generally less familiar and potentially more dangerous thoracic access route is not justifiable.

Morphine as a hydrophilic substance

Morphine is hydrophilic and spreads quickly in the CSF, and it is therefore able to produce analgesia for thoracic procedures even when it is injected into the caudal epidural space. Several studies have shown that lumbar administration of epidural morphine for pain relief after thoracotomy or after high abdominal surgery is just as effective as thoracic administration [9, 33, 74].

Specific complications

Spinal cord injury is among the extremely rare complications with this procedure (see Chapter 41).

Record and checklist

Thoracic catheter epidural anesthesia

Name: _____ Date: _____
Diagnosis: _____
Premedication: ☐ No ☐ Yes _____
Neurological abnormalities: ☐ No ☐ Yes _____

Purpose of block: ☐ Surgical ☐ Treatment (postoperative)
Needle: ☐ Tuohy G ____ ☐ Other ____
i.v. access, infusion: ☐ Yes
Monitoring: ☐ ECG ☐ Pulse oximetry
Ventilation facilities: ☐ Yes (equipment checked)
Emergency equipment (drugs): ☐ Checked
Patient: ☐ Informed

Position: ☐ Lateral decubitus ☐ Sitting
Access: ☐ Median ☐ Paramedian
Injection level: ☐ T _____
Injection technique: ☐ Loss of resistance ☐ Other _____
Epidural space: ☐ Identified
Catheter: ☐ Advanced 3–4 cm cranially
Aspiration test: ☐ Carried out
Catheter end positioned lower than the injection site ☐
Bacterial filter: ☐
Test dose: _____ Epinephrine added: ☐ Yes ☐ No
Check on sensorimotor function after 5 min: ☐ Carried out
Abnormalities: ☐ No ☐ Yes _____
Injection:
☐ Local anesthetic: _____ mL ____ %
  (incremental)
☐ Addition: _____ µg/mg
☐ Additional injection (incremental): _____ mL ____ %

Patient's remarks during injection:
☐ None ☐ Pain ☐ Paresthesias ☐ Warmth
Duration and area: _____
Objective block effect after 20 min:
☐ Cold test ☐ Temperature measurement before ____°C after ____°C
☐ Sensory: L _____ T _____ ☐ Motor

Complications:
☐ None ☐ Radicular symptoms ☐ BP drop ☐ Vascular puncture
☐ Massive epidural anesthesia ☐ Subdural spread ☐ Drop in body temperature
☐ Bladder emptying disturbances ☐ Back pain ☐ Pain ☐ Vasovagal reactions
☐ Dural puncture ☐ Intravascular injection ☐ Total spinal anesthesia
☐ Respiratory disturbance ☐ Muscle tremor ☐ Postdural puncture headache
☐ Neurological complications

Special notes:

© Copyright ABW Wissenschaftsverlag 2004,
Jankovic, Regional nerve blocks and infiltration therapy, 3rd edition

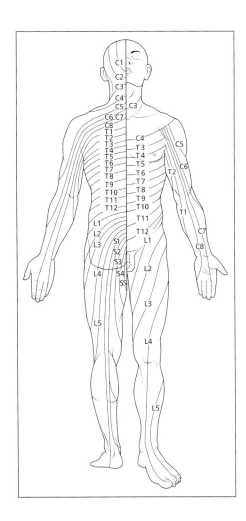

43 Epidural anesthesia in obstetrics

The goal of epidural anesthesia in normal deliveries is sensory block of the desired segments (first stage: T10–T11, L1; second stage: L2–S4/S5), with the lowest possible concentrations of a local anesthetic, opioid, or a combination of the two.

In Cesarean sections, the aim is to achieve adequate anesthesia (T4–6) with larger doses.

Anatomic and physiological changes during pregnancy

Anatomic changes

- During pregnancy, the epidural space narrows due to venous dilation, since some of the blood from the lower extremities is transported via epidural veins to the superior vena cava (see Chapter 35, Fig. 35.18).
  The local anesthetic must therefore be given at a lower dose in pregnant patients.
- There is loosening of the vertebral ligaments and marked pooling of fluid in the tissues.
  This makes it more difficult to identify the epidural space, and there is an increased risk of dural puncture. Particularly during uterine contractions, the negative pressure in the epidural space is lost.

Physiological changes

Respiratory tract
Movement of the diaphragm in the cranial direction increases minute volume by 40%. This causes hyperventilation, with increased oxygen consumption (+ 20%), with peak values during birth (+ 40% in the first stage, up to + 100% during the second stage).

Cardiovascular system
The increase in heart rate and the resulting rise in cardiac output reach a maximum of up to 40% by the 34th gestational week.
This increase is marked in the uteroplacental unit and kidneys. By contrast, arterial blood pressure does not increase.

Gastrointestinal tract
The stomach shifts cranially, resulting in increased intragastric pressure, with a tendency toward reflux, reduced tone, reduced motility and a resultant delay in gastric emptying. The risk of aspiration is increased during tracheal intubation for anesthesia.

Blood volume
Blood volume increases by about 30%.

Labor pain

Two types of labor pain are distinguished, depending on the stage of labor (Fig. 43.1).

First stage
Pain in the first stage of labor primarily results from dilation of the cervix and lower uterine segment and distension of the body of the uterus (10–12 hours in a primipara, 6–8 hours in a multipara). It is characterized by painful uterine contractions.

Visceral dilation pain is caused by uterine contractions and dilation of the cervix and lower segment of the uterus.

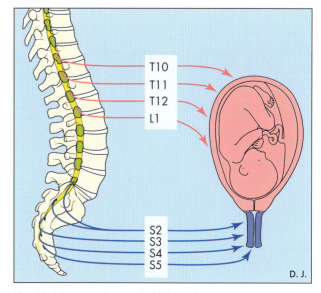

Fig. 43.1 Segmental spread of labor pain

This pain is conducted via unmyelinated C-fibers, which enter the spinal cord through the posterior roots of the spinal nerves – in the early stage at T11–T12 and in the later stage at T10 and L1.

The pain radiates into the lower abdomen, groin, inside of the thighs and dorsally into the lumbar region, hip region and sacrum.

Second stage
This pain covers the period between full dilatation of the cervix (10 cm) and birth of the child. This period lasts 30–40 minutes in a primipara and 20–30 minutes in a multipara.

The pain is caused by dilation of the vagina, vulva and pelvic floor.

Somatic perineal pain in the area innervated by the pudendal nerve is conducted via myelinated A-delta fibers and also includes segments T10 to L1 and L2 to S4–S5 (Fig. 43.1).

Specific risks in obstetric anesthesia

Increased risk of aspiration during intubation for anesthesia

> All patients in late pregnancy are regarded having a full stomach.

Prophylaxis
- 30 mL sodium citrate (0.3 mol/L) about 30 minutes before the start of anesthesia.
- 400 mg cimetidine p.o. (200 mg i.v.) or ranitidine.
- 10 mg metoclopramide i.v.

Aortocaval compression syndrome

At the end of pregnancy, there is pressure from the dilated uterus on the inferior vena cava and lower abdominal aorta when the patient is in the supine position.

Mechanism
A reduction in venous return to the heart, with a decrease in cardiac output and a drop in arterial blood pressure caudal to the compression area. Since the perfusion of the uterine vessels is directly correlated with arterial blood pressure, in untreated cases there may be a risk to the mother or a risk of fetal asphyxia due to reduced blood flow to the uteroplacental unit.

Compensatory mechanism
A collateral circulation occurs via the azygos vein system and sympathetic tone is increased to stimulate venous return to the heart. If the collateral circulation is not sufficient, or if sympathetic tone is canceled out by epidural anesthesia, a dangerous drop in cardiac output and/or arterial blood pressure may occur, with symptoms of shock.

The critical threshold for a drop in blood pressure is 70–80 mmHg, but values between 90 and 100 mmHg over a period of 10–15 minutes can also threaten the fetus if not treated.

Clinical symptoms
Nausea, faintness, pallor, sweating, breathing difficulty.

Prophylaxis
- Left lateral position or at a 15° angle to the left (with a wedge-shaped cushion under the right hip (Fig. 43.2), or using the palm of the hand to displace the uterus to the left (Fig. 43.3).
- Adequate volume load before anesthesia (1000 mL in vaginal delivery, 1500–2000 mL of a balanced electrolyte solution in Cesarean section).
- Give oxygen.
- Vasopressor administration – provided intravascular volume is adequate. The drug of choice is ephedrine 10–20 mg i. v.

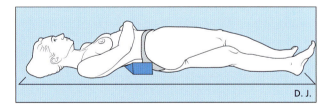

Fig. 43.2 Wedge-shaped cushion under the right hip

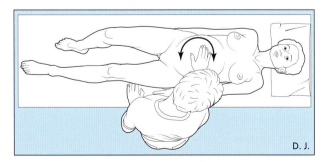

Fig. 43.3 Displacing the uterus to the left

Hypotension

A drop in maternal blood pressure is the most frequent complication of epidural anesthesia. In untreated cases, it leads to reduced blood flow to the uteroplacental unit and fetal asphyxia.

Prophylaxis
- Infusion of a balanced electrolyte solution 20 minutes before the start of anesthesia.
- Prevention of the aortocaval compression syndrome.

Treatment
- Increase in fluid administration.
- Slight Trendelenburg position (10°).
- Give oxygen.
- Vasopressor.

Indications [81]

Maternal
- Labor pain.
- Pulmonary disease (e.g. asthma, upper airway infection).
- Cardiovascular disease.
- Metabolic disease (e.g. diabetes mellitus).
- Neurological diseases (e.g. epilepsy, aneurysms of the cerebral vessels, arteriovenous malformations).
- Pre-eclampsia.

Fetal
- Premature birth.
- Growth retardation.
- Breech presentation.
- Multiple pregnancy.

Obstetric
- Prolonged labor or arrested labor.
- High-risk birth.
- Induction of birth with oxytocin.
- Uncoordinated uterine activity (dystocia).

Anesthesiological
- Anticipated tracheal intubation difficulties.
- Obesity.
- Suspicion or history of malignant hyperthermia.

Contraindications
General
See Chapter 41, p. 306.

Specific
- Placenta previa.
- Prolapse of the umbilical cord.
- Acute fetal asphyxia.

Relative
- Prior Cesarean section (unnoticed uterine rupture).
- Placental abruption (absence of pain).

Procedure

Full prior information for the patient is mandatory.

- Insertion should only be carried out during a pause in labor (the negative epidural pressure is lost during uterine contractions and there is therefore a risk of dural perforation).
- The oxytocin drip should be interrupted during administration of a local anesthetic. Oxytocin administration can only be resumed 15 minutes after the last major dose of a local anesthetic and when the cardiotocogram is normal.
- The membranes should not be ruptured within 30 minutes before or after administration of a major dose of local anesthetic.
- Insertion of an epidural catheter and administration of a local anesthetic can only be carried out if the cervix has opened 5–6 cm in a primipara or 3–4 cm in a multipara.

Preparation and materials
- Check that the emergency equipment is complete and in working order (intubation kit, emergency drugs).
- Strict asepsis.
- Intravenous access, anesthetic machine.
- Ensure adequate intravenous volume load with a balanced electrolyte solution (500–1000 mL).
- Careful monitoring: ECG, BP, pulse oximetry.
- Monitoring of bladder function (atonic bladder during epidural anesthesia!).
- Continuous fetal monitoring.

The use of a purpose-made kit for epidural anesthesia is recommended (e.g. from B. Braun Melsungen).

Patient positioning
The patient is usually placed on the left side; more rarely, a sitting position is adopted – e.g. in obese patients or in those with severe spinal deformities.

Location, skin prep, local anesthesia, skin incision
Location and marking of the puncture site (L2/3 or L3/4) is followed by thorough skin prep, covering with a drape, local anesthesia and skin incision using a hemostylet.

Puncturing the epidural space

Puncture is carried out in the midline using a Tuohy needle (16–18 G) with the bevel directed cranially. The loss-of-resistance technique is used to identify the epidural space (low-friction 10-mL syringe, filled with saline and with a small air bubble; advance with constant pressure on the plunger as far as the epidural space).
The catheter is advanced a maximum of 3–4 cm into the epidural space.
After aspiration, the open end of the catheter is placed below the puncture site on the sterile drape and any escaping fluid (CSF or blood) is noted.

Administration of a test dose

3–4 mL 0.5% ropivacaine, or 0.25% bupivacaine, or 1% mepivacaine with epinephrine added.

The addition of epinephrine in obstetrics is controversial, as it can lead to false-positive reactions and reduced uteroplacental perfusion in about 27% of pregnant patients.
In patients who are receiving beta-blockers, there may be an increase in blood pressure without an increase in the pulse frequency.
As increases in pulse rate and blood pressure often occur spontaneously during birth, a false-positive response is possible.
Many authors therefore recommend using epinephrine-containing test doses only if the situation is uncertain [19, 57, 63].

During the waiting period of 5 minutes, verbal contact with the patient must always be maintained and the spread of the anesthesia must be monitored.

Incremental administration of local anesthetic

If there is no evidence of intravascular or subarachnoid injection, incremental administration of a local anesthetic is now carried out (5 mL each in several test doses), until anesthesia has reached the desired level.
During this phase, particular attention should be given to the patient's position (not supine).
During the following 20–30 minutes, the spread of the sensory block must be monitored.

- Repeated aspiration.
- Use a test dose.
- Select the lowest possible dosage.
- Always inject on an incremental basis (with several test doses).
- Maintain verbal contact.
- Careful monitoring.

Local anesthetic and opioids in obstetrics

Local anesthetics

Due to their physicochemical properties, local anesthetics cross the placenta easily. Independent of the site of injection, amide local anesthetics appear very quickly in the maternal and fetal circulation and produce higher plasma levels.
Concentrations in the umbilical blood after the injection of ropivacaine, bupivacaine, or etidocaine are lower (high protein binding of over 90% in maternal blood) than those of lidocaine and mepivacaine (50–70% binds to plasma proteins).
The elimination half-lives in the newborn are 3 hours for lidocaine, 9 hours for mepivacaine, 8 hours for bupivacaine and 6.5 hours for etidocaine.

Most important local anesthetic in obstetrics

Ropivacaine

Ropivacaine is structurally similar to bupivacaine and it has a similar profile of activity, but it has a much lower cardiotoxic potential.
According to plasma studies in neonates and their mothers, it has a stable and high level of maternal protein binding (94%), so that placental transmission is limited.
In relation to analgesia and motor block, ropivacaine is equivalent to bupivacaine. The onset of effect, duration of effect and anesthetic quality are also comparable to those of bupivacaine [3, 30].
The concentrations used vary from 0.5% to 0.75 (Cesarean section) up to 0.2% (vaginal delivery).
Ropivacaine produces a very good differential sensorimotor block (good analgesic quality with largely preserved motor function – up to 80% of patients have no measurable motor block on the Bromage scale).
At a concentration of 2 mg/mL, ropivacaine is thus the agent of choice for epidural obstetric and postoperative analgesia.

Single-shot injection
Five minutes after administration of the test dose, 10–20 mL 0.2% ropivacaine (20–40 mg) is injected on an incremental basis.
Onset of effect after 10–15 min, duration of effect 30–90 min.

Intermittent epidural analgesia
10–15 mL 0.2% ropivacaine (20–30 mg).

Continuous-infusion epidural analgesia (CIEA)
0.2% ropivacaine, speed 6–10 mL (12–20 mg)/h (max. 37.5 mg/h).

Bupivacaine

Bupivacaine has been used successfully in obstetrics for many years as a long-acting amide local anesthetic. The concentrations used vary from 0.5% (Cesarean section) to 0.25% (vaginal delivery) up to 0.125–0.0625%, usually in combination with opioids.

Low-dose bupivacaine (0.125%) leads to effective analgesia in some 70% of mothers giving birth. Higher concentrations (0.5%) are often associated with a motor block, which is not desirable in a normal delivery. Higher concentrations (0.75%) should be avoided in obstetrics. The cardiotoxicity of bupivacaine must be regarded as a considerable disadvantage [81].

Single-shot injection
After a test dose of 3–4 mL 0.25–0.5% bupivacaine (or 3 mL of a 1% epinephrine-containing mepivacaine solution), 15 mL 0.5% or 20 mL 0.375% bupivacaine (3–5 mL) are injected on an incremental basis.

Intermittent epidural analgesia
After a test dose of 3–4 mL 0.25–0.5% bupivacaine (or 3 mL of a 1% epinephrine-containing mepivacaine solution), injection of an initial dose of 5–8 mL 0.25% (or 0.125%) bupivacaine (titrated in smaller portions) is given until a segmental level of T10 is reached.

Additional injections
Intermittent administration is continued with additional injections of 0.125% (8–16 mL) or 0.25% (5–8 mL) bupivacaine at intervals of 60–90 minutes, or as required.

During the first stage of labor, the local anesthetic dose is injected with one half in the right and left lateral positions, or the full dose with the patient supine (persistent leftward displacement of the uterus).

During the second stage, the patient's trunk should be raised by about 30–60° in order to reach lower segments.

> Every new bolus of a drug involves the same risks as the initial bolus. It is possible to confuse overdose with underdose.

Continuous-infusion epidural analgesia (CIEA)
Five minutes after the administration of the test dose, 5–8 mL 0.25% bupivacaine is injected in smaller increments.

After 30 minutes, if all is well, the continuous infusion can be started: 6 mL 0.25% or 10–15 mL 0.125% bupivacaine per hour.

Careful monitoring of the circulation and checking of the anesthetic spread must be carried out.

Lidocaine

Lidocaine is rarely used for epidural anesthesia in obstetrics, as it produces a marked motor block even at relatively low doses. The duration of effect is 60–90 minutes. Due to its rapid onset, lidocaine is very suitable for short-term augmentation of epidural anesthesia (10–15 mL of a 1.5–2% solution; see also p. 248).

2–3% 2-chloroprocaine

Chloroprocaine is a fast-acting local anesthetic that is toxicologically one of the safest of the ester type, and it has proved its value particularly in emergency situations [81].

It is hydrolyzed to inactive metabolites very quickly even at high dosages (short duration of effect of about 30–60 minutes) and has hardly any effect on the neonate's condition. Chloroprocaine is a very good supplement to bupivacaine, particularly if large amounts of bupivacaine have already been used during a Cesarean section.

Single-shot injection
2% 2-chloroprocaine: 10–15 mL, onset of effect after 4-6 minutes, duration of effect 30–45 minutes.
3% 2-chloroprocaine: 10 mL, onset of effect after 4–6 minutes, duration of effect 45–60 minutes.

The analgesic effect of an opioid injected subsequently (fentanyl) is reduced by antagonism caused by chloroprocaine at the opiate receptor [22]. This local anesthetic is mainly used in the USA, but has recently also been adopted in Switzerland.

Opioids

When opioids alone are used in obstetric anesthesia, adequate analgesia is only achieved in the treatment of visceral pain in the first stage of labor.

Somatic pain in the second stage is more difficult to manage [74, 81].

The rapidly-acting lipophilic opioids sufentanil and fentanyl, which have a duration of effect of 2–3 hours, have replaced the more hydrophilic morphine (duration of effect 8–24 hours).

The agents of choice are low-dose sufentanil or fentanyl in combination with low-dose bupivacaine in the form of an epidural infusion.

Advantages
- Faster onset.
- Longer duration of analgesia.
- Lower total dose of local anesthetic and opioid (about 20–25%).
- Reduced motor block.
- No significant side effects for the mother or child.

Continuous-infusion epidural analgesia (CIEA) [34, 74, 98, 99]

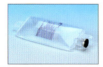

Sufentanil and ropivacaine
After administering a test dose and incremental bolus administration of 15 mL 0.1% ropivacaine and 1–2 µg/mL sufentanil (10–20 µg), the continuous infusion can be started:
0.1% ropivacaine and 0.2–0.3 µg/mL sufentanil.
Speed: 10 mL/h.

Fentanyl and ropivacaine
After administering a test dose and incremental bolus administration of 15 mL 0.1% ropivacaine and 30 µg fentanyl, the continuous infusion can be started:
0.1% ropivacaine and 2 µg/mL sufentanil.
Speed: 10–12 mL/h.

Sufentanil and bupivacaine (levobupivacaine)
After administering a test dose and bolus administration of 10 mL 0.125–0.0625% bupivacaine (0.125–0.0625% levobupivacaine) and 1–2 µg/mL sufentanil (10–20 µg), the continuous infusion can be started after about 30 minutes:
0.0625–0.125% bupivacaine (0.0625–0.125% levobupivacaine)and 0.2–0.3 µg/mL sufentanil.
Speed: 6–10 mL/h.

Fentanyl and bupivacaine (levobupivacaine)
After administering a test dose and bolus administration of 10 mL 0.25% bupivacaine (0.25% levobupivacaine) and 50 µg fentanyl, the continuous infusion can be started after about 30 minutes:
0.0625% bupivacaine (0.0625% levobupivacaine) and 1–2 µg/mL fentanyl.
Speed: 10 mL/h.

Patient-controlled epidural analgesia (PCEA) [34, 74]

Sufentanil and ropivacaine
0.1% ropivacaine and 1 µg/mL sufentanil.
Speed: 5–10 mL/h.
Bolus dose: 5 mL.
Lockout period: 10–20 min.

Fentanyl and ropivacaine
0.1% ropivacaine and 2 µg/mL sufentanil.
Speed: 10 mL/h.
Bolus dose: 10 mL.
Lockout period: 10–20 min.

Sufentanil and bupivacaine (levobupivacaine)
After administering a test dose and bolus administration of 5–10 mL 0.125% bupivacaine (0.125% levobupivacaine) and 10–30 µg/mL sufentanil, the continuous infusion can be started:
0.0625% bupivacaine (0.0625% levobupivacaine) and 1 µg/mL sufentanil.
Basic setting: Speed 5 mL/h (5 µg sufentanil)
Bolus dose 5 mL (5 µg sufentanil)
Lockout period: 20 min.

Fentanyl and bupivacaine (levobupivacaine)
After administering a test dose and bolus administration of 6–10 mL 0.125–0.25% bupivacaine (0.125–0.25% levobupivacaine)and 10 µg fentanyl, incremental until segment T10 is reached, the continuous infusion can be started:
0.125% bupivacaine (0.125% levobupivacaine) and 0.0001% fentanyl [81].
Basic setting: Speed 4 mL/h
Bolus dose 4 mL
Lockout period: 20 min.

Epinephrine addition in obstetrics
Epinephrine has both alpha-adrenergic and beta-adrenergic effects. Adding epinephrine causes a dose-dependent reduction in uterine activity and leads to a delay in delivery. If there is inadvertent intravascular injection of a local anesthetic with epinephrine, adverse circulatory reactions can occur both in the mother (hypertonia, cardiac arrhythmia) and in the child (reduced placental perfusion due to vasoconstriction).
Any addition of epinephrine in obstetrics must therefore be strictly indicated.

Lumbar catheter epidural anesthesia in Cesarean section

When a Cesarean section is to be performed, the spread of the injected local anesthetic must reach segments T4 to T6. The higher the spread of the anesthesia, the greater the risk of severe hypotension. Segments L5, S1 and S2 are not always adequately anesthetized and there is often a delay in anesthesia in this area.

Procedure

Preparation, materials, prerequisites
See Chapter 41, p. 307.

Patient positioning
Left lateral decubitus for L2/3 or L3/4, or sitting (e.g. in obese patients or those with spinal deformities).

Puncture of the epidural space, test dose, incremental administration of local anesthetic

After identification of the epidural space and aspiration, a catheter is placed (see Chapter 41, section on continuous catheter epidural anesthesia, p. 317) and a test dose is administered.

After about 5 minutes, incremental injection of a local anesthetic can be carried out in small increments of up to 5 mL each (several test doses), until adequate anesthesia reaches the desired segmental level of T4 to T6. If the catheter is already in position, there is the following choice: if there has been no injection within the previous 30 minutes, then after testing of the spread of the anesthesia about 12–15 mL 0.75% ropivacaine or 0.5% bupivacaine can be injected on an incremental basis. Alternatively, if an injection has been given shortly before, then initially only 5–10 mL 0.75% ropivacaine or 0.5% bupivacaine is injected.

In a protracted birth with a large total dose of local anesthetic and subsequent Cesarean section or marked fetal acidosis, 2–3% 2-chloroprocaine should be used, due to its fast onset and short half-life in both mother and child.

Additional safety measures

- Supine positioning, with left lateral displacement of the uterus until birth of the child (slight Trendelenburg 10° if appropriate).
- Oxygen administration.
- Careful circulatory monitoring.
- Thorough checking of the spread of anesthesia shortly before the start of surgery.

Local anesthetics for Cesarean section

About 15–30 mL of local anesthetic is necessary for adequate anesthesia up to T4–T6 (Table 43.1).

Adjuvant opioids

The addition of sufentanil or fentanyl to bupivacaine or lidocaine improves analgesia significantly. The following doses can be used:
- Sufentanil: 30–50 µg.
- Fentanyl: 50–100 µg.

Table 43.1 Local anesthetics for Cesarean section

Local anesthetic	Volume (mL)	Onset of effect (min)	Duration of effect (min)
0.75% ropivacaine	15–20	10–20	180–300
0.5% ropivacaine	25–30	10–15	120–150
0.5% bupivacaine	15–30	15–20	120–180
0.5% levobupivacaine	15–30	10–15	120–180
1.5–2% lidocaine	15–25	10–15	45–60
(with the addition of epinephrine 1: 400 000; 0.05 mL in 20 mL of local anesthetic)			
2–3% 2-Chloroprocain	15–25	ca. 10	45–60

Record and checklist

Obstetric catheter epidural anesthesia

Name: _____ Date: _____
Diagnosis: _____
Premedication: ☐ No ☐ Yes _____
Neurological abnormalities: ☐ No ☐ Yes _____

Purpose of block: ☐ Vaginal delivery ☐ Cesarean section
Needle: ☐ Tuohy G ____ ☐ Other ____
i.v. access, infusion: ☐ Yes
Monitoring: ☐ ECG ☐ Pulse oximetry
Ventilation facilities: ☐ Yes (equipment checked)
Emergency equipment (drugs): ☐ Checked
Patient: ☐ Informed
Prerequisites met: ☐ Adequate volume supplementation
☐ Fetal monitoring ☐ No oxytocin drip ☐ No amniotomy
☐ Monitoring of bladder function ☐ Cervix 5–6 cm (primipara)
☐ Cervix 3–4 cm (multipara)

Position: ☐ Left lateral ☐ Sitting
Access: ☐ Median ☐ Paramedian
Injection level: ☐ L3/4 ☐ Other _____
Injection technique: ☐ Loss of resistance ☐ Other _____
Epidural space: ☐ Identified
Catheter: ☐ Advanced 3–4 cm cranially
Aspiration test: ☐ Carried out
Catheter end: ☐ Positioned lower than the injection site
Bacterial filter: ☐
Test dose: _____ Epinephrine added: ☐ Yes ☐ No
Check on sensorimotor function after 5 min: ☐ Carried out
Abnormalities: ☐ No ☐ Yes _____
Injection:
☐ Local anesthetic: _____ mL ____ %
   (incremental)
☐ Addition: _____ µg/mg
☐ Additional injection (incremental): _____ mL ____ %

Patient's remarks during injection:
☐ None ☐ Pain ☐ Paresthesias ☐ Warmth
Duration and area: _____
Objective block effect after 20 min:
☐ Cold test ☐ Temperature measurement before ____ °C after ____ °C
☐ Sensory: L _____ T _____ ☐ Motor

Complications:
☐ None ☐ Radicular symptoms ☐ BP drop ☐ Vascular puncture
☐ Massive epidural anesthesia ☐ Subdural spread ☐ Drop in body temperature
☐ Bladder emptying disturbances ☐ Back pain ☐ Aortocaval compression syndrome ☐ Pain ☐ Vasovagal reactions ☐ Dural puncture ☐ Intravascular injection ☐ Total spinal anesthesia ☐ Respiratory disturbance ☐ Muscle tremor ☐ Postdural puncture headache ☐ Neurological complications

Special notes: _____
_____

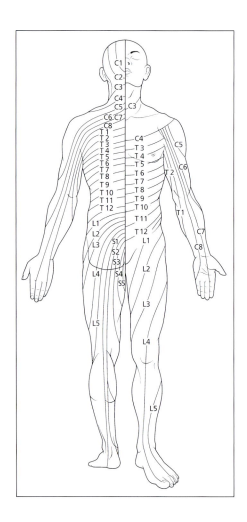

© Copyright ABW Wissenschaftsverlag 2004,
Jankovic, Regional nerve blocks and infiltration therapy, 3rd edition

44 Lumbar epidural anesthesia in children

Advantages
- Better anatomic relationships and thus easier orientation and less time required for puncture.
- Better distribution of the injected local anesthetic than in adults.
- Highly effective anesthesia and analgesia with smaller amounts of local anesthetic.
- Easier passage of the epidural catheter than in the adult.
- Due to immaturity of the sympathetic nervous system, circulatory problems are very rare, particularly in children under eight.
- Very fast recovery phase due to light basic general anesthesia and lack of need for muscle relaxants.
- Stable postoperative phase and sparing of opioids and thus fewer side effects such as nausea, vomiting or urinary retention.
- The need for subsequent postoperative intensive care is reduced.

Disadvantages
- Light general anesthesia is recommended, so that testing of the spread of anesthesia is not possible.

Distinctive features of pediatric anatomy [37, 49]

The following anatomic characteristics must be noted before carrying out epidural puncture in children (Fig. 44.1):
- In the neonate, the spinal cord ends in the area of the L3 segment; at the end of the first year of life, it reaches the L1 segment.
- In the one-year-old child, the dural sac ends in the area of S2 and in the neonate it can even reach as far as the sacral foramina of S3 or S4.
- In infants, the iliac crest line crosses the midline in the area of L5 and at about L5/S1 in neonates.
- Lumbar lordosis has not yet developed in neonates and infants.
- The distance from the skin to the epidural space correlates with the child's age. According to Busoni, measured in millimeters in the L2/L3 segment it is equivalent to 10 mm + (age in years × 2) mm [37].

Characteristics of the pediatric epidural space
See Chapter 48, p. 376.

Indications
Single-shot technique
- All surgical procedures in the region of dermatomes T5–S5 involving operating times of up to 90 minutes – e.g. perineal and perianal procedures, orchidopexy (including undescended testis), hypospadias, inguinal hernia, incarcerated hernia, umbilical hernia, superficial surgical procedures in the lower extremities – e.g. skin grafting, etc.

Continuous technique
- In combination with general anesthesia in more prolonged operations in the upper and lower abdomen, as well as urogenital and orthopedic procedures (dermatomes T5–S5) [28].

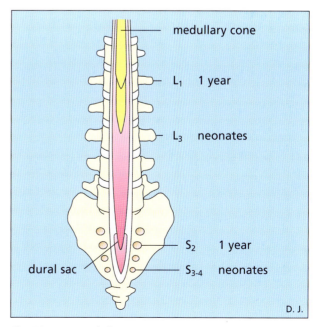

Fig. 44.1 Anatomic features

Advantages
- Shorter recovery time due to sparing of intraoperative drugs.
- Postoperative pain therapy.

Disadvantage
- The dosage is not as reliable as with caudal application.

Contraindications
See Chapter 41, p. 306.

Procedure

Full prior information for the patient and parents is mandatory.

Preparation and materials
These are the same as for epidural anesthesia in adults. Light general anesthesia or more rarely sedation combined with topical application of Emla cream is used for both the single-shot technique and for continuous epidural anesthesia.
- Strict asepsis:
  Thorough, repeated and wide skin prep, drying and covering of the puncture site with a drape.
- Local anesthesia or application of Emla cream.
- Preparation of the drugs:
  Syringe with 1 mL epinephrine-containing local anesthetic (test dose).
  Syringe with the calculated dose of local anesthetic.
- In the continuous technique, the length of the needle should be compared with the marking points on the catheter for better identification of the depth of the catheter after it has been introduced. The ability of the catheter to pass through the needle is tested at the same time.
- Skin incision with a stylet or large needle.

A **precordial stethoscope** is also required. The use of a purpose-designed kit is recommended.

Epidural needles in pediatric patients

Single-shot technique
- Up to four years of age: Tuohy needle with a metal trochar and 0.5 cm calibration marks, 22 G (0.73 × 50 mm) or 20 G (0.9 × 50 mm) – e.g. Perican Paed®, B. Braun Melsungen.
- Over four years of age: Tuohy needle with a plastic trochar and 0.5 cm calibration marks, 18 G (1.3 × 50 mm) – e.g. Perican Paed®, B. Braun Melsungen.

Continuous technique
- Up to four years of age: Tuohy needle with a metal trochar and 0.5 cm calibration marks, 20 G (0.9 × 50 mm), epidural catheter (0.6 mm–75 cm long) with central opening.
- Over four years of age: Tuohy needle with a plastic tochar and 0.5 cm calibration marks, 18 G (1.3 × 50 mm), epidural catheter (0.85 mm–100 cm long) with central opening (e.g. Perifix Paed®, B. Braun Melsungen).

Single-shot technique

Patient positioning
Lateral decubitus, with legs bent.

Finding the epidural space

> Epidural insertion must only be carried out after a preliminary incision with a large needle or stylet, and a needle with a trochar must always be used.

The insertion is carried out in the midline, usually between the spinous processes of L2/3 or L3/4 (Fig. 44.2). A Tuohy needle, with its bevel directed cranially, is advanced through the skin incision at an angle of 90° in neonates or 70° in infants, until it is lying in the interspinous ligament (Fig. 44.3).

- Removal of the trochar and attachment of a low-friction syringe with saline (injection of a maximum of 0.5 mL in the neonate or 3 mL in older children).

> Advancing the catheter further after leaving the interspinous ligament must be carried out gradually and gently, in the direction of the ligamentum flavum.

- Identification of the epidural space is carried out using the loss-of-resistance technique.
- Any fluid escaping from the end of the needle (CSF, blood) should be noted.
- Aspiration test.
- Test dose of 1 mL of an epinephrine-containing local anesthetic.
  During the subsequent waiting period: careful cardiovascular monitoring (plus precordial stethoscope) in order to recognize the development of tachycardia or arrhythmia. However, this test may

lead to unreliable results in anesthetized children [29].

Incremental injection of local anesthetic: after a negative result with the test dose, the calculated dose of local anesthetic is administered on an incremental basis.

Checking the spread of anesthesia

In children who are not under light general anesthesia, the spread of the anesthesia should always be checked.

> Since correct checking of the spread of anesthesia is not possible in anesthetized children, this method should only be used by highly experienced pediatric anesthetists.

Detailed testing of sensory and motor function is conducted postoperatively in the recovery room. The child should only be moved to the ward when he or she can move the legs freely.

Continuous lumbar epidural anesthesia

Comparison with continuous caudal anesthesia

Advantage

Since the risk of contamination of the lumbar epidural catheter is lower (4%) than with a caudally placed catheter (22%) [49], a lumbar epidural catheter is preferable when there is a need for postoperative pain therapy.

Disadvantage

The dosage scheme is less reliable than with the caudal application.

Insertion technique*

A midline insertion in the region of the L5/S1 segment has proved particularly favorable for placing a catheter in the lumbar area (modified Taylor access) [49].
Identification of the epidural space is carried out as described above. After the epidural space has been reached and loss of resistance has been confirmed, an aspiration test is carried out. Before the introduction of a catheter, the needle bevel should be directed cranially.

---

* If technical difficulties arise, the catheter and injection needle are always withdrawn simultaneously. A catheter must never be withdrawn through the injection needle.

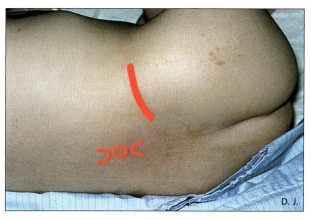

Fig. 44.2 The spinous processes of L3/4 or L2/3 are marked

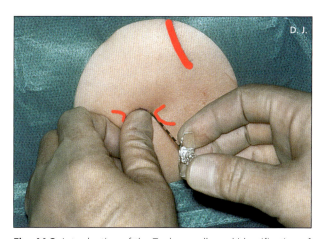

Fig. 44.3 Introduction of the Tuohy needle and identification of the epidural space

The thumb and index finger of the left hand, the side of which rests on the patient's back, secure the epidural needle. Using the thumb and index finger of the right hand, the catheter is advanced to a maximum of 2–3 cm (Fig. 44.4). A catheter must never be advanced against resistance – since this may be created by dura, a nerve or a blood vessel.

After the catheter has been placed in the desired position, the needle is very carefully withdrawn, with the thumb and index finger of the left hand simultaneously securing the catheter at the injection site.
An adapter is attached to the end of the catheter. The patency of the catheter is tested by injecting 1 mL of saline.
After aspiration, the syringe is disconnected and the open end of the catheter is placed on a sterile drape below the level of the puncture site.
Any escaping fluid (CSF, blood) should be noted.

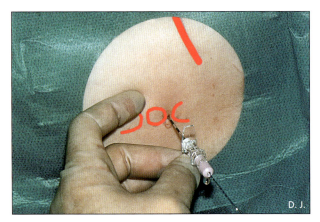

Fig. 44.4 Advancing the catheter

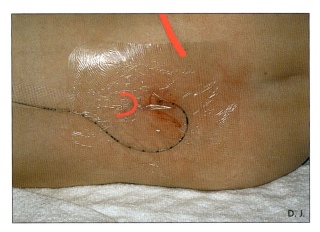

Fig. 44.5 Securing the catheter

A bacterial filter is then placed and the catheter is secured (Fig. 44.5). An epinephrine-containing test dose is administered, followed by incremental injection of local anesthetic.

After a risk–benefit assessment, a catheter for postoperative pain therapy is usually left in place for 48–72 hours. After this period, the risk of infection and migration of the catheter increases.

Local anesthetic and dosage

Age-dependent doses as proposed by Bromage [10] for lumbar epidural administration in adults also apply to pediatric patients. For testing, 2% lidocaine is used (see Chapter 41). This dosage guideline is not suitable for children under the age of four.

Busoni used 2% mepivacaine for testing, and after statistical evaluation developed valuable diagrams that became very popular with anesthetists. However, in comparison with caudal epidural administration (where the local anesthetic only spreads cranially; Fig. 44.6a), these diagrams are less reliable for lumbar epidural administration (in which there is both cranial and caudal spread; Fig. 44.6b) [37].

Another formula was tested with 0.25% bupivacaine: 0.75 mL/kg b.w. (children under eight years of age and under 25 kg) [37]. Yet another [50] is recommended for children under eight years of age: 0.7 mL/kg 1% mepivacaine, 0.25% bupivacaine, or 0.2% ropivacaine. In children over eight years of age, higher concentrations are used at a reduced dosage, based on height and weight as in adults.

> The injection site should be as close as possible to the center of the area to be anesthetized.

Concentration of local anesthetic
- 0.2% ropivacaine.
- 0.25–0.5% bupivacaine.
- 0.25% levobupivacaine.
- 1–1.5% (2%) mepivacaine.
- 1–1.5% (2%) lidocaine.

The concentration of the local anesthetic is based on the location and severity of the procedure. For more extensive abdominal procedures, slightly higher concentrations are required (2% lidocaine, 0.5% bupivacaine and 2% mepivacaine with epinephrine added [37]).

Dosage [51]
Lumbar:
0.2% ropivacaine	1.4 mg/kg b.w.
0.25% bupivacaine	2 mg/kg b.w.
1% mepivacaine	5–7 mg/kg b.w.

Thoracic:
0.2% ropivacaine	0.8–1 mg/kg b.w.
0.25% bupivacaine	1–1.2 mg/kg b.w.
1% mepivacaine	3–5 mg/kg b.w.

Practical recommendations for postoperative pain therapy [49, 51]
Local anesthetics
Initial dose:
0.2% ropivacaine	2 mg/kg b.w.
0.25% bupivacaine	2–2.5 mg/kg b.w.

Lumbar epidural anesthesia in children

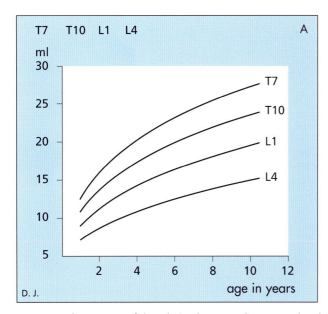
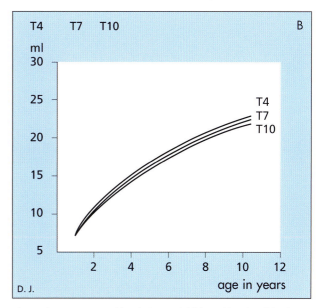

Fig. 44.6a, b Diagram of the relation between dose, spread and age for various segmental levels in caudal (a) and lumbar (b) administration
[adapted from Busoni, in Saint-Maurice C, Schulte-Steinberg O, Armitage E, eds. Regional Anesthesia in Children (Appleton & Lange/Mediglobe, 1990)]

Continuous epidural infusion with 0,1% ropivacaine or 0.125% bupivacaine
Neonates and infants: 0.2 mg/kg/h
Small children: 0.3–0.4 mg/kg/h
Older children: 0.4–0.5 mg/kg/h

Opioids
Morphine 33 µg/kg/every 8–12 h
Fentanyl 0.5 µg/kg/ h
Clonidine 2–3 µg/kg/24 h

Complications
See Chapter 41, section on complications in adults, p. 324.

45 Epidural steroid injection

Introduction

Neuraxial techniques are recognized procedures in diagnostic and therapeutic pain treatment. The first report in Europe describing the administration of steroids in the epidural space was published in 1952 [77]. Since 1961, authors in the United States and the United Kingdom in particular have regularly described lumbar [35, 38] and thoracic [32] epidural administration of methylprednisolone, and since 1986, cervical epidural steroid injections have increasingly been used in treatment-resistant cervical pain conditions [67, 78, 89].

The indications for epidural and intrathecal administration of methylprednisolone in anesthesia, orthopedics, neurology, neurosurgery, and rheumatology have included lumbosacral arachnoiditis, lumbar spine syndrome, multiple sclerosis, brachialgia, cluster headache, diabetic neuritis, post-herpetic neuralgia and causalgia, and Guillain–Barré syndrome.

The focus in neurology has been on intrathecal administration, and the success rates in arachnoiditis, lumbar spine syndrome, cluster headache, multiple sclerosis, and cervicobrachialgia have been estimated at 65% (Cleveland Clinic, 1963: assessment of intrathecal hydrocortisone administration in over 1000 patients [83–86]).

In 1970, a critical study by Goldstein et al. [39] for the first time pointed out the risks of intrathecal administration of methylprednisolone. Experimental studies on the neurotoxic effects of polyethylene glycol, the preservative used in the methylprednisolone preparation Depo-Medrol [59, 87] followed, using animal models. After reports from Australia describing increasing numbers of complications with intrathecal injections, but very rare complications with epidural applications, a reaction set in that led to the withdrawal in 1990 of approval for Depo-Medrol for intrathecal – and consequently also epidural – applications.

This decision was criticized by numerous experienced specialists throughout the world, since epidural administration of methylprednisolone in carefully selected patients had established itself as an effective and safe component of multidisciplinary pain therapy [1, 2, 6, 8, 20, 45, 93, 94, 105].

Even in large groups of patients – both Abram [1, 2] and Delaney et al. [27] reported more than 6000 applications – epidural administration of methylprednisolone was not associated with neurotoxic or meningeal reactions. In our own experience (more than 3000 epidural injections of Depo-Medrol, two-thirds of which were lumbar and one-third cervical), complications were rare and confined to technical problems such as dural puncture.

According to the Australian and British Pain Societies, no evidence has been found that epidural steroid injections are injurious to the patient [41, 101]. "However … the Pain Societies of Great Britain and Australia now feel that a) there is good evidence that epidural steroids are helpful and b) no evidence that epidural steroids are harmful" (J.C.D. Wells, personal communication, 1995) [101].

When epidural steroid injection is carried out correctly by an experienced anesthetist, it is an important and useful component of the treatment of cervical and lumbar pain and is well tolerated by the patient.

Cervical epidural steroid injection

Anatomy
The narrowest sagittal diameter of the epidural space in the cervical region is 1–1.5 mm, but it may enlarge when the neck is flexed [11, 23, 61, 75]. The cervical spinous processes are not angled, and it is therefore advisable to use a midline approach with the patient in a sitting position and with the neck flexed (see also Chapter 41).

Indications
- Acute cervical pain, cervical radicular pain (when surgery is not indicated).
- Acute episodes of chronic cervical pain.
- Treatment-resistant cervicobrachial pain, genuine occipital neuralgia [67], post-herpetic neuralgia [67].
- After whiplash trauma [65].
- After cervical intervertebral disk surgery.
- Compressive lesions [78] and spinal stenoses [89].

Contraindications
See Chapter 41, p. 306.

Relative
- Diabetes mellitus:
  When steroids are administered, regular checking of blood sugar levels must be carried out. The increased risk of infection must be taken into account.
- Neurological disease:
  In individual cases, a strict risk–benefit assessment must be carried out. Epidural injections for surgical and therapeutic purposes have been safely carried out, and are continuing to be carried out safely, in thousands of patients – e.g. after intervertebral disk surgery with stable neurological deficits.

> This block must only be carried out by highly experienced and skilled anesthetists with good training.

Procedure

Full prior information for the patient is mandatory.

Preparation and materials
- Availability and knowledge of all anesthestic facilities.
- Strict indication (risk–benefit assessment).
- Check that the emergency equipment is complete and in working order; sterile precautions, anesthetic machine, intravenous access, BP monitoring, ECG monitoring, pulse oximetry.
- Maintain strict asepsis.

The use of purpose-designed kit for epidural anesthesia is recommended (e.g. from B. Braun Melsungen); disinfectant, endotracheal anesthesia set, emergency drugs.

Puncture needles
See Chapter 41, Fig. 41.3.
Tuohy needle:
The needle most widely used throughout the world is the 18-G Tuohy needle (there are also reports in the literature describing 17-G to 20-G Tuohy needles).
Weiss needle:
This needle (18–20 G) with wings and a blunt tip is preferable for use with the "hanging drop" technique [79].

Spinal needle:
Spinal needles (3½, 20 G) are only used for an epidurogram [99].

Patient positioning
Sitting (this increases the negative epidural pressure, particularly during inspiration), with the neck flexed (this relaxes the cervical muscles, and increases the size of the epidural space), if possible supported by an assistant (Fig. 45.1).
The patient must be informed about the importance of sitting still during the insertion procedure.

Skin prep
In all blocks.

Identifying the epidural space
The epidural space can be identified using either the loss-of-resistance technique (see below), with a subsequent epidurogram if appropriate [101], or using the "hanging drop" technique (see Chapter 41, Fig. 41.11).

Injection technique
For puncture in the C7–T1 and T1–T4 regions, the midline approach is recommended.

Local infiltration
After thorough skin prep (strict asepsis), the puncture area is covered with a sterile drape, and local anesthesia with 1.5 mL 1% prilocaine is given.

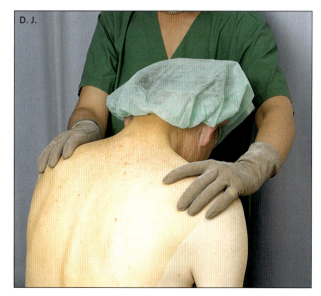

Fig. 45.1 Patient position: sitting, with the neck flexed and supported by an assistant

Cutaneous, subcutaneous, and intraligamentous infiltration is carried out up to a depth of 2 cm (Fig. 45.2).

Reaching the ligamentum flavum
After palpation of the vertebra prominens (nuchal tubercle), the skin between the two spinous processes selected (C7–T1) is incised with a stylet, to make it easier to introduce the Tuohy needle (Fig. 45.3).

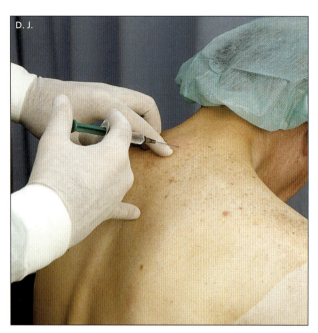

Fig. 45.2 Cutaneous, subcutaneous, and intraligamentous infiltration of the puncture area

The 18-G Tuohy needle, with its bevel directed cranially, is introduced in the midline. Depending on the flexion of the neck, the angle can be about 30° (Fig. 45.4). After about 1.5 cm, it reaches the interspinous ligament. A low-friction syringe filled with 10 mL isotonic saline, and with a small air bubble, is now attached to the needle.

Loss-of-resistance technique
See Chapter 41, Fig. 41.10.
The needle is now advanced very slowly, millimeter by millimeter, with simultaneous pressure on the syringe plunger, using the right hand. The left hand is used to apply braking pressure.

As CSF pressure in the cervical region is very low and the elasticity of the ligamentum flavum is reduced in this area, aspiration must be carried out very frequently. When the epidural space is entered, the contents of the syringe can be injected easily. During the injection, brief paresthesias in the shoulder and arm region and as far as the fingertips are signs that the needle is positioned correctly.

Steroid injection into the epidural space
After this, slow injection of the solution of steroid, saline and local anesthetic can be carried out without a prior test dose [79, 101], as the concentration of local anesthetic in the mixture is very low.

A false loss of resistance often occurs in the cervical region, with the epidural space not being reached. Dur-

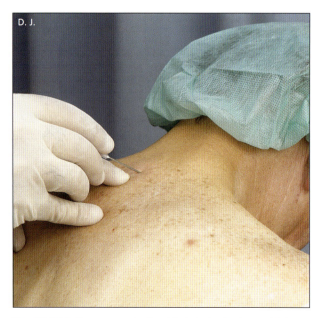

Fig. 45.3 Median approach: the skin is incised using a stylet

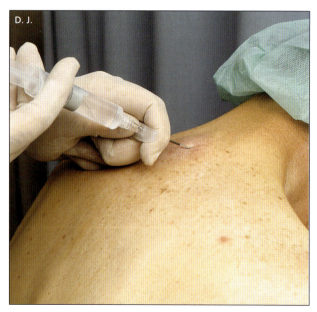

Fig. 45.4 Entering the epidural space using the loss-of-resistance technique. The 18-G Tuohy needle is advanced slowly. The angle is ca. 30°

ing the subsequent saline injection, the patient experiences severe local pain.

Effects of the block and onset
The analgesic and anti-inflammatory effects [52, 104] and resultant relaxation of the tensed neck muscles set in after 1–6 days.

Dosage
Local infiltration of the puncture site
1.5 mL local anesthetic – e.g. 1% prilocaine.

Identification of the epidural space
10 mL isotonic saline.

Injection solution
10 mL total volume: 1.5 mL (60 mg) soluble Volon A (triamcinolone acetonide), mixed with 2 mL 1% mepivacaine and about 6.5 mL isotonic saline. The mixture with saline and local anesthetic dilutes the steroid's preservative to an acceptable level [10]. The total volume guarantees adequate spread of the steroid. These are the reasons why the author prefers this particular injection mixture.

Immediately after the injection, transient fatigue (for about 20 minutes) and brief paresthesias in the shoulder, arm, and hand region are characteristic signs of a successful block.
After the steroid injection, the patient remains lying down for about 1 hour (ECG, pulse oximetry, BP monitoring).
After a further hour, the patient, who should not drive, can be discharged if escorted. During the following 24–48 hours, pain may occur at the injection site.
The risk of an epidural hematoma or abscess developing is extremely low, but it cannot be excluded. The patient must therefore be aware of the need to contact the hospital at the first sign of any complication.

Alternatives
4 mL total volume [79]: 2 mL (50 mg) intralesional Aristocort (triamcinolone diacetate) mixed with 2 mL 1% lidocaine.
4 mL total volume [101]: 2 mL (80 mg) Kenalog (triamcinolone acetonide), mixed with 2 mL 0.25% bupivacaine.

Block series
Patients who are completely free of pain after the first block, and those in whom the first block is not successful, do not receive a second injection [47].
A second or possibly even a third block can only be carried out if there is evidence of improvement in the symptoms [7].
There is no justification for more than three injections at intervals of 1–2 weeks. If the symptoms deteriorate again, periodic single injections are possible after a careful risk–benefit assessment.

Complications
Dural puncture with postdural puncture headache
See Chapter 37, p. 287.

Spinal cord injury
Neurological injuries may occur in all forms of neuraxial regional anesthesia. Spinal cord injury with paraplegia is caused by poor technique, but is extremely rare. Prophylaxis requires extremely cautious advancing of the needle, as well as frequent aspiration. It should be noted that CSF pressure is very low in the cervical region.

Bacterial meningitis
Strict asepsis is always necessary when carrying out this block. In septic diseases and infections in the area of the injection site, the block is contraindicated.

Epidural abscess
No connection has yet been identified between epidural steroid administration and the development of epidural abscesses. Numerous studies [1, 2, 12, 20, 40, 76, 92] report that there is rather evidence of a connection between prior septic disease and the development of abscesses after epidural anesthesia (see Chapter 41, p. 326).

Epidural hematoma
If the patient reports any symptoms of pain or fever, or radicular symptoms, these must be investigated.
Constant contact with the patient is necessary, particularly after outpatient procedures. Immediate investigation (myelography, CT, MRI) and neurosurgical treatment within the first 12 hours are essential to reduce morbidity and mortality (see Chapter 41, p. 326).
During the preliminary examination to exclude contraindications, it should be noted if the patient is receiving any medication that might affect platelet function.
Monotherapy with a platelet aggregation inhibitor does not lead to an increased risk of hemorrhage. In contrast, a combination of different drugs and therapy must be noted.
In connection with anatomic changes or technical difficulties, simultaneous administration of the following preparations can lead to marked risks: Acetylsalicylic acid (ASA, aspirin) or mixed preparations containing ASA, nonsteroidal anti-inflammatory drugs, high-dose antibiotics, propranolol, furosemide, quinidine, heparin, heparinoids, thrombolytics, tricyclic antidepres-

sants, phenothiazine, antilipemic drugs, chemotherapy drugs, dextrans, etc.

An epidural block with steroids should not take place within 5 days of the last intake of acetylsalicylic acid (ASA) and ASA-containing preparations. The last intake of nonsteroidal anti-inflammatory agents should be at least 24 hours previously. There is a lack of controlled studies here, and the topic is a controversial one.

Cushing's syndrome
In extremely rare cases, Cushing's syndrome may manifest as a result of an epidural block with steroids [31]. There is evidence of a reduced plasma cortisol level up to 2 weeks after the injection, even though the usual dosage of 40–80 mg per block is well below the maximum recommended corticosteroid dosage of 3 mg/kg b.w. per injection [96].

Cervical epidural steroid injection
Block no.

Name: _____ Date: _____
Diagnosis: _____
Premedication: ☐ No ☐ Yes
Neurological abnormalities: ☐ No ☐ Yes _____

Purpose of block: ☐ Diagnosis ☐ Pain treatment
Needle: ☐ Tuohy G ____ ☐ Other ____
i.v. access, infusion: ☐ Yes
Monitoring: ☐ ECG ☐ Pulse oximetry
Ventilation facilities: ☐ Yes (equipment checked)
Emergency equipment (drugs): ☐ Checked
Patient: ☐ Informed

Position: ☐ Sitting ☐ Lateral decubitus
Access: ☐ Median ☐ Paramedian
Injection level: ☐ C7/T1 ☐ Other _____
Injection technique: ☐ Loss of resistance ☐ Other _____
Test dose: ☐ No ☐ Yes _____ mL _____ %
Injection mixture: Steroid: _____ mg
                   NaCl 0.9%: _____ mL
                   Local anesthetic: _____ mL ___ %

Patient's remarks during injection:
☐ None   ☐ Pain   ☐ Paresthesias   ☐ Warmth
Duration and area: _____
Objective block effect after 15 min:
☐ Cold test ☐ Temperature measurement before ____°C after ____°C
☐ Sensory   ☐ Motor
Monitoring after block: ☐ <2 h ☐ >2 h
          Time of discharge: _____
          Abnormalities: _____

Complications:
☐ None ☐ Vasovagal reactions ☐ Severe pain ☐ Fever
☐ Dural puncture ☐ Radicular symptoms ☐ Neurological complications

Subjective effects of the block: Duration: _____
☐ None   ☐ Increased pain
☐ Reduced pain   ☐ Relief of pain

VISUAL ANALOG SCALE

|‖‖‖|
0   10   20   30   40   50   60   70   80   90   100

Special notes: _____

© Copyright ABW Wissenschaftsverlag 2004,
Jankovic, Regional nerve blocks and infiltration therapy, 3rd edition

Record and checklist

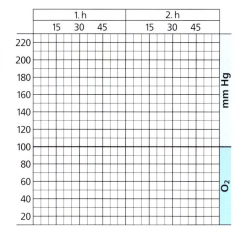

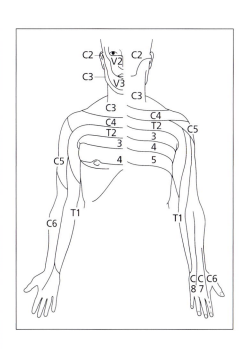

Lumbar epidural steroid injection

This method is not effective in:
Deforming spondylopathy, spondylochondrosis, deforming spondyloarthropathy, spondylolisthesis, spondylarthritis, scoliosis, functional back pain, chronic symptoms.

Indications
- Patients with a short history of pain.
- Unsuccessful intervertebral disk surgery (post-laminectomy syndrome).
- Inflammatory and compressive radiculopathies.
- Intervertebral disk prolapse (not requiring surgery).
- Spinal canal stenosis.
- Post-herpetic neuralgia in the lumbosacral area (best results within 3 months after the start of the disease).

Specific and relative contraindications
See Chapter 41, p. 306 and the section on cervical epidural steroid injection.

> This block must only be carried out by highly experienced and skilled anesthetists with good training.

Procedure

Full prior information for the patient is mandatory.

Preparation and materials
- Strict indication (risk–benefit assessment).
- The patient must be fully informed.
- Check that the emergency equipment is complete and in working order.
- Observe strict asepsis.
- Anesthetic machine, intravenous access, BP monitoring, ECG monitoring, pulse oximetry.

The use of purpose-designed kit for epidural anesthesia is recommended (e.g. from B. Braun Melsungen).

Puncture needles
- Tuohy needle, 17 G or 18 G (see Chapter 41, Fig. 41.3).
- Spinal needles ($3^1/_2$, 20 G) are only used for an epidurogram [101].

Patient positioning
Lateral decubitus with the patient lying on the painful side, or sitting (risk of collapse).

Skin prep, local anesthesia, skin incision, and identification of the epidural space
See Chapter 41, p. 307.

After intervertebral disk surgery, the puncture is carried out about 1 cm above the scar. It can be carried out with a midline or paramedian approach.

Steroid injection into the epidural space
Injection of the steroid, mixed with a local anesthetic, must be carried out slowly.
After the injection, the patient remains in the lateral decubitus position for about 20 minutes.

Effects of the block and onset of effect
See also the section on cervical epidural steroid injection, p. 349.

Immediately after the block, transient fatigue (for about 20 minutes), brief paresthesias, and a sensation of warmth in both legs are characteristic signs of a successful block.
After an injection of steroid combined with local anesthetic, the patient remains recumbent for about 1–2 hours (20 minutes of this lying on the side), until the effect of the local anesthetic has declined.
Monitoring is obligatory during this period.
After a further hour, the patient, who should not drive, can be discharged if escorted. It should be checked and recorded beforehand that the effect of the local anesthetic is no longer present.
During the following 24–48 hours, pain may occur at the injection site. The risk of an epidural hematoma or abscess developing is extremely low, but it cannot be excluded. The patient must therefore be aware of the need to contact the hospital at the first sign of any complication.

Dosage
Injection solution
Test dose: 2 mL 1% lidocaine.
Total volume 10 mL: 2 mL (50 mg) intralesional Aristocort (triamcinolone diacetate), mixed with 2 mL 0.9% NaCl and 6 mL 1% lidocaine [79].
Or:
Test dose: 2 mL 1% lidocaine.
Total volume 10 mL: 2 mL (80 mg) soluble Volon A (triamcinolone acetonide), mixed with 8 mL local anesthetic consisting of equal halves of 1% lidocaine and 0.25 bupivacaine [101].

Block series
See the section on cervical epidural steroid injection, p. 349.

Complications
See Chapter 41, p. 324, and the section on cervical epidural steroid injection, p. 349.

Record and checklist

Lumbar epidural steroid injection
Block no.

Name: _____ Date: _____
Diagnosis: _____
Premedication: ☐ No ☐ Yes
Neurological abnormalities: ☐ No ☐ Yes _____

Purpose of block: ☐ Diagnosis ☐ Pain treatment
Needle: ☐ Tuohy G ____ ☐ Other ____
i.v. access, infusion: ☐ Yes
Monitoring: ☐ ECG ☐ Pulse oximetry
Ventilation facilities: ☐ Yes (equipment checked)
Emergency equipment *(drugs)*: ☐ Checked
Patient: ☐ Informed

Position: ☐ Sitting ☐ Lateral decubitus
Access: ☐ Median ☐ Paramedian
Injection level: ☐ L3/L4 ☐ Other _____
Injection technique: ☐ Loss of resistance ☐ Other _____
Test dose: ☐ No ☐ Yes _____ mL _____ %
Injection mixture: Steroid: _____ mg
NaCl 0.9%: _____ mL
Local anesthetic: _____ mL _____ %

Patient's remarks during injection:
☐ None ☐ Pain ☐ Paresthesias ☐ Warmth
Duration and area: _____
Objective block effect after 15 min:
☐ Cold test ☐ Temperature measurement before _____ °C after _____ °C
☐ Sensory ☐ Motor
Monitoring after block: ☐ < 2 h ☐ > 2 h
Time of discharge: _____
Abnormalities: _____

Complications:
☐ None ☐ Vasovagal reactions ☐ Severe pain ☐ Fever
☐ Dural puncture ☐ Radicular symptoms ☐ Neurological complications

Subjective effects of the block: duration: _____
☐ None ☐ Increased pain
☐ Reduced pain ☐ Relief of pain

VISUAL ANALOG SCALE

|0   10   20   30   40   50   60   70   80   90   100|

Special notes:
_____
_____

© Copyright ABW Wissenschaftsverlag 2004,
Jankovic, Regional nerve blocks and infiltration therapy, 3rd edition

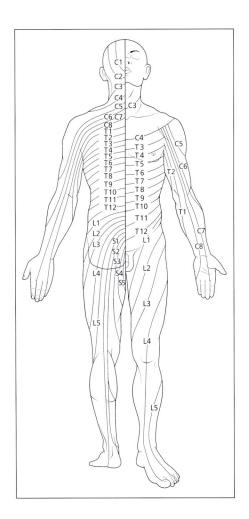

46 Combined spinal and epidural anesthesia (CSE)

Introduction

This combined technique was introduced in neuraxial regional anesthesia in order to exploit as many advantages of both procedures as possible and to minimise their disadvantages.
In CSE, the reliability, fast onset of effect, high success rate, excellent muscle relaxation and low toxicity of spinal anesthesia are combined with the advantages of epidural anesthesia: flexibility, good controllability, ability to prolong the anesthesia as required and potential transition to postoperative pain treatment.
CSE allows better titration and a substantial reduction in the dose of local anesthetic, opioid, or combination of the two.
The advantages of this technique can be used particularly effectively in obstetrics, with results showing a substantial reduction in maternal hypotension during birth.

History

In 1937, the New York surgeon Soresi [90] reported that it was possible to inject procaine first epidurally and then intrathecally through the same needle.
In 1979, Curelaru [26] described the use of CSE in abdominal surgery, urology and orthopedics. After placement of an epidural catheter, a subarachnoid injection was carried out one or two segments below the puncture site.
In 1981, Brownridge [14] reported the use of CSE for cesarean section. He used two different segments for puncture.
A modification of this technique with one-segment puncture ("needle through needle") was used in 1982 by Coates [21] and Mumtaz [64] in orthopedic surgery and in 1984 by Carrie [15] in obstetric surgery.
In 1986, Rawal [70] described the sequential (two-stage) CSE technique for cesarean section.

Indications

Surgical procedures:
- General surgery.
- Outpatient surgery [97].
- Vascular surgery [100].
- Orthopedics [21, 46, 64, 102].
- Gynecology [17].
- Obstetrics [15, 70, 71, 72].
- Urology [26].
- Pediatric surgery [66].
- Postoperative pain therapy.

Contraindications

The contraindications are the same as those for spinal anesthesia (see Chapter 36, p. 272) and epidural anesthesia (see Chapter 41, p. 306).

Procedure

Full prior information for the patient is mandatory.

Preparation and materials
- Check that the emergency equipment is complete and in working order (intubation kit, emergency drugs); anesthetic machine.
- Set up an intravenous infusion and give a volume load (500–1000 mL of a balanced electrolyte solution).
- Careful monitoring: ECG, BP, pulse oximeter.
- Maintain strict asepsis.

The use of purpose-designed kit is recommended – e.g. Espocan from B. Braun Melsungen (Fig. 46.1).

> This procedure must only be carried out by an experienced anesthetist.

Chapter 46

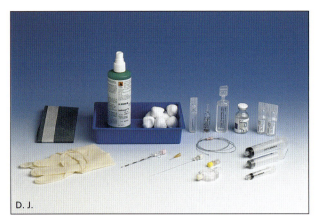

Fig. 46.1 Materials

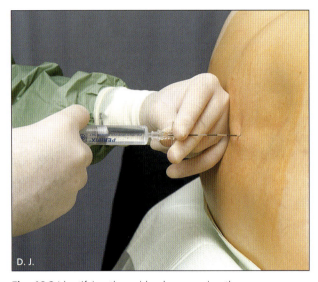

Fig. 46.2 Identifying the epidural space using the loss-of-resistance technique

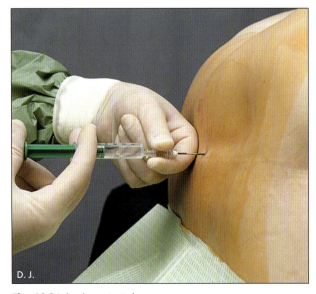

Fig. 46.3 Injecting a test dose

Patient positioning
The puncture is carried out below the L2 segment, with the patient either in the lateral decubitus position (preferable) or sitting.

Injection technique
"Needle through needle"
After locating and marking the puncture site (L2/3 or L3/4), thorough skin prep is carried out, followed by local anesthesia and a skin incision using a stylet.
Insertion is carried out in the midline using an 18-G epidural Tuohy needle, with the bevel directed cranially. Identification of the epidural space is carried out using the loss-of-resistance technique (Fig. 46.2).
After identification of the epidural space and injection of a test dose (Fig. 46.3), a thin 27-G pencil-point spinal needle is carefully advanced through the epidural needle in the direction of the subarachnoid space, until dural perforation is confirmed by a click (Fig. 46.4a).
The adapted form of the Tuohy needle tip, which has a central opening positioned in the needle axis ("back eye"), allows the needle to take a direct path, so that the spinal needle does not need to bend. The plastic coating of the spinal needle expands its outer diameter, so that it fits the epidural needle precisely, maintains its central position as it is advanced and easily passes through the axial opening ("back eye") (Fig. 46.4b).
After careful aspiration of CSF, subarachnoid injection of a local anesthetic, opioid, or a combination of the two is carried out (Fig. 46.5). As this is done, the hub of the spinal needle should be secured with the thumb and index finger of the left hand, which rests on the patient's back. This is the critical phase of the puncture procedure.
The spinal needle is then withdrawn and the epidural catheter is introduced up to a maximum of 3–4 cm (Fig. 46.6).
After aspiration, the open end of the catheter is laid on a sterile surface below the puncture site and any escaping fluid (CSF or blood) is noted (Fig. 46.7).
To test the patency of the catheter, 1–2 mL saline is then injected. The catheter is secured and a bacterial filter is attached (Fig. 46.8).

Combined spinal and epidural anesthesia (CSE)

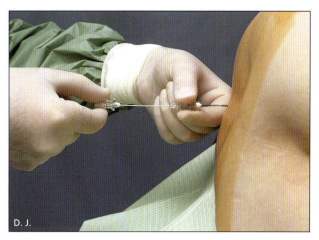

Fig. 46.4a A 27-G pencil-point spinal needle is introduced through the positioned epidural needle

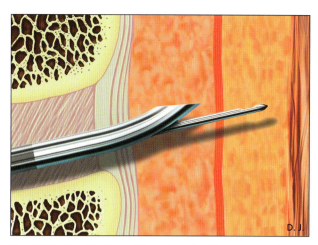

Fig. 46.4b Identification of the subarachnoid space with the dural click

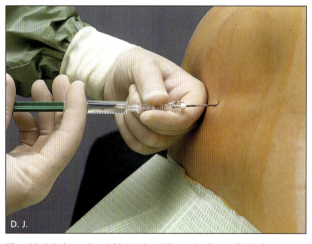

Fig. 46.5 Subarachnoid injection. The spinal needle is then withdrawn

- Repeated aspiration.
- As low a dose as possible.
- Always use incremental injections (several test doses).
- Maintain verbal contact.
- Check the spread of anesthesia carefully.
- Careful monitoring.

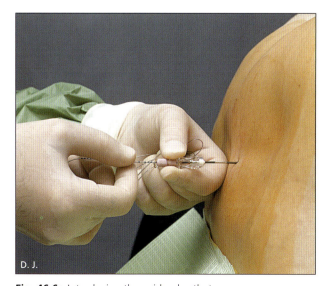

Fig. 46.6a Introducing the epidural catheter

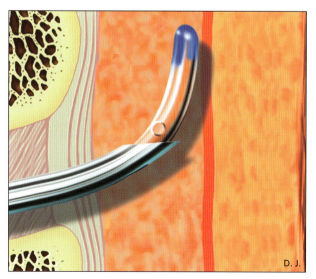

Fig. 46.6b The epidural catheter is advanced by a maximum of 3–4 cm cranially

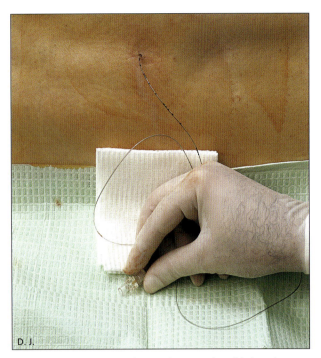

Fig. 46.7 The open end of the catheter is placed below the puncture site

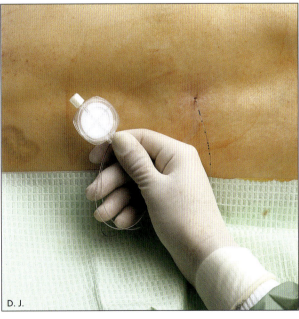

Fig. 46.8 The catheter is secured and a bacterial filter is attached

Problem situations
Specific problems during CSE occur in connection with the administration of a test dose to exclude subarachnoid positioning of the catheter.
As spinal anesthesia is being given, it is not possible to test for incorrect intrathecal positioning of the catheter, and incorrect positioning usually becomes evident through high or total spinal anesthesia.
This technique should therefore only be carried out by experienced anesthetists.
Local anesthetics must only be injected in small incremental amounts (test doses), the spread of the anesthesia must be carefully checked and verbal contact with the patient must be maintained.

Two-segment technique
Puncture is carried out in the midline at the level of L2/3 or L3/4. An 18-G Tuohy needle is used. After identification of the epidural space, the epidural catheter is advanced to a maximum of 3–4 cm. A test dose is then administered. One or two segments lower, conventional spinal anesthesia is then carried out using a 27-G pencil-point needle. The remainder of the procedure is the same as in the "needle-through-needle" technique.

Dosages
in the "needle-through-needle" and two-segment techniques
[69, 70, 74, 98]

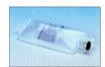

Subarachnoid
- Opioid: 10 μg sufentanil + 1 mL 0.9% saline.
- Local anesthetic:
  0.5% ropivacaine 1–1.5 mL (5–7.5 mg) ± 0.2 mL.
  0.5% hyperbaric bupivacaine 1–1.5 mL (5–7.5 mg) ± 0.2 mL.
- Local anesthetic + opioid:
  0.5% ropivacaine + sufentanil 7.5–10 μg, or
  0.5% ropivacaine + fentanyl 25 μg.
  0.5% hyperbaric bupivacaine 1–2.5 mg + sufentanil 7.5–10 μg, or:
  0.5% hyperbaric bupivacaine 1–2.5 mg + fentanyl 25 μg.

Epidural
- Top-up dose
  After the fixation period for the local anesthetic injected intrathecally (ca. 15 min):
  0.5% ropivacaine, 1.5–2 mL per unblocked segment,
  or
  0.25–0.5% bupivacaine, 1.5–2 mL per unblocked segment.
- Epidural infusion after bolus administration of
  10–15 mL 0.1% ropivacaine + 1–2 µg/mL sufentanil (10–20 µg) or 2 µg/mL fentanyl (30 µg), or:
  10 mL 0.0625–0.125% bupivacaine + 10–20 µg sufentanil, or:
  10 mL 0.125–025% bupivacaine + 50 µg fentanyl.
  Continuous infusion of:
  0.1% ropivacaine + 0.2–0.3 µg/mL sufentanil (2 µg/mL fentanyl) at 10–12 mL/h,
  or:
  0.031–0.0625% bupivacaine + 0.2–0.3 µg/mL sufentanil at 6–10 mL/h, or:
  0.0625% bupivacaine + 1–2 µg/mL fentanyl at 10 mL/h.

Sequential (two-stage) CSE in Cesarean section
This technique has proved particularly useful for Cesarean section, reducing the frequency and severity of maternal hypotension [73].

First stage: procedure in sitting position
- Identification of the epidural space (18-G Tuohy needle).
- Advancing the spinal needle (27-G pencil-point) until dural perforation is achieved (dural click and free CSF flow).
- Intrathecal administration of a local anesthetic and/or opioid. The aim is to reach the segmental level of S5–T9 with as low a concentration as possible (e.g. hyperbaric bupivacaine 1.5 mL ± 0.2 mL).
- Introduction of the epidural catheter.

Second stage: procedure in the supine position (left lateral decubitus)
- 5–20 minute wait until full spread of the subarachnoid local anesthetic is achieved (fixation period).
- After subarachnoid spread of the local anesthetic, incremental epidural injection in small doses (top-up) is carried out through the epidural catheter. Ca. 1.5–2 mL 0.5% bupivacaine is administered for each unblocked segment.

Advantages
The slow, incremental administration of the local anesthetic and/or opioid markedly reduces the risk of severe circulatory reactions during Cesarean section. The sympathetic block is less marked (lowest possible subarachnoid dosage and slow onset of epidural anesthesia). The body has time to activate compensatory mechanisms.
This procedure is particularly suitable for high-risk patients.

Disadvantage
More time-consuming.

Dosage in Cesarean section [69]
Subarachnoid
- 0.5% hyperbaric bupivacaine 1.5 ± 0.2 mL. Block target: S5–T8/9.

Epidural
- Top-up dose in left lateral decubitus position after the fixation period (ca. 15 min) of the local anesthetic injected subarachnoidally: 1.5–2 mL 0.5% bupivacaine per unblocked segment.

Dosage in outpatient obstetrics [69]
Subarachnoid (single-shot)
- 0.5% hyperbaric bupivacaine 1–2.5 mg + 7.5–10 µg sufentanil, or:
  0.5% hyperbaric bupivacaine 1–2.5 mg + 25 µg fentanyl.

Epidural top-up dose (continuous infusion 10 mL/h)
- Bupivacaine 1 mg + 0.075–1.0 µg/mL sufentanil, or:
  Bupivacaine 1 mg + 2 µg fentanyl.

Complications
See Chapter 37, p. 285 and Chapter 41, p. 324.

Chapter 46

Record and checklist

Combined spinal and epidural anesthesia (CSE)

Name: _____ Date: _____
Diagnosis: _____
Premedication: ☐ No   ☐ Yes
Neurological abnormalities: ☐ No   ☐ Yes _____

Purpose of block: ☐ Surgical   ☐ Obstetric   ☐ Postoperative
Needle: Spinal: G _____ Tip _____
               Epidural: Tuohy _____ G   ☐ Other
i.v. access, infusion: ☐ Yes
Monitoring: ☐ ECG   ☐ Pulse oximetry
Ventilation facilities: ☐ Yes (equipment checked)
Emergency equipment (drugs):   ☐ Checked
Patient: ☐ Informed

Position: ☐ Lateral decubitus   ☐ Sitting
Access: ☐ Median   ☐ Paramedian
Injection level: ☐ L3/L4   ☐ L4/L5   ☐ Other _____
Injection technique: ☐ Needle-through-needle ☐ Two-segment
Epidural space: ☐ Identified
Test dose: _____ Epinephrine added: ☐ Yes ☐ No

Subarachnoid:
Injection: ☐ Carried out
CSF aspiration: ☐ Possible   ☐ Not possible
Local anesthetic: _____ mL _____ %
☐ Addition: _____ µg/mg

Epidural:
Epidural catheter: ☐ Advanced 3–4 cm cranially
Aspiration test: ☐ Carried out
Catheter end: ☐ Positioned lower than the puncture site
Bacterial filter: ☐
Local anesthetic: _____ mL _____ %
(incremental)
Abnormalities: ☐ No   ☐ Yes _____

Patient's remarks during injection:
☐ None   ☐ Pain   ☐ Paresthesias   ☐ Warmth
Duration and area: _____
Objective block effect after 20 min:
☐ Cold test ☐ Temperature measurement before _____°C after _____°C
☐ Sensory L _____ T _____   ☐ Motor

Complications:
☐ None ☐ Radicular symptoms ☐ BP drop ☐ Vascular puncture
☐ Massive epidural anesthesia ☐ Subdural spread ☐ Drop in body temperature
☐ Bladder emptying disturbances ☐ Back pain ☐ Aortocaval compression syndrome ☐ Pain ☐ Vasovagal reactions ☐ Dural puncture (epidural needle) or inadvertent dural puncture ☐ Intravascular injection ☐ Total spinal anesthesia ☐ Respiratory disturbance ☐ Muscle tremor ☐ Postdural puncture headache ☐ Neurological complications

Special notes:

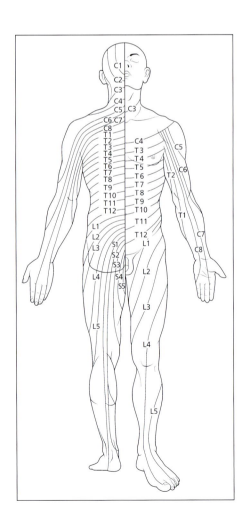

© Copyright ABW Wissenschaftsverlag 2004,
Jankovic, Regional nerve blocks and infiltration therapy, 3rd edition

Caudal epidural anesthesia

47 Caudal anesthesia in adult patients

Definition
Epidural injection of a local anesthetic or a mixture of a local anesthetic and an opioid or steroid through a needle positioned in the sacral canal or through a catheter.

Anatomy

See also Chapter 35, section on the sacral bone, p. 265.

The **sacral hiatus** is located in line with the median sacral crest. Its lateral boundary is formed by the sacral cornua and it is enclosed by the superficial dorsal, deep dorsal and lateral sacrococcygeal ligaments, which pass from the sacrum to the coccyx (Fig. 47.1). The hiatus represents the caudal entrance to the sacral canal.

The **sacral canal** has a diameter of 2–10 mm in an anteroposterior direction and its capacity varies from 12 mL to 65 mL (average 30–34 mL) [19] (Fig. 47.2).

It encloses and protects the dura, arachnoid and subarachnoid space, which in most cases end at the level of the second sacral vertebra, as well as the sacral and coccygeal roots of the cauda equina, the sacral epidural venous plexus, lymphatic vessels and epidural fat.

The **dura** normally ends at the level of the second sacral foramina (1–1.5 cm medial and caudal to the dorsal cranial iliac spines), so that this connecting line externally marks the end of the dural sac (Fig. 47.3).

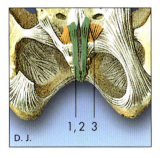

Fig. 47.1 Sacral hiatus, with the sacrococcygeal ligaments.
(1) Superficial dorsal sacrococcygeal ligament,
(2) deep dorsal sacrococcygeal ligament,
(3) lateral sacrococcygeal ligament

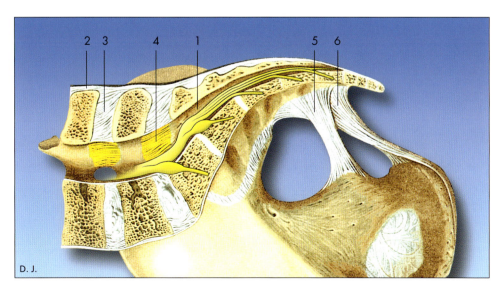

Fig. 47.2 Sacral canal.
(1) Sacral canal,
(2) supraspinous ligament,
(3) interspinous ligament,
(4) ligamentum flavum,
(5) sacrospinous ligament,
(6) sacrotuberal ligament

Anatomic variants are possible (e.g. S2 or S3), so that the distance from the dura to the hiatus can range from 1.6 cm to 7.5 cm (average 4.5 cm). This should be taken into account during insertion [16].

In children under 1 year of age, the dural sac may come up to the level of the fourth sacral vertebra, and particular caution is therefore required during insertion in these patients.

The sacral canal is at its narrowest in the region of the hiatus, and the surrounding area is very well vascularized.

This block should only be carried out by experienced anesthetists or under their supervision.

Indications

Surgical
- Procedures and painful examination in the perineal and perianal area (e.g. hemorrhoids or operations on the prostate, bladder or penis).
- Inguinal and femoral hernias.
- Procedures in the area of the coccyx.
- Superficial procedures on the lower extremities (e.g. skin grafts).

Gynecological
- Procedures and painful examinations (vulva, vagina, cervix, clitoris).

Obstetric
- Pain during the second stage of labor.

Diagnostic and therapeutic
- Various painful conditions in the area of the lumbar spine, pelvis, perineum, genitals, rectum and lower extremities.

Acute pain
- Postoperative and post-traumatic pain.
- Lumbar spine syndrome (only after excluding a surgical cause).
- Post-herpetic neuralgia.
- Vascular insufficiency.
- Ergotism.
- Frostbite.
- Hidradenitis suppurativa.

Chronic pain
- Lumbar radiculopathy.
- Spinal canal stenosis.
- Postlaminectomy syndrome.
- Diabetic polyneuropathy.
- Complex regional pain syndrome, types I and II (sympathetic reflex dystrophy and causalgia).
- Postamputation pain.
- Vasospastic diseases.
- Orchialgia.
- Proctalgia.

Tumor pain
- Genital and rectal, in the pelvis, in the perineum.
- Peripheral neuropathy (after radiotherapy or chemotherapy).

Contraindications

Specific
- Patient refusal.
- Coagulation disorders, anticoagulant therapy.
- Sepsis.
- Local infections (skin diseases) at the puncture site.
- Immune deficiency.
- Severe decompensated hypovolemia, shock.
- Specific cardiovascular diseases of myocardial, ischemic, or valvular origin, if the planned procedure requires higher sensory spread.
- Acute diseases of the brain and spinal cord.
- Increased intracranial pressure.
- A history of hypersensitivity to local anesthetics, without a prior intradermal test dose.

Relative
- Pilonidal cyst.
- Congenital anomalies of the dural sac and its contents.

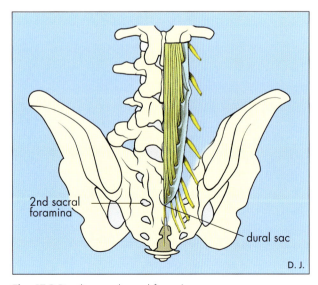

Fig. 47.3 Dural sac and sacral foramina

Procedure

Full prior information for the patient is mandatory.

Preparation and materials
- Check that the emergency equipment is complete and in working order (intubation kit, emergency drugs); sterile precautions, intravenous access, anesthetic machine.
- Intravenous infusion of a balanced electrolyte solution (250–500 mL).
- Careful monitoring: ECG, BP, pulse oximetry.
- Pillow for patient positioning.

The use of a purpose-designed kit is recommended (e.g. from B. Braun Melsungen) Fig. 47.4).

Puncture needles
Single-shot technique
- Plastic indwelling catheter needle with trochar – e.g. Contiplex A plastic indwelling catheter needle 1.3 × 45 mm, 30° bevel.
- Special caudal needle with trochar – e.g. Tuohy: Perican 0.90 × 50 mm 20 G, Perican 1.30 × 50 mm 20 G, Perican 1.30 × 50 mm 18 G × 2″ or Epican, special 32° tip at 0.9 × 50 mm.

Continuous technique
- Tuohy or Crawford or plastic indwelling catheter needle (e.g. Epican, B. Braun Melsungen).

> Current information and standards show that only needles with a trochar should be used, particularly for caudal anesthesia in children.

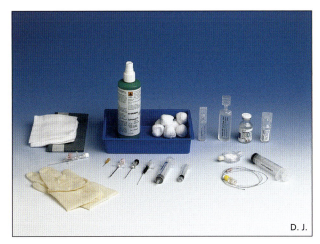

Fig. 47.4 Materials

Single-shot technique

Patient positioning
The puncture is usually carried out with the patient in the prone position, with a pillow under the pelvis and legs spread, so that the heels are turned out and the toes rotated inward. This allows optimal relaxation of the gluteal musculature (Fig. 47.5a). In addition, particularly in obese patients, the gluteal cleft is separated by attaching a broad band of sticky plaster between the skin of the buttocks and the operating table (Fig. 47.5b).
This procedure can also be carried out in the lateral decubitus position (particularly in children and in pregnant patients) or in the knee–elbow position (pregnant patients).

Location, skin prep, local anesthesia, skin incision
Locating and marking the sacral cornua
The sacral cornua or sacral hiatus and sacrococcygeal ligaments are palpated with the thumb and index finger (Fig. 47.6a).

> The thumb and index finger remain in place on the sacral cornua during the entire insertion procedure.

Palpation of the dorsal cranial iliac spines
A triangle is drawn to the sacral cornua (sacral hiatus). About 1–1.5 cm caudal and medial to the dorsal cranial iliac spines lies the second sacral foramen, the connecting line of which indicates the level of the dural sac in most patients. This line must not be reached when the needle is being advanced (Fig. 47.6b).
A swab is placed in the gluteal sulcus to protect the anal and perineal area from disinfectant (Fig. 47.5b).

Chapter 47

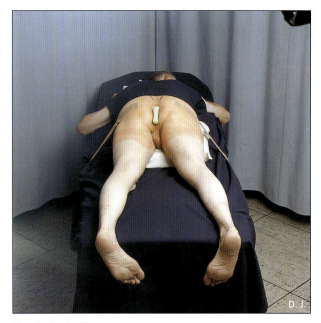

Fig. 47.5a Position

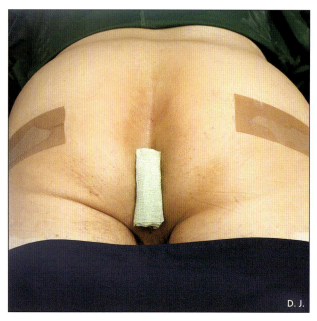

Fig. 47.5b Attachment of a broad adhesive plaster. Placement of a swab in the gluteal cleft

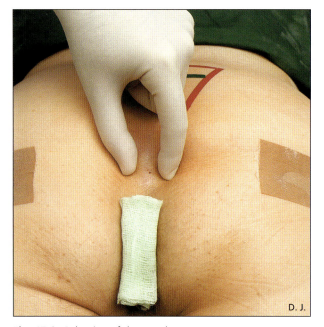

Fig. 47.6a Palpation of the sacral cornua

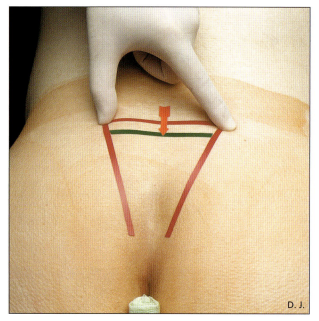

Fig. 47.6b Palpation of the dorsal cranial iliac spines

Strict asepsis
Thorough, repeated wide skin prep, drying and covering of the puncture site with a sterile drape.

Local anesthesia
Local anesthesia with 1% mepivacaine is injected in the subcutaneous tissue over and around the sacral hiatus. The periosteum around the sacral hiatus is particularly sensitive and should also be injected.
The needle is introduced at an angle of 70° to the skin surface of the back of the sacrum (Fig. 47.7)

Preparing the drugs
A syringe with 3–4 mL of an epinephrine-containing local anesthetic (test dose).
A syringe with the calculated dose of local anesthetic.

Skin incision
Using a stylet or large needle (Fig. 47.8).

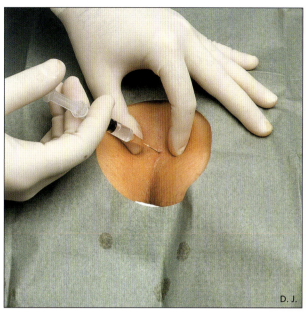

Fig. 47.7 Local anesthesia

Puncture of the caudal epidural space
Puncture
The puncture needle is introduced at an angle of 70° in the direction of the sacral hiatus until bone contact is made (Fig. 47.9a).
The needle is now slightly withdrawn and the anesthetist slowly reduces the angle of the needle (Fig. 47.9b) as far as about 20° in male patients or about 35° in women until perforation of the sacrococcygeal ligament is carried out and the needle can be advanced without resistance parallel to the posterior wall of the sacral canal to a depth of 3 cm [16] (Fig. 47.9c).

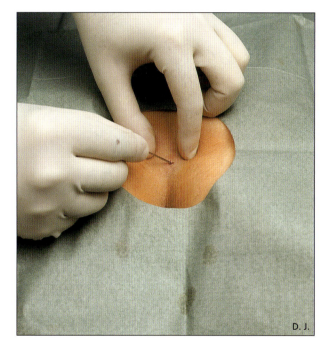

Fig. 47.8 Skin incision

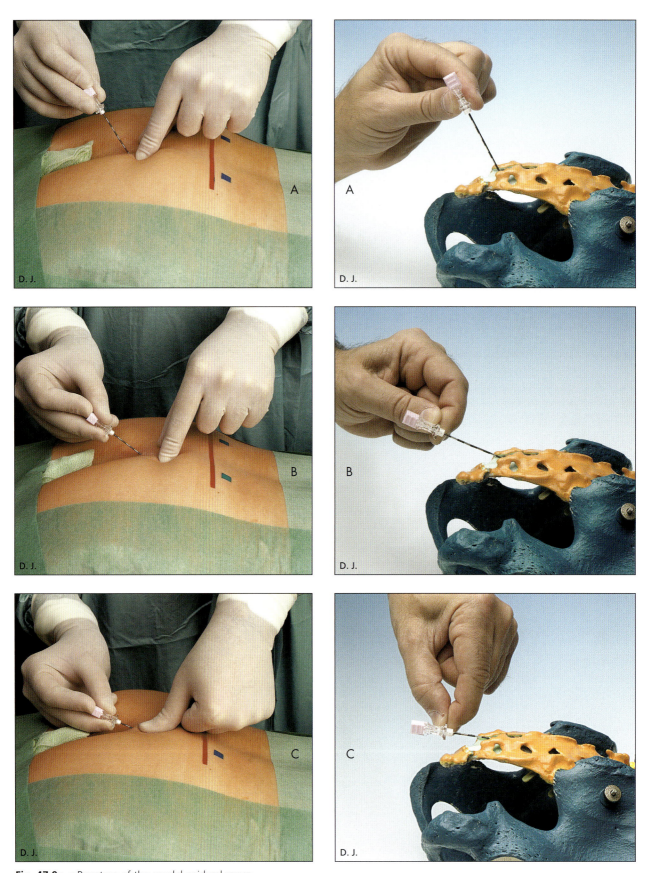

Fig. 47.9a–c Puncture of the caudal epidural space.
a Puncture angle of 70°. **b** Lowering maneuver. **c** Introducing the needle into the sacral canal

Caudal anesthesia in adult patients

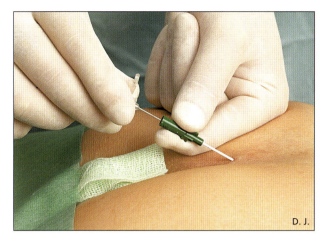

Fig. 47.10 Plastic indwelling catheter needle

When plastic indwelling catheter needles are used, the trochar is withdrawn slightly after the sacral canal has been entered and the plastic part is advanced 2–3 cm (Fig. 47.10).

Checking the position of the needle tip in the dural sac (second sacral foramen)
The trochar is withdrawn and the distance of the needle in the sacral canal checked. This is easily done by placing the trochar on the skin overlying the sacrum (Fig. 47.11).

Checking for escaping fluid (CSF or blood) (Fig. 47.12)

Aspiration test (Fig. 47.13)

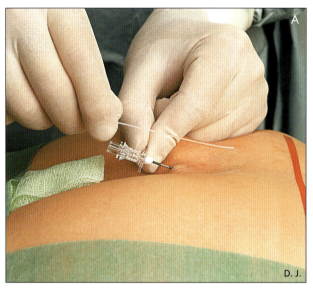 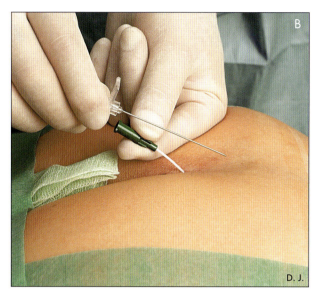

Fig. 47.11a, b Checking the position of the needle tip in the dural sac (second sacral foramen)

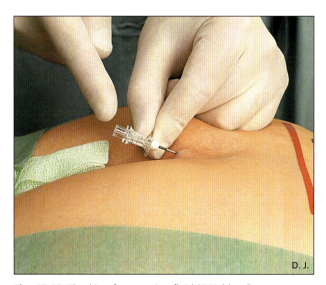 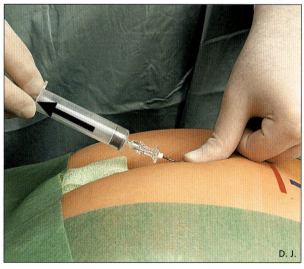

Fig. 47.12 Checking for escaping fluid (CSF, blood)

Fig. 47.13 Aspiration test

Chapter 47

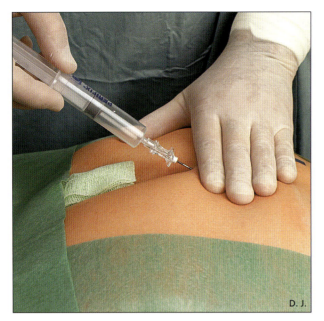

Fig. 47.14 Injection of 5 cm³ of air or 0.9% NaCl

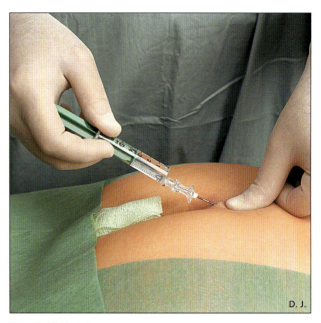

Fig. 47.15 Test dose

Injection of 5 cm³ of air or 0.9% saline
If no blood or CSF escapes, a rapid injection of 5 cm³ of air or 0.9% NaCl is carried out (Fig. 47.14). The patient is then informed that he or she will feel pressure paresthesias in the legs (a sign of correct needle positioning). The anesthetist palpates the surface of the sacrum with the free hand (crepitation, swelling), to exclude the possibility that the catheter is positioned outside the canal.
If pain occurs during this injection, the needle is not correctly positioned.

Test dose
3–4 mL of an epinephrine-containing local anesthetic (Fig. 47.15).

Waiting period
During the 5-minute waiting period, careful cardiovascular monitoring is carried out. Verbal contact must be maintained with the patient.
Five minutes after administration of the test dose, the lower extremities, abdomen and chest are tested for numbness in order to exclude the possibility of inadvertent subarachnoid injection. Extensive spread suggests dural puncture.

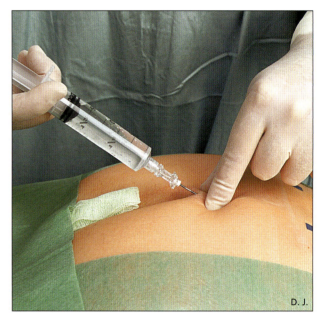

Fig. 47.16 Incremental injection of a local anesthetic

Incremental injection of a local anesthetic
If there is no effect or only a minimal effect, in the form of hypoesthesia in the perineal and perianal area or over the coccyx, and if the patient's sensory function is unchanged and the circulation is stable, then the injection of local anesthetic can be carried out (Fig. 47.16).

Problem situations
Aspiration of blood
- Steel needle or plastic indwelling catheter needle: Reinsert the trochar, then advance by 0.5–1 cm and wait for 2–3 min.
- Steel needle without a trochar: Advance by about 0.5–1 cm, inject 1 mL 0.9% saline and wait for 2–3 min.

If blood is aspirated again, the puncture procedure must be stopped.

Aspiration of CSF
The puncture procedure must be stopped.

Failure
Owing to the highly variable anatomy in the sacral canal, a failure rate of 5–10% can be expected [16]. Experience shows that the sacral hiatus cannot be identified in about 0.5–1% of patients.

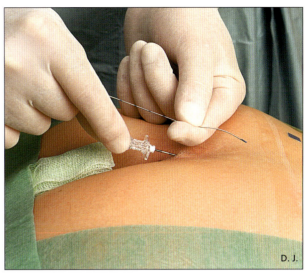

Fig. 47.17 The length of the needle is compared with the calibration marks on the catheter

- The needle must remain in the midline during the puncture procedure.
- The thumb and index finger remain in position on the sacral cornua during the location and injection.
- During the injection of the local anesthetic, the sacral area should be carefully observed for any swelling.
- The local anesthetic should always be injected on an incremental basis.

Continuous caudal anesthesia

Puncture needles
As for the single-shot technique.

Catheter
Atraumatic epidural catheters with a central opening are used.

Before insertion
The length of the needle must be compared with the calibration marks on the catheter to improve assessment of the depth of the catheter after introduction (Fig. 47.17). At the same time, the ability of the catheter to pass through the needle can be tested.
Preparation, puncture and introduction of the needle into the sacral canal are the same as in the single-shot technique.

Further steps
After aspiration at two different levels, the catheter is advanced through the needle to a depth of 3–4 cm.

- If there is any obstruction, the catheter must never be advanced using force, since the obstruction may be caused by the dura, a nerve or a blood vessel.
- The catheter must never be withdrawn through the needle (risk of shearing).

Removing the needle
After the catheter has been positioned as required, the needle is carefully withdrawn, with the catheter being simultaneously secured with the thumb and index finger of the left hand at the injection site (Fig. 47.18).

Checking the patency of the catheter
An adapter is attached to the end of the catheter (Fig. 47.19a) and 1 mL of saline is injected (Fig. 47.19b).

Pain during the injection suggests that the catheter is positioned intraneurally. The injection must be stopped and the position of the catheter must be corrected by withdrawing it minimally.

Chapter 47

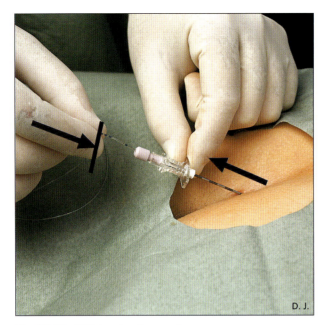

Fig. 47.18a Withdrawing the needle

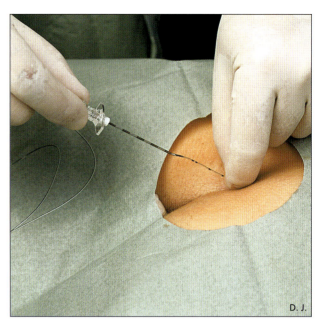

Fig. 47.18b Securing the catheter with the thumb and index finger

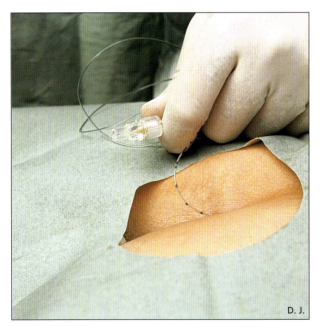

Fig. 47.19a Attaching the adapter

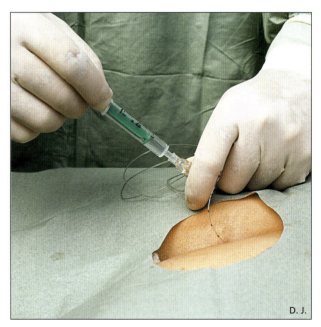

Fig. 47.19b Injection of 1 mL 0.9% NaCl

Caudal anesthesia in adult patients

Aspiration test (Fig. 47.20)

Observe the open end of the catheter carefully
The syringe is disconnected and the open end of the catheter is placed on the sterile drape lower than the puncture site. Any escaping fluid (CSF or blood) is noted (Fig. 47.21).

Test dose
3–4 mL of an epinephrine-containing local anesthetic (Fig. 47.22).

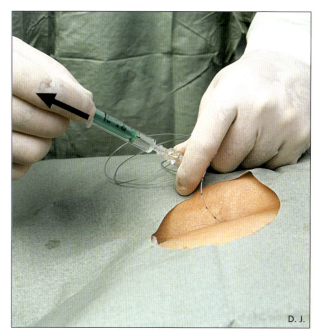

Fig. 47.20 Aspiration test

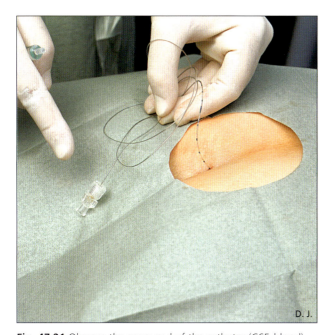

Fig. 47.21 Observe the open end of the catheter (CSF, blood)

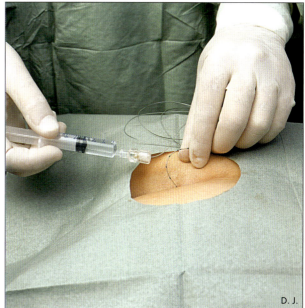

Fig. 47.22 Test dose

Chapter 47

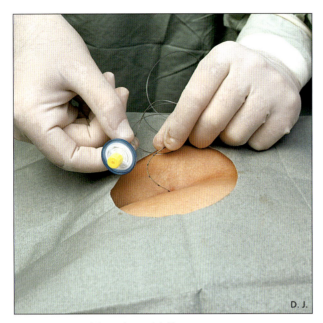

Fig. 47.23 Attaching a bacterial filter

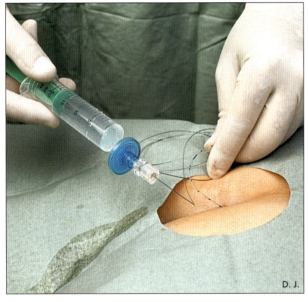

Fig. 47.24 Incremental injection of a local anesthetic

Waiting period
Wait for 5 minutes. During this time, careful cardiovascular monitoring is carried out. Verbal contact must be maintained with the patient.

Five minutes after administration of the test dose, the lower extremities, abdomen and chest are tested for possible numbness, to exclude the possibility of inadvertent subarachnoid injection.

Incremental injection of a local anesthetic
After placement of a bacterial filter (Fig. 47.23), sterile attachment of the catheter and repeated aspiration, incremental injection of local anesthetic is carried out (Fig. 47.24).

Dosages

The same principles apply here as in lumbar epidural anesthesia. Due to the wide variations in the capacity of the sacral canal in the adult, it is difficult to give precise details of the volume of local anesthetic to be injected.

The concentration of local anesthetic determines the intensity of the block. Usually, 20–35 mL of local anesthetic is administered (2–3 mL per segment in the adult). A delay in the onset of effect must be anticipated. The time to onset of effect is shortened and the motor block is intensified when epinephrine is added.

Anesthetic spread (segment)	Local anesthetic (mL)
S5–L2	15–20
S5–T10	25–30

In pregnant patients and obese patients, the dose should be reduced by about 30%.

Local anesthetics
Surgical procedures

Ropivacaine	0.75–1%
Bupivacaine	0.375–0.5% (levobupivacaine 0.375–0.5%)
Prilocaine	2% (contraindicated in obstetrics)
Mepivacaine	1.5–2%
Lidocaine	1.5–2%

Diagnostic and therapeutic blocks
(No addition of epinephrine!)

Block	Sensory	Sympathetic
Ropivacaine	0.375–0.5%	0.2%
Bupivacaine	0.25%	0.125%
Levobupivacaine	0.25%	0.125%
Prilocaine	1%	0.5%
Mepivacaine	1%	0.5%
Lidocaine	1%	0.5%

Pain therapy
Combination of local anesthetic and corticosteroids
- 15 mL 0.2% ropivacaine or 15–20 mL 0.125% bupivacaine (0.125% levobupivacaine) mixed with 40–80 mg triamcinolone acetonide (soluble Volon A) (see Chapter 45).
- In outpatient procedures, 0.5% prilocaine or 0.5% mepivacaine or 0.5% lidocaine can be used as an alternative.

Opioids
Bolus injections
In combination with a local anesthetic:

Sufentanil:	30–50 µg
Fentanyl:	50 µg
Morphine:	2–5 mg

Continuous administration
See Chapter 41, p. 317.

Complications (Fig. 47.25)

- Complications due to poor technique:
  Intraosseous injection into the richly vascularized vertebral bodies.
  Puncture needle lying on the sacrum: crepitation or subcutaneous swelling may be noticed after injection of air, saline or local anesthetic.
  Subperiosteal positioning: this becomes evident through resistance during the injection and associated pain.
  Needle positioned ventral to the sacrum: the needle is located between the sacrum and the coccyx. Advancing it further could lead to perforation of the rectum, or in obstetric anesthesia to injury to the head of the fetus.
  Prophylaxis: strict observation of the midline.
- Infections: in about 0.2% of patients. Strict asepsis is the best form of prophylaxis.
- Intravascular injection (see Chapter 6, p. 65).
- Intrathecal injection, with high or total spinal anesthesia (see Chapter 41, p. 324).
  Prophylaxis: in adults, the puncture needle should not be advanced further than 3.5 cm and in children not more than 1 cm.
  Check the position of the needle tip in relation to the dural sac. Particular care is required in children (the end of the dural sac is often at S3–4).
  Test dose, incremental injection of the local anesthetic, verbal contact with the patient, circulatory monitoring, testing the anesthetic spread.
- Massive epidural anesthesia:
  When attempting to reach segment T10, unpredictable spread of the anesthesia caused by the local anesthetic must be anticipated.
- Hypotension, bradycardia, nausea, vomiting.
- Bladder emptying difficulties.
- Postdural puncture headache (see Chapter 37, p. 287).
- Breaking of the needle or catheter shearing:
  Check the needle before the block and do not advance it over its full length. A catheter must never be withdrawn through the needle.
- Neurological complications:
  These arise very rarely and are usually caused by trauma to the lumbosacral plexus – e.g. by the child's head during delivery or by instruments. The complications include paresthesias, peroneal nerve paralysis or coccygodynia. These complications are not causally connected to the caudal anesthesia.
- Cauda equina syndrome (see Chapter 37, p. 292).
- Epidural abscess (see Chapter 41, p. 326).
- Epidural hematoma (see Chapter 41, p. 326).

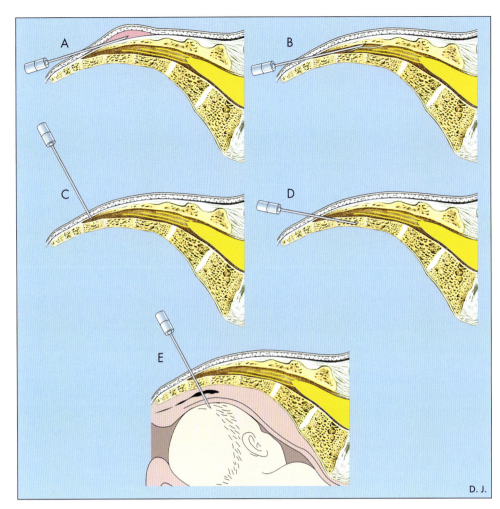

Fig. 47.25a–e Complications due to incorrect technique.
a Outside the sacral canal. **b** Subperiosteal. **c** Into the sacrococcygeal ligament. **d** Spongiosa. **e** Through the sacrum

Caudal anesthesia in adult patients

Caudal anesthesia

Name: _____ Date: _____
Diagnosis: _____
Premedication: ☐ No ☐ Yes
Neurological abnormalities: ☐ No ☐ Yes _____

Purpose of block: ☐ *Surgical* ☐ *Therapeutic* ☐ *Diagnostic*
Needle: ☐ G _____ ☐ *With stylet* ☐ *Without stylet*
i.v. access, infusion: ☐ *Yes*
Monitoring: ☐ *ECG* ☐ *Pulse oximetry*
Ventilation facilities: ☐ *Yes (equipment checked)*
Emergency equipment *(drugs)*: ☐ *Checked*
Patient: ☐ *Informed*

Position: ☐ *Prone* ☐ *Lateral decubitus*
Epidural space: ☐ *Identified*
Checking position of needle tip relative to dural sac (2nd sacral foramen):
☐ *Carried out*
Aspiration test: ☐ *Carried out*
Injection: *(5 cm³ air or 0.9% NaCl)* ☐ *Carried out*
Test dose: _____ Epinephrine added: ☐ *Yes* ☐ *No*
Motor and sensory function check after 5 min: ☐ *Carried out*
Abnormalities: ☐ *No* ☐ *Yes* _____
Injection:
Local anesthetic: _____ mL _____ %
(incremental)
☐ Addition: _____ µg/mg

Patient's remarks during injection:
☐ *None* ☐ *Pain* ☐ *Paresthesias* ☐ *Warmth*
Duration and area: _____
Objective block effect after 20 min:
☐ *Cold test* ☐ *Temperature measurement before* _____ °C *after* _____ °C
☐ *Sensory:* L _____ T _____
☐ *Motor*

Complications:
☐ *None* ☐ *Pain*
☐ *Radicular symptoms* ☐ *Vasovagal reactions*
☐ *BP drop* ☐ *Dural puncture*
☐ *Vascular puncture* ☐ *Intravascular injection*
☐ *Massive epidural anesthesia* ☐ *Total spinal anesthesia*
☐ *Bladder emptying disturbances* ☐ *Respiratory disturbance*
☐ *Coccygeal pain* ☐ *Postdural puncture headache*
☐ *Neurological complications*

Special notes:
_____
_____

© Copyright ABW Wissenschaftsverlag 2004,
Jankovic, Regional nerve blocks and infiltration therapy, 3rd edition

Record and checklist

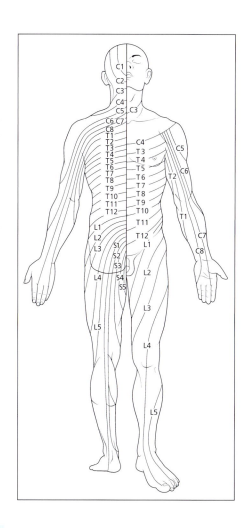

48 Caudal anesthesia in children

In children, the caudal approach is the easiest and safest route to the epidural space.

Advantages [5, 9]
- Better anatomic relationships and thus easier orientation and shorter time required for puncture.
- Perforation of the sacrococcygeal ligament is more easily palpable.
- Better distribution of the injected anesthetic than in the adult.
- Very effective anesthesia and analgesia with small amounts of local anesthetic.
- An 18-G epidural catheter can be used in children of almost any age group.
- It is easier to advance the epidural catheter than in the adult.
- Higher positioning of the catheter is possible, particularly in neonates and infants.
- The immaturity of the sympathetic nervous system means that circulatory problems are extremely rare, particularly up to the age of eight.
- There is a very rapid recovery phase due to the supplementary light general anesthesia and avoidance of muscle relaxants.
- There is a quiet postoperative phase and thus reduced opioids – and therefore fewer side effects such as nausea, vomiting, or urinary retention.
- The need for subsequent postoperative intensive therapy is reduced.

Disadvantages
- Mild light general anesthesia is needed in principle, so that precise testing of the spread of anesthesia is not possible [5]. This problem can sometimes be overcome when Emla cream is used in combination with sedation.
- The risk of contamination with caudal epidural catheters is higher than with lumbar epidural catheters.

Characteristics of the epidural space in children [5]
In children under 1 year of age, the dural sac reaches to the third or even to the fourth sacral foramen. The jelly-like epidural fatty tissue is more permeable and allows the injected local anesthetic to spread much better than in the adult.

When advancing the epidural catheter, hardly any resistance is produced. In neonates and infants up to 6 kg in body weight in particular, it is possible to reach almost any height due to the relatively wide epidural space, which is almost empty and runs parallel to the dura.

In older children, obstruction occurs more often when advancing the catheter, particularly in the area from L2 to L5.

Indications
Single-shot technique
- All surgical procedures below the T10 dermatome with an operating time of up to 90 minutes – e.g. perineal and perianal procedures, orchidopexy (not undescended testis), hypospadias, inguinal hernia, incarcerated hernias.
- Superficial surgical procedures in the lower extremities – e.g. skin grafts, etc.

Contraindications
These correspond to those in caudal anesthesia in the adult (see Chapter 47, p. 362).

Procedure

Full prior information for the patient and parents is mandatory.

Light general anesthesia, or more rarely sedation in combination with local application of Emla cream, is used with both the single-shot technique and continuous caudal anesthesia.

Preparation
- Location and marking of the sacral cornua.
- Palpation of the dorsal cranial iliac spines.
- Strict asepsis (thorough skin prep).
- Local anesthesia or application of Emla cream.

- Preparation of the drugs:
  Syringe with 1 mL epinephrine-containing local anesthetic (test dose).
  Syringe with the calculated quantity of local anesthetic.
- Skin incision using a stylet or large needle.

Materials
These correspond to those for caudal anesthesia in the adult (see Chapter 47, p. 363); a **precordial stethoscope** is also needed.

Caudal needles
A wide variety of needle types are used all over the world for caudal injection in children: normal hypodermic needles, Tuohy or Crawford needles, plastic indwelling catheter needles and in children weighing less than 4 kg, 23-G butterfly needles as well [11].
There are no standardized criteria for assessing these, so that the choice is a matter of personal preference and experience on the part of the anesthetist concerned.

On the basis of numerous publications, the following summary can be given:
the use of puncture needles without a trochar can lead to dangerous transport of free skin particles with epidermal cells into the spinal canal, with later development of epidermoid tumors [3, 10, 12, 18].

For this reason, the following recommendation has been made:
caudal puncture in children should only be carried out after a preliminary skin incision using a large needle or stylet, and a needle with a trochar should always be used [4].
The use of a purpose-designed epidural kit is recommended (e.g. Epican Paed, B. Braun Melsungen).
Pediatric caudal needles:
- Size: 0.53 × 30 mm, 25 G, with 32° short bevel and steel trochar.
- Or 0.73 × 35 mm, 22 G, also with 32° short bevel and steel trochar.
- Or 0.90 × 50 mm, 20 G, also with 32° short bevel and steel trochar.

Single-shot technique

Patient positioning
Lateral decubitus, with the legs bent (Fig. 48.1).

Puncture of the caudal epidural space

> In children younger than 1 year, the dural sac reaches as far as the third or even fourth sacral foramen.

The needle is introduced in a cranial direction at an angle of 60–70°, towards the sacral dorsum (Fig. 48.2). After the very clear sensation of the sacrococcygeal ligament, the needle reaches the sacral canal ("sudden give"). The needle position is not altered any further.
The thumb and index finger remain on the sacral cornua throughout the whole of the location and injection procedure.
Then:
- Withdraw the trochar.
- Check the end of the needle for escaping fluid (CSF, blood).
- Aspirate.
- Inject a test dose of 1 mL of an epinephrine-containing local anesthetic.

During the subsequent waiting period:
Careful cardiovascular monitoring is carried out, along with the precordial stethoscope, to recognize the development of tachycardia or arrhythmia. However, this test can lead to unreliable results in anesthetized children [8].

Incremental injection of local anesthetic
After a negative result with the test dose, the calculated dose of local anesthetic is injected on an incremental basis (Fig. 48.3).
As this is done, the index and middle finger are laid on the surface of the sacrum, so that subcutaneous injection can be recognized quickly.

Checking the spread of anesthesia
The spread of anesthesia should always be checked in children who have not received general anesthesia.
As correct testing of the anesthetic spread is not possible in anesthetized children, this method is reserved only for highly experienced anesthetists.
Postoperatively, a detailed examination of sensory and motor function is carried out. The child should be moved to the normal ward only if he or she is able to move the legs freely.

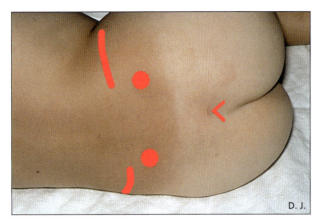

Fig. 48.1 Lateral decubitus position, with the legs bent

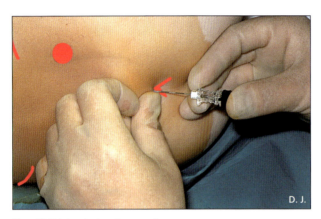

Fig. 48.2 Introducing the needle

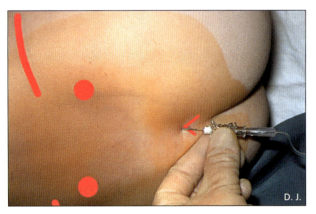

Fig. 48.3 The needle is positioned in the sacral canal. Incremental injection of a local anesthetic

Continuous caudal anesthesia

Indications
In combination with light general anesthesia in longer-duration operations on the upper and lower abdomen, in the urogenital area and on the legs.

Contraindications
See Chapter 47, p. 362.

Disadvantage
Due to the risk of infection (proximity to the anogenital region), the catheter should be withdrawn immediately after the end of the operation.

Preparation, materials, patient positioning
See Chapter 47, p. 363.

Puncture of the caudal epidural space
- Skin incision using a stylet or large needle.
- The plastic indwelling catheter needle (or Tuohy) is advanced at an angle of 60–70° in the direction of the sacrococcygeal ligament. After perforation of the ligament, the needle is advanced 1 cm into the sacral canal, the trochar is removed and the plastic part is advanced a further 0.5 cm.
- After palpation of the iliac crests through the drapes, the catheter should be measured to allow the desired dermatome to be located.
- The catheter is now advanced to the desired dermatome. In neonates, infants and small children, the catheter meets hardly any resistance, so that it is easy to advance it to the upper lumbar or thoracic segments.

> A catheter must never be advanced against resistance, which may be caused by the dura, a nerve or a blood vessel.

Checking the catheter position
- Removal of the plastic indwelling catheter needle.
- Checking the patency of the catheter:
  An adapter is attached to the end of the catheter and 1 mL saline is injected.
- Aspiration.

- The open end of the catheter should be carefully observed.

  The syringe is disconnected, the open end of the catheter is placed on the sterile drape below the level of the puncture and any escaping fluid (CSF or blood) is noted.

Test dose of an epinephrine-containing local anesthetic
During the waiting period: careful circulatory monitoring (ECG, pulse oximetry, precordial stethoscope).

Placement of a bacterial filter, sterile attachment of the catheter

Administration of local anesthetics
- Injection of one-quarter of the calculated dose of local anesthetic.
- When there is no resistance to the injection, the remaining dose can be administered at a speed of 0.7 mL/s.

  Larger amounts of local anesthetic are needed if the injection is carried out more slowly [5].

Dosages
The following parameters are particularly important for the dosage of local anesthetics in neonates, infants and small children:
- Better penetration of the local anesthetic solution takes place due to the incomplete myelinization of the nerves in infants and due to the small diameter of the nerves in small children. This means that lower doses are required.
- Muscle relaxation, particularly in extensive abdominal or orthopedic procedures, can be produced by adding epinephrine.
- The "threshold block" is much more extensive, reaching as far as five dermatomes.
- Surprisingly low plasma concentrations are found in children after administration of the maximum dose of a local anesthetic.
- In comparison with adults, the dosage of local anesthetic is more reliable and precise and is based on the tried and tested parameters of age, weight and height.

The following guidelines may be helpful for the dosage of local anesthetic.

Schulte-Steinberg dose scheme [17]
The age of the child is used according to the following formula:
0.1 mL per segment to be blocked × age in years

The pin-prick test is taken into account here and thin C fibers are blocked.

Busoni and Andreucetti dose scheme [5–7]
For clinical applications, particularly in longer, more extensive surgical procedures, the **age and weight** of the child are used as the parameters, with 1% mepivacaine being tested. Testing of the analgesia is carried out by pinching (thicker A-delta fibers) and pin-pricks (thin C fibers). The anesthesia reaches about four to six dermatomes lower ("threshold block").

In neonates and infants, weight is a reliable parameter; in small children, age has proved to be a better parameter for assessing the required dosage. Experienced anesthetists have found Busoni's diagrams (Fig. 48.4) particularly useful.

Armitage dose scheme [1, 2]
This schema is easy to use and has also proved itself with less experienced anesthetists. The following dosage is recommended:

Lumbosacral block: 0.50 mL/kg b.w.
Thoracolumbar block: 1.00 mL/kg b.w.
Mid-thoracic block: 1.25 mL/kg b. w.

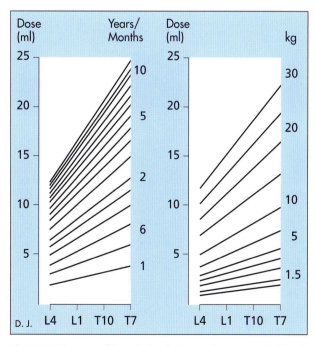

Fig. 48.4 Diagram of the relation between dose, spread of analgesia, age and body weight for various segmental levels.

[Adapted from Busoni, in: Saint-Maurice C, Schulte-Steinberg O, Armitage E (eds.), *Regional Anesthesia in Children* (Appleton & Lange/Mediglobe, 1990]

Concentration of the local anesthetic
Ropivacaine: 0.2%
Bupivacaine: 0.25–0.375%
Levobupivacaine: 0.2%
Mepivacaine: 1%
Lidocaine: 1%

Dosage [13]
Ropivacaine 0.2%: 2 mg/kg b.w.
Bupivacaine 0.25%: 2.5 mg/kg b.w.
Mepivacaine 0.1%: 7–10 mg/kg b.w.

Continuous epidural infusion
Of 0.1% ropivacaine or 0.125% bupivacaine [13]
Neonates and infants: 0.2 mg/kg/h
Small children: 0.3–0.4 mg/kg/h
Older children: 0.4–0.5 mg/kg/h

Opioids
Morphine: 0.03 mg/kg/8 h
Fentanyl: 0.5 µg/kg/h

Clonidine
2–3 µg/kg/24 h

After the volume has been calculated, the maximum dose for the body weight should be calculated and the local anesthetic should be diluted accordingly.
If the calculated quantity of local anesthetic is less than 20 mL, administration of 0.25% bupivacaine, for example, is recommended. If the calculated quantity is over 20 mL, dilution in saline should be carried out until a concentration of 0.19% bupivacaine is reached [9].

Complications
See Chapter 47, section on complications, p. 373.

49 Percutaneous epidural neuroplasty

James E. Heavner, Gabor B. Racz, Miles Day, Rinoo Shah

Introduction

Percutaneous epidural neuroplasty (epidural neurolysis, epidural adhesiolysis) is a form of interventional pain treatment that was first described in 1989 [11]. The method is used at all levels of the spine to treat neuraxial pain conditions or radiculopathies, or both, as well as certain forms of cervicogenic headache.

The development of this procedure and its growing acceptance have been promoted by the following factors: a) new information regarding the importance of epidural and intervertebral structural changes and their role in the development of back pain and radicular pain; b) a better understanding of the structures involved in the origin of pain in the epidural space and its surroundings; c) data on the type and location of pain arising due to stimulation of certain pathological structures in the epidural space and its vicinity; d) the development of reliable percutaneous puncture techniques in the epidural space; e) recognition of epidurography as a valuable method of diagnosis and treatment; f) clear guidelines and theoretical justifications for the procedure and the drugs used in it; g) evidence of the effectiveness of the treatment in patients; and h) recognition of the procedure by qualified physicians.

The aims in percutaneous epidural neuroplasty are:
1. To diagnose pathological changes in the epidural space (e.g. epidural fibrosis) that may prevent administered drugs from reaching these pathological structures. Radiographic contrast media are used to identify the filling defects.
2. To remove all pathological obstructions and scar tissue as potential causes of pain. For this purpose, physiological saline mixed with hyaluronidase is applied to the scar tissue.
3. To determine whether the pathological obstructions causing pain have been removed after a procedure. Radiographic contrast media are again injected for this purpose.
4. To carry out targeted local administration of drugs that lead to the relief or reduction of pain (local anesthetics, steroids and hypertonic saline).

The origins of back pain and sciatica

When conducting surgery under local anesthesia in the lumbar spine, Kuslich et al. [3] found that sciatica could be triggered by irritation of swollen, overextended, or compressed nerve roots. By contrast, back pain could be triggered by stimulation of various tissues in the lumbar region – most frequently in the outer layer of the anulus fibrosus and posterior longitudinal ligament. Roffe [13] showed that both of these structures are richly supplied with nerves connected to the CNS via meningeal branches (sinuvertebral nerves) (Fig. 49.1). By contrast, stimulation of the capsule of the facet joints rarely caused back pain, and never caused sensitivity in the synovial bursa or cartilaginous sur-

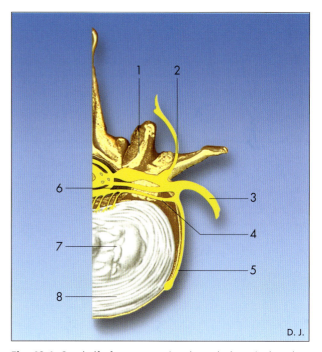

Fig. 49.1 One half of a cross-section through the spinal cord, showing the innervation. As described in the text, the sinuvertebral nerve supplies the anulus fibrosis and the posterior longitudinal ligament – two structures that play an important role in the development of back pain.
(1) Facet, (2) posterior primary ramus, (3) anterior ramus, (4) sinuvertebral nerve, (5) sympathetic, (6) root, (7) nucleus, (8) annulus

faces. In patients who had previously undergone a laminectomy, there were always one or more areas of marked perineural fibrosis. It was never the scar tissue itself that was sensitive; instead, there was often marked irritability in the nerve root. It is suspected that the scar tissue immobilizes the nerve root and thereby favors the development of pain when the nerve root is subject to traction or pressure.

Kusslich et al. concluded that "Sciatica can only be caused by direct pressure or traction on an inflamed, stretched, or compressed nerve root. No other tissue in the spine is able to trigger pain in the leg."

However, nerve roots are exposed not only to mechanical effects, but also to material from degenerated intervertebral disks or facet joints [9].

Pressure (Fig. 49.2)
The effects of pressure on the nerves depend on whether it is high pressure or low pressure (e.g. < 200 mmHg) that is being exerted. High pressure can produce direct mechanical effects on the nerve tissue and can distort the nerve fibers, shift the nodes of Ranvier, or press in the paranodal myelin sheath. Lower pressures lead to tissue changes caused by a reduction in the blood supply to the nerve tissue. In animal experiments, it has been found that when inflation of a balloon attached to the spinal cord makes the pressure on the cauda equina equivalent to arterial pressure, blood flow in the cauda equina is interrupted [9]. Even a pressure of 5–10 mmHg interrupts venous blood flow in some small veins, while a pressure of 10 mmHg reduces the transport of nutrients to the nerve roots by 20–30%. Compression can also cause changes in the permeability or transmural pressure conditions in the endoneural capillaries in the nerve roots, and can lead to edema formation (in the animal experiment, for example, this occurred after 2 min of compression at 50 mmHg).

Intraneural edema due to chronic nerve injury is associated with the development of neural fibrosis, which may contribute to the very slow rate of symptomatic improvement observed in some patients with nerve compression.

Compression of spinal nerves at 10 mmHg for 2 hours by two adjacent balloons (to simulate the clinical conditions occurring in multiple nerve compression) reduced neural conduction and led to a reduction in the recorded amplitudes of action potentials by ca. 65%. By contrast, compression by a single balloon at 50 mmHg for 2 hours did not alter the amplitude of the action potentials. A pressure of 10 mmHg (with incomplete blockage of small veins) only appears to be capable of causing changes in nerve function if the spinal nerve roots are compressed into two segments [9]. Intervertebral disk prolapses or protrusions can cause higher levels of compression pressure than central spinal stenosis.

Chemical irritation (Fig. 49.2)
Some chemical substances have been identified in the nucleus pulposus that can lead to irritation of neighboring structures if tears in the anulus fibrosus lead to them being released into the vertebral canal. These substances, which can cause inflammation of nerve roots and meninges, include lactic acid, glycoprotein, cytokines, and histamine. In addition, it is considered theoretically possible that components of the nucleus pulposus can act as foreign proteins and trigger an autoimmune reaction. This type of chemically caused irritation can arise without any compression by an intervertebral disk.

Structural changes
Intervertebral disk anomalies can manifest as degenerative changes, protrusion, or herniation [1]. Constriction of the intervertebral space due to disk injury is often associated with osteophyte formation and arthrosis of the facet joints, which can lead to increased pressure on the spinal nerves. Stretching of the posterior longitudinal ligament by protruding intervertebral disks initially leads to localized back pain, while more severe protrusions also cause pressure on neighboring nerve roots and can lead to radicular pain.

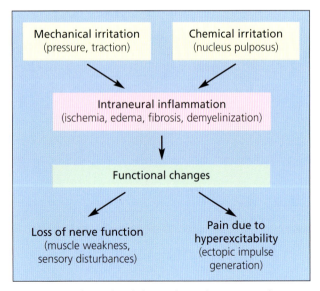

Fig. 49.2 Mechanical and chemical stimulants trigger the development of neuraxial pain and radiculopathy, as well as cervicogenic headache [10]

Theoretical considerations

The current debate has shown that in patients with chronic neuraxial pain and/or radiculopathy or cervicogenic headache, one or more of the following pathological changes may be present (Fig. 49.2):

- Inflammation.
- Edema.
- Fibrosis.
- Venous stasis.
- Mechanical pressure on:
  - Posterior longitudinal ligament
  - Anulus fibrosus
  - Spinal nerve
- Reduced or absent nutrient supply to the spinal nerves or nerve roots.
- Central sensitization.

The inflammatory tissue changes can activate nociceptors or axons that conduct nociceptive information to the CNS. Equally, owing to inflammation, nociceptors or nociceptive axons may react more sensitively to mechanical stimuli. This type of mechanical irritation may be triggered either by pressure stress, as described above, or may be caused by movement-dependent stretching due to entrapment of spinal nerves or nerve roots by fibrous tissue.

Most experience with neuroplasty has been gathered in the treatment of chronic pain conditions. Most of the patients concerned therefore probably have both peripheral and central changes (e.g. central sensitization) contributing jointly to the chronic pain condition.

It is therefore theoretically justifiable to treat back pain with or without radiculopathy by local administration of drugs. Possible forms of treatment include:

- Anti-inflammatory drugs (e.g. corticosteroids).
- Drugs that reduce edema formation (e.g. hypertonic saline 10% and corticosteroids).
- Local anesthetics to block the nerve fibers that conduct pain information to the CNS (hypertonic saline also has a local anesthetic effect).
- Addition of hyaluronidase to remove scar tissue. This makes it possible for the drug being used to reach the target tissue.

Figure 49.3 shows the selection criteria for patients who are candidates for percutaneous epidural neuroplasty; noninvasive, conservative treatment methods should be attempted first. Our technique is described in Table 49.1. Table 49.2 lists the most frequently used injection solutions.

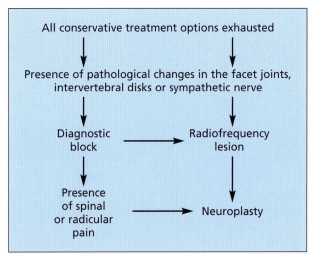

Fig. 49.3 Algorithm for the treatment of neuraxial pain and radiculopathy, as well as cervicogenic headache. Neuroplasty is considered when conservative forms of treatment have proved to be ineffective and the appropriate diagnosis is confirmed

Table 49.1 Overview of neuroplasty

In the operating room:
1. Placement of the epidural needle
2. Injection of contrast and imaging of its spread (epidurogram)
3. If there is a filling defect in the area in which the pain is located, introduction of a Racz catheter into the filling defect (scar)
4. Repeat contrast injection to ensure that the contrast is now also spreading in the area of the filling defect
5. Injection of preservative-free saline, with or without hyaluronidase (Wydase, Hylase)
6. Injection of local anesthetic and corticosteroids
7. Securing the catheter

In the recovery room:
8. 30 min after the injection of a mixture of steroids and local anesthetic, infusion of 10 mL hypertonic saline (10%) over 30 min

On the ward:
9. On each of the two following days, an injection of local anesthetic followed 30 min later by hypertonic saline (10%) is administered
10. The epidural catheter is removed after the final treatment

Table 49.2 Injected solutions according to the spinal cord section (volume in mL) in the injection sequence

Solution	Cervical	Thoracic	Lumbar	Caudal
Iohexol	2–3	4–6	10	10
Iohexol	1–2	2–3	3	3
Saline 0.9% + 1500 IU hyaluronidase	4–6	6–8	10	10
Ropivacaine 0.2% + corticosteroid* (test dose)	2	2	3	3
Ropivacaine 0.2% + cortikosteroid*	2–4	4–6	7	7
Hypertonic saline	4–6	6–8	10	10
Saline 0.9%	2	2	2	2
Then, on each of the following days:				
Ropivacaine 0.2% (test dose)	2	2	3	3
Ropivacaine 0.2%	4	6	7	7
Hypertonic saline	4–6	6–8	10	10
Saline 0.9%	2	2	2	2

* 4 mg dexamethasone oer 40 mg methylprednisolone or triamcinolone

Technique of percutaneous epidural neurolysis

Caudal access route

Procedure

Careful information discussion with the patient before the block
Full prior information for the patient is mandatory. The patient should be informed about all of the potential complications that can occur during and after the procedure (e.g. epidural hematoma, epidural abscess, numbness in the extremities, rectal or bladder emptying disturbances, paralyses, infection, sexual dysfunction, shearing of the epidural catheter, etc.).

Materials
See Chapter 47 on epidural caudal anesthesia.
16-G R-K/15-G RX-Coudé needles – fluoropolymer-coated epidural catheter made of stainless steel with a spiral tip (Racz-Tun-L-Kath/24; Epimed International, Inc. Irving, Texas, USA).

Preparations
See Chapter 47 on epidural caudal anesthesia.
Intravenous access is required in order to treat potential adverse events (e.g. total spinal anesthesia, subdural injection, intravascular injection, etc.), as well as to administer analgesia and sedation during the procedure and antibiotics postoperatively.
Analgesia and sedation are recommended before the procedure (e.g. 1–2 mg midazolam + 25–50 µg fentanyl), as the injection is usually painful in patients with epidural adhesions. The injection pain is probably caused by stretching of the nerve roots affected, and it spreads in the corresponding cutaneous innervation area. The patient should not receive deep sedation. The patient needs to be capable of cooperating during the procedure to ensure that any signs of spinal cord compression are not overlooked. (The patient has to be able to move the extremity affected and report any weakness or paralysis during the procedure).
All procedures are conducted under fluoroscopic guidance, using a C-arm with a storage function (reduced radiation exposure). Fluoroscopic guidance optimizes the results of the procedure (correct needle positioning, easier identification of the defect, ability to check the spread of the contrast and correct positioning of the catheter). The usual protective measures for staff are obligatory.

Selection of drugs
■ Radiographic contrast media
To exclude inadvertent subarachnoid injection, a water-soluble contrast medium is used. In our experience, the presence of epidural adhesions increases the risk of subarachnoid injections. Subarachnoid injection of a contrast medium that is not water-soluble can lead to serious complications (spinal cord irritation, spinal cramp or clonus, arachnoiditis, paralysis, and death).

■ Local anesthetic
E.g. 0.2% ropivacaine.

■ Corticosteroids
The choice of the corticosteroid to be used (Table 49.2) mainly depends on which agents are available. Long-acting steroid emulsions have a particle size of ca. 20 µm and it is therefore not possible to inject them through bacterial filters.

■ Hypertonic saline (10%)
The local anesthetic effect of hypertonic saline is used to prolong the intended pain relief so that the patient can receive physiotherapy twice a day.

■ Antibiotics
30 min before the start of the procedure, 1 g ceftriaxone (Rocephin) is administered intravenously. During the hospital stay, the same dose is administered every 24 hours. Patients who are allergic to penicillin receive 500 mg ciprofloxacin (Ciprobay) or levofloxacin orally 1 hour before the procedure, as well as over the following 5 days (500 mg cefalexin or ciprofloxacin every 12 hours, or 500 mg levofloxacin every 12 hours).

Technique
Patient position
The patient is placed in the prone position on the fluoroscopy table (see Chapter 47, p. 364).

Landmarks
The sacral region is prepared and covered with sterile drapes, and the sacral cornua and sacral hiatus are palpated. The puncture site is located in the gluteal cleft **opposite the affected side**, approximately 1 cm lateral to and 2.5 cm below the sacral hiatus. From this point, it is easier to guide the needle and catheter towards the affected side. The lateral access reduces the risk of the needle or catheter penetrating the dural sac or subdural space.

Local anesthesia
Infiltration of the puncture site with 1% lidocaine is carried out.

Puncture
After a skin incision with a stylet, an epidural needle (preferably a 16-G R-K or 15-G RX-Coudé needle; Fig. 49.5) is introduced into the sacral hiatus.

> Tuohy needles should not be used.

The needle is introduced caudal to the S3 foramen. Lateral fluoroscopy is used to check that the needle is positioned inside the osseous canal. This radiographic check is particularly important when there are unusual anatomical features in the sacral bone. Anteroposterior radiography is used to check that the needle tip is directed toward the affected side. A check is then made for escaping fluid (CSF or blood), and an aspiration test is carried out. After a negative aspiration test, 10 mL Iohexol (Omnipaque 240) is injected under fluoroscopic guidance. When injected into the epidural space, the contrast forms a **Christmas-tree–shaped distribution pattern**. The presence of epidural adhesions prevents the contrast from spreading in this characteristic pattern, with the affected nerve roots being omitted.

Problem situations
■ Subarachnoid needle location
If the puncture needle is in a subarachnoid location, the contrast medium spreads in a central and cranial direction. If it is in a subdural position, the contrast spreads in a similar fashion, but not as far as with a subarachnoid injection. Despite this, the contours of the nerve roots and dura are visible, since the contrast spreads into the less resistant subdural space.
Injection of a local anesthetic into the subarachnoid or subdural space leads to a motor block that is much stronger and has a much faster onset of effect than injection into the epidural space.

■ Aspiration of blood
When blood is aspirated, the needle position should be carefully corrected until no more blood is aspirated.

■ Aspiration of CSF
If CSF is aspirated, it is best to halt the procedure and repeat it on the following day.

■ Allergic reactions
When the patient has an allergic reaction to an iodine-containing contrast agent, it is best to continue the rest of the procedure without radiographic guidance after confirming fluoroscopically that the needle is in the correct position.

Introducing the epidural catheter (Fig. 49.4)
Radiopaque catheters with soft tips are used in the injections of local anesthetics, corticosteroids, and hypertonic saline described below. For this purpose, a fluoropolymer-coated epidural catheter made of stainless steel, with a spiral tip (Racz-Tun-L-Kath/24) or a less flexible Racz-Tun-Kath XL (Fig. 49.5) is introduced into the adhesions through the needle. The beveled side of the needle should be directed toward the ventrolateral side of the caudal canal, since this position – together with a 15–30° bend about 2.5 cm below the catheter

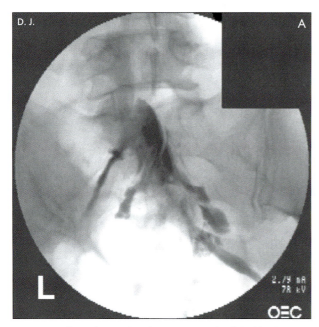 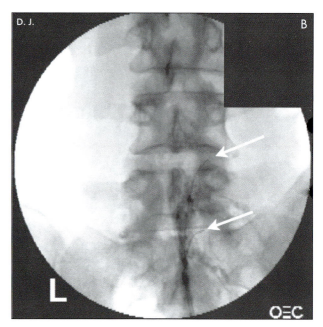

Fig. 49.4a, b Radiographs of a patient with "failed back surgery syndrome" and bilateral sciatica in the region of L2–L5. The pain was more severe on the right than on the left. **a** Epidurogram at the start of the procedure. The contrast has not spread beyond the iliosacral joint, and a filling defect is seen on the right. **b** After catheter placement and injection of the solutions (see text). The tips of two catheters were placed in the intervertebral spaces in L4–L5 and L5–S1

tip – makes it easier for the catheter tip to reach the desired anterolateral position and reduces the risk of catheter shearing. As the epidural adhesions are usually irregularly distributed, several corrections of the catheter position may be needed to achieve the correct position of the catheter in the desired area. For this reason, it is recommended to use a 16-G R-K or 15-G RX-Coudé epidural catheter, or an SCA catheter introducer, to make it easier to carry out the necessary corrections of the catheter's position.

Contrast injection
After the catheter tip has been placed in the correct position and after a negative aspiration test, contrast is injected again (Table 49.2). Previously recognizable filling defects along the targeted spinal nerves or nerve roots should now fill.

Injection of the local anesthetic and corticosteroid
Following a repeated aspiration test, 0.2% ropivacaine and 40 mg triamcinolone acetate is now injected through the catheter (Table 49.2). The areas in which epidural adhesions had developed and were dissolved should be documented.

Injection of hypertonic saline
30 min later, after a negative aspiration test, the patient is placed in the lateral decubitus position on the painful side for the following 30–60 min. 10 mL of a hypertonic saline solution (10%) is injected epidurally via an infusion pump over 30 min. The indwelling catheter is then rinsed with 0.9% saline (Table 49.2). Hypertonic saline has a reversible weak-

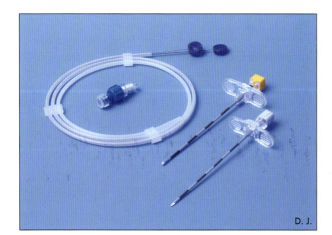

Fig. 49.5 Materials. 16-G R-K-/15-G RX-Coudé needles; fluoropolymer-coated epidural catheters made of stainless steel with spiral tips (Racz-Tun-L-Kath/24, Epimed International, Inc. Irving, Texas, USA)

ly anesthetic effect and reduces edema formation in previously scarred or inflamed nerve roots. However, the injection of hypertonic solutions into the epidural space is extremely painful if no local anesthetics have been administered beforehand. Consequently, if the hypertonic saline spreads beyond the segment in which local anesthesia was previously applied, it is possible that the patient may experience extreme pain requiring intravenous administration of sedatives or an additional epidural dose of local anesthetic. However, the pain rarely lasts for more than 5 min.

If iodine-containing radiographic contrast is not used when the patient has a known history of allergy, the procedure is carried out in the same way without it. To exclude a subarachnoid or subdural position of the needle or catheter, a test dose of local anesthetic is administered. In this case, the patient experiences pain in the skin area corresponding to the scarred epidural region. As the catheter is advanced, resistance is felt when contact is made with adhesions. It is necessary to advance the catheter slowly to avoid penetrating the subarachnoid or subdural space.

After the procedure
Securing the catheter
When the procedure has been completed, the catheter is firmly secured with a skin suture. The exit point is generously covered with antibiotic ointment (triple combination) and covered with two slit compresses (5 × 5 cm). Benzoin tincture is spread on the surrounding skin. Fixation with a transparent Tegaderm plaster (10 × 5 cm) is then carried out. Finally, fixation with four strips of a porous elastic Hypafix plaster is carried out, so that the patient cannot "sweat off" the plaster over the course of the 3 days.

An injection syringe adapter and a bacterial filter are attached to the catheter. The free end of the catheter is attached to the patient's side. During the hospital stay, prophylactic antibiotic treatment continues to be administered to prevent bacterial colonization (which is favored by steroid administration). After discharge, antibiotics are prescribed for a further 5 days.

Technique for subsequent injections
The indwelling catheter remains attached for the following 3 days. Further injections are given on the second and third days. After each negative aspiration test and administration of a test dose, as described above, a local anesthetic and then after ca. 30 min hypertonic 10% saline are slowly injected. On the third day, the catheter is removed ca. 10 min after the last injection. The patient should keep the insertion site as dry as possible for as long as the catheter is in place. We also recommend our patients to keep the area dry for a further 48 hours after removal of the catheter in order to reduce the risk of infection.

Epidural adhesiolysis usually leads to a significant improvement in pain symptoms and motor function. After this, it is important to start intensive physiotherapy in order to improve muscle strength and muscle tone.

Due to their size, existing epidural adhesions cannot always be fully dissolved. The procedure can be repeated if necessary. A 3-month pause is recommended between each treatment (due to the steroids used). During this period, intensive physiotherapy must be carried out, with targeted muscle training.

Percutaneous epidural neuroplasty in the cervical, thoracic and lumbar regions

The technique has to be modified for percutaneous epidural neuroplasty in the cervical, thoracic and lumbar regions, in order to ensure that the needle is located in the epidural space and to avoid compression of the spinal cord during subsequent injections.

Technique of cervical epidural neuroplasty
The patient is placed in the left lateral position on the fluoroscopy table. The "3D" technique (direction, depth, direction) is used.

Cervical placement of the epidural catheter using the 3D technique
Preoperative
- Examination of the patient and identification of the puncture area.
- Laboratory tests to asses the usual parameters that are important when carrying out neuraxial blocks.

Intraoperative
- The patient is placed in the left lateral position.
- Preparation and draping.
- Puncture site: C7–T1 or T1–T2.
- Access: paramedian, 1 cm or less lateral to the midline, one intervertebral space below the planned epidural access.
- Epidural puncture is carried out with a 16-G R-K or 15-G R-K-Coudé needle.
- Anteroposterior fluoroscopy to assess the puncture direction.
- Lateral fluoroscopy to assess the injection depth.
- Anteroposterior fluoroscopy to assess again and if necessary correct the puncture direction.
- The needle is advanced to the base of the spinous process. The injection depth corresponds to the po-

sition of the lamina of the vertebral arch in the vicinity of the posterior epidural space.
- Removal of the trochar.
- Attach a pulsator syringe (low-friction) filled with 4 mL 0.9% NaCl and 2 mL air.
- Identification of the epidural space is carried out using the loss-of-resistance technique.
- Optimal positioning of the needle in the midline.
- Injection of 1–2 mL radiographic contrast (for the cervical epidurogram).
- Introduction of the catheter through the epidural needle in the direction of the targeted nerve root in the lateral epidural space. Lateral positioning of the catheter is important because the nociceptors are concentrated in the lateral space. Repeated aspiration is important.
- Injection of 1500 IU hyaluronidase mixed with 4–6 mL NaCl 0.9%.
- Incremental injection of the local anesthetic and corticosteroid (in 2–3 mL portions).
- The needle is removed under fluoroscopic guidance.
- Attachment of a bacterial filter.
- The catheter is secured with a skin suture, an antibacterial and antimycotic ointment is applied, followed by a dressing.

Postoperative (recovery room)
- Careful monitoring of the patient for at least 30min after the procedure, checking the spread of the anesthesia to exclude the ever-present risk of inadvertent subarachnoid or subdural injection.
- Administration of 6 mL hypertonic 10% saline through the epidural catheter using an infusion pump.
- Rinsing of the catheter with 2 mL of preservative-free 0.9% saline.

On the following two postoperative days (pain treatment unit)
- Aspiration test before the injection.
- Injection of a test dose of 2 mL 0.2% ropivacaine through the catheter. After 5 min – after excluding a subarachnoid or subdural injection – a further 4 mL 0.2% ropivacaine is administered.
- Wait 20 min.
- Infusion of 6 mL hypertonic 10% saline using an infusion pump, over 30 min.
- Rinsing of the catheter with 2 mL 0.9% saline.
- Removal of the catheter.

The patient must be informed about the risk of infection (e.g. meningitis after a latency period of 2–4 weeks, as the injected corticosteroids have a long-lasting effect).

Larkin et al. [4] recently described a technique of epidural steroid injection in which the catheter is used as a monopolar stimulation electrode for better localization of the cause of the pain.

Percutaneous thoracic epidural neuroplasty

A paramedian access route is also used for catheterization of the thoracic epidural space (percutaneous thoracic neuroplasty). The procedure is carried out in the same sequence of steps as that described for lumbosacral and cervical neuroplasty. The dosages for the drugs injected are listed in Table 49.2.

Placement of the catheter in the anterior epidural space or in an intervertebral foramen

Drugs that are injected into the posterior or posterolateral epidural space do not reach possible pathological changes in the intervertebral foramina or anterior epidural space. It may therefore be necessary to place the catheter in these areas. The catheter's direction is checked a) by introducing the R-K epidural needle or SCA catheter introducer in the target direction; b) by bending the catheter tip to make it easier to guide the catheter in the desired direction. When neuroplasty is being carried out through the sacral hiatus in order to place the catheter in the anterior lumbosacral area, the catheter should reach this area below S3. The transforaminal access route should be used for all other segments.

Complications

The potential side effects and complications of percutaneous epidural neuroplasty include:
- Inadvertent subarachnoid or subdural injection of local anesthetics or hypertonic 10% saline. A subarachnoid injection of hypertonic saline can lead to cardia arrhythmia, paralyses, or loss of sphincter function.
- Epidural abscess (see Chapter 41, p. 326).
- Epidural hematoma (see Chapter 41, p. 326).
- Paralyses.
- Disturbances of bladder or rectal function.
- Infections (corticosteroid administration leads to immune suppression, with the resulting risk of infection; strictly aseptic conditions should therefore be observed).
- Catheter shearing.

It is possible in some circumstances for septation to occur, or for fluid to collect in a separate compartment of the epidural space. This is associated with a substantial increase in epidural pressure, which can lead to local damage or even – when the pressure is transferred via the subarachnoid space – to injury to the central nervous system [12].

Undiagnosed neurogenic bladder and rectal disturbances

The problem of preoperatively unrecognized neurogenic bladder disturbances in patients with "failed back surgery syndrome" or spinal cord injuries led to distrust both of practicing physicians and of the technique. It is therefore important to carry out and document the necessary urological examinations before neuroplasty. This prevents previously existent micturition disturbances or rectal disturbances from being incorrectly attributed to injury after a neuroplasty procedure has been carried out. This type of examination is particularly important in patients with constrictive arachnoiditis, as this not infrequently leads to disturbances of rectal and bladder function, and of sexual function as well in men.

Spinal cord compression

As discussed above, all injections should be carried out slowly. Fast injections into the epidural space can in some circumstances create a strong increase in CSF pressure, with the risk of cerebral hemorrhage, visual disturbances, headache and disturbances of the blood supply to the spinal cord.

Infection

Patients are informed that epidural infections can occur in the first 2–6 weeks after the procedure – both due to the procedure itself and due to the steroid-related immunosuppression it involves. Until proved otherwise, any occurrence of nausea, vomiting, stiffness in the neck, severe pain, weakness, numbness, or paralysis must therefore be regarded as due to the procedure and correspondingly treated.

Patients should be advised to contact the physician who conducted the procedure, or their general practitioner, immediately if any of these symptoms arise. Appropriate in-patient treatment must be immediately instituted (see Chapter 41, epidural anesthesia, complications). No cases of epidural abscess have so far been observed among the patients we have treated. However, due to the potentially extremely serious sequelae of unrecognized and untreated epidural abscesses, extreme attentiveness and careful patient information are indispensable.

Hyaluronidase hypersensitivity

In a follow-up study by Moore [8] including 1520 patients who underwent epidural hyaluronidase administration, hyaluronidase hypersensitivity was observed in 3% of the patients. The fact that this 3% incidence was not observed with the technique described here may possibly be due to the injection of a corticosteroid in the same site at which the hyaluronidase was injected. The steroid remains in the epidural space for longer than the hyaluronidase, and may provide protection against allergic reactions.

The reduction in the incidence of treatment-resistant pain conditions obtained with this procedure entirely justifies the use of hyaluronidase; however, very careful attention must be given to any signs of hypersensitivity.

Experience at the Texas Tech University Health Sciences Center (TTUHSC)

At our center, the epidural adhesiolysis technique described here has been carried out in more than 4000 patients. Only a few complications were observed. Subarachnoid or subdural injection of the local anesthetic is extremely rare. Two of the patients developed meningitis after epidural adhesiolysis and were quickly and effectively treated with antibiotics. No cases of paralysis were observed in any of the patients; one patient developed transient motor weakness (caudal access). There were no significant, longer-lasting cases of rectal or bladder dysfunction, although a few patients developed mild micturition or defecation disturbances during the first 2 weeks after the procedure. There was a report of transient numbness in the perineal area, which resolved again after 1–2 months.

Additional aspects

This chapter describes a procedure involving a 3-day course of injection treatment based on the results of a randomized, prospective double-blind study [2]. However, Manchikanti et al. [6] have shown that one-day treatments are also effective. The pain reduction is more persistent, however, when more frequent and repeated injections are carried out [5]. There is evidence that the epidural neuroplasty procedure is also suitable for pain treatment in cases of spinal canal stenosis. Previously disturbed motor function also improves after treatment in some patients [7].

Summary

Percutaneous epidural neuroplasty is an interventional procedure in the treatment of pain caused by structures in the epidural space or its vicinity and in the intervertebral foramina in all segments of the spine. Adequate scientific justification for the procedure appears to be provided by the current state of knowledge regarding the pathogenesis of back pain and radiculopathy. To ensure the safety of the procedure and achieve the best possible results, it is recommended that the details of the procedure described here (regarding technique and patient selection) should be followed precisely.

50 Adjuncts to local anesthesia in neuraxial blocks

Opioids, vasopressors, clonidine (an alpha-2-adrenoceptor antagonist), ketamine and – in subarachnoid administration in particular – glucose can be used as adjuncts to a neuraxially administered local anesthetic.

Glucose

In the hyperbaric spinal anesthesia technique, glucose is mixed at concentrations of 5–10% with a local anesthetic in order to produce a density higher than that of CSF.

Vasopressors

Vasopressors that can be used to prolong the duration of effect of a local anesthetic include:
- Phenylephrine (Neo-Synephrine)
  0.5–5 mg (0.05–0.5 mL in a 1% solution), with which the duration of effect of the local anesthetic is extended by 30–100% [31].
- Epinephrine (adrenaline)
  0.2–0.5 mg (0.2–0.5 mL, 1 : 1000 in solution), with which the duration of effect of the local anesthetic can be extended by 40–50% [31].

Advantages and disadvantages of phenylephrine/epinephrine
The addition of a vasopressor leads to slower vascular resorption of the local anesthetic. This slows down contact with neural tissue, while at the same time reducing systemic toxicity.
Reservations regarding the possible association of added vasopressors with spinal cord ischemia, with subsequent neurological complications, have not been clinically confirmed [10, 23].
The causes of neurological injury are fairly multifactorial, and include the technique, equipment and injected drugs. In addition, the patient's individual situation and possible distinctive anatomic features play a role. However, this topic continues to be a controversial one [31].

Opioids [13, 27, 28, 42]

Neuraxial administration of an opioid – as a single agent, or in combination with a low-dose local anesthetic – produces very good analgesia during surgery and in the postoperative period.
Central or systemic side effects are seen very rarely.
The receptors specific for opioids are located alongside areas in the brain and particularly in the substantia gelatinosa of the spinal cord. Their concentration there is at its most dense.
In comparison with a local anesthetic, an opioid injected in the vicinity of the spinal cord has a selective effect – i.e. it produces pure analgesia, without sensory or motor block and with only a slight sympathetic block.
In comparison with systemic administration, opioids are very potent and have a marked segmental effect, a long duration and a low tendency to produce side effects.
The following characteristics of opioids are important for optimal effectiveness:
- **High affinity with the receptor** and thus **high analgesic** potency.
- **High lipophilia,** causing acceleration of their passage through the dura and CSF to the spinal cord. At the same time, however, there is a high rate of elimination, which is reflected in a short duration. Agents such as sufentanil or fentanyl, for example, remain in the CSF for only a very short time and are quickly absorbed by the lipid-rich structures of the spinal cord. They are characterized by a steep gradient of effect, but also by a short duration.
- **Low hydrophilia** and thus a short period of persistence in the CSF.

The strongly hydrophilic opioids – the main representative being morphine – remain in the CSF for a longer period, so that a larger proportion is transported to the brain before binding with opioid receptors can take place.
The consequences of this are slow systemic resorption, a slower gradient of effect, a long duration of effect, a low elimination rate and the risk of cranial diffusion.

Due to the slow circulation of CSF, the patient is at risk of **respiratory depression** even after several hours. This applies particularly to hydrophilic substances – so that after morphine administration, depending on the dosage, respiratory depression can be expected after even 18–24 hours.
- **Long receptor binding and thus a long duration of effect** (e.g. buprenorphine).
- **Low tendency for tolerance to develop.**

Pharmacokinetic data for the most frequently used opioids

Administration of an opioid can be carried out intrathecally or epidurally. It is mainly pure opioid agonists that are used.

Strongly lipophilic opioids
- **Sufentanil**
  High lipophilia, high receptor affinity, ca. 1000 times more effective than morphine – the drug of the future in neuraxial applications.
  Suitable for acute pain therapy.
  Epidural:
  Dosage 30–50 µg, onset 10 min, duration 4–5 h.
  Subarachnoid:
  Dosage 7.5–10 µg, onset 2–10 min, duration 1–3 h.
- **Fentanyl**
  Strongly lipophilic and 75 times more effective than morphine. Suitable for acute pain therapy.
  Epidural:
  Dosage 50–100 µg, onset 5–10 min, duration 2–3 h.
  Subarachnoid:
  Dosage 25–50 µg, onset 2–10 min, duration 30–120 min.

Strongly hydrophilic opioids
- **Morphine**
  Epidural:
  Dosage:
  Adults: 2–5 mg morphine sulfate (only after appropriate dilution with 10–15 mL isotonic saline), onset ca. 30–60 min, duration 8–22 h.
  Children: 0.01 mg/kg b.w.
  Subarachnoid:
  Dosage:
  Adults: 0.2–0.5 mg morphine sulfate (only after appropriate dilution with 1–4 mL isotonic saline), onset 10–20 min, duration 8–24 h.
  Children: 0.001 mg/kg b.w.

Combinations

In some clinical situations, the effect of opioids alone is not adequate. A combination of opioids and local anesthetics leads to an additive or multiplied analgesic effect, characterized by faster onset, longer duration and reduced motor block. The blocking of pain takes place at various sites – at the neural axon and via the opioid receptors in the spinal cord.

The use of such combinations is becoming more and more routine.

Types of application [27]

Epidural bolus injection
The lowest possible volume should be selected, with volumes of 5–10 mL normally being preferred.

Epidural infusion
A bolus dose of 10 mL bupivacaine (0.0625–0.125%) in combination with 1–2 µg/mL sufentanil is followed by infusion of a mixture of bupivacaine (0.031%) and sufentanil (0.2–0.3 µg/mL) at a speed of 6–10 mL/h. These low dosages are used in obstetrics in particular.

Patient-controlled epidural anesthesia (PCEA)
This mode of application leads to a significant reduction in the total dose, by up to 30%.
A bolus dose of 10–30 µg sufentanil is followed by a baseline infusion rate of 5 µg/h. The maximum single dose is 5 µg, with a lockout time of 10–20 minutes.

Factors influencing epidural infusion

Important factors that influence the opioid/local anesthetic dosage in epidural infusions are:
- The location and type of surgery.
- Pain type (obstetric, post-traumatic).
- Opioid type and its initial dosage.
- Injection volume.
- Concentration of the local anesthetic.
- Patient characteristics (age, obesity, concomitant diseases).
- Intraoperative blood loss.
- Pharmacokinetics of the injected opioid.
- Position of the catheter tip in the epidural space.

Complications and side effects [13, 28]

Respiratory depression
This is the most feared complication, particularly after subarachnoid administration.
The cause is either overdose, or systemic absorption of the opioid. Respiratory depression occurs relatively

soon after administration, or may be delayed by slow rostral diffusion to the respiratory center. Delayed respiratory depression is particularly seen after morphine administration, since its marked hydrophilia leads to larger amounts remaining in the slowly circulating CSF and spreading towards the respiratory center. Slowly circulating CSF takes 6–10 hours to pass from the lumbar subarachnoid space to the fourth ventricle.

Low levels of respiratory depression are possible even after the administration of lipophilic opioids [16, 34]. Monitoring of respiration after giving both hydrophilic and lipophilic opioids is therefore strongly recommended. Despite the binding of lipophilic opioids to the receptors in the spinal cord, the analgesic effect of these agents is mainly systemic rather than spinal. Thus, the same quality of analgesia can be achieved independently of the catheter position (lumbar or thoracic, after a thoracotomy: see Chapter 42, p. 331).

The following measures are regarded as effective forms of prophylaxis to reduce the risk of respiratory depression:
- Careful monitoring of respiration and circulation.
- Use of lipophilic opioids.
- Individual dose adjustment and dose reduction by titration.
- Low volumes.
- Dose reduction in older patients, pregnant patients and obese patients.
- If the patient becomes somnolent, it is a warning signal.
- Particular caution should be used when there is intraoperative blood loss and a drop in blood pressure.
- Lumbar injection and epidural infusion are preferable.
- Possible catheter dislodgement should be carefully monitored.
- Avoid the use of intravenous supplementation (opioids or sedatives).

Therapy
Naloxone 0.1–0.2 mg i.v. as a bolus, or as infusion 5–10 µg/h
Nalbuphine 5–10 mg i.v.

Pruritus

This is a harmless side effect, which can be observed in a large proportion of patients (40%) after administration of an initial dose. In most cases, it resolves spontaneously after 10–20 minutes without any treatment being needed.

In resistant cases, treatment with nalbuphine 5–10 mg i.v. or naloxone is recommended.

Alternatively, propofol (10–20 mg) and antihistamines can be used.

Urinary retention

This is often observed after spinal administration of opioids.
Treatment: carbachol (Doryl) i.m. or catheterization.

Nausea/vomiting

These side effects are often seen after the administration of pethidine.
Treatment: metoclopramide 10–20 mg i.v. nalbuphine 5–10 mg i.v. or propofol 10–20 mg i.v. A final alternative is naloxone 0.2–0.4 mg.

Drop in blood pressure

Occurs in 11.5% of cases [13].

Bradycardia

Occurs in 1.6% of cases [13].

Muscle relaxation

Occurs in 7% of cases [13].

Clonidine

Clonidine, a derivative of imidazoline, binds to alpha-2-adrenoceptors.

The alpha-2-adrenoceptors are mainly found in the intermediomedial nucleus (preganglionic sympathetic cells of origin for T4–L2/3), in the intermediolateral nucleus (preganglionic parasympathetic cells of origin for the sacral spinal cord) and in the substantia gelatinosa of the dorsal horn.

The receptor density in the sacral cord is 50% greater than in the thoracic and lumbar spinal cord [29, 30]. Clonidine's high lipid solubility and low plasma protein binding (20%) allows it to pass the blood–brain barrier more quickly.

Its analgesic effect is segmental. Maximum CSF levels are observed 30 minutes after epidural administration of clonidine, and these are about 100 times higher than the simultaneous plasma levels.

The elimination half-life in CSF is about 80 minutes and in plasma 12 ± 7 hours. The elimination is mainly renal.

Hemodynamic side effects

As clonidine is a potent hypotensive drug, bradycardia, hypotension, or sedation can be expected after epidural or subarachnoid application. Administration of clonidine in patients with cardiac insufficiency or hypovolemia is therefore contraindicated.

Nerve injury in the form of ischemia due to vasoconstriction has not as yet been observed after epidural or subarachnoid administration of clonidine.

Combination with local anesthetics or opioids

Clonidine has a very good additive effect when combined with local anesthetics or opioids.

Subarachnoid administration
Subarachnoid administration of clonidine (150 µg) combined with a local anesthetic leads to a prolonged duration of effect and prolonged motor block in spinal anesthesia, due to its additive effect.
The dose required for adequate effect in subarachnoid injection is about one-third of the epidural dose.
In subarachnoid combination with a local anesthetic, clonidine does not lead to more severe circulatory depression in comparison with pure spinal anesthesia with a local anesthetic.
Long-term subarachnoid administration of clonidine in pain therapy has been reported [18].

Epidural administration
The combination of clonidine with a local anesthetic or an opioid leads to a significant improvement in the quality and duration of analgesia.
This has been reported in particular in orthopedics [12], obstetrics [21], pediatric anesthesia [17] and in long-term pain therapy [20].

Dosage recommendations for clinical application

If opioids and alpha-2-agonists are being used in neuraxial analgesia procedures, it can be assumed that antinociception undergoes an additive effect, if not a synergistic one.
This is associated with a doubling of the duration of effect and has been reported for combinations of clonidine with morphine, fentanyl and sufentanil.

Suggested dosages
- Subarachnoid:
  Clonidine 150 µg in combination with a local anesthetic.
- Epidural:
  Clonidine 2–4 µg/kg b.w. + morphine 30–50 µg/kg b.w. [29].
  Clonidine 4 µg/kg b.w. + fentanyl 2 µg/kg b.w. + 0.25% bupivacaine ad 50 mL, infusion at 0.05 mL/kg/h [29].
  Clonidine 150 µg + fentanyl 100 µg [29].
  Clonidine 150 µg + sufentanil 10 µg [36].

Clonidine 2–4 µg/kg b.w. + sufentanil 0.2–0.3 µg/mL + 0.125% bupivacaine ad 50 mL, infusion at 6–10 mL/h.

Ketamine

Ketamine was synthesized in 1963 and is structurally related to the addictive hallucinogen phencyclidine (PCP, "angel dust").
It is used as an analgesic, narcotic and for tracheal intubation in status asthmaticus.
It has a firmly established place in anesthesia, intensive care medicine and in emergency medicine. Its importance as a low-dose co-analgesic drug in neuraxial applications is growing. In particular, intravenous or epidural administration of the stereoisomer S-(+)-ketamine is likely to become more important. In comparison with the racemate form, it has double the analgesic and anesthetic potency, an equally fast onset of effect, shorter recovery times and a wider range of therapeutic application [2–4].

Mechanism of effect [2–4]

Ketamine is a nonspecific N-methyl-D-aspartate (NMDA) receptor antagonist.
The most important binding site for the analgesic effect of ketamine is the NMDA-sensitive glutamate receptor channel.
The NMDA receptors belong to the excitatory amino acid system (EAA) of the central nervous system. Glutamate is the most important excitatory neurotransmitter in the vertebrate central nervous system. PCP receptor agonists such as ketamine inhibit the effect of glutamate at the NMDA receptor channels noncompetitively and thus prevent calcium transport into the cells. The analgesic effect of ketamine is mainly produced by this process.
The local anesthetic effect of ketamine, in contrast, is based on sodium ion channel inhibition, with raised concentrations being found at the site of application.
At low dosages, the local anesthetic effect (in the spinal cord) is very low. Ketamine is also thought to have a neuroprotective effect in the context of NMDA receptor antagonism [3].
There is an affinity with other receptors, but the significance of these in mediating the effect has not yet been fully clarified: opioid receptors, nicotinic (nACh) and muscarinic (mACh) acetylcholine receptors, dopamine receptors (indirectly), serotonin receptors (indirectly), adrenoceptors (indirectly), ion channel block (voltage-operated channels, particularly Na^+, K^+, Ca^{++}), GABA

receptor A binding (modulation of the chloride channel).

Neuraxial use of ketamine

The use of ketamine in combination with an opioid or local anesthetic (rarely as a monoanalgesic) has proved its value in the following areas:
- Postoperative pain therapy.
- Various chronic pain syndromes that are treatment resistant.
- Cancer pain.

A combination of subanalgesic doses of ketamine and morphine synergistically enhances the effect of morphine and interaction with various receptors. This leads to the following advantages:
- Very good analgesia, comparable with that of high-dose morphine administration [40].
- A substantial reduction in the rate of adverse side effects, particularly respiratory depression, resulting from the reduced dosage of morphine.
- Prophylaxis against developing opioid tolerance.
  In cases of morphine tolerance, ketamine is a good way of potentiating the effect through an additional attack at the NMDA receptor.

Subarachnoid application

Subarachnoid administration of ketamine as a co-analgesic (rarely as a single agent) is **not recommended,** due to the **neurotoxicity** of the preservative benzethonium chloride that is contained in ketamine preparations.
Ketamine may only be used exceptionally and in the form of a preservative-free solution for subarachnoid applications [14, 15, 37, 40].

Cancer pain
Treatment-resistant cancer pain is the principal indication for the subarachnoid administration of ketamine as a co-analgesic with morphine [41], or as an addition to clonidine and a local anesthetic [24] in the form of a continuous infusion.
The potentiating effect of ketamine leads to a substantial reduction in the morphine dosage and thus a reduction in the risk of adverse side effects.

Anesthesiology
The use of ketamine as a single agent in anesthesiology has not as yet proved successful.
The reasons for this are the high dosages required (0.7–0.95 mg/kg), the short duration of effect and its dose-dependent central sympathomimetic side effects [15].

Epidural application

The first publications reporting the epidural use of ketamine date from 1982.
The administration of ketamine as a co-analgesic, usually with morphine (more rarely as a single drug) leads to very good postoperative analgesia, particularly when administered pre-emptively.
The nociceptors are blocked to an extent such that a subsequent pain stimulus does not lead to increased sensitivity in its effects on the nerve cell. Pain-related central adaptation processes, which increase postoperative pain, are thereby prevented.
Ketamine should be used without a preservative substance and at a concentration of 0.1–0.3% [15, 37, 40].

Surgical indications
- Gynecological procedures [1, 19].
- Upper abdominal procedures via a thoracic catheter [9].
- General surgery [8].
- Cholecystectomy [25].
- Orthopedic prostheses [37, 38].
- Pediatric surgery (orchidopexy) via caudal administration [11, 32].

The epidural dosage of ketamine is 20–50 mg [14].

Indications in pain therapy
- Post-herpetic neuralgia [39].
- Complex regional pain syndrome (CRPS), types I and II [22, 35].
  A dose of 7.5–10 mg in combination with 0.75–1 mg morphine and 0.1% bupivacaine is recommended here.
- For continuous epidural infusion, a dose of 25 µg/kg/h is recommended [35].
- Phantom pain [26].
- Cancer pain.

Specific contraindications
- Poorly adjusted or untreated arterial hypertension.
- Pre-eclampsia and eclampsia.
- Manifest hyperthyroidism.

Relative contraindications
- Unstable angina pectoris.
- Myocardial infarction within the previous 6 months.

- Raised intracranial pressure without adequate ventilation.
- Glaucoma and perforating eye injuries.

Interactions
Combined application with thyroid hormones leads to severe hypertension and tachycardia.

References

Chapter 1: Regional nerve blocks and infiltration therapy in clinical practice

1. Baranowski, A. P., De Courcey, J., Bonelle, E.: A trial of intravenous lidocaine on the pain and allodynia of postherpetic neuralgia. J Pain Symptom Manage 17 (6) (1999) 429–433
2. Basler, H.-D., Ernst, A., Flöter, Th., Gerbershagen, H.-U., Hankemeier, U., Jungck, D., Müller-Schwefe, G., Zimmermann, M.: Gemeinsame Richtlinien der Deutschen Gesellschaft zum Studium des Schmerzes e.V. (DGSS) und des SCHMERZtherapeutischen Kolloquiums e.V. (StK) für die Zusatzweiterbildung zum Algesiologen DGSS/STK. SCHMERZtherapeutisches Kolloquium 11 (1995) 3–5
3. Bonica, J. J., Buckley, P. F.: Regional analgesia with local anesthetics. In: Bonica, J. J. (ed.): Management of Pain. (2nd ed.) Lea & Febiger, Philadelphia – London (1990)
4. Borchard, U., Niesel, H. C.: Grundlagen der Pharmakologie der Lokalanästhetika. In: Niesel, H. C. (Hrsg.): Regionalanästhesie, Lokalanästhesie, Regionale Schmerztherapie. Georg Thieme Verlag, Stuttgart – New York (1994)
5. Campbell, J. N., Raja, S. N., Cohen, R. H., Manning, D. C., Khan, A. A., Meyer, R. A.: Peripheral neural mechanisms of nociception. In: Wall, P. D., Melzack, R. (eds.): Textbook of Pain. (2nd ed.) Churchill Livingstone, Edinburgh (1989)
6. Devor, M.: Central changes mediating neuropathic pain. In: Dubner, R., Gebhart, G. F., Bond, M. R. (eds.): Proceedings of the Vth World Congress on Pain. Pain Research and Clinical Management. Elsevier, Amsterdam (1988)
7. Galer, B. S., Rowbotham, M. C., Perander, J.: Topical lidocaine patch relieves postherpetic neuralgia more effectively than a vehicle topical patch: results of an enriched enrollment study. Pain 80 (1999) 533–538
8. Gammaitoni, A. R., Alvarez, N. A., Galer, B. S.: Safety and tolerability of the lidocaine patch 5 %, a targeted peripheral analgesic: a review of the literature. J Clin Pharmacol 43 (2) (2003) 111–117
9. Groban, L., Deal, D. D., Vernon, J. C. James, R. L., Butterworth, J.: Cardiac Resuscitation after Incremental Overdoeage with Lidocaine, Bupivacaine, Levobupivacaine, and Ropivacaine in Anesthetized Dogs. Anesth Analg 2001; 92; 37–43
10. Hildebrandt, A. G. (Bundesgesundheitsamt): Bekanntmachung über die Zulassung und Registrierung von Arzneimitteln. Abwehr von Arzneimittelrisiken, Stufe II – Lidocain- und Etidocain-haltige Arzneimittel (Ausgenommen sind Lidocain-haltige Arzneimittel, die zur anti-arrhythmischen Therapie angewendet werden). Bundesanzeiger Nr. 149, Jahrgang 45 (1993) 7494
11. Jankovic, D.: New approaches to chronic pain: Nerve blocks in the head. In: Van Zundert, A., Rawal, N. (eds): Highlights in Regional Anesthesia and Pain Therapy. XI (Special Edition: World Congress on Regional Anaesthesia and Pain Therapy, Barcelona (2002) 258–269
12. Rowbotham, M. C., Davies, P. S., Fields, H. L.: Topical lidocaine gel relieves postherpetic neuralgia. Ann Neurol 37 (1995) 246–253
13. Rowbotham, M. C., Davies, P. S., Galer, B. S.: Multicenter, double-blind, vehicle-controlled trial of long term use of lidocaine patches for postherpetic neuralgia (abstract). In: 8th World Congress on Pain. IASP Press, 274 (1996)
14. Rowbotham, M. C., Davies, P. S., Verkempinck, C.: Lidocaine patch: double-blind controlled study of a new treatment method for postherpetic neuralgia. Pain 65 (1996) 39–44
15. Rowbotham, M. C., Reisner-Keller, L. A., Fields, H. L.: Both intravenous lidocaine and morphine reduce the pain of postherpetic neuralgia. Neurology (41) (1991) 1024–1028
16. Tryba, M.: Lokalanästhetika. In: Zenz, M., Jurna, I. (Hrsg.): Lehrbuch der Schmerztherapie. Grundlagen, Theorie und Praxis für Aus- und Weiterbildung. Wissenschaftliche Verlagsgesellschaft, Stuttgart (1993)
17. Weninger, E.: Pharmakodynamik der Lokalanästhetika. Anästhesiologie & Intensivmedizin 5 (37) (1996) 249–267
18. Zimmermann, M.: Physiologie von Nozizeption und Schmerz. In: Zimmermann, M., Handwerker, H. O. (Hrsg.): Schmerz-Konzepte und ärztliches Handeln. Springer-Verlag, Berlin (1984)

19. Zink, W. et al.: Bupivacaine but not Ropivacaine Induces Apoptosis in Mammalian Skeletal Muscle Fibers. Poster Discussion, Local Anesthesia and Pain, Basic Science II, ASA 2002: A-971

Chapter 2: Regional anesthesia in ophthalmology
(André van Zundert, Danilo Jankovic)

1. Budd, J., Hardwick, M., Barber, K., Prosser, J.: A single-centre study of 1000 consecutive peribulbar blocks. Eye 15 (2001) 464–468
2. Gills, J. P., Hustead, R. F., Sanders, D. R.: Ophthalmic Anesthesia. Slack Incorporated, USA (1993)
3. Guise, P. A.: Sub-Tenon anesthesia – A prospective study of 6000 blocks. Anesthesiology 98 (2003) 964–968
4. Habib, N. E., Balmer, H. G., Hocking, G.: Efficacy and safety of sedation with propofol in peribulbar anesthesia. Eye 16 (2002) 60–62
5. Kahle, W.: Nervensystem und Sinnesorgane. Im Taschenatlas der Anatomie. 7. Auflage. Thieme Verlag, Stuttgart – New York
6. Kallio, H., Paloheimo, M., Maunuksela, E. L.: Hyaluronidase as an adjuvant in bupivacain-lidocaine mixture for retrobulbar/peribulbar block. Anesth Analg 91 (2000) 934–937
7. Karampatiakis, V., Natsis, K., Gigis, P., Stangos, N. T.: Orbital depth measurements of human skulls in relation to retrobulbar anesthesia. Eur J Opthalmol 8 (1998) 118–120
8. Koller, K.: Über die Verwendung des Cocains zur Anästhesierung am Auge. Med. Wochenschr. 34 (1884) 1276–1278, 1309–1311
9. Konstantatos, A. Anticoagulation and cataract surgery: a review of the current literature. Anaesth Intensive Care 29 (2001) 11–18
10. Kumar, C. M., Dodds, C., Fanning, G. L.: Ophthalmic Anesthesia. Swetz & Zeitlinger Publishers, Netherlands (2002)
11. Kumar, C. M., Dodds, C.: Evaluation of the Greenbaum sub-Tenon's block. Br J Anaesth 87 (2001) 631–633
12. Nicol, M.: Anesthesia for Ophthalmic Surgery. In: Aitkenhead, A. R., Rowbotham, D. J., Smith, G. (eds), Textbook of Anesthesia. Churchill Livingstone, UK, (2001) 594–605
13. Prasad, N., Kumar, C. M., Patil, B. B., Dowd, T. C.: Subjective visual experience during phacoemulsification cataract surgery under sub-Tenon's block. Eye 17 (2003) 407–409
14. Rewari, V., Madan, R., Kaul, H. L., Kumar, L.: Remifentanil and propofol sedation for retrobulbar nerve block. Anaesth Intensive Care 30 (2002) 433–437
15. Ruschen, H., Bremner, F. D., Carr, C.: Complication after sub-Tenon's eye block. Anesth Analg 96 (2003) 273–277
16. Wadood, A. C., Dhillon, B., Singh, J.: Inadvertent ocular perforation and intravitreal injection of an anesthetic agent during retrobulbar injection. J Cataract Refract Surg 28 (2002) 562–565

Chapter 3: Occipital nerves

1. Bonica, J. J.: Block of cranial nerves. In: Bonica, J. J. (ed.): The management of Pain. (2nd ed.) Lea & Febiger, Philadelphia (1990)
2. Murphy, T. M.: Somatic blockade of head and neck. In: Cousins, M. J., Bridenbaugh, P. O. (eds.): Neural Blockade. (2nd ed.) Lippincott, Philadelphia (1988)
3. Netter, F. H.: Anatomie. In: Firbas, W. (Hrsg.): Farbatlanten der Medizin (Band 7). Bewegungsapparat I: Anatomie, Embryologie, Physiologie und Stoffwechselkrankheiten. Georg Thieme Verlag, Stuttgart – New York (1992)
4. Steenks, M. H., deWijer, A.: Kiefergelenksfehlfunktionen aus physiotherapeutischer und zahnmedizinischer Sicht. Quintessenz, Berlin (1991)
5. Tilscher, H., Eder, M.: Infiltrationstherapie. Hippokrates, Stuttgart (1994)
6. Travell, J. G., Simons, D. G.: Myofascial Pain and Dysfunction. The Trigger Point Manual. Williams & Wilkins, Baltimore – London (1983)

Chapter 4: Trigeminal nerve

1. Amster, L. J.: Sphenopalatine ganglion block for the relief of painful vascular and muscular spasm with special reference to lumbosacral pain. NY State J. Med. 48 (1948) 2475–2480
2. Auberger, H. G., Niesel, H. C.: Gesichtsschädel: Proximale Leitungsanästhesie im Bereich des N. trigeminus. In: Auberger, H. G., Niesel, H. C. (Hrsg.): Praktische Lokalanästhesie. (4. Auflage) Georg Thieme Verlag, Stuttgart – New York (1982)
3. Berger, J. J., Pyles, S. T., Saga-Rumley, S. A.: Does topical anesthesia of the sphenopalatine ganglion with cocaine or lidocaine relieve low back pain? Anesth. Analg. 65 (1986) 700–702
4. Bonica, J. J.: Block of cranial nerves. In: Bonica, J. J. (ed.): The management of Pain. (2nd ed.) Lea & Febiger, Philadelphia (1990)
5. Byrd, H., Byrd, W.: Sphenopalatine phenomena: Present status of knowledge. Arch. Intern. Med. 46 (1930) 1026–1038
6. Devogel, J. C.: Cluster headache and sphenopalatine block. Acta Anesth. Belg. 32 (1981) 101–107

7. Jenkner, F. L.: Nervenblockaden auf pharmakologischem und auf elektrischem Weg. Springer, Wien (1980)
8. Lebovits, A. H., Alfred, H., Lefkowitz, M.: Sphenopalatine ganglion block: Clinical use in the pain management clinic. Clin. J. Pain 6 (1990) 131–136
9. Moore, D. C.: Regional Block. (4th ed.) Charles Thomas, Springfield (1976)
10. Murphy, T. M.: Somatic Blockade of Head and Neck. In: Cousins, M. J., Bridenbaugh, P. O. (eds.): Neural Blockade. (2nd ed.) Lippincott, Philadelphia (1988)
11. Netter, F. H.: Nervengeflechte und periphere Nerven. In: Krämer, G. (Hrsg.): Farbatlanten der Medizin. (Band 5). Nervensystem I: Neuroanatomie und Physiologie. Georg Thieme Verlag, Stuttgart – New York (1987)
12. Prasanna, A., Murthy, P. S. N.: Sphenopalatine ganglion block and pain of cancer. J. of Pain 8 (3) (1993) 125
13. Petren, T.: Anatomie des Nervus trigeminus. In: Eriksson, E. (Hrsg.): Atlas der Lokalanästhesie. (2. Auflage) Springer-Verlag, Berlin – Heidelberg – New York (1980)
14. Reder, M., Hymanson, A. S., Reder, M.: Sphenopalatine ganglion block in treatment of acute and chronic pain. In: Hendle, N. H., Long, D. M., Wise, T. N. (eds.): Diagnosis and treatment of chronic pain. John Wright, Boston (1982)
15. Rosen, S., Shelesnyak, M. C., Zacharias, L. R.: Nasogenital relationship II. Pseudopregnancy following extirpation of sphenopalatine ganglion in rat. Endocrinology 27 (1940) 463–468
16. Ruskin, A. P.: Sphenopalatine (nasal) ganglion: Remote effects including „psychosomatic" symptoms, rage reaction, pain and spasm. Arch. Phys. Med. Rehabil. 60 (1979) 353–358
17. Ruskin, S. L.: The neurologic aspects of nasal sinus infections. Headaches and systemic disturbances of nasal ganglion origin. Arch. Otolaryng. 4 (10) (1929) 337–382
18. Saade, E., Paige, G. B.: Patient administrated sphenopalatine ganglion block. Reg. Anesthesia 21 (1) (1996) 68–70
19. Sluder, G.: Injection of the nasal ganglion and comparison of methods. In: Nasal Neurology, Headaches and Eye disorders. CV Mosby, St. Louis (1918)
20. Waldman, S. D.: Sphenopalatine ganglion block – 80 years later. Reg. Anesthesia 18 (1993) 274–276
21. Zacharias, L. R.: Further studies in naso-genital relationship: Anatomical studies of perihypophyseal region in rat. J. Comp. Neurol. 74 (1941) 421–445

Chapter 5: Infiltration of trigger points in the muscles of mastication

1. Laskin, D. M.: Myofascial Pain Dysfunction Syndrome. In: Sarnat, B. G., Laskin, D. M.(eds): The Temporomandibular Joint. Charles Thomas, Springfield (1980) Chapter 14
2. Tilscher, H., Eder, M.: Infiltrationstherapie. Hippocrates, Stuttgart (1994)
3. Travell, J. G., Simons, D. G.: Myofascial Pain and Dysfunction. The Trigger Point Manual. Williams & Wilkins, Baltimore – London (1983)

Chapter 6: Cervicothoracic ganglion (stellate ganglion)

1. Abram, S. E., Boas, R. A.: Sympathetic and visceral nerve blocks. In: Benumof, L. J. (ed.): Clinical procedures in anesthesia and intensive care. Lippincott, Philadelphia (1992)
2. Bonica, J. J.: Cervicothoracic sympathetic block. In: Bonica, J. J. (ed.): Management of Pain. (2nd ed.) Lea & Febiger, Philadelphia-London (1990)
3. Carron, H., Litwiller, R.: Stellate ganglion block. Anesth. Analg. 54 (1975) 567–570
4. Colding, A.: The effect of regional sympathetic blocks in the treatment of herpes zoster. Acta Anesth. Scand. 13 (1969) 133–141
5. Dan, K., Higa, K., Noda, B.: Nerve block for herpetic pain. In: Fields, H. L. et al. (eds.): Advances in Pain Research and Therapy (Vol. 9.) Raven Press, New York (1985)
6. Davies, R. M.: Stellate ganglion block: A new approach. Anesthesia 7 (1952) 151–153
7. Dukes, R. R., Leroy, A. A.: Transient locked-in syndrome after vascular injection during stellate ganglion block. Reg. Anesthesia 18 (1993) 378–380
8. Fine, P. G., Ashburn, M. A.: Effect of stellate ganglion block with fentanyl on postherpetic neuralgia with a sympathetic component. Anesth. Analg. 67 (1988) 897–899
9. Floyd Jr., J. B.: Traumatic cerebral edema relieved by stellate ganglion anesthesia. South Med. J. 80 (1987) 1328
10. Ganz, H., Klein, H.: Verläufe und Spätergebnisse beim Hörsturz. HNO 16 (11) (1968) 334–339
11. Goto, F., Fujita, T., Kitani, Y., Kano, M.: Hyperbaric oxygen and stellate ganglion blocks for idiopathic sudden hearing loss. Acta Otorinolaring. 88 (1979) 335–342
12. Hardy, P. A. J., Wells, J. C. D.: Extent of sympathetic blockade after stellate ganglion block with bupivacaine. Pain 36 (1989) 193–196

13. Haug, O., Draper, W. L., Haug, S. A.: Stellate ganglion blocks for idiopathic sensorineural hearing loss. Arch. Otorinolaring. 102 (1) (1976) 5–8
14. Hickey, R.: Lokalanästhetikumstoxizität. In: Ramamurthy, S., Rogers, J. N. (Hrsg.): Schmerztherapeutische Entscheidungen. Ullstein Mosby, Berlin – Wiesbaden (1995)
15. Jankovic, D.: Die Effektivität der Ganglion stellatum Blockade bei Kopf- und Gesichtsschmerzen. Speyerer-Tage: Zeitgemäße Diagnostik und Therapie von Kopf-, Gesichts- und Schulterschmerzen, Speyer (1993)
16. Katz, J., Renck, H.: Stellatumblockade. In: Katz, J., Renck, H. (Hrsg.): Thorakoabdominale Nervenblockaden. Edition Medizin, Weinheim (1988)
17. Lang, J.: Klinische Anatomie der Halswirbelsäule. Thieme, Stuttgart – New York (1991)
18. Lang, J.: Einige Befunde zur Anatomie des Halssympathikus. Med. Orth. Tech. 112 (1992) 194–200
19. Löfström, B. J., Cousins, M. J.: Sympathetic neural blockade of upper and lower extremity. In: Cousins, M. J., Bridenbaugh, P. O. (eds.): Neural Blockade. (2nd ed.) Lippincott, Philadelphia (1988)
20. Malmquist, R. N., Bengtsson, M., Sörensen, J.: Efficacy of stellate ganglion block: A clinical study with bupivacaine. Reg. Anesthesia 17 (1992) 340–347
21. Matsuoka, H., Tokutomi, Y., Muteki, T., Yokoyama, M. M.: Influence of stellate ganglion block on the immune system. Masui Jap. J. Anesthesiology 34 (7) (1985) 917–923
22. Mays, K. S., North, W. C., Schnapp, M.: Stellate ganglion blocks with morphine in sympathetic type pain. J. Neurol. Neurosurg. Psychiat. 44 (1981) 189–190
23. Milligan, N. S., Nash, T. P.: Treatment of postherpetic neuralgia. A review of 77 consecutive cases. Pain 23 (1985) 381–386
24. Miyazaki, H., Tashiro, M., Kakiuchi, Y.: The effect of drug therapy and stellate ganglion block with or without oxygen inhalation on sudden hearing loss. Masui Jap. J. Anesthesiology 40 (8) (1991) 1251–1255
25. Moore, D. C.: Anterior (paratracheal) approach for block of the stellate ganglion. In: Moore, D. C. (ed.): Regional Block. (4th ed.) Charles Thomas, Springfield (1976)
26. Nabil, M. K. A.: Does sympathetic ganglionic block prevent postherpetic neuralgia? Reg. Anesthesia 20 (3) (1995) 227–233
27. Naveira, F. A., Morales, A.: Treatment of persistent cough after stellate ganglion block. Reg. Anesthesia 18 (1993) 312–314
28. Netter, F. H.: Autonomes Nervensystem. Autonome Innervation von Kopf und Hals. In: Krämer, G. (Hrsg.): Farbatlanten der Medizin (Band 5). Nervensystem I: Neuroanatomie und Physiologie. Georg Thieme Verlag, Stuttgart – New York (1987)
29. Olson, E. R., Ivy, H. B.: Stellate block for trigeminal zoster. J. Clin. Neuro-Ophth. 1 (1) (1981) 53–55
30. Scott, D. B.: Stellate ganglion block. In: Scott, D. B. (ed.): Techniques of Regional Anesthesia. Mediglobe, Singapore (1989)
31. Stannard, C. F., Glynn, C. J., Smith, S. P.: Dural puncture during attempted stellate ganglion block. Anesthesia 15 (1990) 952–954
32. Tenicella, R., Lovasik, D., Eaglstein, W.: Treatment of herpes zoster with sympathetic blocks. Clin. J. Pain 1 (1985) 63–67
33. Thompson, G. E., Brown, D. L.: Stellate block. In: Nunn, J. F., Utting, J. E., Brown Jr., B. R. (eds.): General Anesthesia. (5th ed.) Butterworths, London (1989)
34. Umeda, S., Hasihida, T., Kakita, T.: Clinical application of stellate ganglion morphine infiltration for chronic pain relief. Masui Jap. J. Anesthesiology 31 (1982) 1403–1406
35. Waldman, S. D., Waldman, K.: Reflex sympathetic dystrophy of the face and neck: Report of six patients treated with stellate ganglion block. Reg. Anesthesia 12 (1987) 15–17
36. Winnie, A. P., Hartwell, P. W.: Relationship between time of treatment of acute herpes zoster with sympathetic blockade and prevention of postherpetic neuralgia: Clinical support for a new theory of the mechanism by which sympathetic blockade provides therapeutic benefit. Reg. Anesthesia 18 (1993) 277–282

Chapter 7: Superior cervical ganglion

1. Amar, A. P., Heck, C. N., Levy, M. L. et al.: An institutional experience with cervical vagus nerve trunk stimulation for medically refractory epilepsy: Rationale, tecnique and outcome. Neurosurgery 43 (1998) 1265–1280
2. Ben-Menacham, E., Manon-Espaillat, R., Ristanovic, R. et. al.: Vagus nerve stimulation for treatment of partial seizures: A controlled study of effect on seizures. Epilepsia 35 (1994) 616–626
3. Glassmann, A. H.: Depression, cardiac death and the central nervous system. Neuropsychobiology 37 (1998) 80–83
4. Gross, D.: Therapeutische Lokalanästhesie des Halsgrenzstranges. In: Gross, D. (Hrsg.): Therapeutische Lokalanästhesie. Hippokrates, Stuttgart (1972)

5. Harder, H. J.: Die Behandlung der Migraine Blanche und Ophthalmique mit Blockaden des Ganglion cervicale superius. Regional-Anaesthesie 4 (1981) 1–9
6. Jenkner, F. L.: Blockade des Ganglion cervicale superius. In: Jenkner, F. L. (Hrsg.): Nervenblockaden auf pharmakologischem und auf elektrischem Weg. Springer, Wien (1980)
7. Kirchner, A., Birklein, F., Stefan, H., Handwerker, H. O.: Vagusstimulation – Eine Behandlungsoption für chronische Schmerzen? Schmerz 15 (2001) 272–277
8. Lang, J.: Klinische Anatomie der Halswirbelsäule. Thieme, Stuttgart-New York (1991)
9. Lang, J.: Einige Befunde zur Anatomie des Halssympathikus. Med. Orth. Techn. 112 (1992) 194–200
10. Matsuoka, H., Tokutomi, Y., Muteki, T., Yokojama, M. M.: Influence of stellate ganglion block on the immune system. Masui, Jap. J. Anesthesiology 34 (7) (1985) 917–923
11. Netter, F. H.: Nervengeflechte und periphere Nerven. In: Krämer, G. (Hrsg.): Farbatlanten der Medizin (Band 5). Nervensystem I: Neuroanatomie und Physiologie. Georg Thieme Verlag, Stuttgart-New York (1987)
12. Olfson, M., Marcus, S., Sackeim, H. A. et al.: Use of ECT for the inpatient treatment of reccurent major depression. Am J Psychiatry 155 (1998) 22–29
13. Rosenbaum, J. F., Heninger, G.: Vagus nerve stimulation for treatment-resistant depression. Biol Psychiatry 47 (2000) 273
14. Rush, A. J., George, M. S., Sackeim, H. A. et al.: Vagus nerve stimulation (VNS) for treatment-resistant depressions: A multicenter study. Biol Psychiatry 47 (2000) 277–286
15. Vaugh, B. V., D'Cruz, O. F.: Effect of vagal nerve stimulation on sleep (abstract). Epilepsia 40 (1999) 137

Chapter 8: Deep (and superficial) cervical plexus

1. Castresana, E. J., Shaker, I. J:, Castresana, M. R.: Incidence of shunting during carotid endarterectomy: Regional versus general anesthesia. Reg. Anesthesia 22 (2, Suppl.) (1997)
2. Davies, M. J., Silbert, B. S., Scott, D. A., Cook, R. J., Mooney, P. H., Blyth, C.: Superficial and deep cervical plexus block for carotid artery surgery: A prospective study of 1000 blocks. Reg. Anesthesia 22 (5) (1997) 442–446
3. Moore, D. C.: Block of the cervical plexus. In: Moore, D. C. (ed.): Regional Block. (4th ed.) Charles Thomas, Springfield (1976)
4. Murphy, T. M.: Somatic blockade of head and neck. In: Cousins, M. J., Bridenbaugh, D. L. (eds.): Neural Blockade. (2nd ed.) Lippincott, Philadelphia (1988)

Chapter 9: Brachial plexus

1. Allesio, J. G., Rosenblum, M., Shea, K., Freitas, D.: A retrospective comparison of interscalene block and general anesthesia for ambulatory surgery and shoulder arthroscopy. Reg. Anesthesia 20 (1) (1995) 62–68
2. Barutell, C., Vidal, F., Raich, M., Montero, A.: A neurological complication following interscalene brachial plexus block. Anesthesia 35 (1980) 365–367
3. Blanchard, J., Ramamurthy, S.: Brachial plexus. In: Benumof, L. J. (ed.): Clinical procedures in anesthesia and intensive care. Lippincott, Philadelphia (1992)
4. Bridenbaugh, D. L.: The upper extremity: Somatic blockade. In: Cousins, M. J., Bridenbaugh, D. L. (eds.): Neural Blockade. (2nd ed.) Lippincott, Philadelphia (1988)
5. Büttner, J., Kemmer, A., Argo, A., Klose, R., Forst, R.: Axilläre Blockade des Plexus brachialis. Reg. Anaesth. 11 (1988) 7
6. Cockings, E., Moore, P. L., Lewis, R. C.: Transarterial brachial plexus blockade using high doses of 1,5% mepivacaine. Reg. Anesthesia 12 (1987) 159–164
7. Cooper, K., Kelley, M. N., Carrithers, J.: Perceptions of side effects following axillary block used for outpatient surgery. Reg. Anesthesia 20 (3) (1995) 212–216
8. De Jong, R. H.: Axillary block of the brachial plexus. Anesthesiology 22 (1961) 215–225
9. De Jong, R. H.: Modified axillary block. Anesthesiology 26 (1965) 615
10. De Jong, R. H., Wagman, I. H.: Physiological mechanisms of peripheral nerve block by local anesthetics. Anesthesiology 24 (1963) 684–727
11. Durrani, Z., Winnie, A. P.: Brainstem toxicity with reversible locked-in syndrome after interscalene brachial plexus block. Anesth. Analg. 72 (1991) 249–252
12. Fletcher, D., Kuhlman, G., Samii, K.: Addition of fentanyl to 1,5% lidocaine does not increase the success of axillary plexus block. Reg. Anesthesia 19 (3) (1994) 183–188
13. Gentili, M. E., Le foulon-Gourves, M., Mamelle, J. C.: Acute respiratory failure following interscalene block: Complications of combined general and regional anesthesia. Reg. Anesthesia 19 (4) (1994) 292–293
14. Gologorsky, E., Leanza, R. F.: Contralateral anesthesia following interscalene block. Anestn Analg 75 (1992) 311–312

15. Greene Jr., E. R.: Intravascular injection of local anesthetics after veni puncture of axillary vein during attempted brachial plexus block. Anesth. Analg. 65 (1986) 421
16. Groh, G. I., Gainor, J. B., Jeffries, J. T., Brown, M.: Pseudoaneurysm of the axillary artery with median-nerve deficit after axillary block anesthesia. Bone Joint Surg. 72 (1990) 1407–1408
17. Haasio, J., Tuominen, M. K., Rosenberg, P. H.: Continuous interscalene brachial plexus block during and after shoulder surgery. Ann. Chir. Gynaecol. 79 (1990) 103–107
18. Hickey, R., Rogers, J., Hoffman, J., Ramamurthy, S.: Comparison of the clinical efficacy of three perivascular techniques for axillary brachial plexus block. Reg. Anesthesia 18 (1993) 335–338
19. Hirschel, G.: Anästhesierung des Plexus brachialis bei Operationen an der oberen Extremität. Münchn. med. Wschr. 58 (1911) 1555–1556
20. Jankovic, D.: Blockadetechniken des Plexus brachialis. Eine prospektive klinische Studie über 430 Blockaden. Inauguraldissertation. Mainz (1981)
21. Kardash, K., Schools, A., Concepcion, M.: Effects of brachial plexus fentanyl on supraclavicular block. Reg. Anesthesia 20 (4) (1995) 311–315
22. Kilka, H., Geiger, P., Mehrkens, H. H.: Infraclavicular vertical brachial plexus blockade. A new method for anesthesia of the upper extremity. An anatomical and clinical study. Anaesthesist 44 (1995) 339–344
23. Kulenkampff, D.: Die Anästhesierung des Plexus brachialis. Dtsch. med. Wschr. 38 (1912) 1878–1880
24. Kumar, A., Battit, G. E., Froese, A. B., Long, M. C.: Bilateral cervical and thoracic epidural blockade complicating interscalene brachial plexus block: Report of two cases. Anesthesiology 35 (1971) 650–652
25. Lanz, E., Theiss, D., Jankovic, D.: The extent of blockade following various techniques of brachial plexus block. Anesth. Analg. 62 (1983) 55–58
26. Lennon, R. L., Stinson Jr., L. W.: Continuous axillary brachial plexus catheters. In: Morrey, B. F. (ed.): The Elbow and its Disorders. (2nd ed.) W. B. Saunders, Philadelphia (1993)
27. Löfström, B., Wennberg, A., Widen, L.: Late disturbances in nerve function after block with local anesthetic agents. Acta Anesth. Scand. 10 (1966) 111–122
28. Lombard, T. P., Couper, J. L.: Bilateral spread of analgesia following interscalene brachial plexus block. Anesthesiology 58 (1983) 472–473
29. Mehler, D., Otten, B.: Ein neuer Katheterset zur kontinuierlichen axillären Plexusanaesthesie. Regional-Anaesthesie 6 (1983) 43–46
30. Mehrkens, H. H., Geiger, P. K.: Continuous brachial plexus blockade via the vertical infraclavicular approach. Anaesthesia 53 (S2) (1998) 19–20
31. Meier, G., Bauereis, C., Heinrich, C.: Der interskalenäre Plexuskatheter zur Anästhesie und postoperativen Schmerztherapie. Anaesthesist 46 (1997) 715–719
32. Moore, D. C.: Supraclavicular (axillar) approach for block of the Brachial plexus. In: Moore, D. C. (ed.): Regional Block. (4th ed.) Charles Thomas, Springfield (1976)
33. Neil, R. S.: Postoperative analgesia following brachial plexus block. Br. J. Anaesth. 50 (1978) 379–382
34. Netter, F. H.: Nervengeflechte und periphere Nerven. In: Krämer, G. (Hrsg.): Farbatlanten der Medizin (Band 5). Nervensystem I: Neuroanatomie und Physiologie. Georg Thieme Verlag, Stuttgart – New York (1987)
35. Neuburger, M., Landes, H., Kaiser, H.: Pneumothorax bei der Vertikalen Infraklavikulären Blockade des Plexus brachialis. Anaesthesist 49 (2000) 901–904
36. Ott, B., Neuberger, L., Frey, H. P.: Obliteration of the axillary artery after axillary block. Anesthesia 44 (1989) 773–774
37. Pere, P.: The effect of continuous interscalene brachial plexus block with 0,125% bupivacaine plus fentanyl on diaphragmatic motility and ventilatory function. Reg. Anesthesia 18 (1993) 93–97
38. Pippa, P., Cominelli, E., Marinelli, C., Aito, S.: Brachial plexus block using the posterior approach. Eur J Anaesth 7 (1990) 411–420
39. Poeck, K.: Therapie der peripheren Nervenschädigungen. In: Poeck, K. (Hrsg.): Neurologie. (9. Aufl.) Springer, Berlin-Heidelberg-New York (1994)
40. Postel, J., März, P.: Elektrische Nervenlokalisation und Kathetertechnik. Ein sicheres Verfahren zur Plexus brachialis Anaesthesie. Regional-Anaesthesie 7 (1984) 104–108
41. Raj, P. P., Montgomery, S. J., Nettles, D., Jenkins, M. T.: Infraclavicular brachial plexus block – A new approach. Anesth. Analg. 52 (1973) 897–904
42. Rodrigues, J., Barcena, M., Rodrigues, V., Aneiros, F., Alvarez, J.: Infraclavicular brachial plexus block effects on respiratory function and extent of the block. Reg Anesth and Pain Med. 23 (6) (1998) 564–568
43. Ross, S., Scarborough, C. D.: Total spinal anesthesia following brachial plexus block. Anesthesiology 39 (1973) 458
44. Rucci, F. S., Pippa, P., Barbagli, R., Doni, L.: How many interscalenic blocks are there? A comparison between the lateral and posterior approach. Eur J Anesth 10 (1993) 303–307

45. Sada, T., Kobayashi, T., Murakami, S.: Continuous axillary brachial plexus block. Can. Anaesth. Soc. J. 30 (1983) 201
46. Selander, D.: Catheter technique in axillary plexus block. Acta Anesth. Scand. 21 (1977) 324–329
47. Selander, D., Dhuner, K. G., Lundborg, G.: Peripheral nerve injury due to injection needles used for regional anesthesia. Acta Anesth. Scand. 21 (1977) 182–188
48. Selander, D., Brattsand, R., Lundborg, G., Nordborg, C., Olsson, Y.: Local anesthetics: Importance of mode of application, concentration and adrenaline for the appearance of nerve lesions. Acta Anesth. Scand. 23 (1979) 127–136
49. Selander, D., Edshage, S., Wolff, T.: Paraesthesiae or no paraesthesiae? Acta Anesth. Scand. 23 (1979) 27–33
50. Siler, J. N., Liff, P. I., Davis, J. F.: A new complication of interscalene brachial plexus block. Anesthesiology 38 (6) (1973) 590–591
51. Silverstein, W. B., Moin, U., Saiyed, M. D., Brown, A. R.: Interscalene block with a nerve stimulator: A deltoid motor response is a satisfactory endpoint for successful block. Reg Anesth and Pain Med 25 (4) (2000) 356–359
52. Sims, J. K.: A modification of landmarks for infraclavicular approach to the brachial plexus block. Anesth Analg 56 (1977) 554
53. Stan, T. C., Krantz, M. A., Solomon, D. L.: The incidence of neurovascular complications following axillary brachial plexus block using a transarterial approach. Reg. Anesthesia 20 (6) (1995) 486–492
54. Stark, P., Watermann, W. F.: Die Anwendung des Nervenstimulators zur Nervenblockade. Regional-Anaesthesie 1 (1978) 16–19
55. Stinson Jr. L. W., Lennon, R. L., Adams, R. A., Morrey, B. F.: The technique and efficacy of axillary catheter analgesia as an adjunct to distraction elbow arthroplasty: A prospective study. J. Shoulder Elbow Surg. 2 (1993) 182–189
56. Tetzlaff, J. E., Yoon, H. J., Brems, J.: Interscalene brachial plexus block for shoulder surgery. Reg. Anesthesia 19 (5) (1994) 339–343
57. Tetzlaff, J. E., Yoon, H. J., Dilger, J., Brems, J.: Subdural anesthesia as a complication of an interscalene brachial plexus block. Reg. Anesthesia 19 (5) (1994) 357–359
58. Theiss, D., Robbel, G., Theiss, M., Gerbershagen, H. U.: Experimentelle Bestimmung einer optimalen Elektrodenanordnung zur elektrischen Nervenlokalisation. Anaesthesist 26 (1977) 411–417
59. Thiagarajah, S., Lear, E., Azar, I., Salzer, J., Zeiligson, E.: Bronchospasm following interscalene brachial plexus block. Anesthesiology 61 (1984) 759–761
60. Travell, J. G., Simons, D. G.: Myofascial Pain and Dysfunction. The Trigger Point Manual. (Vol. 1) Williams & Wilkins, Baltimore (1983)
61. Urban, M. K., Urquhart, B.: Evaluation of brachial plexus anesthesia for upper extremity surgery. Reg. Anesthesia 19 (3) (1994) 175–182
62. Urmey, W. F.: Interscalene Block: The truth about twitches. Reg Anesth and Pain Med 25 (4) (2000) 340–342
63. Urmey, W. F., Talts, K. H., Sharrock, N. E.: One hundred percent incidence of hemidiafragmatic paresis associated with interscalene brachial plexus anesthesia as diagnosed by ultrasonography. Anesth Analg 72 (1991) 498–503
64. Viel, E. J., Eledjam, J. J., de la Coussage, J. E., D'Athis, F.: Brachial plexus block with opioids for postoperative pain relief: Comparison between buprenorphine and morphine. Reg. Anesthesia 14 (1989) 274–278
65. Vranken, J. H., van der Vegt, M. H., Zuurmond, W. A., Pijl, A. J., Dzoljic, M.: Continuous brachial plexus block at the cervical level using a posterior approach in the management of neuropathic cancer pain. Reg Anesth and Pain Med 26 (6) (2001) 572–575
66. Wall, J. J.: Axillary nerve blocks. Am. Fam. Physician 11 (1975) 135–142
67. Whiffler, K.: Coracoid block-A safe and easy technique. Br J Anaesth 53 (1981) 845
68. Winchell, S. W., Wolf. R.: The incidence of neuropathy following upper extremity nerve blocks. Reg. Anesthesia 10 (1985) 12–15
69. Winnie, A. P.: An „immobile needle" for nerve blocks. Anesthesiology 31 (1969) 577–578
70. Winnie, A. P.: Interscalene brachial plexus block. Anesth. Analg. 49 (1970) 455–466
71. Winnie, A. P.: Regional Anesthesia. Surg. Clin. North America 54 (1975) 861–881
72. Winnie, A. P.: Does the transarterial technique of axillary block provide a higher success rate and a lower complication rate than a paresthesia technique? Reg. Anesthesia 20 (6) (1995) 482–485
73. Winnie, A. P., Collins, V. J.: The subclavian perivascular technique of brachial plexus anesthesia. Anesthesiology 25 (1964) 353–363
74. Winnie, A. P., Radonjic, R., Akkineni, S. R., Durrani, Z.: Factors influencing distribution of local anesthetics injected into the brachial plexus sheath. Anesth. Analg. 58 (1979) 225–234

75. Zipkin, M., Backus, W. W., Scott, B.: False aneurysm of the axillary artery following brachial plexus block. J. Clin. Anesth. 3 (1991) 143–145

Chapter 10: Suprascapular nerve
Chapter 11: Subscapular nerve blocks
  Infiltration of subscapular muscle trigger points
Chapter 12: Rotator cuff muscles
  Injection techniques in the myofascial trigger points
Chapter 13: Shoulder region: intra-articular injections
  Intra-articular injection

1. Batemann, J. E.: The Shoulder and Neck. W. B. Saunders, Philadelphia (197) 134, 145–146, 149, 284–290
2. Bonica, J. J., Buckley, P. F.: Regional analgesia with local anesthetics. In: Bonica, J. J. (ed.): Management of Pain. (2nd ed.) Lea & Febiger, Philadelphia – London (1990)
3. Cailliet, R.: Shoulder Pain. 3rd ed. Davis Company, Philadelphia (1991) 105–123, 193–226
4. Cailliet, R.: Soft Tissue Pain and Disability. F. A. Davis, Philadelphia (1977) 161–162
5. Dursun, E., Dursun, N., Ural, C. E., Cakci, A.: Glenohumeral joint subluxation and reflex sumpathetic dystrophy in hemiplegic patients. Arch Phys Med Rehabil (2000) 81 (7) 944–946
6. Ekelund, A.: New knowledge of the mysterious „frozen shoulder". Surgical treatment can accelerate the recovery in more serious cases. Lakartidningen (1998) 95 (48) 5472–5474
7. Hecht, J. S.: Subscapular nerve block in the painful hemiplegic shoulder. Arch Phys Med Rehabil (1992) 73 (11) 1036–1039
8. Kopell, H. P., Thompson, W. L.: Pain and the frozen shoulder. Surg Gynecol Obstet (1959) (109) 92–96
9. Mc Laughlin, H. L.: Lesions of the musculotendinous cuff of the shoulder. J Bone Joint Surg (1944) (26) 31
10. Mercadante, S., Sapio, M., Villari, P.: Suprascapular nerve block by catheter for breakthrough shoulder cancer pain. Reg. Anesthesia 20 (4) (1995) 343–346
11. Moore, D. C.: Block of the suprascapular nerve. In: Moore, D. C. (ed.): Regional Block. (4th ed.) Charles Thomas, Springfield (1976)
12. Muller, L. P., Muller, L. A., Happ, J., Kerschbaumer, F.: Frozen shoulder: a sympathetic dystrophy? Arch Orthop Trauma Surg (2000) (120) (1–2) 84–87
13. Mumenthaler, M.: Der Schulter-Arm-Schmerz. Huber, Bern – Stuttgart – Wien (1980)
14. Netter, F. H.: Nervengeflechte und periphere Nerven. In: Krämer, G. (Hrsg.): Farbatlanten der Medizin (Band 5). Nervensystem I: Neuroanatomie und Physiologie. Georg Thieme Verlag, Stuttgart – New York (1987)
15. Travell, J. G., Simons, D. G.: Myofascial Pain and Dysfunction. The Trigger Point Manual. (Vol. 1) Williams & Wilkins, Baltimore (1983)

Chapter 14: Peripheral nerve blocks in the elbow region
Chapter 15: Peripheral nerve blocks in the wrist region

1. Bridenbaugh, D. L.: The upper extremity: Somatic blockade. In: Cousins, M. J., Bridenbaugh, D. L. (eds.): Neural-Blockade. (2nd ed.) Lippincott, Philadelphia (1988) 405–416
2. Brown, D. L.: Distal upper extremity blocks. In: Atlas of Regional Anesthesia. W. B. Saunders (1992) 48–54
3. Covic, D.: Blockaden peripherer Nerven im Ellenbogenbereich. Blockade peripherer Nerven im Handwurzelbereich. In: Hoerster, W., Kreuscher, H., Niesel, H. C, Zenz, M. (Red.): Regionalanaesthesie. Gustav Fischer Verlag, Stuttgart (1989) 86–101
4. Löfström, B.: Blockade der peripheren Nerven des Armes in der Ellenbeuge. Blockade der peripheren Nerven des Armes in der Handwurzelgegend. In: Eriksson, E. (Hrsg.): Atlas der Lokalanaesthesie. (2. Auflage) Springer (1980) 86–92
5. Netter, F. H.: Nervengeflechte und periphere Nerven. In: Krämer, G. (Hrsg.): Farbatlanten der Medizin (Band 5). Nervensystem I: Neuroanatomie und Physiologie. Georg Thieme Verlag, Stuttgart – New York (1987)

Chapter 16: Elbow and wrist
  Infiltration of myofascial trigger points and intra-articular injections

1. Huber, M., Heck, G.: Spastikbehandlung mit Botulinumtoxin A. Schulter-Arm-Hand. Pocket Atlas. Band 1. Saentis Verlag – Dr. Heck (2202)
2. Tilscher, H., Eder, M.: Infiltrationstherapie. Hippocrates, Stuttgart (1994)
3. Travell, J. G., Simons, D. G.: Myofascial pain and Dysfunction. The Trigger Point Manual. (Vol. 1). Williams & Wilkins, Baltimore (1983)

Chapter 17: Intravenous regional anesthesia (IVRA)
Chapter 18: Intravenous sympathetic block with guanethidine (Ismelin®)

1. Armstrong, P., Power, I., Wildsmith, J. A.: Addition of fentanyl to prilocaine for intravenous regional anesthesia. Anaesthesia 46 (1991) 278–280
2. Erciyes, N., Akturk, G., Solak, M.: Morphine/prilocaine combination for intravenous regional anesthesia. Acta Anaesthesiol Scand 39 (1995) 845–846
3. Gorgias, N., Maidatsi, P., Kyriakidis, A. et al.: Clonidine versus Ketamine to prevent tourniquet pain during intravenous anesthesia with lidocaine. Reg Anesth and Pain Med 26 (6) (2001) 512–517
4. Hannington-Kiff, J.: Intravenous regional sympathetic block with guanethidine. Lancet I, (1974) 1010–1020
5. Hannington-Kiff, J.: Antisympathetic drugs in limbs. In: Wall, P. D., Melzack, R. (eds.): Textbook of Pain. Churchill Livingstone, London (1984)
6. Holmes, C.: Intravenous Regional Nerve Blockade. In: Cousins, M. J., Bridenbaugh, D. L. (eds) Neural Blockade (3rd ed.) Lippincott-Raven, Philadelphia – New York (1998) 395–409
7. Pitkänen, M. T.: Intravenous regional anesthesia. In: Rosenberg, P. (ed.): Local and Regional Anesthesia. BMJ Books (2000) 55–56
8. Simgen, W. L. A.: Intravenöse Regionalanästhesie. In: Hörster, W., Zenz, M., Niesel, H. C., Kreuscher, H. (Redaktion): Regionalanästhesie. Gustav Fischer, Stuttgart – New York (1989) 82–85
9. Wahren, K. L., Gordh, T., Torebjörk, E.: Effects of regional intravenous guanethidine in patients with neuralgia in the hand, a follow up study over a decade. Pain 62 (1995) 379–385

Chapter 19: Thoracic spinal nerve blocks
Chapter 20: Lumbar paravertebral somatic nerve block
Chapter 21: Lumbar sympathetic block
Chapter 22: Celiac plexus block
Chapter 23: Iliolumbosacral ligaments

1. Brown, D. L.: Intercostal Block. In: Brown, D. L. (ed.): Atlas of Regional Anesthesia. W. B. Saunders Company (1992) 211–217
2. Buy, J. N., Moss, A. A., Singler, R. C.: CT guided celiac plexus and splanchnic nerve neurolysis. J. Comput. Ass. Tomogr. 6 (1982) 315
3. Galizia, E. J., Lahiri, S. K.: Paraplegia following coeliac plexus block with phenol. Br. J. Anaesth. 46 (1974) 539
4. Gerbershagen, H. U., Panhans, C., Waisbrod, H., Schreiner, K.: Diagnostische Lokalanaesthesie zur Differenzierung des Kreuzschmerzursprungs. Teil I, Kreuzschmerz bei ilio-lumbo-sakraler Bänderinsuffizienz. Rohrer GmbH, Bielefeld (1986)
5. Hegedues, V.: Relief of pancreatic pain by radiography-guided block. Am. J. Roentgenol. 133 (1979) 1101
6. Jenkner, F. L.: Blockade der Interkostalnerven; Blockade der thorakalen Spinalnerven (paravertebral). In: Jenkner, F. L.: Nervenblockaden auf pharmakologischen und auf elektrischem Weg. Springer Verlag, Wien (1980)
7. Katz, J., Renck, H.: Thorakale paravertebrale Blockade (S. 130); Interkostale Nervenblockade (S. 132–134). In: Katz, J., Renck, H. (Hrsg.): Thorakoabdominale Nervenblockaden. Edition Medizin, Weinheim (1988)
8. Kirvelä, O., Antila, H.: Thoracic paravertebral block in chronic postoperative pain. Reg. Anesth. 17 (1992) 348–350
9. Klein, S. M., Greengrass, R. A., Weltz, C., Warner, D. S.: Paravertebral somatic nerve block for outpatient inguinal herniorrhaphy: An expanded case report of 22 patients. Reg. Anesth. and Pain Med. 23 (3) (1998) 306–310
10. Moore, D. C.: Intercostal Nerve Block; Paravertebral thoracic somatic Nerve Block. In: Moore, D. C. (ed.): Regional Block. (4th ed.) Charles Thomas, Springfield (1976) 163–166, 200–204
11. Netter, F. H.: Nervengeflechte und periphere Nerven. In: Krämer, G. (Hrsg.): Farbatlanten der Medizin (Band 5). Nervensystem I: Neuroanatomie und Physiologie. Georg Thieme Verlag, Stuttgart – New York (1987)
12. Sayed, I., Elias, M.: Acute chemical pericarditis following celiac plexus block. Middle East J. Anesthesiol. 14 (3) (1997) 201–205
13. Thompson, G. E., Moore, D. C.: Celiac plexus, intercostal and minor peripheral blockade. In: Cousins, M. J., Bridenbaugh, D. L. (eds.): Neural Blockade. (2nd ed.) Lippincott, Philadelphia (1988)
14. Wassef, M. R., Randazzo, T., Ward, W.: The paravertebral nerve root block for inguinal herniorrhaphy – A comparison with the field block approach. Reg. Anesth. and Pain Med. 23 (5) (1998) 451–456
15. Wong, G. Y., Brown, D. L.: Transient paraplegia following alcohol celiac plexus block. Reg. Anesth. 20 (4) (1995) 352–355

Chapter 24: Ganglion impar (Walther ganglion) block

1. Kahle, W.: Nervensystem und Sinnesorgane. In: Taschenatlas der Anatomie. 7. vollständig überarbeitete Auflage. Georg Thieme Verlag. Stuttgart – New York, 2001
2. Nebab, E. G., Florence, I. M.: An alternative needle geometry for interruption of the ganglion impar. Anesthesiology 86 (1997) 1213–1214
3. Netter, F. H.: Nervengeflechte und periphere Nerven. In: Krämer, G. (Hrsg.): Farbatlanten der Medizin (Band 5). Nervensystem I. Neuroanatomie und Physiologie. Georg Thieme Verlag, Stuttgart – New York (1987)
4. Patt, R. B., Plancarte, R.: Neurolytic blocks of the sympathetic axis. In: Patt, R. B. (ed.): Cancer pain. JB. Lippincott, Philadelphia (1993)
5. Patt, R. B., Plancarte, R.: Superior hypogastric plexus and ganglion impar. In: Hahn, M. B., McQuillan, P. M., Sheplock, G. J. (eds.): Regional Anesthesia, Mosby (1996)
6. Plancarte, R., Amescua, C., Patt, R. B. et al: Presacral blockade of Walther (ganglion impar). Anesthesiology 73 (1990) A 751

Chapter 25: Infiltration of the piriform trigger points ("piriform syndrome")

1. Beaton, L. E., Anson, B. J.: The sciatic nerve and the piriformis muscle: Their interrelation a possible cause of coccygodynia. The Journal of Bone and Joint Surgery. 20 (3) (1938): 686–688
2. Durani, Z., Winnie, A.: Piriformis muscle syndrome: An underdiagnosed cause of sciatica. J of Pain and Symptom Management 6 (6) (1991): 373–379
3. Fishmann, S. M., Caneris, O. A., Bandmann, T. B., Audette, J. F., Borsook, D.: Injection of the piriformis muscle by fluoroscopic and electromyographic guidance. Reg Anesth and Pain Med 23 (6) (1998): 554–559
4. Hanania, M., Kitain, E.: Perisciatic injection of steroid for the treatment of sciatica due to piriformis syndrome. Reg Anesth and Pain Med 23 (2) (1998): 223–228
5. Hanania, M.: New technique for piriformis muscle injection using a nerve stimulator. Reg Anesth 22 (1997): 200–202
6. Jankovic, D.: Commonly overlooked pain syndromes responsive to simple therapy. Esra Winter Forum. „Regional Anesthesia Pearls". Davos 2003
7. Karl, R. D., Yedinak, M. A., Hartshorne, M. F. et al.: Scintigraphic appearance of the piriformis muscle syndrome. Clinical Nuclear Medicine. 10 (10) (1985): 361–363
8. Kirkaldy-Willis, W. H., Hill, R. J.: A more precise diagnosis for low-back pain. Spine 4 (2) (1979): 102–109
9. Netter, F. H.: Anatomie. In: Firbas, W.(Hrsg.): Farbatlanten der Medizin (Band 7). Bewegungsapparat I: Anatomie, Embryologie, Physiologie und Stoffwechselkrankheiten. Georg Thieme Verlag, Stuttgart – New York (1992)
10. Pace, B. J.: Commonly overlooked pain syndromes responsive to simple therapy. Postgraduate Medicine. 58 (4) (1975): 107–113
11. Retzlaff, E. W., Berry, A. H., Haight, A. S. et al.: The piriformis muscle syndrome. J of AOA 73 (1974): 799–807
12. Solheim, L. F., Siewers, P., Paus, B.: The piriformis muscle syndrome. Acta Orthop Scand 52 (1981): 73–75
13. Thiele, G. H.: Coccygodynia and pain in the superior gluteal region. JAMA 109, (1937): 1271–1275
14. Travell, J. G., Simons, D. G.: Myofascial Pain and Dysfunction. The Trigger Point Manual. Williams & Wilkins, Baltimore – London (1983)
15. Wyant, G. M.: Chronic Pain Syndromes and Treatment III. The Piriformis Syndrome. Canad Anesth Soc J 26 (1979): 305–308
16. Yue, S. K.: Morphological findings of asymmetrical and dystrophic psoas and piriformis muscles in chronic lower back pain during CT guided botulinum toxin injections. Reg Anesth and Pain Med 23 (3), (1998) May–June Suppl

Chapter 26: Inguinal femoral paravascular block ("three-in-one" block)
Chapter 27: Psoas compartment block (Cheyen access)
Chapter 28: Sciatic nerve block
Chapter 29: Femoral nerve
Chapter 30: Lateral femoral cutaneous nerve
Chapter 31: Obturator nerve
Chapter 32: Ilioinguinal and iliohypogastric nerves
Chapter 33: Blocking peripheral nerves in the knee joint region
Chapter 34: Blocking peripheral nerves in the ankle joint region

1. Berkowitz, A., Rosenberg, H.: Femoral block with mepivacaine for muscle biopsy in malignant hyperthermia patients. Anesthesiology 62 (1985) 651–652

2. Bridenbaugh, P. O.: The lower extremity: Somatic blockade. In: Cousins, M. J., Bridenbaugh, D. L. (eds.): Neural Blockade in Clinical Anesthesia and Management of Pain. (2nd ed.) Lippincott, Philadelphia (1988) 417–441
3. Chayen, D., Nathan, H., Clayen, M.: The psoas compartment block. Anesthesiology 45 (1976) 95–99
4. Di Benedetto, P., Bertini, L., Casati, A., Borghi, B., Albertin, A., Fanelli, G.: A new posterior approach to the sciatic nerve block. A prospective, randomized comparison with the classical posterior approach. Anaesth Analg 93 (2001): 1040–1044
5. Elmas, C., Atanassoff, P.: Combined inguinal paravascular (3 in 1) and sciatic nerve blocks for lower limb surgery. Reg. Anesth. 18 (1993) 88–92
6. Frerk, C. M.: Palsy after femoral nerve block. Anaesthesia 43 (1988) 167–168
7. Hirst, G. C., Lang, S. A., Dust, W. N., Cassidy, D., Yip, R. W.: Femoral nerve block. Single injection versus continuous infusion for total knee arthroplasty. Reg. Anesth. 21 (4) (1996) 292–297
8. Hoerster, W.: Blockaden peripherer Nerven im Bereich des Kniegelenkes; Blockaden im Bereich des Fußgelenkes (Fußblock). In: Hoerster, W., Kreuscher, H., Niesel, H. C., Zenz, M. (Red.): Regionalanaesthesie. Gustav Fischer Verlag, Stuttgart (1989) 124–139
9. Kofoed, H.: Peripheral nerve blocks at the knee and ancle in operations for common foot disorders. Clin. Orthop. 168 (1982) 97–101
10. Lynch, J.: Prolonged motor weakness after femoral nerve block with bupivacaine 0,5 %. Anaesthesia 45 (1990) 421
11. McCutcheon, R.: Regional anesthesia for the foot. Can. Anaesth. Soc. J. 12 (1995) 465
12. Misra, U., Pridie, A. K., McClymont, C., Bower, S.: Plasma concentrations of bupivacaine following combined sciatic and femoral 3 in 1 nerve blocks in open knee surgery. Br. J. Anaesth. 66 (1991) 310–313
13. Moore, D. C.: Regional Block. (4th ed.) Charles Thomas, Springfield (1976)
14. Ringrase, N. H., Cross, M. J.: Femoral nerve block in knee joint surgery. Am. J. Sports Med. 12 (1984) 398–402
15. Rooks, M., Fleming, L. L.: Evaluation of acute knee injuries with sciatic femoral nerve blocks. Clin Orthop. 179 (1983) 185–188
16. Rorie, D. K., Beyer, D. E., Nelson, D. O.: Assessment of block of the sciatic nerve in popliteal fossa. Anesth. Analg. 59 (1980) 371–376
17. Singelyn, F. J., Gouverneur, J. M.: The continuous „3-in-1" block as postoperative pain treatment after hip, femoral shaft or knee surgery: A large scale study of efficacy and side effects. Anesthesiology 81 (1994) 1064
18. Smith, B. E., Fischer, A. B. J., Scott, P. U.: Continuous sciatic nerve block. Anaesthesia 39 (1984) 155–157
19. Winnie, A. P., Ramamurthy, S., Durani, Z.: The inguinal paravascular technic of lumbar plexus anesthesia: The „3-in-1" block. Anesth. Analg. 52 (1973) 989–996

Chapter 35: Neuraxial anatomy
Chapter 36: Spinal anesthesia
Chapter 37: Complications of spinal anesthesia
Chapter 38: Continuous spinal anesthesia (CSA)
Chapter 39: Continuous spinal anesthesia (CSA) in obstetrics
Chapter 40: Chemical intraspinal neurolysis with phenol in glycerol

1. Abboud, T. K., Raya, J., Noueihed, R., Daniel, J.: Intrathecal morphine for relief of labor pain in parturient with severe pulmonary hypertension. Anesthesiology 59 (1983) 477–479
2. Abouleish, E., de la Vega, S., Blendinger, I., Tio, T.: Long-term follow up of epidural blood patch. Anaesth. Analg. 54 (1975) 459–463
3. Aguilar, J. L., Sierra, J. C.: Transient neurologic symptoms following spinal anaesthesia. Choice of local anaesthetics. In: Van Zundert, A., Rawal, N. (eds.): Highlights in Regional Anaesthesia and Pain Therapy. XI (Special Edition: World Congress on Regional Anaesthesia And Pain Therapy, Barcelona (2002) 301–306, Cyprint Ltd, Cyprus
4. Arkoosh, V.: Continuous spinal analgesia and anesthesia in obstetrics. Reg. Anesth. 18 (1993) 402–405
5. Armstrong, L. A., Littlewood, D. G., Chambers, W. A.: Spinal anesthesia with tetracaine – the effect of added vasoconstrictors. Anaesth. Analg. 62 (1983) 793
6. Atulkumar, M. K., Foster, P. A.: Adrenocorticotropic hormone infusion as a novel treatment for postdural puncture headache. Reg. Anesth. 22 (5) (1997) 432–434
7. Bannister, R.: Brain's clinical neurology. (6th ed.) Oxford University Press (1985) 52
8. Barash, P. G., Cullen, B. F., Stoelting, R. K. In: Barash, P. G., Cullen, B. F., Stoelting, R. K. (eds.): Clinical Anesthesia. Lippincott Comp, Philadelphia (1989) 778–780
9. Baxter, A.: Continuous spinal anesthesia: The Canadian perspective. Reg. Anesth. 18 (1993) 414–418

10. Beards, S. C., Jackson, A., Griffiths, A. G., Horsman, E. L.: Magnetic resonance imaging of extradural blood patches: Appearances from 30 min to 18 h. Br. J. Anaesth. 71 (1993) 182–188
11. Bergmann, H.: Komplikationen, Fehler und Gefahren der Spinalanaesthesie. In: Nolte, H., Meyer, J. (Hrsg.): Die rückenmarksnahen Anaesthesien. Georg Thieme Verlag, Stuttgart (1972) 45
12. Bevacqua, B.: Continuous spinal anesthesia: Operative indication and clinical experience. Reg. Anesth. 18 (1993) 394–401
13. Bolton, V. E., Leicht, C. H., Scanlon, T. S.: Postpartum seizure after epidural blood patch and intravenous caffeine sodium benzoate. Anesthesiology 70 (1989) 146–149
14. Bridenbaugh, P. O., Greene, N.: Spinal (subarachnoid) Neural Blockade. In: Cousins, M. J., Bridenbaugh, P. O. (eds.): Neural Blockade. (2nd ed.) Lippincott, Philadelphia (1988)
15. Brizgys, R. V., Shnider, S. M.: Hyperbaric intrathecal morphine analgesia during labor in a patient with Wolff-Parkinson-White syndrome. Obstet. Gynecol. 64 (3) (1984) 44–46
16. Caldwell, C., Nielsen, C., Baltz, T., Taylor, P.: Comparison of high dose epinephrine and phenylephrine in spinal anesthesia with tetracaine. Anesthesiology 62 (1995) 804
17. Camann, W. R., Murray, R. S., Mushlin, P. S., Lambert, D. H.: Effects of oral caffeine on postdural puncture headache: a double-blind, placebo-controlled trial. Anesth. Analg. 70 (1990) 181–184
18. Carp, H., Singh, P. J., Vahera, R., Jayaram, A.: Effects of the serotonin-receptor agonist sumatriptan on postdural puncture headache: Report of six cases. Anesth. Analg. 79 (1994) 180–182
19. Carrie, L. E. S.: Postdural puncture headache and extradural blood patch. Br. J. Anaesth. 71 (1993) 179
20. Casati, A., Fanelli, G., Aldegheri, G., Colnaghi, E., Cedrati, V.: Frequency of hypotension during conventional or asymmetric hyperbaric spinal block. Reg Anesth Pain Med 24 (1999) 214–219
21. Casati, A., Fanelli, G., Cappelleri, G. L., Aldegheri, G. et al: Effects of spinal needle type on lateral distribution of 0.5 % hyperbaric bupivacaine. A doubleblind study. Anest Analg 87 (1998) 355–359
22. Casati, A., Fanelli, G., Cappelleri, G. L. Borghi, B. et al: Low dose hyperbaric bupivacaine for unilateral spinal anesthesia: evaluation of solution concentration. Can J Anaesth 45 (1998) 850–854
23. Cass, W., Edelist, G.: Postspinal headache. JAMA 227 (1974) 786–787
24. Chambers, W. A., Littlewood, D. G., Logan, M. R., Scott, D. B.: Effect of added epinephrine on spinal anesthesia with lidocaine. Anesth. Analg. 60 (1981) 417
25. Chambers, W. A., Littlewood, D. G., Scott, D. B.: Spinal anesthesia with bupivacaine: Effect of added vasoconstrictors. Anesth. Analg. 61 (1982) 49
26. Charsley, M., Abram, S.: The injection of intrathecal normal saline reduces the severity of postdural puncture headache. Reg Anesth Pain Med 26 (4) (2001) 301–305
27. Chibber, A. K., Lustik, S. J.: Unexpected neurologic deficit following spinal anesthesia. Reg. Anesth. 21 (4) (1996) 355–357
28. Clayton, K. C.: The incidence of Horner's syndrome during lumbar extradural for elective caesarean section and provision of analgesia during labour. Anaesthesia 38 (1983) 583–585
29. Collier, B. B: Treatment for dural puncture headache. Br. J. Anaesth. 72 (1994) 366
30. Concepcion, M., Maddi, R., Francis, D.: Vasoconstrictors in spinal anesthesia. A comparison of epinephrine and phenylephrine. Anesth. Analg. 63 (1984) 134
31. Craft, J. B., Epstein, B. S., Coakley, C. S.: Prophylaxis of dural-puncture headache with epidural saline. Anesth. Analg. 52 (1973) 228–231
32. Crul, B. J., Gerritse, B. M., van Dongen, R. T., Schooderwaldt, H. C.: Epidural fibrin glue injection stops persistent postdural puncture headache. Anesthesiology 91 (1999) 576–577
33. Dahlgren, N., Törnebrandt, K.: Neurological complications after anaesthesia. A follow-up of 18 000 spinal and epidural anaesthetics performed over three years. Acta. Anaesth. Scand. 39 (1995) 872–880
34. Day, C. J., Schutt, L. E.: Auditory, ocular and facial complications of central neural block. A review of possible mechanisms. Reg. Anesth. 21 (3) (1996) 197–201
35. Di Giovanni, A. J., Dunbar, B. S.: Epidural injections of autologous blood for postlumbar-puncture headache. Anesth. Analg. 49 (1970) 268–271
36. Drasner, K.: Cauda equina syndrome and continuous spinal anesthesia (Letter). Anesthesiology 78 (1993) 215–216
37. Drasner, K.: Models for local anesthetic toxicity from continuous spinal anesthesia. Reg. Anesth. 18 (1993) 424–438
38. Dripps, R. D., Vandam, L. D.: Long-term follow-up of patients who received 10098 spinal anesthetics. I. Failure to discover major neurological sequelae. JAMA 156 (1954) 1486

39. Dunteman, E., Turner, S. W., Swarm, R.: Pseudo-spinal headache. Reg. Anesth. 21 (4) (1996) 358–360
40. Enk, D.: Unilateral spinal anaesthesia: gadget or tool? Curr Opin Anaesthesiol 11 (1998) 511–515
41. Enk, D., Prien, T., Van Acken, H., Mertes, N. et al: Success rate of unilateral spinal anesthesia is dependent on injection flow. Reg Anesth Pain Med 26 (5) (2001) 420–427
42. Errando, C. L.: Transient neurologic syndrome, transient radicular irritation, or postspinal musculosceletal symptoms: Are we describing the same „syndrome" in all patients. Reg Anesth Pain Med 26 (2) (2001) 178–179
43. Ford, C. D., Ford, D. C., Koenigsberg, M. D.: A simple treatment of post-lumbar-puncture headache. J. Emerg. Med. 7 (1989) 29–31
44. Freye, E.: Peridurale Analgesie mit Opioiden. In: Freye, E. (Hrsg): Opioide in der Medizin. Wirkung und Einsatzgebiete zentraler Analgetika. Springer (1995)
45. Gazmuri, R. R., Ricke, C. A., Dagnino, J. A.: Trigeminal nerve block as a complication of epidural anesthesia. Reg. Anesth. 17 (1992) 50–51
46. Gentili, M.: Epidural fibrin glue injection stops postdural puncture headache in patients with long term intrathecal catheterization. Reg Anest Pain Med 28 (1) (2003) 70
47. Gerbershagen, H. U., Baar, H. A., Kreuscher, H.: Langzeitnervenblockaden zur Behandlung schwerer Schmerzzustände. Die intrathekale Injektion von Neurolytika. Anaesthesist 21, Springer (1972) 112–121
48. Gerritse, B. M., van Dongen, R. T., Crul, B. J.: Epidural fibrin glue injection stops persistent cerebrospinal fluid leak during long-term intrathecal catheterization. Anesth Analg 84 (1997) 1140–1141
49. Giering, H., Glözner, F. L., Pock, H. G.: Persistierendes Querschnittsyndrom nach Spinalanaesthesie. Anaest. Intensivmed. 10 (38) (1997) 505–508
50. Gogarten, W., Van Aken, H., Wulff, H., Klose, R., Vandermeulen, E., Harenberg, J.: Rückenmarksnahe Regionalanaesthesien und Thromboembolieprophylaxe/Antikoagulation. Empfehlung der Deutschen Gesellschaft für Anaesthesiologie und Intensivmedizin. Anaesth. Intensivmed. 12 (38) (1997) 623–628
51. Gonsales-Carrasco, J., Nogues, S., Aguilar, J. L., Vidal-Lopez, F., Llubia, C.: Pneumocephalus after accidental dural puncture during epidural anesthesia. Reg. Anesth. 18 (1993) 193–195
52. Harrington, T. M.: An alternative treatment for spinal headache. J. Fam. Pract. 15 (1982) 172–177
53. Hawkins, J. L.: Wet tap during labor – now what? Am. Soc. Reg. Anesth. 12th Annual Meeting, Syllabue (1995) 259–270
54. Heavner, J. R., De Jong, R. H.: Lidocaine blocking concentration for B and C nerve fibers. Anaesthesiology 40 (1974) 228–233
55. Hönig, O., Winter, H., Baum, K. R., Schöder, P., Winter, P.: Sectio caesarea in Katheter-Spinalanästhesie bei einer kardiopulmonalen Hochrisikopatientin. Anaesthesist 47, Springer Verlag (1998) 685–689
56. Hurey, R.: Continuous spinal anesthesia: A historical perspective. Reg. Anesth. 18 (1993) 390–393
57. Jaradeh, S.: Cauda equina syndrome: A neurologist's perspective. Reg. Anesth. 18 (1993) 473–480
58. Jarvis, A. P., Greenawalt, J. W., Fagraeus, L.: Intravenous caffeine for postdural puncture headache. Anesth. Analg. 65 (1986) 316–317
59. Kalichman, M.: Physiologic mechanisms by which local anesthetics may cause injury to nerve and spinal cord. Reg. Anesth. 18 (1993) 448–452
60. Kubina, P., Gupta, A., Oscarsson, A., Axelsson, K., Bengstsson, M.: Two cases of cauda equina syndrome following spinal-epidural anesthesia. Reg. Anesth. 22 (5) (1997) 447–450
61. Kuusniemi, K. S., Pihlajamäki, K. K., Pitkänen, M.: A low dose of plain or hyperbaric bupivacine for unilateral spinal anesthesia. Reg Anesth Pain Med 25 (6) (2000) 605–610
62. Larsen, R.: Spinalanaesthesie. In: Larsen, R. (Hrsg): Anaesthesie. (4. Auflage) Urban & Schwarzenberg (1985)
63. Lehmann, L. J., Hacobian, A., De Sio, M.: Successful use of epidural blood patch for postdural puncture headache following lumbar sympathetic block. Reg. Anesth. 21 (4) (1996) 347–349
64. Leicht, C. H., Evans, D. E., Durkan, W. J., Noltner, S.: Sufentanil versus fentanyl intrathecally for labor analgesia. Anesth Analg 72 (1991) 159
65. Le Polain, B., De Kock, M., Scoltes, J. L., Vanleirde, M.: Clonidine combined with sufentanil and bupivacaine with adrenaline for obstetric analgesia. Br. J. Anaesth. 71 (1993) 657–660
66. Levinson, G.: Spinal Anesthesia. In: Benumof, J.: Clinical procedures in anesthesia and intensive care. Lippincott, Philadelphia (1992) 645–661
67. Lowe, D. M., Mc Cullough, A. M.: 7th nerve palsy after extradural blood patch. Br. J. Anaesth. 65 (1990) 721–722
68. Lund, P. C.: Principles and practise of spinal anesthesia. IL Charles Thomas, Springfield (1971)
69. Maher, R., Mehta, M.: Spinal (intrathecal) and extradural analgesia. In: Lipton, S. (ed.): Persistant pain. Modern methods of treatment. (Vol. 1) Academic Press, London (1977)

70. Möllmann, M., Auf der Landwehr, U.: Post-operative Analgesia following continuous Spinal Anesthesia (CSA). B. Braun Satellite Symposium: Continuous Regional post-operative Analgesia: Breaking up some taboos. 17 ESRA Congress Geneva, (Sept. 1998)
71. Möllmann, M.: St. Franziskus Hospital Münster. Persönliche Mitteilung (1998)
72. Netter, F. H.: Knöcherne Bedeckung des Gehirns und des Rückenmarks; Makroskopische Anatomie des Gehirns und des Rückenmarks. In: Krämer, G. (Hrsg.): Farbatlanten der Medizin (Band 5). Nervensystem I. Neuroanatomie und Physiologie. Thieme Verlag, Stuttgart – New York (1987)
73. Norris, M. C., Leighton, B. L.: Some useful information for obstetrical anesthesia. In: Physician Education Program in Regional Anesthesia. (Volume 2) Becton & Dickinson, (1994)
74. Paech, M. J.: Unexplained neurologic deficit after uneventful combined spinal and epidural anesthesia for ceasarean delivery. Reg. Anesth. 22 (5) (1997) 479–482
75. Palmer, C. M.: Early respiratory depression following intrathecal fentanyl-morphine combination. Anesthesiology 74 (1991) 1153–1155
76. Perez, M., Olmos, M., Garrido, J.: Facial nerve paralysis after epidural blood patch. Reg. Anesth. 18 1(1993) 96–198
77. Pittoni, G., Toffoletto, F., Calcarella, G. et al: Spinal anaesthesia in out patients knee surgery: 22-gauge versus 25-gauge Sprotte needle. Anaesth Analg 81 (1995) 73–79
78. Poeck, K.: Die wichtigsten neurologischen Syndrome. In: Poeck, K. (Hrsg.): Neurologie. (9. Aufl.) Springer Verlag, Berlin-Heidelberg-New York (1994)
79. Pollock, J. E.: Lidocaine spinal anaesthesia: Extent of the problem and clinical picture. In: van Zundert, A., Rawal, N. (eds): Highlights in Regional Anaesthesia and Pain Therapy. XI (Special Edition: World Congress on Regional Anaesthesia and Pain Therapy, Barcelona, 2002) 290–300, Cyprint Ltd, Cyprus
80. Ravindran, R. S., Bond, V. K., Tasch, M. D., Gupta, C. D., Leurssen, T. G.: Prolonged neural blockade following regional anesthesia with 2-chloroprocaine. Anesth. Analg. 59 (1980) 447–454
81. Rawal, N.: Klinischer Einsatz der rückenmarksnahen Opioidanalgesie. Teil 1. Der Schmerz 10, Springer Verlag (1996) 176–189
82. Rawal, N.: Klinischer Einsatz der rückenmarksnahen Opioidanalgesie. Teil 2. Der Schmerz 10, Springer Verlag (1996) 226–236
83. Ray, B. S., Hindey, J. C., Geohegan, W. A.: Preservations of the distribution of the sympathetic nerves to the pupil and upper extremity as determined by stimulation of the anterior nerve roots in man. Ann. Surg. 118 (1943) 647–655
84. Renck, H.: Neurological complications of central nerve blocks. Acta. Anaesth. Scand. 39 (1995) 859–868
85. Rigler, M. L., Drasner, K., Krejcie, T. C., Yelich, S. J., Scholnick, F. T., De Fontes, J., Bohner, D.: Cauda equina syndrome after continuous spinal anesthesia. Anesth. Analg. 72 (1991) 275–281
86. Schneider, M., Hampl, K., Petersen-Felix, S.: Controversies in clinical practice of regional anaesthesia. In: Rosenberg, P. (ed): Local and Regional Anaesthesia BMJ Books (2000) 124–134
87. Sechzer, P. H., Abel, L.: Post-spinal anesthesia headache treated with caffeine: evaluation with demand method. Part I. Curr. Ther. Res. 24 (1978) 307–312
88. Sechzer, P. H.: Post-spinal anesthesia headache treated with caffeine, part II: intracranial vascular distention, a key factor. Curr. Ther. Res. 26 (1979) 440–448
89. Shigematsu, T., Wang, H., Nagano, M.: Trigeminal nerve palsy after lumbar epidural anesthesia. Anaesth. Analg. 64 (1985) 653
90. Spencer, H.: Postdural puncture headaches: what matters in technique. Reg. Anesth. and Pain Med. 23 (4) (1998) 374–379
91. Spivey, D. L.: Epinephrine does not prolong lidocaine spinal anesthesia in term parturients. Anaesth. Analg. 64 (1985) 468
92. Sprung, J., Haddox, J. D., Maitra-D'Cruze, A. M.: Horner's syndrome and trigeminal nerve palsy following epidural anesthesia for obstetrics. Can. J. Anesth. 38 (1991) 767–771
93. Srinivasa, V., Eappen, S., Schlossmacher, M., Gerner, P.: Seizures after epidural blood patch. Reg Anesth Pain Med 28 (1) (2003) 71
94. Stevens, D. S., Peeters-Asdourian, C.: Treatment of postdural puncture headache with epidural dextran patch. Reg. Anesth. 18 (1993) 324–325
95. Tanasichuk, M. A., Schulz, E. A., Matthews, J. H., Van Bergen, F.: Spinal hemianalgesia: An evaluation of a method, ist applicability and influence on the incidence of hypotension. Anesthesiology 22 (1961) 74–85
96. Tetzlaff, J., O'Hara, J., Bell, G., Grimm, K., Yoon, H.: Influence of baricity on the outcome of spinal anesthesia with bupivacaine for lumbar spine surgery. Reg. Anesth. 20 (6) (1995) 533–537

97. Thomas, P. K.: Other cranial nerves. In: D. J., Ledingham, J. G. G., Warell, D. A. (eds.): Weatherall, Oxford Textbook of Medicine 21. (2nd ed.) Oxford University Press, Oxford (1988) 92

98. Usubiaga, J. E.: Neurological complications following epidural anesthesia. Int. Anaesth. Clin. 13 (1975) 33–96

99. Van Zundert, A.; Transient neurologic symptoms prevention and treatment. In: Van Zundert, A., Rawal, N. (eds): Highlights in Regional Anaesthesia and Pain Therapy. XI (Special Edition: World Congress on Regional Anaesthesia and Pain Therapy. Barcelona (2002) 307–309, Cyprint Ltd, Cyprus

100. Zenz, M., Donner, B.: Regionale Opioidanalgesie. In: Niesel, H. C. (Hrsg.): Regionalanaesthesie, Lokalanaesthesie, Regionale Schmerztherapie. Thieme Verlag (1994)

101. Zoys, T. N.: An overview of postdural puncture headaches and their treatment. In: ASRA Supplement of the American Society of Regional Anesthesia (1996)

Chapter 41: Lumbar epidural anesthesia
Chapter 42: Thoracic epidural anesthesia
Chapter 43: Epidural anesthesia in obstetrics
Chapter 44: Lumbar epidural anesthesia in children
Chapter 45: Epidural steroid injection
Chapter 46: Combined spinal and epidural anesthesia (CSE)

1. Abram, S. E.: Perceived dangers from intraspinal steroid injections. Arch. Neurol. 46 (1989) 719–720

2. Abram, S. E., O'Connor, T.: Complications associated with epidural steroid injections. Reg. Anesth. 21 (2) (1996) 149–162

3. Bachmann-Mennenga, B.: Epidurale Analgesie in der Geburtshilfe. In: Van Aken, H. (Hrsg.): Regionalanaesthesiologische Aspekte, Band 10. Ein neues Lokalanaesthetikum – Naropin. Arcis Verlag, (1997)

4. Badner, N. H., Sandler, A. N., Koren, G.: Lumbar epidural fentanyl infusions for post-thoracotomy patients: analgesic, respiratory, and pharmacokinetic effects. J. Cardiothorac. Anesth. 4 (1990) 543

5. Baker, A. S., Ojemann, R. G., Schwarz, M. N., Richardson, E. P.: Spinal epidural abscess. N. Engl. J. Med. 293 (1975) 463–468

6. Beilin, Y., Arnold, I., Telfeyan, C. et al: Quality of analgesia when air versus saline is used for identification of the epidural space in the parturient. Reg Anesth Pain Med 25 (6) (2000) 596–599

7. Benzon, H. R.: Epidural injections for low back pain and lumbosacral radiculopathy. Pain 24 (1986) 277–295

8. Bogduk, N.: Back pain: Zygapophysial blocks and epidural steroids. In: Cousins, M. J., Bridenbaugh, P. O. (eds.): Neural Blockade. (2nd ed.) Lippincott, Philadelphia (1988) 935–954

9. Brodsky, J. B., Kretzschmar, M., Mark, J. B. D.: Caudal epidural morphine for post-thoracotomy pain. Anesth. Analg. 67 (1988) 409

10. Bromage, P. R.: Diagnostic and therapeutic applications. In: Bromage, P. R. (ed.): Epidural Block. Saunders, Philadelphia (1978) 601–643

11. Bromage, P. R.: Anatomy. In: Bromage, P. R. (ed.): Epidural Block. Saunders, Philadelphia (1978) 8–67

12. Bromage, P. R.: Spinal extradural abscess: Pursuit of vigilance. Br. J. Anesth. 70 (1993) 471–473

13. Bromage, P., Benumof, J.: Paraplegia following intracord injection during attempted epidural anesthesia under general anesthesia. Reg. Anesth. and Pain Med. 23 (1) (1998) 104–107

14. Brownridge, P.: Epidural and subarachnoid analgesia for elective caesarean section. Anaesthesia 36 (1981) 70

15. Carrie, L. E. S., O'Sullivan, G: Subarachnoid bupivacaine 0,5% for caesarean section. Eur. J. Anaesth. 1 (1984) 275–283

16. Castagnera, L., Maurette, P., Pointillart, V., Vital, J., Erny, P., Senegas, J.: Long-term results of cervical epidural steroid injection with and without morphine in chronic cervical radicular pain. Pain 58 (1994) 239–243

17. Cherng, Y. G., Wang, Y. P., Liu, C. C., Shi, J. J., Huang, S. C.: Combined spinal and epidural anesthesia for abdominal hysterectomy in a patients with myotonic dystrophy. Reg. Anesth. 19 (1994) 69–72

18. Cherry, D. A.: Epidural depotcorticosteroids. Med. J. Austr. 2 (1983) 420

19. Chestnut, D. H., Owen, C. L., Brown, C. K., Vandewalker, G. E., Weiner, C. P.: Does labor affect the variability of maternal heart rate during induction of epidural anesthesia? Anesthesiology 68 (1988) 622

20. Cicala, R. S., Turner, R., Morgan, B. S. et al.: Methylprednisolone acetate does not cause inflammatory changes in the epidural space. Anesth. Analg. 72 (1990) 556–558

21. Coates, M.: Combined subarachnoid and epidural techniques. A single space technique for surgery of the hip and lower limb. Anaesthesia 37 (1982) 89

22. Coda, B., Bausch, S., Haas, M., Chavkin, C.: The hypothesis that antagonism of fentanyl analgesia by 2-chloroprocaine is mediated by direct action on opioid receptors. Reg. Anesth. 22 (1) (1997) 43–52

23. Cousins, M. J., Bromage, P. R.: Epidural Neural Blockade. In: Cousins, M. J., Bridenbaugh, P. O. (eds.): Neural Blockade. (2nd ed.) Lippincott, Philadelphia (1988) 253–274
24. Cousins, M. J., Bromage, P. R.: Epidural Neural Blockade. In: Cousins, M. J., Bridenbaugh, P. O. (eds.): Neural Blockade. (2nd ed.) Lippincott, Philadelphia (1988) 341
25. Covino, B. G., Scott, B. D.: Epidurale Anästhesie und Analgesie. Lehrbuch und Atlas. Edition Medizin, Weinheim (1987)
26. Curelaru, I.: Long duration subarachnoid anaesthesia with continuous epidural block. Prakt. Anästh. 14 (1979) 71–78
27. Delaney, T. J., Rowlingson, J. C., Carron, H., Butler, A.: Epidural steroid effects on nerves and meninges. Anesth. Analg. 58 (1980) 610–614
28. Delleur, M. M.: Continuous lumbar epidural block. In: Saint-Maurize, C., Schulte-Steinberg, O., Armitage, E. (eds.): Regional Anaesthesia in Children. Appleton & Lange, Mediglobe (1990) 106–109
29. Desparmet, J., Mateo, J., Ecoffey, C., Mazoit, X.: Efficacy of an epidural test dose in children anesthetized with halothane. Anesthesiology 72 (1990) 249
30. Eddleston, J. M., Holland, J. J., Griffin, R. P., Corbett, A., Horsman, E. L., Reynolds, F.: A double-blind comparison of 0,25 % ropivacaine and 0,25 % bupivacaine for extradural analgesia in labour. Br. J. Anaesth. 76 (1996) 66–71
31. Edmonds, C. L., Vance, L. M., Hughes, M.: Morbidity from paraspinal depot corticosteroid injections for analgesia: Cushing's syndrome and adrenalin suppression. Anesth. Analg. 72 (1991) 820–822
32. Forrest, J.: The response to epidural steroids in chronic dorsal root pain. Can. Anesth. Soc. J. 27 (1980) 40–46
33. Fromme, G. A., Steidl, L. J., Danielson, D. R.: Comparison of lumbal and thoracic epidural morphine for relief of postthoracotomy pain. Anesth. Analg. 64 (1985) 454
34. Gambling, D. R., Yu P. Cole, McMorland, G. H., Palmer, L.: A comparative study of patient controlled epidural analgesia (PCEA) and continuous infusion epidural analgesia (CIEA) during labour. Can. J. Anaesth. 35 (1988) 249–254
35. Gardner, W. J., Goebert, H. W., Sehgal, A. D.: Intraspinal corticosteroids in the treatment of sciatica. Trans. Am. Neurol. Assoc. 86 (1961) 214–215
36. Gianferrari, P., Clara, M. E., Borghi, B., Marzullo, A. et al: Sufentanil vs morphine combined with ropivacaine for epidural anaesthesia. Minerva Anesthesiol 67 (9–S 1) (2001) 115–119
37. Giaufre, E.: Single shot lumbar epidural block. In: Saint-Maurize, C., Schulte Steinberg, O., Armitage, E. (eds.): Regional Anaesthesia in Children. Appleton & Lange, Mediglobe (1990) 98–105
38. Goebert, H. W., Jallo, S. J., Gardner, W. J., Asmuth, C. E.: Painful radiculopathy treated with epidural injections of procaine and hydrocortisone acetate. Results in 113 patients. Anesth. Analg. 140 (1961) 130–134
39. Goldstein, N. P., McKenzie, B. F., McGuckin, W. F., Mattox, V. R.: Experimental intrathecal administration of methylprednisolone acetate in multiple sclerosis. Trans. Am. Neurol. assoc. 95 (1970) 243–244
40. Goucke, C. R., Graziotti, P.: Extradural abscess following local anaesthetic and steroid injection for chronic low back pain. Br. J. Anaesth. 65 (1990) 427–429
41. Gronow, D. W., Mendelson, G.: Epidural injection of depot corticosteroids. Position Statement. Med. J. Austr. 157 (1992) 417–420
42. Guinard, J. P., Mulroy, M. F., Carpenter, R. L., Knopes, K. D.: Test doses optimal epinephrine content with and without acute beta-adrenergic blockade. Anesthesiology 73 (1990) 386
43. Guinard, J. P., Mulroy, M. F., Carpenter, R. L.: Aging reduces the reliability of epidural epinephrine test doses. Reg. Anesth. 20 (1995) 193
44. Harik, S. I., Raichle, M. E., Reis, D. J.: Spontaneously remitting spinal epidural hematoma in a patient on anticoagulants. N. Engl. J. Med. 284 (1971) 1355
45. Haynes, G., Melinda, K. B., Davis, S., Mahaffey, J. E.: Use of methylprednisolone in epidural analgesia. Arch. Neurol. 46 (1989) 1167–1168
46. Holmström, B., Laugaland, K., Rawal, N., Hallberg, S.: Combined spinal epidural block versus spinal and epidural block for orthopedic surgery. Can. J. Anaesth. 40 (1993) 601–606
47. Hopwood, M. B., Abram, S. E.: Factors associated with failure of lumbar epidural steroids. Reg. Anesth. 18 (1993) 238–243
48. Hurford, W. E., Dutton, R. P., Alfille, P. H., Clement, D., Wilson, R. S.: Comparison of thoracic and lumbar epidural infusions of bupivacaine and fentanyl for post-thoracotomy analgesia. J. Cardiothorac. Vasc. Anesth. 7 (1993) 521
49. Ivani, G.: Continuous epidural techniques for postoperative pain relief in paediatric use. B. Braun Satellite Symposium: Continuous Regional postoperative Analgesia: Breaking up some taboos. 17. ESRA Congress Geneva (Sept. 1998)
50. Ivani, G. (Head dept. of Anaesth. & Intensive Care, Regina Margherita Children's Hospital, Turin, Italy). Persönliche Mitteilung (1998)

51. Ivani, G., Conio, A., Papurel, G., Gilberto, F., et al: 1000 consecutive blocks in a children's hospital: How to manage them safely. Reg Anesth Pain Med 26 (1) (2001) 93–94
52. Johansson, A., Hao, J., Sjolund, B.: Local corticosteroid application blocks transmission in normal nociceptive C-fibers. Acta Anesth. Scand. 34 (1990) 335–338
53. Katz, J., Renck, H.: Thorakoabdominale Nervenblockaden. Lehrbuch und Atlas. Edition Medizin, Weinheim (1988)
54. Krane, E., Dalens, B. J., Murat, I., Murell, D.: The safety of epidurals placed during general anesthesia. Editorial. Reg. Anesth. and Pain Med. 23 (5) (1998) 433–438
55. Kumar, C.: Combined subarachnoid and epidural block for caesarean section. Can. J. Anaesth. 34 (1987) 329–330
56. Lee, B., Ngan, K. W., Griffith, J.: Vertebral osteomyelitis and psoas abscess occuring after obstetric epidural anesthesia. Reg Anesth Pain Med 27 (2) (2002) 220–224
57. Leighton, B. L., Norris, M. C., Sosis, M., Epstein, R., Chayen, B., Larijani, G. E.: Limitations of epinephrine as a marker of intravascular injection in laboring women. Anesthesiology 66 (1987) 688–691
58. Liu, S. L., Carpenter, R. L.: Hemodynamic responses to intravascular injection of epinephrine containing epidural test doses in adults during general anesthesia. Anesthesiology 84 (1996) 81
59. McKinnon, S. E., Hudson, A. R., Gentili, F.: Peripheral nerve injury with steroid agents. Plast. Reconstr. Surg. 69 (1982) 482–489
60. Melendez, J. A., Cirella, V. N., Delphin, E. S.: Lumbar epidural fentanyl analgesia after thoracic surgery. J. Cardiothorac. Anesth. 3 (1989) 150
61. Mense, S., Kaske, A. (Institut für Anatomie und Zellbiologie, Ruprecht-Karls-Universität Heidelberg). Persönliche Mitteilung (1995)
62. Moore, D. C., Batra, M. S.: The components of an effective test dose prior to epidural block. Anesthesiology 55 (1981) 693
63. Mulroy, M. F.: The epinephrine test dose for epidural anesthesia – Is it necessary? In: ASRA Supplement of the American Society of Regional Anesthesia (1996)
64. Mumtaz, M. H., Daz, M., Kuz, M.: Combined subarachnoid and epidural techniques. Anaesthesia 37 (1982) 30
65. Nelson, D. A.: Intraspinal therapy using methylprednisolone acetate – 23 years of clinical controversy. Spine 18 (2) (1993) 278–286
66. Peutrell, J., Hughes, D. G.: Combined spinal and epidural anaesthesia for inguinal hernia repair in babies. Pediatric Anaesth. 4 (1994) 221–227
67. Purkis, I. E.: Cervical epidural steroids. The Pain Clinic 1 (1986) 3–7
68. Rao, A. K., Carvalho, A. C. A.: Aquired qualitative platelat defects. In: Colman, R. W., Hirsh, J., Marder, V. J., Salzman, E. W. (eds.): Hemostasis and Thrombosis. (3rd ed.) Lippincott, Philadelphia (1994)
69. Rawal, N.: The combined spinal-epidural technique. Permanyer, S. L. Publications, (1997)
70. Rawal, N.: Single segment combined spinal-epidural block for caesarean section. Can. Anaesth. Soc. J. 33 (1986) 254–255
71. Rawal, N.: Combined spinal-epidural anesthesia. In: Van Zundert, A., Ostheimer, G. W. (eds.): Pain relief and anaesthesia in obstetrics. Churchill Livingstone, New York (1996) 413–426
72. Rawal, N., Schollin, J., Wesström, G.: Epidural versus combined spinal-epidural block for caesarean section. Acta Anaest. Scand. 32 (1998) 61–66
73. Rawal, N., Van Zundert, A., Holmström, B., Crowhurst, J.: Combined spinal-epidural technique. Reg. Anesth. 22 (5) (1997) 406–423
74. Rawal, N.: Klinischer Einsatz der rückenmarknahen Opioidanalgesie. Teil 1. Der Schmerz 10 (1996) 176–189
75. Reisner, L. S., Ellis, J.: Epidural and caudal puncture. In: Benumof, L. J. (ed.): Clinical procedures in anesthesia and intensive care. Lippincott, Philadelphia (1992) 663–679
76. Reisner, L. S., Ellis, J.: Epidural and caudal puncture. In: Benumof, L. J. (ed.): Clinical procedures in anesthesia and intensive care. Lippincott, Philadelphia (1992) 691
77. Robecci, A., Capra, R.: L'idrocortisone (composto F): Prime esperience cliniche in campo reumatologico. Minerva Med. 43 (1952) 1259–1263
78. Rowlingson, J. C., Kirchenbaum, L. P.: Epidural analgesic techniques in the management of cervical pain. Anesth. Analg. 65 (1986) 938–942
79. Rowlingson, J. C. (Health Sciences Center, University of Virginia). Persönliche Mitteilung (1995)
80. Saberski, L. R., Kondamuri, S., Osinubi, O. Y. O.: Identification of the epidural space: Is loss of resistance to air safe technique? A review of the complications related to the use of air. Reg. Anesth. 22 (1) (1997) 3–15
81. Schneider, M. C., Alon, E.: Die geburtshilfliche Epiduralanalgesie. Anaesthesist 45 Springer Verlag, (1996) 393–409
82. Scott, D. B.: Identification of the epidural space: Loss of resistance to air or saline? Editorial. Reg. Anesth. 22 (1) (1997) 1–2

83. Seghal, A. D., Gardner, W. J.: Corticosteroids administrated intradurally for relief of sciatica. Cleveland Clin. Quart. 27 (1960) 198–201
84. Seghal, A. D., Gardner, W. J., Dohn, D. F.: Pantopaque arachnoiditis treatment with subarachnoid injection of corticosteroids. Cleveland Clin. J. Med. 29 (1962) 177–178
85. Seghal, A. D., Gardner, W. J.: Place of intrathecal methylprednisolone acetate in neurological disorders. Trans Am. Neurol. Assoc. 88 (1963) 275–276
86. Seghal, A. D., Tweed, D. E., Gardner, W. J., Foote, M. K.: Laboratory studies after intrathecal corticosteroids: Determination of corticosteroids in plasma and cerebrospinal fluid. Arch. Neurol. 9 (1963) 64–68
87. Selby, R.: Complications from Depo-Medrol. Surg. Neurol. 19 (1983) 393–394
88. Shenouda, P., Cunningham, B.: Assessing the superiority of saline versus air for use in epidural loss of resistance technique: A literature review. Reg Anesth Pain Med 28 (1) (2003) 48–53
89. Shulman, M.: Treatment of neck pain with cervical epidural steroid injection. Reg. Anesth. 11 (1986) 92
90. Soresi, A.: Episubdural anesthesia. Anesth. Analg. 16 (1937) 306–310
91. Sreerama, V., Ivan, L. P., Dennery, J. M., Richard, M. T.: Neurosurgical complications of anticoagulant therapy. Can. Med. Assoc. J. 108 (1973) 305
92. Strong, W. E.: Epidural abscess associated with epidural catheterisation: A rare event? Anesthesiology 74 (1991) 943–946
93. Strong, W. E., Wesley, R., Winnie, A. P.: Epidural steroids are safe and effective when given appropriately. Arch. Neurol. 48 (1991) 1012
94. Sugar, O.: Steroid injections. Surg. Neurol. 19 (1983) 91
95. Tanaka, M., Yamamoto, S., Ashimura, H., Iwai, M., Matsumiya, N.: Efficacy of an epidural test dose in adult patients anesthetized with isoflurane: lidocaine containing 15 mcg epinephrine reliably increases arterial blood pressure, but not heart rate. Anesth. Analg. 80 (1995) 310
96. Tuel, S., Meythaler, M., Cross, L.: Cushing's syndrome from epidural methylprednisolone. Pain 40 (1990) 81–84
97. Urmey, W. F., Stanton, J., Peterson, M., Sharrock, N. E.: Combined spinal epidural anesthesia for outpatient surgery. Dose-response characteristic of intrathecal isobaric lidocaine using a 27-gauge Whitacre needle. Anesthesiology 83 (1995) 528–534
98. Vassiliev, D., Nystrom, E., Leicht, G.: Combined spinal and epidural anesthesia for labor and cesarean delivery in patient with Guillain-Barre syndrome. Reg Anesth and Pain Med 26 (2) (2001) 174–176
99. Velickovic, I., Leicht, G.: Patient-controlled epidural analgesia for labor and delivery in a parturient with chronic inflammatory demyelinating polyneuropathy. Reg Anesth and Pain Med 27 (2) 217–219
100. Vercauteren, M. P., Geernaert, K., Vandeput, D. M., Adriansen, H.: Combined continuous spinal-epidural anaesthesia with a single interspace, double catheter technique. Anaesthesia 48 (1993) 1002–1004
101. Wells, J. C. D. (Director Pain Relief Center, Walton Hospital, Liverpool). Persönliche Mitteilung (1995)
102. Wilhelm, S., Standl, T.: CSA vs. CSE bei Patienten in der Unfallchirurgie. Anaesthesist 46 (1997) 938–942
103. Williams, K. N., Jackowski, A., Evans, P. J. D.: Epidural hematoma requiring surgical decompression following repeated cervical steroid injections for chronic pain. Pain 42 (1990) 197–199
104. Winnie, A. P., Hartman, J. T., Meyers, H. L., Ramamurthy, S., Barangan, V.: Pain clinic II: Intradural and extradural corticosteroids for sciatica. Anesth. Analg. 51 (1972) 990–999
105. Zimmermann, G.: The epidural space: The „Carbage Can" or „Gold Mine" in anesthesia. In: ASRA Supplement of the American Society of Regional Anesthesia (1995)

Chapter 47: Caudal anesthesia in adult patients
Chapter 48: Caudal anesthesia in children

1. Armitage, E. N.: Caudal block in children. Anaesthesia 34 (1979) 396
2. Armitage, E. N.: Regional Anaesthesia in pediatrics. Clinics in Anaesthesiology 3 (1985) 555
3. Boyd, H. R.: Iatrogenic intraspinal epidermoid. J. Neurosurg. 24 (1966) 105–107
4. Broadman, L. M.: Where should advocacy for pediatric patients end and concerns for patients safety begin? Editorial. Reg. Anesth. 22 (3) (1997) 205–208
5. Busoni, P.: Continuous caudal block. In: Saint-Maurice, C., Schulte Steinberg, O., Armitage, E. (eds.): Regional Anaesthesia in Children. Appleton & Lange, Mediglobe (1990) 88–96
6. Busoni, P., Andreucetti, T.: The spread of caudal analgesia in children: a mathematical model. Anaesth. Intens. Care 14 (1986) 140

7. Busoni, P., Sarti, A.: Sacral intervertebral epidural block. Anesthesiology 67 (1987) 993
8. Desparmet, J., Mateo, J., Ecoffey, C., Mazoit, X.: Efficacy of an epidural test dose in children anesthetized with halothane. Anesthesiology 72 (1990) 249
9. Giaufre, E.: Single shot caudal block. In: Saint-Maurize, C., Schulte Steinberg, O., Armitage, E. (eds.): Regional Anaesthesia in Children. Appleton & Lange, Mediglobe (1990) 81–87
10. Gibson, T., Norris, W.: Skin fragments removed by injection needles. Lancet 2 (1958) 983–985
11. Greenscher, J., Mofenson, H. C., Borofsky, L. G., Sharma, R.: Lumbar puncture in the neonate: A simplified techique. J. Pediatr. 78 (1971)1034
12. Halcrow, S. J., Crawford, P. J., Craft, A. W.: Epidermoid spinal cord tumour after lumbar puncture. Arch. Dis. Child. 60 (1985) 978–979
13. Ivani, G., Conio, A., Papurel, G., Gilberto, F. et al: 1000 consecutive blocks in a children's hospital: How to manage them safely. Reg Anesth Pain Med 26 (1) (2001) 93–94
14. Moore, D. C.: Single-dose caudal block. In: Moore, D. C. (ed.): Regional Block. (4th ed.) Charles Thomas, Springfield (1976)
15. Netter, F. H.: Knöcherne Bedeckung des Gehirns und des Rückenmarks. In: Krämer, G. (Hrsg.): Farbatlanten der Medizin (Band 5). Nervensystem I: Neuroanatomie und Physiologie. Georg Thieme Verlag, Stuttgart – New York (1987)
16. Reisner, L., Ellis, J.: Epidural and caudal puncture. In: Benumof, L. J. (ed.): Clinical procedures in anesthesia and intensive care. Lippincott, Philadelphia (1992) 681
17. Schulte Steinberg, O.: Kaudalanästhesie – transsacrale Anästhesie – sacral-intervertebrale Epiduralanästhesie. In: Niesel, H. C. (Hrsg.): Regionalanästhesie, Lokalanästhesie, Regionale Schmerztherapie. Georg Thieme Verlag, Stuttgart – New – York (1994)
18. Shaywitz, B.: Epidermoid spinal cord tumors and previous lumbar punctures. J. Pediatr. 80 (1972) 638–640
19. Willis, R.: Caudal epidural blockade. In: Cousins, M. J., Bridenbaugh, P. O. (eds.): Neural Blockade. (2nd ed.) Lippincott, Philadelphia (1988) 361–383

Chapter 49: Percutaneous epidural neuroplasty
(James E. Heavner, Gabor B. Racz, Miles Day, Rinoo Shah)

1. Benzon, H. T.: Epidural steroid injection for low back pain and lumbosacral radiculopathy. Pain 1986; 24: 277–295
2. Heavner, J. E., Racz, G. B., Raj, P.: Percutaneous epidural neuroplasty: prospective evaluation of 0.9 % NaCl versus 10 % NaCl with or without hyaluronidase. Reg Anesthesia Pain Med 1999; 24: 202–7
3. Kuslich, S. D., Ulstrom, C. L., Michael, C. J.: The tissue origin of low back pain and sciatica. Orthopaedic Clin NA 1991; 22: 181–7
4. Larkin, T. M., Carragee, E., Cohen, S.: A novel technique for delivery of epidural steroids and diagnosing the level of nerve root pathology. J Spinal Disorders Techniques 2003; 16: 186–92
5. Manchikanti, L., Pakanati, R. R., Bakhit, C. E., Pampati, V.: Role of adhesiolysis and hypertonic saline neurolysis in management of low back pain: evaluation of modification of the Racz protocol. Pain Digest 1999; 9: 91–6
6. Manchikanti, L., Pampati, V., Fellows, B., Rivera, J., Beyer, C. D., Damron, K. S.: Role of one day epidural adhesiolysis in management of chronic low back pain: a randomized clinical trial. Pain Physician 2001; 4: 153–166
7. Manchikanti, L., Pampati, V., Fellows, B., Rivera, J., Beyer, C. D., Damron, K. S., Cash, K. A.: Effectiveness of percutaneous adhesiolysis with hypertonic saline neurolysis in refractory spinal stenosis. Pain Physician 2001; 4: 366–73
8. Moore, D. C.: The use of hyaluronidase in local and nerve block analgesia other than the spinal block. 1520 cases. Anesthesiology 1951; 12: 611–26
9. Olmarker, K., Rydevik, B.: Pathophysiology of sciatica. Orthopedic Clin NA 1991; 22: 223–33
10. Racz, G. B., Heavner, J. E., Diede, J. H.: Lysis of epidural adhesions utilizing the epidural approach. In: Waldman SD, Winnie AP, (eds). Interventional pain management text. Dannemiller Memorial Educational Foundation, Philadelphia, W. B. Saunders Company, 1986. 339–51
11. Racz, G. B., Holubec J. T.: Lysis of adhesions in the epidural space. In: Racz, G. B. (ed): Techniques of neurolysis. Boston, Kluwer Academic, 1989. 57–72
12. Rocco, A. G., Philip, J. H., Boas, R. A., Scott, D.: Epidural space as a Starling resistor and elevation of inflow resistance in a diseased epidural space. Reg Anesthesia 1997; 22: 167–77
13. Roffe, P. G.: Innervation of the annulus fibrosus and posterior longitudinal ligament. Arch Neurol Psychiatry 1040; 44: 100

Chapter 50: Adjuncts to local anesthesia in neuraxial blocks

1. Abdel-Ghaffar, M. E. Abdulatif, M. A., al Ghamdi, A., Mowafi, H., Anwar, A.: Epidural ketamine reduces postoperative epidural PCA consumption of fentanyl/bupivacaine. Can. J. Anaesth. 45 (2) (1998) 103–109
2. Adams, H. A., Werner, C.: Vom Razemat zum Eutomer: (S)-Ketamin. Renaissance einer Substanz? Anaesthesist 46 (1997) 1026–1042
3. Bastigkeit, M.: S(+)-Ketamin: Mehr Wirkung – weniger Nebenwirkung. Rettungsdienst 2 (1998) 114–119
4. Bastigkeit, M.: Ketamin: Chirales Pharmakon mit vielen Facetten. Pharmazeutische Zeitung 4 (1997) 40–47
5. Borgbjerg, F., M., Svensson, B. A., Frigast, C., Gordh, T.: Histopathology after repeated intrathecal injections of preservative-free ketamine in rabbit: A light and electron microscope examination. Anesth. Analg. 79 (1994) 105–111
6. Chambers, W. A., Littlewood, D. G., Logan, M. R., Scott, D. B.: Effect of added epinephrine on spinal anesthesia with lidocaine. Anesth. Analg. 60 (1981) 417
7. Chambers, W. A., Littlewood, D. G., Scott, D. B.: Spinal anesthesia with bupivacaine: Effect of added vasoconstrictors. Anesth. Analg. 61 (1982) 49
8. Chia, Y. Y., Liu, K., Liu, Y. C., Chang, H. C., Wong, C. S.: Adding ketamine in a multimodal patient-controlled epidural regimen reduces postoperative pain and analgesic consumption. Anesth. Analg. 86 (6) (1998) 1245–1249
9. Choe, H., Choi, Y. S., Kim, Y. H., Ko, S. H., Choi, H. G., Han, Y. J., Song, H. S.: Epidural morphine plus ketamine for upper abdominal surgery: improved analgesia from preincisional versus postincisional administration. Anesth. Analg. 84 (3) (1997) 560–563
10. Dripps, R. D., Vandam, L. D.: Long term follow-up of patients who recieved 10098 spinal anesthetics. I. Failure to discover major neurological sequelae. JAMA 156 (1954) 1486
11. Findlow, D., Aldridge, L. M., Doyle, E.: Comparison of caudal block using bupivacaine and ketamine with ilioinguinal nerve block for orchidopexy in children. Anaesthesia 52 (11) (1997) 1110–1113
12. Fogarty, D. J., Carabine, U. A., Milligan, K. R.: Comparison of the analgesic effects of intrathecal clonidine and intrathecal morphine after spinal anesthesia in patients undergoing total hip replacement. Br. J. Anaesth. 71 (1993) 661–664
13. Freye, E.: Peridurale Analgesie mit Opioiden. In: Freye, E.: Opioide in der Medizin. Wirkung und Einsatzgebiete zentraler Analgetika. Springer Verlag (1995)
14. Gebhardt, B.: Pharmakologie und Klinik der periduralen und intrathekalen Anwendung von Ketamin. Anaesthesist. 43 (2) (1994) 34–40
15. Hawksworth, C., Serpell, M.: Intrathecal anesthesia with ketamine. Reg. Anesth. and Pain Med. 23 (3) (1998) 283–288
16. Hays, R. L., Palmer, C. M.: Respiratory depression after intrathecal sufentanil during labor. Anesthesiology 81 (1994) 511–512
17. Jamali, S., Monin, S., Begon, C., Dubousset, A. M., Ecoffey, C.: Clonidine in pediatric caudal anesthesia. Anesth. Analg. 78 (1994) 663–666
18. Kabeer, A. A., Hardy, P. A.: Long-term use of subarachnoid clonidine for analgesia in refractory sympathetic dystrophy. Case report. Reg. Anesth. 21 (3) (1996) 249–252
19. Kawana, Y., Sato, H., Shimada, H., Fujita, N., Hayashi, A., Araki, Y.: Epidural ketamine for postoperative pain relief after gynecologic operations: a double-blind study and comparison with epidural morphine. Anesth. Analg. 66 (8) (1987) 735–738
20. Knight, B.: Comment on case report of Kabeer and Hardy. Reg. Anesth. 22 (5) (1997) 485–486
21. Le Polain, B., De Kock, M., Scoltes, J. L., Vanleirde, M.: Clonidine combined with sufentanil and bupivacaine with adrenaline for obstetric analgesia. Br. J. Anesth. 71 (1993) 657–660
22. Lin, T. C., Wong, C. S., Chen, F. C., Lin, S. Y., Ho, S. T.: Long-term epidural ketamine, morphine and bupivacaine attenuate reflex sympathetic dystrophy neuralgia. Can. J. Anaesth. 45 (2) (1998) 175–177
23. Lund, P. C.: Principles and practice of spinal anesthesia. IL. Charles Thomas, Springfield (1971)
24. Muller, A., Lemos, D.: Cancer pain: Beneficial effect of ketamine addition to spinal administration of morphine-clonidine-lidocaine mixture. Ann. Fr. Anesth. Reanim 15 (3) (1996) 271–276
25. Naguib, M., Adu-Gyamfi, Y., Absood, G. H., Farag, H., Gyasi, H. K.: Epidural ketamine for postoperative analgesia. Can. Anaesth. Soc. J. 33 (1) (1986) 16–21
26. Nikolajsen, L., Hansen, C. L., Nielsen, J., Keller, J., Arendt-Nielsen, L., Jensen, T. S.: The effect of ketamine on phantom pain: A central neuropathic disorder maintained by peripheral input. Pain 67 (1) (1996) 69–77
27. Rawal, N.: Klinischer Einsatz der rückenmarksnahen Opioidanalgesie. Teil 1. Der Schmerz 10 (1996) 176–189

28. Rawal, N.: Klinischer Einsatz der rückenmarksnahen Opioidanalgesie. Teil 2. Der Schmerz 10 (1996) 226–236
29. Rockemann, M. G., Seeling, W.: Epidurale und intrathekale Anwendung von alpha-2-Adrenozeptor-Agonisten zur postoperativen Analgesie. Der Schmerz 10 (1996) 57–64
30. Rockemann, M. G., Seeling, W., Georgieff, M: Stellenwert der alpha-2-Agonisten in Anästhesie und Intensivmedizin. Anästh. Intensivmed. 35 (1994) 176–184
31. Rowlingson, J.: Toxicity of local anesthetic additives. Reg. Anesth. 18 (1993) 453–460
32. Semple, D., Findlow, D., Aldridge, L. M., Doyle, E.: The optimal dose of ketamine for caudal epidural blockade in children. Anaesthesia 51 (12) (1996) 1170–1172
33. Spivey, D. L.: Epinephrine does not prolong lidocaine spinal anesthesia in term parturients. Anaesth. Analg. 64 (1985) 468
34. Stevens, R. A., Petty, R. H., Hill, H. F., Kao, T. C., Schaffer, R., Hahn, M. B., Harris, P.: Redistribution of sufentanil to cerebrospinal fluid and systemic circulation after epidural administration in dogs. Anesth. Analg. 76 (1993) 323–327
35. Takahashi, H., Miyazaki, M., Nanbu, T., Yanagida, H., Morita, S.: The NMDA-receptor antagonist ketamine abolishes neuropathic pain after epidural administration in a clinical case. Pain 75 (2–3) (1998) 391–394
36. Vercauteren, M., Lauwers, E., Meese, G., de Heert, S., Adriaensen, H.: Comparison of epidural sufentanil plus clonidine with sufentanil alone for postoperative pain relief. Anaesthesia 45 (1990) 531
37. Wong, C. S., Liaw, W. J., Tung, C. S., Su, Y. F., Ho, S. T.: Ketamine potentiates analgesic effect of morphine in postoperative epidural pain control. Reg. Anesth. 21 (6) (1996) 534–541
38. Wong, C. S., Lu, C. C., Cherng, C. H., Ho, S. T.: Pre-emptive analgesia with ketamine, morphine and epidural lidocaine prior to total knee replacement. Can. J. Anaesth. 44 (1) (1997) 31–37
39. Wong, C. S., Shen, T. T., Liaw, W. J., Cherng, C. H., Ho. S. T.: Epidural coadministration of ketamine, morphine and bupivacaine attenuates postherpetic neuralgia – a case report. Acta Anaesth. Sin. 34 (4) (1996) 151–155
40. Yaksh, T. L.: Epidural Ketamine: A useful, mechanistically novel adjuvant for epidural morphine. Reg. Anesth. 21 (6) (1996) 508–513
41. Yang, C. Y., Wong, C. S., Chang, J. Y., Ho, S. T.: Intrathecal ketamine reduces morphine requirements in patients with terminal cancer pain. Can. J. Anaesth. 43 (4) (1996) 379–383
42. Zenz, M., Donner, B.: Regionale Opioidanalgesie. In: Niesel, H. C.: Regionalanaesthesie, Lokalanaesthesie, Regionale Schmerztherapie. Thieme Verlag (1994)

Subject index

Page numbers in **bold** represent tables, those in *italics* represent figures.

A

acromioclavicular joint
–, intra-articular injection 139–40, *140*
–, *see also* shoulder joint
adductor pollicis muscle 156, *156*, 157
anesthetic machine 4
angulus oculi medialis 19
ankle joint blocks 254–9
–, anatomy 254–6, *254*, *255*
–, contraindications 256
–, deep peroneal nerve block *257*
–, definition 254
–, documentation *259*
–, indications 256
–, posterior tibial nerve block 256, *257*, *258*
–, procedure *256*
–, saphenous nerve block 257–8, *257*, *258*
–, sural nerve and superficial peroneal nerve block 257, *258*
anterior longitudinal ligament 265
anterior scalene syndrome 60
anterior spinal artery 269
anterior spinal artery syndrome 292
aortocaval compression syndrome *334*
arachnoid granulations 271
arachnoid mater 266, 268, *268*
arterial pial network 270
auriculotemporal nerve 34
axillary block 106–22, 120–2
–, advantages 118
–, continuous 114–17
– –, contraindications 114
– –, documentation 117
– –, dosage 115
– –, indications 114
– –, maintenance dose 115–16
– –, procedure 114–15, *114*, *115*
– –, side effects and complications 116
–, disadvantages 118
–, single-shot technique 106–13, *106*, *107*
– –, block series 111
– –, complications 111–12
– –, contraindications 106–7
– –, distribution of block 110–11, *111*
– –, distribution of local anesthetic 109–10, *110*
– –, documentation 113
– –, dose 110
– –, indications 106
– –, injection technique 107–8, *108*, *109*
– –, needle position 108–9, *108*
– –, procedure *107*
– –, side effects 111

B

back pain 290
–, origins of 381–4, *381*
– –, chemical irritation *382*
– –, pressure *382*
– –, structural changes *382*
bacterial meningitis 325, 349
benzocaine 6
biceps femoris muscle 232
blood-brain barrier 271
blood patch 288, *289*
body temperature, reduction in 286
brachial plexus 82–122
–, anatomy 82–3, 82, *83*, *84*
brachial plexus blocks
–, axillary block 106–22, *120–2*
–, catheter technique 119
–, interscalene block 83–95
–, supraclavicular perivascular (subclavian perivascular) block 96–9
–, vertical infraclavicular block 99–105
buccal nerve 34
bupivacaine 14, **300**
–, caudal epidural anesthesia 373
–, Cesarean section **339**
–, chemical structure 6
–, epidural anesthesia **322**, 323
– –, obstetric 337, 338
– –, thoracic 331
–, pediatric epidural anesthesia 344, *345*
–, physicochemical/pharmacological properties **7**
–, potency **7**
–, spinal anesthesia **280**
–, toxicity **8**

419

C

caffeine sodium benzoate 288
carpal tunnel syndrome 156, 158, *158*
carticaine *6*
caruncula lacrimalis 19
catheter shearing 325
cauda equina syndrome 292, 297
caudal epidural anesthesia 361–75
–, anatomy 361–2, *361*, *362*
–, (in) children 376–80
– –, advantages 376
– –, contraindications 376
– –, disadvantages 376
– –, indications 376
– –, procedure 376–9, *378*
–, complications 373, *374*
–, continuous 369, *369–72*, 371–2
–, contraindications 362
–, definition 361
–, documentation 375
–, dosages 372–3, 379–80, *379*
–, ailure 369
–, indications 362
–, problem situations 369
–, procedure 363
– –, puncture of caudal epidural space 365–8, *365–8*
– –, single shot 363–5, *363–5*
celiac plexus block 199–205
–, anatomy 199, *200*
–, complications 204
–, contraindications 199
–, definition 199
–, documentation 205
–, dosage 203
–, indications 199
–, injection technique 202–3, *202*, *203*, *204*
–, procedure 199–201, *201*
–, side effects 204
central retinal artery 19
cerebrospinal fluid 270–1
cervical ganglia *59*
cervical plexus block 76–81
–, anatomy 76–8, *76*, *77*
–, block series 80
–, complications 80
–, documentation 81
–, dosage 80
–, effects of 80
–, indications 78
–, injection technique 79–80, *79*
–, procedure 78–9, *78*, *79*
–, side effects 80
cervicothoracic ganglion block 59–68
–, anatomy *59*, *60*, *61*
–, block series 64
–, complications 65–7, *65–7*
–, contraindications 61
–, documentation 68
–, dosage 64
–, effect of 63–4, *63*
–, indications 60–1
–, injection technique *63*
–, materials *62*
–, side effects 64–5, *64*
Cesarean section 338–9
–, local anesthetics **339**
Chassaignac's tubercle 87
chemical intraspinal neurolysis 301–4
–, complications 303
–, contraindications 301
–, documentation 304
–, indications 301
–, observations after 303
–, procedure 301–3, *301–3*
children
–, caudal epidural anesthesia 376–80
– –, advantages 376
– –, contraindications 376
– –, disadvantages 376
– –, indications 376
– –, procedure 376–9, *378*
–, lumbar epidural anesthesia 341–5
– –, advantages 341, 342
– –, anatomy *341*
– –, concentration of local anesthetic 344
– –, continuous 343–4, *344*
– –, disadvantages 341, 342
– –, dosage 344, *345*
– –, epidural needles 342
– –, indications 341
– –, single shot 342–3
– –, spread of anesthetic 343
chloroprocaine 11
–, Cesarean section **339**
–, chemical structure *6*
–, epidural anesthesia, obstetric 337
choroid plexus 270
ciliary arteries 19
clonidine 393–4
CNS toxicity *66*, 93
cocaine *6*
coccygeal plexus anatomy 218, *219*
combined spinal/epidural anesthesia 355–60
–, contraindications 355
–, documentation 360
–, dosage 358–9
–, history 355
–, indications 355

–, injection technique 356–8, *356–8*
–, procedure 355–6
common peroneal (fibular) nerve 230, 248, *248, 249*
–, block 252–3, *252*
conus medullaris 266, *267*
coracobrachialis muscle **129**
cornea 19
costal angle block 178–80, *178–80*
costal pleura 172
crystalline lens 19
Cushing's syndrome 350

D

deep peroneal (fibular) nerve *255*
–, block *257*
deltoid muscle **129**
dental pain 57
diagnostic blocks 3
distal sciatic nerve block 250–2, *250, 251*
documentation 15
–, ankle joint block 259
–, axillary block 113, 117
–, caudal epidural anesthesia 375
–, celiac plexus block 205
–, cervical plexus block 81
–, cervicothoracic ganglion block 68
–, chemical intraspinal neurolysis 304
–, combined spinal/epidural anesthesia 360
–, continuous spinal anesthesia 297
–, epidural obstetric anesthesia 340
–, epidural steroid injection 351, 354
–, ganglion impar (Walther ganglion) block 213
–, Gasserian ganglion block 54
–, intercostal nerve block 178
–, interscalene block 94–5
–, intravenous regional anesthesia 163
–, intravenous sympathetic block with guanethidine 168
–, lumbar epidural anesthesia 316, 320
–, lumbar paravertebral somatic nerve block 190
–, lumbar sympathetic block 198
–, mandibular nerve block 49
–, maxillary nerve block 44
–, ophthalmology 29
–, sciatic nerve block 237
–, spinal anesthesia 284
–, superior cervical ganglion block 75
–, thoracic epidural anesthesia 332
–, thoracic paravertebral somatic nerve block 176
–, thoracic spinal nerves, posterior branches 185
–, vertical infraclavicular block 104–5
dorsal primary rami 171
dorsal rami of thoracic nerves 171

drugs
–, (for) emergency treatment *4*
–, *see also* local anesthetics; and individual drug names
Dupuytren's contracture 128, 152–3, *153*
dura 361
dura mater 266, *268*
dural puncture 287–90, 324–5
–, *see also* postdural puncture headache

E

effective pain therapy *1*
elbow blocks 143–5, 149–56
–, anatomy 143–4, *143*
–, complications 145
–, contraindications 144
–, dosage 145
–, finger extensors 150–1, *151*
–, flexor carpi radialis and ulnaris muscles 152–4, *152–4*
–, hand extensors 149–50, *149, 150*
–, indications 144
–, intra-articular injection 154, *154, 155*
–, medial epicondyle 152
–, palmaris longus muscle 152–3, *153*
–, procedure *144*
–, pronator teres muscle *152*
–, supinator muscle 151–2, *151, 152*
–, technique 144–5, *144, 145*
electrostimulator *5*
emergency equipment *3, 4*
endothoracic fascia 172
epidural abscess 326, 349
epidural anesthesia
–, caudal *see* caudal epidural anesthesia
–, lumbar *see* lumbar epidural anesthesia
–, obstetric *see* obstetric epidural anesthesia
–, thoracic *see* thoracic epidural anesthesia
–, *see also* combined spinal/epidural anesthesia
epidural hematoma 326, 349–50
epidural injection 92–3
epidural steroid injection 346–54
–, cervical 346–9
– –, anatomy 346
– –, complications 349–50
– –, contraindications 347
– –, documentation 351
– –, dosage 349
– –, indications 346
– –, injection technique 347–9, *347, 348*
– –, procedure 347
– –, puncture needles 347
–, lumbar 352–4
– –, documentation 354

– –, dosage 353
– –, effect of block 352
– –, indications 352
– –, onset of effect 352
– –, procedure 352
esophageal perforation 67
etidocaine
–, chemical structure 6
–, epidural anesthesia **322**
–, physicochemical/pharmacological properties 7
–, potency 7
extensor carpi radialis brevis muscle 149
extensor carpi radialis longus muscle 149
extensor carpi ulnaris muscle 149, *150*
extensor digitorum muscle 149, 150, *151*
extensor indicis muscle 150
external intercostal muscles 172
extraconal space 19
eye *see* ophthalmology
eyelids *19*
–, facial nerve block 26–8, *26*, *27*

F
facial nerve block 26–8, *26*, *27*
–, Atkinson method *27*, 28
–, Nadbath-Rehmann method *27*, 28
–, O'Brien method *27*, 28
–, Van Lint method *27*, 28
fascial clicks 108
fasciculus lateralis 82
femoral nerve block 238–40
–, anatomy *238*
–, definition 238
–, dosage 240
–, indications 238
–, injection technique 239–40, *239*, *240*
–, procedure 239
fentanyl **300**, 323, 331, 338, 373, 392
finger extensors 150–1, *151*
flexor carpi radialis muscle 152–4, *152–4*
frontal nerve 33
frozen shoulder 128

G
ganglion impar (Walther ganglion) block 210–13
–, anatomy *210*
–, complications 212
–, contraindications 210
–, definition 210
–, documentation 213
–, dosage 212
–, indications 210
–, injection technique *212*
–, procedure *211*

Gasserian ganglion block 50–2, *50*
–, complications 52
–, contraindications 50
–, documentation 54
–, dosage 52
–, indications 50
–, needle insertion technique 51–2, *51*
–, procedure 50–1, *51*
genitofemoral nerve 246
glucose 391
gluteus maximus muscle 232
golfer's elbow 152
great auricular nerve 76
guanethidine, intravenous sympathetic block 164–8
–, complications 167
–, contraindications 164
–, documentation 168
–, dosage 167
–, indications 164
–, procedures 164–5, *164–6*
–, side effects 167

H
"hand behind the back" position *134*
hand extensors 149–50, *149*, *150*
hanging drop technique
–, lumbar epidural anesthesia 310, *312*
–, thoracic epidural anesthesia *329*
high spinal anesthesia 285–6
Horner's syndrome 43, 63–4, *63*, 286
hyaluronidase hypersensitivity 389
hypotension, in pregnancy 335

I
iliohypogastric nerve block 246–7
–, anatomy *247*
–, definition 246
–, dosage 247
–, indications 247
–, injection technique *247*
–, procedure *247*
ilioinguinal nerve block 246–7
–, definition 246
–, dosage 247
–, indications 247
–, injection technique *247*
–, procedure *247*
iliolumbar ligament 206
iliolumbosacral ligament 266, *266*, *267*
–, block 206–9
– –, anatomy 206–7, *206*
– –, complications 209
– –, contraindications 207
– –, definition 206

– –, dosage 209
– –, indications 207
– –, injection technique *208*
– –, procedure 207–8, *207*
indications for regional anesthesia 1
inferior alveolar nerve 34
inferior descending cervical nerve 78
inferior hypogastric plexus 210
inferior oblique muscle 19
inferior rectus muscle 19
infraorbital nerve 53
–, block 36–8
– –, dosages 37–8
– –, indications 36
– –, injection techniques *37*
– –, procedure 37
– –, side effects 38
infraspinatus muscle **129**, 135–6, *135*, *136*
infusion solutions 4
inguinal femoral paravascular ("three-in-one") block 220–5
–, advantages 220
–, complications *225*
–, contraindications 221
–, definition 220, *221*, *222*
–, disadvantages 220
–, dosage 224
–, indications 220–1
–, injection technique 222–4, *222*, *223*, *224*
–, procedure 221–2, *222*
intercostal nerve block 177–82
–, contraindications 177
–, costal angle 178–80, *178–80*
–, definition 177
–, documentation 178
–, dorsal *181*
–, indications 177
–, procedure *177*
intercostal vessels 172
internal intercostal muscles 172
interscalene block 83–95
–, advantages 118
–, complications 92–3, *92*
–, continuous
– –, anterior technique 89–90, *89*
– –, posterior technique 90–2, *90–2*
–, contraindications 85
–, disadvantages 118
–, distribution of blocks 92
–, documentation 94–5
–, indications 83–4
–, side effects *92*
–, Winnie's anterior route
– –, dosage 88–9

– –, electrostimulation 88
– –, single shot 85–8, *85–8*
interspinous ligament 265
intertransverse ligaments 265
intra-articular injection *see* acromioclavicular joint; shoulder joint
intraconal space 19
intracranial vascular response 287
intravascular injection *65*, *73*, 74, *92*
intravenous regional anesthesia 159–63
–, advantages 162
–, complications 162
–, disadvantages 162
–, documentation 163
–, dosage 162
–, indications *159*
–, procedure 159, *160*
–, technical procedure 160, *160*, *161*
intravenous sympathetic block *see* guanethidine
Iohexol **384**
iris 19

K
ketamine 394–6
knee joint blocks 248–53
–, anatomy 248–9, *248*, *249*, *250*
–, common peroneal (fibular) nerve block 252–3, *252*
–, contraindications 250
–, distal sciatic nerve block 250–2, *250*, *251*
–, indications 249
–, procedure *250*
–, saphenous nerve block *253*
–, tibial nerve block *252*

L
lacrimal gland 19, *20*
lateral femoral cutaneous nerve block 241–2
–, anatomy *241*
–, contraindications 241
–, definition 241
–, dosage 242
–, indications 241
–, injection technique *242*
–, procedure 241–2, *241*
lateral pterygoid muscle *57*, *58*
latissimus dorsi muscle **129**
lesser occipital nerve 76
levator palpebrae superioris muscle 19
levobupivacaine 14
–, Cesarean section **339**
–, chemical structure 6
–, epidural anesthesia **322**, 323
–, physicochemical/pharmacological properties **7**
–, potency **7**

Subject index

–, thoracic epidural anesthesia 331
–, toxicity **8**
lidocaine **10**, 11–12
–, caudal epidural anesthesia 373
–, Cesarean section **339**
–, chemical structure 6
–, epidural anesthesia **322**
– –, obstetric 337
–, physicochemical/pharmacological properties **7**
–, potency **7**
–, spinal anesthesia **280**
–, toxicity **8**
ligamentum flavum *266*, *305*
lingual nerve 34
local anesthetics 5–15
–, allergic potential 9–10
–, block profile 7, **8**
–, chemical requirements **8**
–, chemical structure 5, **6**
–, dosage 321–3, **322**
–, duration of effect 6
–, (in) epidural space 321
–, equipotency 7
–, incompatibility 7
–, long-acting 13–14
–, medium-term 11–13
–, onset of effect 6
–, physicochemical properties 5, **6**, **7**
–, potency 4–5
–, selection of 10
–, short-acting 10–11
–, side effects and systemic effects 7–10, **8**, **9**, **10**
–, subarachnoid space 278–80, **280**
–, *see also individual drugs*
locked-in syndrome 66
loss-of-resistance technique
–, lumbar epidural anesthesia *310*
–, thoracic epidural anesthesia *329*
lumbar epidural anesthesia 305–26
–, anatomy 305–6, *305*
–, (in) children 341–5
– –, advantages 341, 342
– –, anatomy *341*
– –, concentration of local anesthetic 344
– –, continuous 343–4, *344*
– –, disadvantages 341, 342
– –, dosage 344, *345*
– –, epidural needles 342
– –, indications 341
– –, procedure 342
– –, single shot 342–3
– –, spread of anesthetic 343
–, complications 324–6
– –, bacterial meningitis 325

– –, catheter shearing 325
– –, cranial and cervical nerve involvement 325
– –, dural puncture 324–5
– –, early *324*
– –, epidural abscess 326
– –, epidural hematoma 326
– –, intravascular injection 325
– –, massive epidural anesthesia 325
– –, spinal cord injury 325
–, continuous 317–20
– –, documentation 320
– –, problem situations *319*
– –, procedure *317–19*
–, contraindications 306–7
–, dose of local anesthetic 321–3, **322**
–, indications 306
–, local anesthetics in epidural space 321
–, procedure *307*
–, single shot 308–16
– –, advantage 310
– –, aspiration test *313*
– –, disadvantages 310
– –, documentation 316
– –, escaping blood *314*
– –, escaping CSF *315*
– –, escaping fluid *314*
– –, hanging drop technique 310, *312*
– –, local anesthetic injection *314*
– –, loss-of-resistance technique 310
– –, median approach 308–11, *308–11*
– –, paramedian (paraspinal) approach 315
–, *see also* Spinal anesthesia
lumbar paravertebral somatic nerve block 186–90
–, anatomy 186
–, complications 189
–, contraindications 186
–, definition 186
–, documentation 190
–, dosage 189
–, indications 186
–, injection technique 187–8, *188*
–, procedure 186–7, *187*
lumbar plexus
–, anatomy 218, *219*
–, blocks
– –, femoral nerve 238–40
– –, ilioinguinal and iliohypogastric nerves 246–7
– –, inguinal femoral paravascular ("three-in-one") block 220–5
– –, lateral femoral cutaneous nerve 241–2
– –, obturator nerve 243–5
– –, psoas compartment block (Cheyen approach) 226–9

lumbar sympathetic block 191–8
–, anatomy 191, *192*, *193*
–, complications 197
–, contraindications 192
–, definition 191
–, documentation 198
–, dosage 197
–, indications 191
–, injection technique 194–5, *195*, *196*
–, neurolytic block 197
–, procedure 192–4, *193*, *194*
lumbosacral trunk 218

M
mandibular nerve 34, *53*
–, block 46–9
– –, block distribution *48*
– –, block series 48
– –, complications 48
– –, contraindications 46
– –, documentation 49
– –, dosage 48
– –, indications 46
– –, injection technique 46–8, *47*
– –, procedure 46, *47*
– –, side effects 48
masseter muscle 55–7, *55*
–, dosage 57
–, injection technique 55, *56*
–, procedure 55
maxillary nerve 34, *53*
–, block 39–43, *39*
– –, block series 42
– –, complications 43
– –, contraindications 40
– –, documentation 44
– –, dosage 42
– –, extraoral technique 41–2, *42*
– –, indications 40
– –, injection technique *41, 42*
– –, intraoral technique *41*
– –, procedure 40–1, *41*
– –, side effects *43*
medial epicondyle 152
medial rectus muscle 19
median nerve 143, 146, *147*
–, block *145, 148*
median sacral crest *264*, 265
Ménière's disease 60
meninges 266, 268, *268*
mental nerve 34, *53*
–, block 38–9
– –, complications 39
– –, indications 38

– –, injection techniques 38–9
– –, procedure *38*
– –, side effects 39
mepivacaine **10**, 12
–, caudal epidural anesthesia 373
–, chemical structure *6*
–, epidural anesthesia **322**
–, pediatric epidural anesthesia 344, *345*
–, physicochemical/pharmacological properties **7**
–, potency **7**
–, spinal anesthesia **280**
–, toxicity **8**
monitoring 4, *5*
morphine **300**, 323, 373, 392
multimodal treatment approach 3

N
nerve blocks *2*
–, *see also individual nerve blocks*
nerve fibers **10**
neuraxial anatomy 261–71
–, cerebrospinal fluid 270–1
–, iliolumbosacral ligaments 266, *266*, *267*
–, sacrum *264*, *265*
–, spinal cord 266, *267*, 268–9, *268*, *269*
–, spinal cord arteries 269–70, *269*, *270*
–, spinal ligaments 265–6, *265*, *266*
–, spine 263–4, *263*, *264*
–, veins of the spinal cord and vertebrae 270, *271*
neurogenic bladder 389

O
obstetric anesthesia
–, continous spinal 299–300
–, epidural 333–40
– –, Cesarean section 338–9, **339**
– –, documentation 340
– –, indications 335
– –, local anesthetics 336–8
– –, procedure 335–6
– –, risks 334–5, *334*
obturator nerve block 243–5
–, anatomy *243*
–, complications 245
–, contraindications 243
–, definition 243
–, dosage 245
–, indications 243
–, injection technique 244–5, *244*, *245*
–, procedure 243, *244*
occipital nerve 30–2
–, anatomy *31*
–, block 30–2, *32*
– –, complications 32

– –, dosage 32
– –, indications 30–1
– –, injection techniques *31*, *32*
– –, procedure 31–2, *31*
occipital neuralgia 31
oculopressor *22*
ophthalmic artery 19, *21*
ophthalmic nerve *33*, *52*
ophthalmology 19–29
–, anatomy of eye 19–21, *19*, *20*
–, anticoagulation and ocular block 25
–, documentation 29
–, facial nerve block 26–8, *26*, *27*
–, local/surface anesthesia 26
–, peribulbar block 23–4
–, retrobulbar block 22–3
–, sub-Tenon block 24–5
opioids 337–8, 391–3
–, complications and side effects 392–3
–, pharmacokinetics 392
–, *see also individual drugs*
opponens pollicis muscles 156, *156*, *157*
orbicularis oculi muscle 19
otic ganglion 34
–, block *see* mandibular nerve block

P
pain 1–2
–, chronic 2, 3
palmaris longus muscle 152–3, *153*
patient preparation 15
patient-controlled epidural analgesia (PCEA) 338
pediatric *see* children
percutaneous epidural anaplasty 381–90
–, anterior epidural space/intervertebral foramen 388
–, caudal access route 384–7, *386*
–, cervical 387–8
–, complications 388–9
– –, hyaluronidase hypersensitivity 389
– –, infection 389
– –, neurogenic bladder and rectal disturbances 389
– –, spinal cord compression 389
–, injection solutions **384**
–, origins of back pain and sciatica 381–4, *381*
– –, chemical irritation *382*
– –, pressure *382*
– –, structural changes *382*
–, percutaneous thoracic 388
peribulbar block 23–4
–, complications 24
–, disadvantages 24
–, dosage 24
–, injection technique *24*
–, materials 24

pethidine **300**
pharaoh posture 125, 184
phenol injection 301–4
phrenic nerve 78
pia mater 266, *268*
pincer-grip palpation 55, *56*
piriform syndrome 214–16
piriform trigger points 214–16
–, anatomy 214–15, *214*, *215*
–, complications 216
–, dosage 216
–, mechanism of pain 214
–, pace transgluteal injection technique 216
–, procedure *215*
–, symptoms 214–15
–, transgluteal injection technique *216*
pneumothorax *67*, *93*, *99*, *103*, *127*
popliteal fossa 250, *251*
post-laminectomy syndrome 215
postdural puncture headache 287–90, 297
–, associated symptoms 287
–, clinical symptoms 287
–, CSF hypotension syndrome 287, *288*
–, differential diagnosis 288
–, etiology 287
–, frequency 287
–, location 287
–, mechanism 287
–, therapy 288–90, *289*
posterior longitudinal ligament 265
posterior spinal arteries 269, 270
posterior tibial nerve block 256, *257*, *258*
preconditions 3
pregnancy
–, anatomic changes 333
–, labor pain 333–4, *333*
–, physiological changes 333
–, *see also* obstetric anesthesia
prilocaine **10**, 12–13
–, caudal epidural anesthesia 373
–, chemical structure *6*
–, epidural anesthesia **322**
–, physicochemical/pharmacological properties **7**
–, potency **7**
–, spinal anesthesia **280**
–, toxicity **8**
procaine 10–11
–, chemical structure *6*
–, physicochemical/pharmacological properties **7**
–, potency **7**
prognostic blocks 3
pronator teres muscle *152*
psoas compartment block (Cheyen approach) 226–9
–, advantages 226

–, complications 229
–, contraindications 226
–, definition 226
–, disadvantages 226
–, dosage 229
–, indications 226
–, injection technique 228–9, *229*
–, preliminary puncture 227
–, procedure *227*
pterygopalatine ganglion block
–, nasal 45–6, *45*, *46*
–, see also maxillary nerve block
pterygopalatine (sphenopalatine) ganglion 34
pulse oximetry 4, *5*
pupil 19

Q
quadriceps femoris muscle 228

R
radial nerve 143–4, 146, *147*
–, block *145*
rami communicantes 69
Raynaud-Burger syndrome 60
regional anesthesia 1–16
 –, indications 1
–, intravenous see intravenous regional anesthesia
    retrobulbar block 22–3
–, dosage 23
–, indications 22
–, injection technique 22, *23*
–, materials *22*
–, patient positioning 22
–, side effects and complications 23
rima palpebrarum 19
ropivacaine 13–14
–, caudal epidural anesthesia 373
–, Cesarean section **339**
–, chemical structure *6*
–, epidural anesthesia **322**, 323
– –, obstetric 336–7, 338
– –, thoracic 331
–, pediatric epidural anesthesia 344, *345*
–, percutaneous epidural neuroplasty **384**
–, physicochemical/pharmacological properties **7**
–, potency **7**
–, spinal anesthesia **280**
–, toxicity **8**
rotator cuff muscles 128, 133–7

S
sacral canal 361
sacral hiatus 265, 361
sacral plexus anatomy 218, *219*

sacral splanchnic nerves 210
sacroiliac joint 206
sacroiliac ligaments 206
sacrospinous ligament 206
sacrotuberous ligament 206
sacrum *264*, *265*
saphenous nerve 249, *250*, *255*, 256
–, block *253*, 257–8, *257*, *258*
sciatic line 234
sciatic nerve block 230–7
–, anatomy *230*
–, anterior approach 233, *234*
–, continuous subgluteal 235–6, *235*, *236*
–, contraindications 231
–, definition 230
–, Di Benedetto-Borghi subgluteal access route
    234–5, *234*, *235*
–, documentation 237
–, dorsal transgluteal (Labat) technique 231–3, *232*,
    233, *234*
–, indications 230–1
–, procedure *231*
sciatica see back pain
semimembranosus muscle 232
semitendinosus muscle 232
shoulder joint, intra-articular injection 138–9
–, dorsal route access 138–9, *138*, *139*
–, indications 138
–, injection techniques *138*
Sims position *215*, *231*
solar plexus 199
spinal anesthesia 272–84
–, advantages 272
–, complications 285–92
– –, back pain 290
– –, collapse 285
– –, early postoperative phase 286–7
– –, gastrointestinal tract disturbances 286
– –, high total spinal anesthesia 285–6
– –, hypotension 285
– –, (during) injection 285
– –, (immediately after) injection 285–6
– –, late 287–92
– –, neurological 290–1
– –, postdural puncture headache 287–90
– –, reduced body temperature 286
– –, respiratory disturbance 286
– –, subdural spread 286
– –, transient neurologic symptoms 290–1
– –, urinary retention 286–7
–, continuous 293–8
– –, advantages 293, 295
– –, contraindications 294
– –, disadvantages and complications 297

– –, documentation 298
– –, dosage 295, 297
– –, history 293
– –, indications 294
– –, injection technique 294–5, *295*, *296*
– –, (in) obstetrics 299–300
– –, procedure *294*
–, contraindications 272–3
–, disadvantages 272
–, documentation 284
–, hyperbaric 278
–, hypobaric 278
–, indications 272
–, injection technique
– –, median approach 276–8, *276*, *277*
– –, paramedian approach 278, *279*
– –, Taylor's approach 278, *279*
–, isobaric 278
–, local anesthetics 270, 278–80, **280**
–, patient position 273–5, *274*, *275*
–, procedure 272–3, *272*, *273*
–, spread and duration 281, *282*, *283*
–, unilateral 280–1
–, *see also* combined spinal/epidural anesthesia; epidural anesthesia
spinal cord 266, *267*, 268–9, *268*, *269*
–, arteries 269–70, *269*, *270*
–, compression 389
–, injury 349
–, meninges 266, 268, *268*
–, veins 270, *271*
spinal dermatomes *268*, *269*
spinal ganglion 171
spinal ligaments 265–6, *265*, *266*
spinal nerves 268–9, *268*
spine 263–4, *263*, *264*
stellate ganglion *see* cervicothoracic ganglion
sub-Tenon block 24–5
–, advantages 25
–, complications 25
–, disadvantages 25
–, dosage 25
–, materials *24*, 25
–, procedure 25
subarachnoid injection 92–3
subarachnoid space 270, 278–80, **280**
subcostal nerve 171
subdural injection 286
subscapular nerve block 128–32
–, anatomical insertions 129
–, anatomy *128*, 129
–, block series 131
–, complications 132
–, dosage 131, **132**

–, injection technique 130–1, *130*, *131*
–, innervation and function **129**
–, procedure *130*
–, side effects 132
–, symptoms 130
–, technique *130*
subscapularis muscle **129**
sufentanil **300**, 323, 331, 338, 373, 392
superficial peroneal (fibular) nerve *254*, *255*
–, block 257, *258*
superior cervical ganglion block 69–75
–, anatomy 69, *69*, *70*
–, block series 72
–, complications 73–4, *73*
–, contraindications 70
–, documentation 75
–, dosage 72
–, effects of 72
–, indications 70
–, injection technique 71, *72*
–, pain therapy 74
–, procedure 70–1, *71*
–, side effects 72–3
superior oblique muscle 19
superior rectus muscle 19
supinator muscle 151–2, *151*, 152
supraclavicular nerves 77
supraclavicular perivascular (subclavian perivascular) block 96–9
–, advantages 118
–, complications 99
–, contraindications 96
–, definition 96
–, disadvantages 118
–, distribution of block 98, *99*
–, dosage 98
–, electrostimulation *98*
–, indications 96
–, problem situations 98
–, procedure 96
–, side effects 98–9
–, technique 96–8, *97*, *98*
supraorbital nerve 33
–, block 35–6
– –, complications 36
– –, indications 35
– –, injection techniques 35–6, *35*, *36*
– –, procedure 35
– –, side effects 36
suprascapular nerve block 125–7
–, anatomy *125*, *126*
–, complications *127*
–, contraindications 125
–, dosage 127

–, indications 125
–, intrainjection technique *127*
–, procedure 125, *126*
–, side effects 127
supraspinatus muscle **129**, *133*, *134*
supraspinous ligaments 265
supratrochlear nerve *33*
–, block 35–6
– –, complications 36
– –, indications 35
– –, injection techniques 35–6, *35*, *36*
– –, procedure 35
– –, side effects 36
sural nerve *255*
–, block 257, *258*
surgical blocks 3

T

technical requirements 3–5
temperature sensor *5*
temporal headache 57
temporal muscle *57*
temporomandibular joint *57*
–, pain-dysfunction syndrome 55
tennis elbow 149, 151–2, *151*, *152*
teres major muscle **129**
teres minor muscle **129**, 136–7, *137*
tetracaine 11
–, chemical structure *6*
–, spinal anesthesia **280**
therapeutic blocks 3
thoracic epidural anesthesia 327–35
–, advantages 327
–, anatomy 327–8, *327*
–, complications 331
–, contraindications 328
–, disadvantages 327
–, documentation 332
–, dosages 331
–, epidural needles 328, *329*
–, hanging drop technique *329*
–, indications **328**
–, loss-of-resistance technique *329*
–, midline insertion in sitting position 328–9
–, paramedian insertion 329, *330*, 331
–, procedure 328
thoracic paravertebral somatic nerve block 172–6
–, block series 173
–, complications 175
–, contraindications 173
–, definition 172
–, documentation 176
–, dosage 175
–, indications 173

–, injection technique 174–5, *174*, *175*
–, procedure 173–4, *173*, *174*
thoracic spinal nerve blocks 171–85
–, anatomy 171–2, *171*, *172*
–, intercostal nerve block 177–82
–, posterior branches 183–5
– –, anatomy *183*
– –, documentation 185
– –, dosage 184
– –, effect of block 184
– –, indications 183
– –, procedure 183–4, *184*
– –, side effects 184
–, thoracic paravertebral somatic nerve block 172–6
three-in-one block *see* inguinal femoral paravascular block
thrombophlebitis 60
tibial nerve 230, 248, *248*, *249*, *254*
–, block 252
total spinal anesthesia 285–6
tracheal perforation *67*
transverse cervical nerve *77*
trigeminal nerve 33–54
–, analgesic zones *52*, *53*
–, anatomy 33–4, *33*, *34*
trigeminal nerve palsy 286
tunica conjunctiva *19*

U

ulnar nerve 143, 146, *147*
–, block *144*, 147, *148*
ulnaris muscle 152–4, *152–4*
urinary retention 286–7

V

vasopressors 391
vasovagal syncope 285
ventral primary rami 171
ventral rami of thoracic nerves 171
vertebrae *264*
–, veins 270, *271*
vertebral ganglion *59*
vertebral venous plexuses 270, *271*
vertical infraclavicular block 99–105
–, complications *103*
–, continuous technique *102*
–, distribution of block *102*
–, documentation 104–5
–, dosage 103
–, indications and contraindications 99
–, procedure 99–100, *100*
–, side effects 103
–, technique 101, *101*, *102*

vitreous body 19
Volkmann's ischemic contracture 60

W

Walther ganglion block *see* ganglion impar (Walther ganglion) block
weeder's thumb 156, *156*, *157*
wrist blocks 146–8, 156–8
–, adductor pollicis and opponens pollicis muscles 156, *156*, *157*
–, anatomy 146, *147*
–, carpal tunnel syndrome 156, 158, *158*
–, complications 148
–, contraindications 146
–, dosage 148
–, indications 146
–, procedure 146, *148*
–, technique 147–8, *148*